Today and Tomorrow of Parkinson's Disease

Today and Tomorrow of Parkinson's Disease

Editor: Helena Shelton

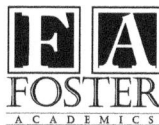

FA
FOSTER
ACADEMICS

www.fosteracademics.com

www.fosteracademics.com

FA
FOSTER
ACADEMICS

Cataloging-in-Publication Data

Today and tomorrow of Parkinson's disease / edited by Helena Shelton.
  p. cm.
Includes bibliographical references and index.
ISBN 978-1-63242-951-3
1. Parkinson's disease. 2. Brain--Diseases. I. Shelton, Helena.
RC382 .T63 2020
616.833--dc23

© Foster Academics, 2020

Foster Academics,
118-35 Queens Blvd., Suite 400,
Forest Hills, NY 11375, USA

ISBN 978-1-63242-951-3 (Hardback)

Contents

Preface

This book aims to highlight the current researches and provides a platform to further the scope of innovations in this area. This book is a product of the combined efforts of many researchers and scientists, after going through thorough studies and analysis from different parts of the world. The objective of this book is to provide the readers with the latest information of the field.

Parkinson's disease (PD) is a degenerative disorder of the central nervous system that significantly affects the motor system. A set of symptoms known as Parkinsonism, including tremor, rigidity, bradykinesia and postural instability, are commonly exhibited. Non-motor symptoms such as behavioral and thinking problems also occur in individuals with this disease. Parkinson's disease is a prevalent disorder, affecting nearly 1% of the world's population above the age of 60. Several theories pertaining to the cause of PD suggest the death of dopamine-producing neurons in the central nervous system, due to oxidative stress. Such oxidative stress is attributed to metabolism and the production and accumulation of free radicals. Drugs like levodopa and dopamine agonists can moderate the symptoms of the disease. However, these medications become ineffective when multiple dopamine-producing cells have been destroyed. Research is being undertaken to investigate the link between dietary patterns and Parkinson's. The potential of stem cell transplantation, gene therapy and neuroprotective agents in the management of PD is also being explored. This book unravels the recent studies in Parkinson's disease. It brings forth the fundamental as well as modern approaches of its management. The extensive content of this book provides the readers with a thorough understanding of this disease.

I would like to express my sincere thanks to the authors for their dedicated efforts in the completion of this book. I acknowledge the efforts of the publisher for providing constant support. Lastly, I would like to thank my family for their support in all academic endeavors.

Editor

Coping with Cognitive Impairment in People with Parkinson's Disease and their Carers

Rachael A. Lawson [ID],[1] Daniel Collerton,[1] John-Paul Taylor,[1] David J. Burn,[1] and Katie R. Brittain[2]

[1]Institute of Neuroscience, Newcastle University, Newcastle upon Tyne, UK
[2]Department of Nursing, Midwifery and Health, Northumbria University, Newcastle upon Tyne, UK

Correspondence should be addressed to Rachael A. Lawson; rachael.lawson@ncl.ac.uk

Academic Editor: Hélio Teive

Cognitive impairment is common in Parkinson's disease (PD). However, the psychosocial impact of living and coping with PD and cognitive impairment in people with PD and their carers have not been explored. This paper draws on a qualitative study that explores the subjective impact of cognitive impairment on people with PD and their carers. Thirty-six one-to-one interviews were completed; people with PD were from three groups: normal cognition, mild cognitive impairment, and dementia. Data collection and analysis were iterative, and verbatim transcripts were analysed using thematic analysis. Themes were interpreted in consultation with coping and adaptation theory. The analysis revealed four main themes: threats to identity and role, predeath grief and feelings of loss in carers, success and challenges to coping in people with PD, and problem-focused coping and finding meaning in caring. Our data highlight how cognitive impairment can threaten an individual's self-perception; the ostensible effects of cognitive impairment depended on the impact individual's perceived cognitive impairment had on their daily lives. For carers, cognitive impairment had a greater emotional impact than the physical symptoms of PD. The discussion that developed around protective factors provides possible opportunities for future interventions, such as psychological therapies to improve successful adjustment.

1. Introduction

Cognitive impairment in Parkinson's disease (PD) is a common nonmotor symptom, with up to 80% of people with PD developing dementia (PDD) [1]. Previous quantitative studies have shown that cognitive impairment can be detrimental to the quality of life of people with PD and their informal caregivers [2, 3]. However, these studies could not explain the mechanism or what aspects of cognitive impairment affected people with PD and their carers. In-depth qualitative studies may be more suitable to address these questions.

Qualitative aspects of the carer experience associated with dementia have been thoroughly explored [4–10]. Spousal carers of people with dementia or cognitive impairment experience high levels of burden; they have related feeling stressed, anxious and depressed, and neglected self-care [11]. However, few qualitative studies explore the effects of cognitive impairment on people with PD and/or their carers. Birgersson and Edberg [12] more broadly investigated the experience of support in people with PD and their carers. People with PD may have high perceived support and experience a sense of solidarity and community but may also feel humiliated, excluded, or misunderstood. For carers, they may be recognised for the support they give but may themselves feel neglected, uncertain about the future, and isolated [12]. The perception that PD was taking over the person was a theme in a study by Williamson et al. [13], which was similar to findings in other studies [12, 14, 15]. Conversely, Chiong-Rivero et al. [16] found that both carers and people with PD found a new appreciation for life and that meaningful relationships with loved ones were strengthened.

Research into coping and adjustment in the context of chronic illness is heterogeneous; there are multiple complex conceptualisations, theoretical frameworks, contributing factors, and measures of adjustment across chronic illnesses [17–20]. Theories of coping and adjustment postulate that maintaining good quality of life requires successful coping and adjustment skills in response to stressors from a chronic illness. However, not all people with chronic illness successfully adjust; those who do not can experience psychological disturbances such as fear, anger, distress, and depression [17, 18]. Adjustment and coping heavily rely on individuals having the cognitive reserve necessary to implement successful strategies outlined in the models [21]. Hurt et al. [22] found that even mild to moderate cognitive impairment in subjects with PD can contribute to reduced task-oriented coping strategies. Similarly, Kudlicka et al. [23] suggested that executive dysfunction could contribute to ineffective strategies to overcome limitations of PD or ineffective coping strategies relating to psychological distress.

Therefore, PD may affect emotional well being, independence, and sense of self in both people with PD and their carer. Previous research has shown that there are numerous ways to cope with illness-related stressors, but that cognition plays a role in adjustment and cognitive impairment may make successful adjustment more difficult. What is not understood is the role that cognitive impairment associated with PD has, how it is experienced, and how it is managed from both the perspectives of the person with PD and their carer. We sought to understand whether cognitive impairment affected coping with PD and caring for someone with PD, and if so what the impact of cognitive impairment was. We also sought to understand how individuals interpreted cognitive impairment and associated symptoms, such as hallucinations. Finally, we wanted to deepen the understanding of the relationship between carers and people with PD, in terms of their needs and priorities that may be unrecognised.

2. Method

This exploratory study used a qualitative design as part of a mixed-methods study. A partially mixed concurrent equal status design was used, where quantitative and qualitative data were collected in parallel to address the same overarching aims and hypotheses [24]. The rational for this approach is that this design is complementary and seeks to gain a deeper, richer, and more complete understanding of a phenomenon by utilising the different methods to investigate either overlapping phenomena or different aspects of a single phenomenon [25]. This paper draws on the findings from the qualitative component of the study.

The study was approved by the Newcastle and North Tyneside Research Ethics Committee. All participants provided written informed consent and had the capacity to give informed consent. Participants were invited to take part by a letter and detailed information sheet informing them of the aims of the study, that participation was voluntary, they could withdraw at any time, and that data would be treated confidentially. Any identifiable information was removed from transcripts, such as first names or surnames mentioned during interviews, to ensure the anonymity of the interviewee.

2.1. Sample. All participants lived in the North East of England and were interviewed between October 2012 and January 2015. Inclusion criteria for people with PD were as follows: a diagnosis of PD made by a movement disorders expert and fulfilled Queen's Square Brain Bank criteria [26] and required an informal caregiver to help with daily activities. Informal carers were spouses, partners, adult family members, or friends who were the primary caregiver of the person with PD.

Purposeful sampling was used to ensure a range of participants and balance between people with PD disease without cognitive impairment, people with PD and mild cognitive impairment, people with PDD, and PD disease severity. Informal carers were sampled based on the PD diagnosis of the care recipient. These three groups were chosen to explore the impact of PD and cognitive impairment across the different diagnoses and to explore whether there were differences in coping and adjustment between groups. PD participants were diagnosed as mild cognitive impairment using Movement Disorder Society Level II classification [27] based on their results on the neuropsychological tests, as described by Yarnall et al. [28]. PDD was diagnosed using Movement Disorder Society criteria [29].

2.2. Data Collection and Analysis. For consistency, all interviews were carried out and analysed by the same researcher (RAL), a research assistant and PhD student working on the study and known to the PD participants and carers. One-to-one interviews were carried out at the research unit so that both the PD participants and their carer might speak more freely about their experiences. Interviews were recorded on a digital device. Semistructured interviews were used to allow the researcher to cover the issues or topics relating to the aims of the study in-depth while enabling them to also explore novel subjects or themes as they arose. An interview schedule was developed by RAL, with guidance from KRB, based on a review of the literature (Table 1).

NVivo 11 software was used to aid analysis. The interviews were transcribed verbatim and these texts formed the basis for analysis. Data collection and analysis was an interactive process and continued until saturation was reached, and RAL and KRB agreed no new themes were emerging from the data. Additional interviews were conducted to ensure an equal distribution of participants between the three cognitive groups and to confirm data saturation. The interview content was analysed using thematic analysis as detailed by Braun and Clarke [30] in Figure 1. Open coding by RAL and KRB was at first used in detail, which allowed the early formation of themes and concepts; RAL was the primary coder. Each code was analysed across participants by reviewing all extracts relating to that code; this allowed for a deeper understanding of the codes. A coding frame was derived from the data that included subthemes (Table 2); DC, JPT, and DJB reviewed these conceptually. Differences or inconsistencies in coding and concepts were discussed and were resolved by consensus. The coding frame was used to identify and collate extracts from the interview transcripts from each theme derived from

TABLE 1: Semistructured interview schedule.

Life before you/they were diagnosed with Parkinson's.

Experience of diagnosis.

How have thins changed?

What does quality of life mean and has this changed?

Discussion on cognitive problems (memory/making decisions/concentrating).

Understanding of dementia in Parkinson's. Discussion on coping.

What helps you to cope with these changes?

Discussion on relationships.

Feelings about the future.

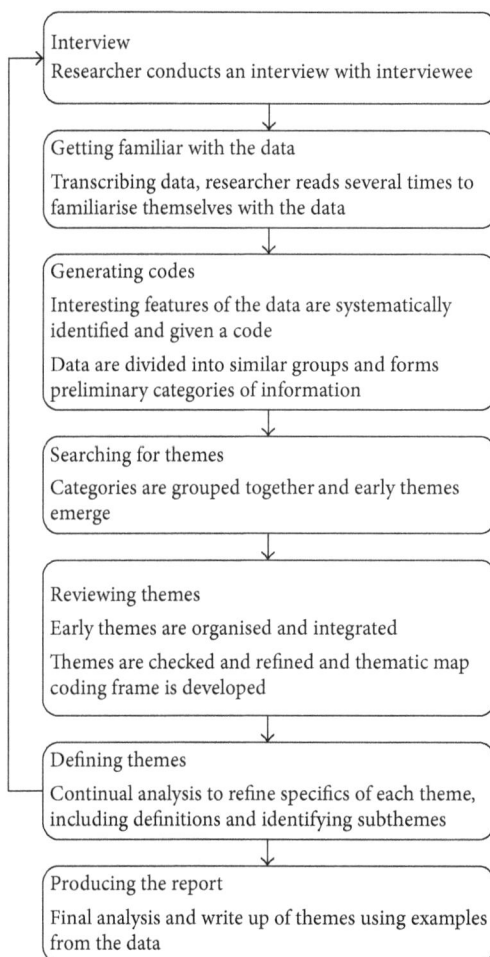

FIGURE 1: Phases of thematic analysis described by Braun and Clarke [30].

the data [30]. Themes were interpreted in consultation with theory of coping and adaptation [19]. Extracts were reviewed and interrogated as to how they related back to the aims of this study. Selected quotations supporting the analysis and interpretations of results were included in this report.

Rigour of data analysis was ensured by several means. The research team comprised multidisciplinary members, a health psychologist (RAL), a clinical neuropsychologist (DC), an old age psychiatrist (JPT), a neurologist (DJB), and a social gerontologist (KRB). This allowed for investigator and theoretical triangulation of data analysis and interpretation.

We referred to consolidated criteria for reporting qualitative studies (COREQ) [31] and reflected on these to ensure methodological rigour and trustworthiness.

3. Findings

Thirty-six people were interviewed comprising 18 people with PD and 18 carers (Table 3). The majority of PD participants were male; most caregivers were spousal, with one carer being an adult child of the person with PD and another who was an acquaintance of the person with PD who became an informal carer through mutual agreement.

The qualitative analysis of the participants' interviews revealed a number of themes. Four principal themes emerged in relation to the aims of this study: (1) cognitive impairment as a threat to perceived identity and role, (2) predeath grief and feelings of loss in carers of people with PD and cognitive impairment, (3) success and challenges to coping in people with PD, and (4) problem-focused coping and finding meaning in caring. Additional quotes to support these findings are presented in Supplementary Table 1.

3.1. Cognitive Impairment as a Threat to Perceived Identity and Role. This theme related to challenges coping with cognitive impairment in PD. Having PD and cognitive impairment was a threat to participants' perception of themselves and their role within familial and social groups, which was a source of distress.

Participants with mild cognitive impairment and PDD discussed how they were not the same person and that their image of themselves had changed as a result. Being diagnosed with PD to many participants was a life-changing event that split their lives into "before" and "after." The uncertainty of PD and the awareness of how they had changed physically and mentally, from challenging day-to-day tasks they previously took for granted, were frequent reminders of PD. Their previous self-image was no longer congruent with their physical and mental state, which forced them to construct a new self-image which incorporated PD. Participants grieved for the part of themselves that PD took away.

I almost had a breakdown because I couldn't remember who I used to be, I literally couldn't, I found that whatever was going on in my life it all revolved around Parkinson's, even when I dream now I've got Parkinson's, to me it's as if it's always been like this ... I think what a lot had been

TABLE 2: Coding frame.

Main themes	Subthemes	Descriptors
Cognitive impairment stressors	Cognitive impairment as a threat to perceived identity and role	Loss of sense of self Parent/child relationship Diminished Becoming a carer Loss of partner
	Predeath grief: feelings of loss in carers	Not the same person Taken from me Loss of mutuality and marriage
Coping and adjustment	Success and challenges to coping in people with Parkinson's disease	Successful adjustment Acceptance: I just cope Maintaining independence Uncertain future Perceived helplessness Avoidance Catastrophizing
	Between helplessness and survival in carers coping with cognitive impairment	Sacrificing own needs Isolation Struggling with cognitive symptoms Finding meaning

TABLE 3: Demographics of participants with Parkinson's and their carers.

	Age	Sex	People with Parkinson's disease Occupation	Pseudonym	Relationship with carer	Age	Sex	Carer Occupation	Pseudonym
Parkinson's disease	62	Male	Retired engineer	Harry	Partner	66	Female	Retired care assistant	Pamela
	69	Male	Retired housing director	David	Spouse	70	Female	Homemaker	Evelyn
	74	Female	Retired dinner lady	Claire	Husband	74	Male	Retired electrical engineer	Frank
	75	Male	Retired air traffic controller	Will	Spouse	67	Female	Retired air traffic controller	Heather
	80	Male	Retired medical lab technician	Mike	Spouse	69	Female	Retired nurse	Kate
	81	Male	Retired doctor	Peter	Spouse	78	Female	Retired radiographer	Ruth
Mild cognitive impairment	65	Male	Retired HGV driver	Ted	Spouse	64	Female	Retired physiotherapist	Opal
	66	Male	Retired solicitor	George	Spouse	61	Female	Solicitor	Frances
	66	Male	Retired nurse	Steve	Carer/friend	—	Female	Retired PA	Nina
	67	Female	Retired catering technician	Denise	Spouse	71	Male	Retired maintenance electrician	Jack
	67	Male	Semiretired sound recording engineer	Edward	Spouse	64	Female	Audio services	Val
	68	Male	Retired salesman	Kevin	Spouse	67	Female	Retired psychiatric nurse	Anne
Parkinson's dementia	67	Male	Retired fitter	Nigel	Spouse	66	Female	Retired shop assistant	Joyce
	70	Female	Retired lab technician	Sylvia	Spouse	77	Male	Retired boiler plater	Owen
	72	Male	Retired labourer	Rob	Spouse	72	Female	Retired care assistant	Gwen
	79	Female	Retired shop assistant	Ingrid	Mother/Daughter	52	Female	Carer	Liz
	69	Male	Retired local government officer	Alan	Spouse	56	Female	Teacher	Barbra
	87	Male	Retired salesman	Colin	Partner	68	Female	Retired	Mary

wrong with me too was I think I was grieving for somebody I'd lost, which was myself, I found a lot of similarities in grieving the things that you feel. (Steve, man with Parkinson's and mild cognitive impairment)

For some people with PD, the threat to their perceived identity came from a change in their perceived role in their family. Participants with PD and cognitive impairment felt unimportant or less significant compared to before they had PD. They described feeling redundant and that their roles had been assumed by someone else, often the caregiver. As a result, their self-confidence was diminished, and they felt dissatisfied with their new perceived role within the family environment. The feeling of not being in control of their lives, or control being taken from them, was identified as contributing to this change in identity.

I used to you know I felt head of the family, not that that means, I didn't wield a stick but you know I couldn't I could never do that, but I felt as though I had a position in the family, but now I don't, I feel downgraded a bit, whether that's paranoia setting in or not I don't know but I just feel a lesser person . . . I feel as though she's the boss now, really and it's quite rightly is too because she's got me to put up with, so there you are. (Kevin, man with Parkinson's and mild cognitive impairment)

In contrast to the people with PD and cognitive impairment, those without any cognitive problems did not experience the same threats to their sense of self. They did not describe changes in their perception of themselves, their relationship with their partner, or their place in the family unit. Instead, they described fewer threats to their emotional equilibrium from illness stressors:

. . . there wasn't sort of a dividing line where that's pre-PD and post-PD it seemed to be from my point of view it seemed to be a gradual thing . . . I know I've been diagnosed but nothing dramatic has happened, I think that's what I've been trying to tell the tale throughout I can't see any dramatic change yet. (David, man with Parkinson's)

Change in role of the carers was also a key issue. Becoming a carer was something they had to incorporate into their own identity and sense of self, although some saw it part of their spousal duty. Part of this was driven by an increase in responsibilities in terms of physical tasks, such as housework, gardening, getting dressed, talking on the telephone, and driving. Carers of people with PD and cognitive impairment also had additional caring activities and responsibilities due to the care recipient not having the cognitive capacity to carry them out, for example, handling household affairs, finances, and decision making. For many, this was a reversal in roles they previously had with PD participants. Carers also perceived their needs were less important than those of PD participants, particularly those with cognitive impairment, and assumed the role of person in charge and protector, which reinforced the role change.

I never had children and I never wanted children but now I have two children. i.e., my mam and dad . . . I think that's probably one of the hardest things is that your parents don't become your parents you become the parent and they become the child. (Liz, daughter of woman with Parkinson's dementia)

3.2. Predeath Grief: Feelings of Loss in Carers of People with Parkinson's and Cognitive Impairment. For carers, dissatisfaction centred on changes in their perceived role and feelings of loss. Carers found that cognitive changes in the person with PD were more challenging to deal with emotionally compared to the physical changes. Some carers, predominantly those with partners with PDD, spoke of feelings of loss and grief, both in terms of who the person with PD was and the change in life expectations. Perceptions of people with PD were altered by dementia; a key issue was how the person with PD was no longer themselves, particularly those who also had dementia.

He was just totally different, he just you'd think he'd been unplugged, it's the only way I could describe it, he was it just wasn't Nigel at all, he was totally different. (Joyce, wife of man with Parkinson's dementia)

Cognitive impairment had a bigger emotional impact on carers compared to the physical impact of the motor symptoms. The grief centred on how PD and cognitive impairment was taking their loved one from them; some carers referred to that person as already gone. The person they were left caring for was someone they did not recognise. The sense of emotional loss in carers was evident, owing to a mourning of their planned future, restricted social life, and their relationship with the person with PD.

I suppose they make me feel a little bit depressed at time because I feel as if I'm losing him a bit . . . I know we've still got a wonderful relationship we've always had a great relationship, sometimes I feel, oh it sounds horrible, as if I'm love, living with an old man which has never been Colin, so I do get depressed over it yes. (Mary, partner of man with Parkinson's dementia)

For some carers, it was the loss of mutuality as a result of cognitive impairment in PD. The grief encompassed interpersonal loss for their partner, where they had become the sole carer rather than having a mutually beneficial relationship. In addition, the carers had lost their source of social support; they provided increasing support for the person with PD while having no support to cope with their own feelings of anxiety, grief, and powerlessness.

It's that change from that dual partnership of having that rock beside you to being the carer really and it changes the balance obviously in the relationship which you will know from everybody else, that's hard actually to deal with and try, not to mask it but to try, you use up a lot of energy trying to make things better, to try and regain that balance, you know, and sort of refocus it, to try and help self-esteem and keep trying to keep, almost maintain the status quo, but it's not. (Barbra, wife of man with Parkinson's dementia)

Only one carer whose husband had PD but no cognitive impairment expressed similar feelings. Although there were no cognitive problems, apathy and depression in the participant with PD were barriers to mutuality and perpetuated feelings of loss and emotional distress in the carer.

I feel like I've lost my partner, he's become very self-absorbed, it feels like life revolves around him now, it feels like he's living so much in a bubble that he has stopped noticing how things impact on me completely... I actually just feel really lonely . . . I can't quite find the words to describe how much it's changed our relationship really, I feel like I've lost him in lots of ways (Crying). (Heather, wife of man with Parkinson's)

3.3. Success and Challenges to Coping in People with Parkinson's Disease.

This theme centred on the issues around coping and adjustment to PD and cognitive impairment in participants with PD. Some participants coped and adjusted to having cognitive impairment and/or PD better than others. This theme explored the facilitators and barriers to successful coping. Participants with PD and no cognitive impairment generally showed good psychosocial adjustment. They used cognitive and behavioural strategies that facilitated good adjustment when faced with PD-related challenges, such as seeking social support, acceptance of their illness, appropriate expression of emotions, and maintaining their activity levels despite the possible limitations due to having PD.

I can talk about it now, I found that I couldn't talk about it when I got diagnosed I don't know why like, it's just I didn't want to talk about it as well like you know, but now I can talk to people about it like you know and mainly to say look I've got Parkinson's but I get on with life and I'm doing fine. (Harry, man with Parkinson's)

Some participants with PD and cognitive impairment had coped better than others. Those that showed good psychosocial adjustment used problem-focused coping strategies to help overcome symptoms of cognitive impairment. Alarms or pill boxes were used to help participants regulate their own medication; some used calendars regularly to remind them about important events and appointments. These coping methods allowed them to maintain some of their activities and independence; it was evident that participants who used problem-focused coping strategies had accepted changes, both physically and cognitively, and had some perceived control over these changes.

I've got to write on the calendar or, or I just wouldn't I just wouldn't attend like half of them I wouldn't be here . . . and I'm always checking them to see if I've put the right dates

on like you know, just checking and checking and checking just to make sure. (Rob, man with Parkinson's dementia)

In contrast, some participants with PD and cognitive impairment found coping challenging. For some, their future had changed from something they had control over, to something that was unknown and uncertain. This was difficult to adjust to for some participants. The negative illness representations that some PD participants had, particularly concerning dementia and the possibility of developing dementia in the future, were barriers to high positive affect. Instead, these participants were distressed and had low positive affect:

...the dementia frightens me more than Parkinson's I think, Parkinson's I've got sewn up, well I'm not going to say sewn up, the other one is the unknown quantity really. (Nigel, man with Parkinson's dementia)

Rather than using an appropriate expression of emotion, some PD participants vented their emotions. Participants talked about how their condition was unfair, that they felt bitter and angry. This was partly driven by perceived helplessness or low perceived social support. Participants were frustrated by the necessity of being cared for. Some participants described how they "bottled things up" and did not feel they were able to talk to their family about their feelings and the difficulties they experienced. Sometimes this was because they did not want to worry their loved ones, whereas other individuals described themselves as having always been less inclined to seek social support. These participants had low perceived social support and repressed their emotions.

Sometimes I say, "you take all my independence away from me," the little bit I try to build up because he is a mother hen, he likes to do things and he thinks he is doing right, I say, "you are not Jack, you are not helping me by being like this," I feel like I am fighting him and I am fighting the Parkinson's and it is just a vicious circle. (Denise, woman with Parkinson's and mild cognitive impairment)

PD and cognitive impairment was a disruption to everyday activities in several participants. Some participants had reduced or even avoided activities where they perceived difficulties or potentially distressing situations. The apprehension of being seen as stupid or less than they once were by others was upsetting for some participants, which perpetuated their wish for avoidance or people or certain situations.

I'm told I am nobody notices but it's knocked my confidence for going up to the shops, going into the town a little bit on my own, and then I worry about getting the money getting out of the, I go shopping and I can pick say a dress up or some shoes and then I start to worry about getting to the counter and getting my money out and getting my card out, I feel as if I'm being slow. (Sylvia, woman with Parkinson's dementia)

A small number of participants had dysfunctional cognitions and bias. These participants would catastrophize, where small issues with memory or their future would escalate into serious issues. This can be a barrier to good psychosocial adjustment. These participants had low self-esteem, low positive affect, and negative illness perceptions.

Well, I get frustrated with myself, the worst part about it, as you know, is I'm losing stuff, I just lose so much now, I mean money glasses keys, you name it, they'll just disappear in thin air, that upsets me a bit because I worry about doing something that's going to harm others, I might forget to turn the gas off and leave the water running and stuff like that, that bothers me, as I say. (Steve, man with Parkinson's and mild cognitive impairment)

3.4. Problem-Focused Coping and Finding Meaning in Caring. Coping and adjustment varied between the three groups of carers. Most carers who cared for someone without cognitive impairment had good psychosocial adjustment, where they were able to cope well with illness stressors. Carers of participants with PD without cognitive impairment were able to be more independent that those who cared for someone with PD and cognitive impairment. These carers had increasing responsibilities due to physical disability in the person with PD; however, they identified the importance of not sacrificing their own needs to those of their partner or family member. This was partly motivated by the awareness that the well-being of their partner or family member was dependent on the maintenance of their well-being. Respite from caring facilitated coping in these carers as they were able to rest, seek social support from other sources, and time to gain fresh perspective through the implementation of problem-focused coping strategies.

I end up doing a lot of things by myself as well because I want to see things too and I'm not going to sit back ... I would say no this is my life as well, I've still got to keep it you know otherwise if I go and anything goes wrong with me then Kevin would be in a worse state than ever, so I've got to look after my own interests too without being seen to be selfish you know. (Anne, wife of man with Parkinson's and mild cognitive impairment)

In contrast, there was tension between the needs of carers and coping with cognitive impairment and PD in their partner or family member. Carers of participants with PDD found it more difficult to cope well with cognitive impairment, and to a lesser extent some mild cognitive impairment carers also found good psychosocial adjustment difficult. These carers had high perceived stress, perceived helplessness, and repressed their emotions; these manifested as self-blame, wishful thinking, venting of negative emotions, and catastrophizing. As a result, carers felt unsupported, isolated, and unable to cope:

the Parkinson's you think, a piece of cake, the dementia is the real tricky one actually it's that rollercoaster with the dementia ... I blame him and that's really not coping because it's not his fault, and I know it's not his fault and I say to myself, "it's the illness," but sometimes still you want to blame him for your change in life and that's completely wrong and cruel. (Crying) So that's really not coping and, you know, just being less than kind, you feel horrible. (Barbra, wife of man with Parkinson's dementia)

In addition to increased responsibilities as a result of physical and cognitive disability, there were challenging symptoms and behavioural problems that they also had to cope with. Hallucinations, delusions, and outburst of aggression were not recognised by the person with PD; however, they were evidently distressing for the carers and challenging to cope with. These were very salient intrusions to the lives of the carers and caused disruptions which were unpredictable and distressing. This was exacerbated by carers' feeling they were helpless to both cope with these symptoms and that the person with PDD was not aware of the distress they were causing their partner. This made it difficult for carers to implement problem-focused coping strategies:

...there's nothing much I can do about it, you see it's difficult because say if you hurt your foot I could help you with your foot and say oh I'll put a bandage on or whatever but if it's something mental the mind you don't know how to cope with that, you can talk to and I'm talking to you I can talk to her and sometimes you see well it's not getting through to her you know because it keeps happening all the time ... how do you cope with that, you know? (Owen, husband of woman with Parkinson's dementia)

Conversely, some carers found meaning and purpose in being a carer, which facilitated good psychosocial adjustment and coping. There was increased appreciation for their family member and expressed an enrichment to their lives from caring. Carers who found meaning and purpose exhibited positive personal growth, where they became more patient, understating, and resilient as a result of caring for their loved one. They further observed gains in the relationship, where the relationship improved with the person with PD.

When she's come out the shower and I wrap her in the towel and I dry and she's like, "oh you're angel I don't know what I'd do without you," and that's like more than if you'd won the lottery to be honest ... it makes you a better person, that's what I believe, it's made me a better person, it's enriched my life, yeah without a doubt. (Liz, daughter of woman with Parkinson's dementia)

4. Discussion

This qualitative study is the first to explore the impact of cognitive impairment in people with PD and their carers. The findings highlight that for some participants with PD, cognitive impairment negatively impacted on their quality of life and caused emotional distress, but this was not the case for all. It seemed that if PD participants did not have an awareness of any cognitive impairment, and it was not intrusive to their daily lives, then their emotional equilibrium was not disturbed [19]. In carers, however, we found that cognitive impairment has a greater emotional impact than the physical symptoms associated with PD. Central to emotional distress in carers were feelings of loss of their loved one, helplessness, and feeling overwhelmed by cognitive impairment and associated symptoms.

While recent quantitative studies have found that cognitive impairment is associated with poorer quality of life in both patients and their carers [2, 3, 32, 33], they have been unable to determine the impact it has on individuals and how they cope with its effects. We were able to explore this in our study. Our data showed that cognitive impairment threatened emotional equilibrium [19] and affected a range of aspects of their daily lives: social participation, leisure activities, independence, daily activities, mood, and identity.

Challenges to identity and perceived role were important issues, where participants described feeling less confident or insignificant, and PD patients reversed roles with their carer. Through living with PD and cognitive impairment, their previous self-image and social identity were no longer congruent with their current physical and mental state; PD participants suggested that periodic deteriorations caused a crisis which disrupted their emotional equilibrium [19, 34]. Such crises have been proposed to trigger a grief-like mourning period, where individuals grieve for the person they were and their past life before the disease [35]. Parallels can be drawn from other chronic diseases, where this has been coined as 'chronic sorrow' [36] and has been observed in a previous study in PD [15]. Comparably, role reversal and dissatisfaction has been described previously in carers and people with dementia [37] but has not previously been investigated in PD. Previous studies have illustrated that people with PD who have to accept care and support can feel humiliated and excluded, as well as excluded socially and misunderstood, while partners who were the source of support felt neglected and isolated [12]. This suggests that needing support and becoming that source of support is a potential stressor and could result in poor psychosocial outcomes without the implementation of successful coping strategies [19].

We have extended existing knowledge of cognition and coping in PD. Our findings show that periodically, all PD participants described coping difficulties including uncertain futures, depression, worry, fear, guilt, and anger, which are indicative of poor psychosocial adjustment [19]. Those with cognitive impairment found successful coping difficult and used unhelpful strategies such as wishful thinking, catastrophizing, venting, and negative illness representations; these have been described as emotion-focused strategies by the stress and coping model of adjustment [38]. PD participants without cognitive impairment used problem-focused coping to implement cognitive and behavioural factors to successful adjust more often than those with cognitive impairment [38]. This may be due to participants with PD having insufficient cognitive reserve to implement appropriate

coping techniques to facilitate good psychosocial adjustment. Cognitive reserve has been previously suggested as necessary to instigate effective coping strategies [21]. Two quantitative studies proposed that mild cognitive dysfunction could impair the implementation of helpful coping strategies [22], causing difficulties with positive reappraisal, goal setting, and adjusting expectations [23].

We found that carers of people with PD and cognitive impairment experienced greater emotional distress due to the cognitive symptoms compared to the physical symptoms; carers of PDD participants expressed the greatest emotional distress and coping difficulty. Parkinson's dementia carers also described feelings of predeath grief towards their spouses or partners with cognitive impairment, where the person with PDD is no longer cognitively or emotionally present, which was emotionally upsetting for carers. They also grieved for their change in circumstances and for the loss of their planned futures. Predeath grief, also referred to as latent grief or social death, has previously reported that cognitive change was the biggest predictor of carer grief in PD [39].

Parkinson's dementia carers in our study described feeling overwhelmed with cognitive changes and challenging behaviours associated with delusions and hallucinations. Neuropsychiatric symptoms in PDD have previously been associated with increased carer distress [40], similar to the findings of our study. A qualitative study by Williamson, Simpson, and Murray [13] conveyed diverse ways in which spousal carers and people with PD adapted to neuropsychiatric symptoms, with varying success and distress. We found carers expressed difficulty coping and adjusting to hallucinations and delusions our study in comparison to Williamson et al. [13]. Perhaps, this is because the participants in our study were more recently diagnosed with PD, and neuropsychiatric symptoms had first occurred relatively [19].

Our study found that a good mutual relationship between the carer and the patient was protective, with some carers suggesting that they experienced positive personal growth as a result of caregiving. Comparisons can be found in dementia studies; Netto et al. found informal familial carers of people with dementia exhibited positive personal growth, where they become more patient, understating, and resilient as a result of caring for a loved one [41]. Our participants further observed gains and improvement in the relationship with the care recipient. Lyons et al. showed that mutuality was protective of role strain in carers over a 10-year period [42]; it has also been associated with better mental health, lower carer burden, and better carer quality of life [43].

The strengths of this study include the comparatively large number of participants, rigorous methodology, and purposefully sampled participants using theoretical criteria to give a representative sample of carers and people with PD across cognitive groups. Extensive quotations have been presented to ensure the credibility of the analysis. We have also drawn parallels of our findings from other chronic diseases, which denote the validity of our findings. This study was part of a larger mixed-methods study and was able to address the disparities that the quantitative arm of the study. There are several limitations to this study. First, the gender ratio of PD participants and carers were both uneven, with more male PD participants and more female carers taking part. However, this reflects the reality of the disease, where proportionally more men are diagnosed with PD, and that society relies on female care provision [44, 45]. Similarly, most of the carers were the spouse or partner of the person with PD; thus, the experiences of other relatives, such as adult children as carers, are underrepresented. Finally, only PD participants were used in this study; it would be of interest to include carers and patients from other neurodegenerative diseases, such as Alzheimer's disease. Future studies should include a wider range of relationships to the care recipient and should also compare the experiences of patients and carers with different types of dementias.

5. Conclusion

This study has highlighted that coping and adjustment to PD and cognitive impairment varies among patients and their carers. Cognitive impairment can threaten an individual's self-perception and their perceived role among family and friends. However, the ostensible effects of cognitive impairment and PD depended on the impact individual's perceived cognitive impairment to have on their daily lives. For carers, cognitive impairment in their partner or family member had a greater emotional impact compared to the physical symptoms of PD, where carers experienced predeath grief. The discussion which developed around protective factors provides possible opportunities for future psychological interventions, such as therapies to improve mood and successful adjustment. By promoting protective factors to enhance existing coping mechanisms, better quality of life for both carers and the person with PD may be achieved to prevent longer term decline and untimely nursing home placement.

Disclosure

This manuscript is formed part of a doctoral thesis (https://theses.ncl.ac.uk/dspace/).

Authors' Contributions

Rachael A. Lawson was involved with study design, coordination of the study, participant recruitment, and data collection, analysis, and interpretation and drafted the manuscript. Daniel Collerton, John-Paul Taylor, and David J. Burn were involved with study design, data interpretation, and manuscript revision. Katie R. Brittain was involved with study design, data analysis and interpretation, and manuscript revision. All coauthors have seen and approved the contents of the manuscript.

Acknowledgments

ICICLE-PD was funded by Parkinson's UK (J-0802, G-1301), who played no role in the design, execution, analysis and interpretation of the data, or writing of the study. The research was supported by the Lockhart Parkinson's Disease Research Fund and the National Institute for Health Research (NIHR) Newcastle Biomedical Research Unit based at Newcastle upon Tyne Hospitals NHS Foundation Trust and Newcastle University. The authors would like to thank all participants for their contribution towards this study.

References

[1] M. A. Hely, W. G. Reid, M. A. Adena, G. M. Halliday, and J. G. Morris, "The Sydney multicenter study of Parkinson's disease: the inevitability of dementia at 20 years," *Movement Disorders*, vol. 23, no. 6, pp. 837–844, 2008.

[2] R. Lawson, A. Yarnall, G. Duncan et al., "Cognitive decline and quality of life in incident Parkinson's disease: the role of attention," *Parkinsonism & Related Disorders*, vol. 27, pp. 47–53, 2016.

[3] R. A. Lawson, A. J. Yarnall, F. Johnston et al., "Cognitive impairment in Parkinson's disease: impact on quality of life of carers," *International Journal of Geriatric Psychiatry*, vol. 32, no. 12, pp. 1362–1370, 2017.

[4] F. Bunn, C. Goodman, K. Sworn et al., "Psychosocial factors that shape patient and carer experiences of dementia diagnosis and treatment: a systematic review of qualitative studies," *PLoS Medicine*, vol. 9, no. 10, p. e1001331, 2012.

[5] L. Robinson, A. Gemski, C. Abley et al., "The transition to dementia–individual and family experiences of receiving a diagnosis: a review," *International Psychogeriatrics*, vol. 23, no. 7, pp. 1026–1043, 2011.

[6] E. Gruffydd and J. Randle, "Alzheimer's disease and the psychosocial burden for caregivers," *Community Practitioner*, vol. 79, no. 1, pp. 15–18, 2006.

[7] J. Murray, J. Schneider, S. Banerjee, and A. Mann, "EUROCARE: a cross-national study of co-resident spouse carers for people with Alzheimer's disease: II—a qualitative analysis of the experience of caregiving," *International Journal of Geriatric Psychiatry*, vol. 14, no. 8, pp. 662–667, 1999.

[8] J. Paton, K. Johnston, C. Katona, and G. Livingston, "What causes problems in Alzheimer's disease: attributions by caregivers. A qualitative study," *International Journal of Geriatric Psychiatry*, vol. 19, no. 6, pp. 527–532, 2004.

[9] L. Todres and K. Galvin, "Caring for a partner with Alzheimer's disease: intimacy, loss and the life that is possible," *International Journal of Qualitative Studies on Health and Well-being*, vol. 1, no. 1, pp. 50–61, 2006.

[10] J. Wuest, P. K. Ericson, and P. N. Stern, "Becoming strangers: the changing family caregiving relationship in Alzheimer's disease," *Journal of Advanced Nursing*, vol. 20, no. 3, pp. 437–443, 1994.

[11] H. D. Davies, L. A. Newkirk, C. B. Pitts et al., "The impact of dementia and mild memory impairment (MMI) on intimacy and sexuality in spousal relationships," *International Psychogeriatrics*, vol. 22, no. 4, pp. 618–628, 2010.

[12] A. M. B. Birgersson and A. K. Edberg, "Being in the light or in the shade: persons with Parkinson's disease and their partners'

experience of support," *International Journal of Nursing Studies*, vol. 41, no. 6, pp. 621–630, 2004.

[13] C. Williamson, J. Simpson, and C. D. Murray, "Caregivers' experiences of caring for a husband with Parkinson's disease and psychotic symptoms," *Social Science & Medicine*, vol. 67, no. 4, pp. 583–589, 2008.

[14] J. H. Hodgson, K. Garcia, and L. Tyndall, "Parkinson's disease and the couple relationship: a qualitative analysis," *Families, Systems, & Health*, vol. 22, no. 1, pp. 101–118, 2004.

[15] C. L. Lindgren, "Chronic sorrow in persons with Parkinson's and their spouses," *Scholarly Inquiry for Nursing Practice*, vol. 10, no. 4, pp. 351–366, 1996.

[16] H. Chiong-Rivero, G. W. Ryan, C. Flippen et al., "Patients' and caregivers' experiences of the impact of Parkinson's disease on health status," *Patient Related Outcome Measures*, vol. 2011, no. 2, pp. 57–70, 2011.

[17] D. de Ridder, R. Geenen, R. Kuijer, and H. van Middendorp, "Psychological adjustment to chronic disease," *The Lancet*, vol. 372, no. 9634, pp. 246–255, 2008.

[18] R. Moos and C. Holahan, "Adaptive tasks and methods of coping with illness and disability," in *Coping with Chronic Illness and Disability*, E. Martz, H. Livneh, and B. Wright, Eds., pp. 107–126, Springer US, 2007.

[19] R. Moss-Morris, "Adjusting to chronic illness: time for a unified theory," *British Journal of Health Psychology*, vol. 18, no. 4, pp. 681–686, 2013.

[20] A. L. Stanton, T. A. Revenson, and H. Tennen, "Health psychology: psychological adjustment to chronic disease," *Annual Review of Psychology*, vol. 58, no. 1, pp. 565–592, 2007.

[21] J. V. Hindle, A. Martyr, and L. Clare, "Cognitive reserve in Parkinson's disease: a systematic review and meta-analysis," *Parkinsonism & Related Disorders*, vol. 20, no. 1, pp. 1–7, 2014.

[22] C. S. Hurt, S. Landau, D. J. Burn et al., "Cognition, coping, and outcome in Parkinson's disease," *International Psychogeriatrics*, vol. 24, no. 10, pp. 1656–1663, 2012.

[23] A. Kudlicka, L. Clare, and J. V. Hindle, "Quality of life, health status and caregiver burden in Parkinson's disease: relationship to executive functioning," *International Journal of Geriatric Psychiatry*, vol. 29, no. 1, pp. 68–76, 2014.

[24] J. W. Creswell and V. L. Plano Clark, *Designing and Conducting Mixed Methods Research*, SAGE, Thousand Oaks, CA, USA, 2nd edition, 2011.

[25] A. Tashakkori and C. Teddlie, *Sage Handbook of Mixed Methods in Social & Behavioral Research*, SAGE, Thousand Oaks, CA, USA, 2010.

[26] A. J. Hughes, S. E. Daniel, L. Kilford, and A. J. Lees, "Accuracy of clinical diagnosis of idiopathic Parkinson's disease: a clinico-pathological study of 100 cases," *Journal of Neurology, Neurosurgery, and Psychiatry*, vol. 55, no. 3, pp. 181–184, 1992.

[27] I. Litvan, J. G. Goldman, A. I. Tröster, B. A. Schmand, and D. Weintraub, "Diagnostic criteria for mild cognitive impairment in Parkinson's disease: Movement Disorder Society Task Force guidelines," *Movement Disorders*, vol. 27, no. 3, pp. 349–356, 2012.

[28] A. J. Yarnall, D. P. Breen, G. W. Duncan et al., "Characterizing mild cognitive impairment in incident Parkinson disease: the ICICLE-PD study," *Neurology*, vol. 82, no. 4, pp. 308–316, 2014.

[29] M. Emre, D. Aarsland, R. Brown et al., "Clinical diagnostic criteria for dementia associated with Parkinson's disease," *Movement Disorders*, vol. 22, no. 12, pp. 1689–1707, 2007.

[30] V. Braun and V. Clarke, "Using thematic analysis in psychology," *Qualitative Research in Psychology*, vol. 3, no. 2, pp. 77–101, 2006.

[31] A. Tong, P. Sainsbury, and J. Craig, "Consolidated criteria for reporting qualitative research (COREQ): a 32-item checklist for interviews and focus groups," *International Journal for Quality in Health Care*, vol. 19, no. 6, pp. 349–357, 2007.

[32] I. Leroi, K. McDonald, H. Pantula, and V. Harbishettar, "Cognitive impairment in Parkinson disease: impact on quality of life, disability, and caregiver burden," *Journal of Geriatric Psychiatry and Neurology*, vol. 25, no. 4, pp. 208–214, 2012.

[33] D. Morley, S. Dummett, M. Peters et al., "Factors influencing quality of life in caregivers of people with Parkinson's disease and implications for clinical guidelines," *Parkinson's Disease*, vol. 2012, Article ID 190901, 6 pages, 2012.

[34] R. H. Moos and J. A. Schaefer, *The Crisis of Physical Illness, Coping with Physical Illness*, Springer, Berlin, Germany, 1984.

[35] H. Livneh and R. F. Antonak, "Psychosocial adaptation to chronic illness and disability: a primer for counselors," *Journal of Counseling & Development*, vol. 83, no. 1, pp. 12–20, 2005.

[36] B. H. Davis, "Disability and grief," *Social Casework*, vol. 68, no. 6, pp. 352–357, 1987.

[37] N. F. Toepfer, J. L. H. Foster, and G. Wilz, "The good mother and her clinging child": patterns of anchoring in social representations of dementia caregiving," *Journal of Community & Applied Social Psychology*, vol. 24, no. 3, pp. 234–248, 2014.

[38] R. S. Lazarus and S. Folkman, *Stress, Appraisal, and Coping*, Springer Publishing Company, New York, NY, USA, 1984.

[39] J. H. Carter, K. S. Lyons, A. Lindauer, and J. Malcom, "Predeath grief in Parkinson's caregivers: a pilot survey-based study," *Parkinsonism & Related Disorders*, vol. 18, no. 3, pp. S15–S18, 2012.

[40] D. Aarsland, K. Brønnick, U. Ehrt et al., "Neuropsychiatric symptoms in patients with Parkinson's disease and dementia: frequency, profile and associated care giver stress," *Journal of Neurology, Neurosurgery & Psychiatry*, vol. 78, no. 1, pp. 36–42, 2007.

[41] N. R. Netto, G. Y. N. Jenny, and Y. L. K. Philip, "Growing and gaining through caring for a loved one with dementia," *Dementia*, vol. 8, no. 2, pp. 245–261, 2009.

[42] K. S. Lyons, B. J. Stewart, P. G. Archbold, and J. H. Carter, "Optimism, pessimism, mutuality, and gender: predicting 10-year role strain in Parkinson's disease spouses," *Gerontologist*, vol. 49, no. 3, pp. 378–387, 2009.

[43] H. Tanji, K. E. Anderson, A. L. Gruber-Baldini et al., "Mutuality of the marital relationship in Parkinson's disease," *Movement Disorders*, vol. 23, no. 13, pp. 1843–1849, 2008.

[44] J. M. Glozman, "Quality of life of caregivers," *Neuropsychology Review*, vol. 14, no. 4, pp. 183–196, 2004.

[45] D. Santos-Garcia and R. de la Fuente-Fernandez, "Factors contributing to caregivers' stress and burden in Parkinson's disease," *Acta Neurologica Scandinavica*, vol. 131, no. 4, pp. 203–210, 2015.

Reliability and Validity of the Geriatric Depression Scale in Italian Subjects with Parkinson's Disease

Perla Massai,[1] Francesca Colalelli,[1] Julita Sansoni [ID],[2] Donatella Valente,[3] Marco Tofani [ID],[1] Giovanni Fabbrini [ID],[3,4] Andrea Fabbrini,[3] Michela Scuccimarri,[1] and Giovanni Galeoto [ID][2]

[1]*Sapienza University of Rome, Rome, Italy*
[2]*Department of Public Health and Infection Disease, Sapienza University of Rome, Rome, Italy*
[3]*Department Human Neurosciences, Sapienza University of Rome, Rome, Italy*
[4]*IRCSS Neuromed Institute, Pozzilli, IS, Italy*

Correspondence should be addressed to Giovanni Galeoto; giovanni.galeoto@uniroma1.it

Academic Editor: Aristide Merola

Introduction. The Geriatric Depression Scale (GDS) is commonly used to assess depressive symptoms, but its psychometric properties have never been examined in Italian people with Parkinson's disease (PD). The aim of this study was to study the reliability and validity of the Italian version of the GDS in a sample of PD patients. *Methods.* The GDS was administered to 74 patients with PD in order to study its internal consistency, test-retest reliability, construct, and discriminant validity. *Results.* The internal consistency of GDS was excellent ($\alpha = 0.903$), as well as the test-retest reliability (ICC = 0.941 [95% CI: 0.886–0.970]). GDS showed a strong correlation with instruments related to the depression ($\rho = 0.880$) in PD ($\rho = 0.712$) and a weak correlation with generic measurement instruments ($-0.320 < \rho < -0.217$). An area under the curve of 0.892 (95% CI 0.809–0.975) indicated a moderate capability to discriminate depressed patients to nondepressed patient, with a cutoff value between 15 and 16 points that predicts depression (sensitivity = 87%; specificity = 82%). *Conclusion.* The GDS is a reliable and valid tool in a sample of Italian PD subjects; this scale can be used in clinical and research contexts.

1. Introduction

Parkinson disease (PD) is characterized by motor and nonmotor symptoms. Bradykinesia, tremor at rest, and rigidity are the cardinal motor manifestations of PD [1]. Nonmotor symptoms include gastrointestinal dysfunctions, sleep disorders, cognitive disorders, and neuropsychiatric disturbances. Depression has been found to be more frequent in PD patients than in age-matched healthy controls or in patients with other chronic medical conditions [2, 3]. For example, major depression may be found in up to 20% of PD patients [4]. To measure the level of depression, it is crucial that clinicians and researchers have access to reliable and valid instruments. A recent systematic review about depression tools in PD patients recommended the use of the Hamilton Depression Inventory as a rating scale, which takes into consideration the judgment of the clinician or the

caregiver, and the Geriatric Depression Scale (GDS), that considers the patient's point of view, for the screening and measurement of the degree of perceived depression in patients with PD [5].

The GDS [6], composed by 30 items, was developed to evaluate the level of depressive symptoms over the past week. It was transculturally adapted in several languages [7–9], and it has proven to be reliable and valid in subjects with dementia [10–13], stroke [14–17], rheumatoid arthritis [18], and psychiatric disorders [19, 20]. In PD, several studies showed that GDS has good psychometric properties, a high internal consistency (Cronbach's alpha = 0.92) [21], an excellent test-retest reliability (intraclass correlation coefficient = 0.89 [95% CI 0.83–0.93]), and a minimal detectable change of 5.4 points [22]. Taking into account the validity, the GDS showed good correlations with the Beck Depression Inventory ($r_s = 0.62$, $p < 0.05$) and with mood related items of the Unified Parkinson's Disease Rating Scale ($r_s = 0.38$, $p < 0.05$) [23], and moderate correlations with the 17-item Hamilton Depression Rating Scale ($r = 0.54$, $p < 0.001$) [24]. Recently, the GDS was used in an Italian sample of geriatric patients, and this study confirmed the good psychometric properties of GDS [25]. As the measurement properties of an instrument are affected by the disease investigated and by the contextual factors, for a reliable and valid use of the instrument in Italian subjects, the GDS should be validated also in the target population to which the questionnaire will be administered. No study has assessed the psychometric properties of GDS in Italian patients with PD. Therefore, the aim of this study is to assess the reliability and the validity of the GDS in a sample of Italian PD patients, using the Classical Theory Test.

2. Methods

2.1. Subjects. Seventy-four (older than 18 years) patients with clinically diagnosed PD were consecutively recruited through a convenience sample in the Rehabilitation Unit of San Giovanni Battista Hospital, Polyclinic Italia, and in the Department of Neurosciences, Sapienza University of Rome. Patients with cognitive impairment (Mini-Mental State Examination score <23 points) and problems with reading and understanding the Italian language were excluded. All subjects gave their informed consent [26, 27] to participate in the study, and the research was conducted according to the principles of Declaration of Helsinki.

2.2. Outcome Measures

2.2.1. Geriatric Depression Scale. This scale assesses the depressive symptoms [6]. The version used in this study was composed by 30 items that investigated different aspects of the depression over the last week. Each item is rated by a dichotomous score (yes = 1; no = 0), and some items (Item numbers 1, 5, 7, 9, 15, 19, 21, 27, 29, and 30) presented a reverse score (yes = 0; no = 1). The total score is given adding the item scores, and it ranged from 0 (no depression) to 30 (maximum depression) points. The Italian version used in this study demonstrated to be reliable and valid [25].

2.2.2. Hospital Anxiety and Depression Scale. This scale measures the level of depression and anxiety [28]. It is composed by 14 items divided in two subscales: 7 items investigate depressive symptoms, and the other 7 measure anxious symptoms. Subjects respond to each item on four-level ordinal score (0 = no symptoms; 3 = maximum symptoms); therefore, the total scores may vary between 0 and 21 points for each subscale. The Italian version of the scale was used in this study [29].

2.2.3. Parkinson Disease Questionnaire. This questionnaire assesses the impact of parkinsonian symptoms in the life of these patients in the past month [30]. It contains 39 items that examine 8 domains through separately scored subscales: mobility (10 items), activities of daily living (6 items),

emotional well-being (6 items), stigma (4 items), social support (3 items), cognition (4 items), communication (4 items), and bodily discomfort (3 items). A 5-point level score is attributed to each item (0 = never; 1 = occasionally/rarely; 2 = sometimes; 3 = often; 4 = always). A total score ranging from 0 (indicating best health status) to 100 (indicating worst health status) was calculated by summing the score of each item, both for the 8 subscores and for the total score. The Italian version used in this study was recently evaluated [31] and revealed good psychometric properties.

2.2.4. Short Form 36-Health Survey Questionnaire (SF-36). This is a 36-item questionnaire measuring the patient's health status in the past four weeks [32]. The total score ranges from 0 to 100 with higher scores indicating a better condition. The Italian version is considered to be a valid and reliable tool [33].

2.2.5. Barthel Index. This well-known test measures the disability on the ADLs [34]. It is composed of 10 items including feeding, bathing, grooming, dressing, bowel and bladder control, toilet use, transfers (bed to chair and back), mobility, and stairs climbing. Three ordinal level scores are attributed to each item (0, 5, or 10; 15 points for items regarding transfers and mobility) to assess whether the patient can perform the various activities independently, with assistance or whether they are totally dependent from others. The total score is generated summing each score, and it varies from 0 (total dependence) to 100 (total independence). The Italian version was administered in this study [35, 36].

2.3. Procedures. Four clinicians (three occupational therapists and one physical therapist) screened all patients for their recruitment. Once enrolled, these clinicians collected demographic and clinical variables and administered the outcome measure to all patients. In order to study the test-retest reliability, the GDS was readministered after seven days. To assess the discriminant validity, a physician diagnosed the depression in this sample. According to DSM-5, patients were diagnosed with depression if they had at least five depressive symptoms including "depressed mood" and "loss of interest or pleasure" for at least two weeks [37].

2.4. Statistical Analysis. Descriptive statistics was used to analyze the sample characteristics; in particular, mean ± standard deviation (SD), median with 25th and 75th percentiles, and frequency with percentage were calculated for intervallic, ordinal, and categorical data, respectively.

The reliability of GDS was assessed in terms of internal consistency and test-retest reliability. Internal consistency was determined calculating Cronbach's alpha [38]: for values closer to 1, the internal consistency is higher. Alpha was considered excellent if >0.9, good if >0.8, and acceptable if >0.7 [39]. Test-retest reliability was calculated by the intraclass correlation coefficient (ICC) with a 95% confident interval (CI). ICC values greater than 0.75 are a minimum requirement to use the instrument in group measurements [40]; ICC values greater than 0.90 are considered essential for the use of the instrument in individual measurements [41].

The construct validity of the GDS was studied calculating the Pearson correlation coefficient (ρ) when comparing the GDS with the other administered instruments. The following ranges were considered in order to interpret the results: $\rho > 0.70$ = strong correlation, $0.50 < \rho < 0.70$ = moderate correlation, and e $\rho < 0.50$ = weak correlation [42].

In order to study the discriminant validity, the receiving operating characteristic (ROC) curve was created, and the area under the curve (AUC) was calculated. The closer the AUC value is to 1.0, the greater the instrument's ability to distinguish depressed and nondepressed patients. An AUC higher than 0.75 confers to the tool a moderate discriminative validity; while an excellent one is demonstrated by a value ≥0.90.

For all statistical analyses, the α value was set at 0.05, and SPSS statistical software program, version 18.0 for Windows (SPSS Inc., Chicago, IL, USA), was used.

3. Results

3.1. Sample Characteristics. Seventy-four patients (44 males; 30 females) with PD were included in this study. The demographic and clinical characteristics of the patients studied are reported in Table 1.

3.2. Internal Consistency. The internal consistency for the total GDS score was excellent ($\alpha = 0.903$).

3.3. Test-Retest Reliability. Test-retest reliability was assessed in a subsample of 35 patients. Excellent reliability was observed for the GDS total score (ICC = 0.941 [95% CI: 0.886–0.970]).

3.4. Validity. Pearson's correlation coefficient values are reported in Table 2. Taking into account the comparisons between GDS and the other instrument related to depression (HADS) and PD (PDQ-39), Pearson coefficient ranged between 0.712 and 0.880, indicating a strong correlation. On the other hand, regarding the comparisons between GDS and generic measurement instrument (Barthel Index and SF-36), the correlation coefficient varied from −0.320 to −0.217, showing a weak correlation.

Regarding the discriminant validity, the AUC showed a value of 0.892 (95% CI 0.809–0.975), indicating a moderate capability to discriminate depressed patients to nondepressed patient. The score with the best sensibility and specificity that predicts depression is between 15 and 16 (sensitivity = 87%; specificity = 82%) (Figure 1).

4. Discussion

The use of a reliable and valid instrument is essential in clinical practice and when measuring specific outcomes [43]. Several questionnaires are available to measure depression in patients with PD [5]. The psychometric properties of GDS

TABLE 1: Main demographic and clinical characteristics of the sample ($N = 74$).

Variables	Values
Age (years)[a]	66.9 ± 9.7
Gender[b]	
(i) Male	44 (59.5%)
(ii) Female	30 (40.5%)
Depression[b]	
(i) Presence	23 (31.1%)
(ii) Absence	51 (68.9%)
Medications prescribed to depressed subjects (N=23)[b]	
(i) Antidepressant	11 (47.8%)
(ii) Anxiolytic	10 (43.5%)
(iii) No medications	2 (8.7%)
Educational level[b]	
(i) Primary	9 (12.2%)
(ii) Secondary	17 (23%)
(iii) High school	33 (44.6%)
(iv) Degree	13 (17.6%)
(v) Not reported	3 (4.1%)
Employment[b]	
(i) Employed	13 (17.6%)
(ii) Not employed	4 (5.4%)
(iii) Retired	57 (77%)
Marital status[b]	
(i) Married	56 (75.6%)
(ii) Unmarried	17 (23%)
(iii) Not reported	1 (1.4%)
Time since PD diagnosis (years)[a]	7.8 ± 5.6
Hoehn and Yahr stage[c]	3 (2; 3)
Setting[b]	
(i) Department	20 (27%)
(ii) Ambulatory	53 (71.6%)
(iii) Day-hospital	1 (1.4%)
MMSE score[c]	29 (27.25; 30)
HADS-A score[c]	7 (4; 10)
HADS-D score[c]	7 (4; 10)
HADS total score[c]	15 (10; 20)
GDS total score[c]	13 (6; 19)
PDQ-39 subscale score[c]	
(i) Mobility	17.5 (7.5; 25.75)
(ii) Activities of daily living	10 (4; 15.75)
(iii) Emotional well-being	9 (5; 14)
(iv) Stigma	4 (2; 8)
(v) Social support	1 (0; 3.75)
(vi) Cognition	5 (2; 8)
(vii) Communication	3 (1.25; 6)
(viii) Bodily discomfort	4 (2; 7)
PDQ-39 total score[c]	59 (31.25; 76)
SF-36[c]	95 (86.25; 102)
Barthel Index[c]	85 (75; 95)

Data are expressed as [a]mean ± standard deviation, [b]frequency with percentage, or [c]median with 25th and 75th percentiles. MMSE: Mini-Mental State Examination; HADS-A: Hospital Anxiety and Depression Scale of Anxiety; HADS-D: Hospital Anxiety and Depression Scale of Depression; GDS: Geriatric Depression Scale; PDQ-39: Parkinson's Disease Questionnaire; SF-36: Short Form 36-Health Survey Questionnaire.

have been extensively studied in different pathologies and in different settings. To our knowledge, however, no study assessed the psychometric properties of GDS in Italian

TABLE 2: Pearson's correlation coefficient for each comparison.

	HADS-A	HADS-D	Total HADS	PDQ	SF-36	Barthel Index
GDS	0.799*	0.800*	0.880*	0.712*	−0.320**	−0.217

*$p < 0.01$; **$p \leq 0.5$. HADS-A: Hospital Anxiety and Depression Scale of Anxiety; HADS-D: Hospital Anxiety and Depression Scale of Depression; GDS: Geriatric Depression Scale; PDQ-39: Parkinson's Disease Questionnaire; SF-36: Short Form 36-Health Survey Questionnaire.

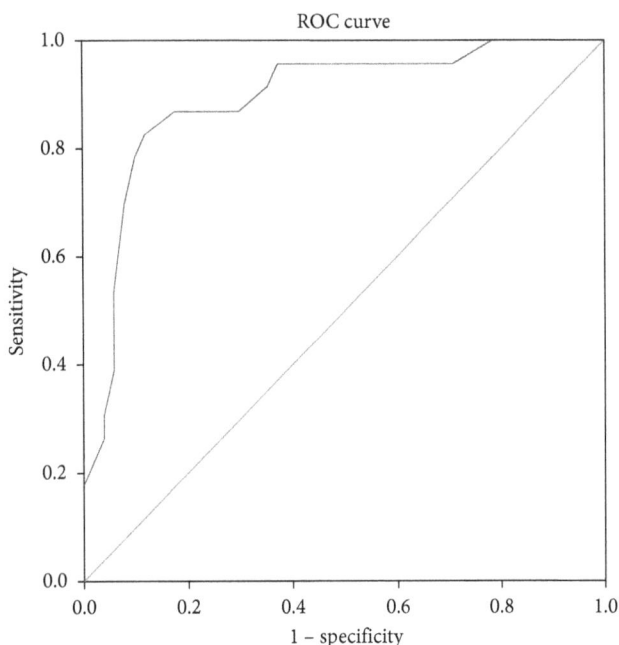

FIGURE 1: Receiving operating characteristic curve.

patients with PD. Studying the measurement properties in the context in which the instrument will be administered is crucial because these properties can be influenced by various contextual, social, and environmental factors [44]. The results of our study show that GDS is a reliable and valid instrument in Italian patients with PD.

The internal consistency assessed by calculating Cronbach's alpha (equal to 0.903) was excellent. The results obtained in the PD patients we studied are similar to those obtained in patients with different clinical conditions. For example, Cronbach's alpha was found to be 0.876 in a study on 294 geriatric patients [45] and 0.90 in 888 depressed and nondepressed elderly subjects [46].

We demonstrated an excellent test-retest reliability of the questionnaire (ICC = 0.941). The results obtained in our sample of PD patients are similar to those found in a cohort of 75 Chinese subjects with PD (ICC = 0.89 [95% CI 0.83–0.93]) [22].

The construct validity was investigated through the correlations between the GDS and other validated questionnaires. In particular, a strong construct validity was obtained through correlations with HADS (both with anxiety and depression) and PDQ-39. On the other hand, a weak correlation was found when the GDS was compared with the Barthel Index and the SF-36. The strong correlations between GDS and HADS can be explained because these two scales intend to measure the same variable, that is, the depression; these results are in line with previous studies that obtained similar correlations with questionnaires related to depression—Beck Depression Inventory ($r_s = 0.62$, $p < 0.05$) [23] and Hamilton Depression Rating Scale at 17 items ($r = 0.54$, $p < 0.001$) [24]. Conversely, the low correlation found with SF-36 and Barthel Index may be explained because both the Barthel Index and the SF-36 are generic instruments.

Finally, the discriminating validity was studied through the ROC curve in order to identify the best sensitivity and specificity of the cutoff value that can distinguish depressed and nondepressed patients. The cutoff value of 15–16 points showed a sensitivity of 87% and a specificity of 82%. Comparing our results with those obtained in other studies is not easy considering the different patient populations and the different settings; for example, the study by McDonald et al. showed a cutoff value of 9–10 points [24] and the study by Ertan et al. [7] a cutoff value of 13–14.

This study presents limitations that need to be taken into account. The design of the study did not allow the assessment of some fundamental psychometric properties such as content validity and responsiveness.

In conclusion, this study shows that GDS can be used in clinical practice as a valid measurement instrument in order to quantify depression in patients with PD.

Disclosure

All authors have no commercial associations or disclosures that may pose or create a conflict of interest with the information presented within this manuscript.

References

[1] R. B. Postuma, D. Berg, M. Stern et al., "MDS clinical diagnostic criteria for Parkinson's disease," *Movement Disorders*, vol. 30, no. 12, pp. 1591–1601, 2015.

[2] D. Aarsland and M. G. Kramberger, "Neuropsychiatric symptoms in Parkinson's disease," *Journal of Parkinson's Disease*, vol. 5, no. 3, pp. 659–667, 2015.

[3] A. H. V. Schapira, K. R. Chaudhuri, and P. Jenner, "Non-motor features of Parkinson disease," *Nature Reviews Neuroscience*, vol. 18, no. 7, pp. 435–450, 2017.

[4] J. S. Reijnders, U. Ehrt, W. E. Weber, D. Aarsland, and A. F. Leentjens, "A systematic review of prevalence studies of

depression in Parkinson's disease," *Movement Disorders*, vol. 23, no. 2, pp. 183–189, 2008.

[5] E. Torbey, N. A. Pachana, and N. N. Dissanayaka, "Depression rating scales in Parkinson's disease: a critical review updating recent literature," *Journal of Affective Disorders*, vol. 184, pp. 216–224, 2015.

[6] J. A. Yesavage, T. L. Brink, T. L. Rose et al., "Development and validation of a geriatric depression screening scale: a preliminary report," *Journal of Psychiatric Research*, vol. 17, no. 1, pp. 37–49, 1982.

[7] T. Ertan and E. Eker, "Reliability, validity, and factor structure of the geriatric depression scale in Turkish elderly: are there different factor structures for different cultures?," *International Psychogeriatrics*, vol. 12, no. 2, pp. 163–172, 2000.

[8] J. Martínez de la Iglesia, M. C. Onís Vilches, R. Dueñas Herrero, C. Aguado Taberné, C. Albert Colomer, and M. C. Arias Blanco, "Abbreviating the brief. Approach to ultra-short versions of the Yesavage questionnaire for the diagnosis of depression," *Atención Primaria*, vol. 35, no. 1, pp. 14–21, 2005.

[9] G. G. Gottfries, S. Noltorp, and N. Nørgaard, "Experience with a Swedish version of the Geriatric Depression Scale in primary care centres," *International Journal of Geriatric Psychiatry*, vol. 12, no. 10, pp. 1029–1034, 1997.

[10] W. N. Havins, P. J. Massman, and R. Doody, "Factor structure of the Geriatric Depression Scale and relationships with cognition and function in Alzheimer's disease," *Dementia and Geriatric Cognitive Disorders*, vol. 34, no. 5-6, pp. 360–372, 2012.

[11] R. Lucas-Carrasco, "Spanish version of the Geriatric Depression Scale: reliability and validity in persons with mild-moderate dementia," *International Psychogeriatrics*, vol. 24, no. 8, pp. 1284–1290, 2012.

[12] H. W. Lach, Y. P. Chang, and D. Edwards, "Can older adults with dementia accurately report depression using brief forms? reliability and validity of the Geriatric Depression Scale," *Journal of Gerontological Nursing*, vol. 36, no. 5, pp. 30–37, 2010.

[13] H. Debruyne, M. Van Buggenhout, N. Le Bastard et al., "Is the geriatric depression scale a reliable screening tool for depressive symptoms in elderly patients with cognitive impairment?," *International Journal of Geriatric Psychiatry*, vol. 24, no. 6, pp. 556–562, 2009.

[14] E. Y. Sivrioglu, K. Sivrioglu, T. Ertan et al., "Reliability and validity of the Geriatric Depression Scale in detection of poststroke minor depression," *Journal of Clinical and Experimental Neuropsychology*, vol. 31, no. 8, pp. 999–1006, 2009.

[15] J. S. Cinamon, L. Finch, S. Miller, J. Higgins, and N. Mayo, "Preliminary evidence for the development of a stroke specific geriatric depression scale," *International Journal of Geriatric Psychiatry*, vol. 26, no. 2, pp. 188–198, 2011.

[16] W. K. Tang, S. S. Chan, H. F. Chiu et al., "Can the Geriatric Depression Scale detect poststroke depression in Chinese elderly?," *Journal of Affective Disorders*, vol. 81, no. 2, pp. 153–156, 2004.

[17] J. Chau, C. R. Martin, D. R. Thompson, A. M. Chang, and J. Woo, "Factor structure of the Chinese version of the Geriatric Depression Scale," *Psychology, Health and Medicine*, vol. 11, no. 1, pp. 48–59, 2006.

[18] K. L. Smarr and A. L. Keefer, "Measures of depression and depressive symptoms: Beck Depression Inventory-II (BDI-II), Center for Epidemiologic Studies Depression Scale (CES-D), Geriatric Depression Scale (GDS), Hospital Anxiety and Depression Scale (HADS), and Patient Health Questionnaire-9 (PHQ-9)," *Arthritis Care and Research*, vol. 63, no. 11, pp. S454–S466, 2011.

[19] A. C. Chan, "Clinical validation of the Geriatric Depression Scale (GDS): Chinese version," *Journal of Aging and Health*, vol. 8, no. 2, pp. 238–253, 1996.

[20] J. N. Bae and M. J. Cho, "Development of the Korean version of the Geriatric Depression Scale and its short form among elderly psychiatric patients," *Journal of Psychosomatic Research*, vol. 57, no. 3, pp. 297–305, 2004.

[21] F. S. Ertan, T. Ertan, G. Kiziltan, and H. Uygucgil, "Reliability and validity of the Geriatric Depression Scale in depression in Parkinson's disease," *Journal of Neurology, Neurosurgery and Psychiatry*, vol. 76, no. 10, pp. 1445–1447, 2005.

[22] S. L. Huang, C. L. Hsieh, R. M. Wu, and W. S. Lu, "Test-retest reliability and minimal detectable change of the Beck Depression Inventory and the Taiwan Geriatric Depression Scale in patients with Parkinson's disease," *PLoS One*, vol. 12, no. 9, Article ID e0184823, 2017.

[23] V. Tumas, G. G. Rodrigues, T. L. Farias, and J. A. Crippa, "The accuracy of diagnosis of major depression in patients with Parkinson's disease: a comparative study among the UPDRS, the geriatric depression scale and the Beck depression inventory," *Arquivos de Neuro-Psiquiatria*, vol. 66, no. 2A, pp. 152–156, 2008.

[24] W. M. McDonald, P. E. Holtzheimer, M. Haber, J. L. Vitek, K. McWhorter, and M. Delong, "Validity of the 30-item geriatric depression scale in patients with Parkinson's disease," *Movement Disorders*, vol. 21, no. 10, pp. 1618–1622, 2006.

[25] G. Galeoto, J. Sansoni, M. Scuccimarri et al., "A psychometric properties evaluation of the Italian version of the Geriatric Depression Scale," *Depression Research and Treatment*, vol. 2018, p. 7, 2018.

[26] G. Galeoto, R. De Santis, A. Marcolini, A. Cinelli, and R. Cecchi, "The informed consent in occupational therapy: proposal of forms," *Giornale Italiano di Medicina del Lavoro ed Ergonomia*, vol. 38, no. 2, pp. 107–115, 2016.

[27] G. Galeoto, R. Mollica, O. Astorino, and R. Cecchi, "Informed consent in physiotherapy: proposal of a form," *Giornale Italiano di Medicina del Lavoro Ergonomia*, vol. 37, no. 4, pp. 245–254, 2014.

[28] A. S. Zigmond and R. P. Snaith, "The hospital anxiety and depression scale," *Acta Psychiatrica Scandinavica*, vol. 67, no. 6, pp. 361–370, 1983.

[29] F. Mondolo, M. Jahanshahi, A. Granà, E. Biasutti, E. Cacciatori, and P. Di Benedetto, "The validity of the hospital anxiety and depression scale and the geriatric depression scale in Parkinson's disease," *Behavioural Neurology*, vol. 17, no. 2, pp. 109–115, 2006.

[30] C. Jenkinson, R. Fitzpatrick, V. Peto, R Greenhall, and N. Hyman, "The Parkinson's disease questionnaire (PDQ-39): development and validation of a Parkinson's disease summary index score," *Age and Ageing*, vol. 26, no. 5, pp. 353–357, 1997.

[31] G. Galeoto, F. Colalelli, P. Massai et al., "Quality of life in Parkinson's disease: Italian validation of the Parkisnon's disease questionnaire (PDQ-39-IT)," *Neurological Sciences*, In press.

[32] J. E. Ware Jr. and C. D. Sherbourne, "The MOS 36-item short-form health survey (SF-36). I. Conceptual framework and item selection," *Medical Care*, vol. 30, no. 6, pp. 473–483, 1992.

[33] G. Apolone and P. Mosconi, "The Italian SF-36 Health Survey: translation, validation and norming," *Journal of Clinical Epidemiology*, vol. 51, no. 11, pp. 1025–1036, 1998.

[34] F. I. Mahoney and D. W. Barthel, "Functional evaluation: the Barthel index," *Maryland State Medical Journal*, vol. 14, pp. 61–65, 1965.

[35] G. Galeoto, A. Lauta, A. Palumbo et al., "The Barthel index: Italian translation, adaptation and validation," *International Journal of Neurology and Neurotherapy*, vol. 2, no. 2, pp. 1–7, 2015.

[36] S. F. Castiglia, G. Galeoto, A. Lauta et al., "The culturally adapted Italian version of the Barthel Index (IcaBI): assessment of structural validity, inter-rater reliability and responsiveness to clinically relevant improvements in patients admitted to inpatient rehabilitation centers," *Functional Neurology*, vol. 32, no. 4, p. 221, 2017.

[37] F. Edition, *Diagnostic and Statistical Manual of Mental Disorders*, American Psychiatric Publishing, Arlington, VA, USA, 2013.

[38] J. M. Bland and D. G. Altman, "Cronbach's alpha," *BMJ*, vol. 314, no. 7080, p. 572, 1997.

[39] D. George and P. Mallery, *SPSS for Windows Step by Step: A Simple Guide and Reference, 11.0 Update*, Allyn & Bacon, Boston, MA, USA, 2003.

[40] M. W. Post, "What to do with "moderate" reliability and validity coefficients?," *Archives of Physical Medicine and Rehabilitation*, vol. 97, no. 7, pp. 1051-1052, 2016.

[41] L. G. Portney and M. P. Watkins, *Foundations of Clinical Research: Applications to Practice*, Vol. 2, Prentice-all, Prentice-all, Upper Saddle River, NJ, USA, 2000.

[42] B. Munro, *Statistical Methods for Health Care Research*, J. B. Lippincott, Philadelphia, PA, USA, 2000.

[43] A. A. Küçükdeveci, A. Tennant, G. Grimby, and F. Franchignoni, "Strategies for assessment and outcome measurement in physical and rehabilitation medicine: an educational review," *Journal of Rehabilitation Medicine*, vol. 43, no. 8, pp. 661–672, 2011.

[44] D. L. Streiner and G. R. Norman, *Health Measurement Scales: A Practical Guide to Their Development and Use*, Oxford University Press, Oxford, UK, 4th edition, 2008.

[45] K. B. Adams, H. C. Matto, and S. Sanders, "Confirmatory factor analysis of the geriatric depression scale," *Gerontologist*, vol. 44, no. 6, pp. 818–826, 2004.

[46] J. Y. Kim, J. H. Park, J. J. Lee et al., "Standardization of the Korean version of the geriatric depression scale: reliability, validity, and factor structure," *Psychiatry Investigation*, vol. 5, no. 4, p. 23, 2008.

3

Drosophila Mutant Model of Parkinson's Disease Revealed an Unexpected Olfactory Performance: Morphofunctional Evidences

Francescaelena De Rose,[1] Valentina Corda,[2] Paolo Solari,[1]
Patrizia Sacchetti,[3] Antonio Belcari,[3] Simone Poddighe,[1] Sanjay Kasture,[4] Paolo Solla,[5]
Francesco Marrosu,[5] and Anna Liscia[1]

[1]*Department of Biomedical Sciences, University of Cagliari, Cagliari, Italy*
[2]*Department of Life and Environmental Sciences, University of Cagliari, Cagliari, Italy*
[3]*Department of Agricultural Biotechnology, Section of Plant Protection, University of Florence, Firenze, Italy*
[4]*Pinnacle Biomedical Research Institute, Bhopal, India*
[5]*Department of Public Health, Clinical and Molecular Medicine, University of Cagliari, Cagliari, Italy*

Correspondence should be addressed to Anna Liscia; liscia@unica.it

Academic Editor: Jan Aasly

Parkinson's disease (PD) is one of the most common neurodegenerative diseases characterized by the clinical triad: tremor, akinesia, and rigidity. Several studies have suggested that PD patients show disturbances in olfaction as one of the earliest, nonspecific nonmotor symptoms of disease onset. We sought to use the fruit fly *Drosophila melanogaster* as a model organism to explore olfactory function in LRRK *loss-of-function* mutants, which was previously demonstrated to be a useful model for PD. Surprisingly, our results showed that the LRRK mutant, compared to the wild flies, presents a dramatic increase in the amplitude of the electroantennogram responses and this is coupled with a higher number of olfactory sensilla. In spite of the above reported results, the behavioural response to olfactory stimuli in mutant flies is impaired compared to that obtained in wild type flies. Thus, behaviour modifications and morphofunctional changes in the olfaction of LRRK *loss-of-function* mutants might be used as an index to explore the progression of parkinsonism in this specific model, also with the aim of studying and developing new treatments.

1. Introduction

The olfactory system represents the most common and ancient sensory system within the animal kingdom, from single-celled organisms through higher animals [1], and one of the most important sensory modalities, due to its crucial role in conveying information about the external world to the nervous system. In this respect, dysfunctions of the olfactory system may have negative effects on the quality of life [2] and in some cases it has been associated with a higher mortality risk [3]. Several studies have demonstrated the connection between smell dysfunctions and Parkinson's disease (PD) [4–9]. Although PD is usually considered as a movement disorder, several studies have shown that PD

nonmotor symptoms may have greater impact on quality-of-life measures, institutionalisation rates, or health economics (for a review, see [10]). Moreover, among PD nonmotor disorders, olfactory disturbances may often precede motor symptoms, representing a potential predicting marker for PD [11]. Indeed, the same presence of Lewy bodies in the substantia nigra [12], strictly related to the onset of typical PD motor symptoms, is a later step in the progression of the pathology. Indeed, initial presence of Lewy bodies has been clearly observed in the medulla oblongata and in the olfactory bulb, thus preceding the successive involvement of midbrain, diencephalic nuclei, and neocortex [13].

Although it is now clear that PD is associated with a combination of risk factors, including environmental noxious agents and genetic predisposition [14], which of the many risk factors may be associated with the timing of disease onset is not known.

Furthermore, regarding genetic predisposition, only a limited percentage is due to monogenic forms of the disease [15]. Among the several genetic mutations implicated in PD aetiology, those associated with the leucine-rich repeat kinase 2 gene (LRRK2) are actually known as responsible for the most common familial and sporadic disorder cases [16–18]. Two more common variations in the *LRRK2* gene have been described: G2019S and G2385R [19]. Among them, the most common (G2019S) accounts for 3–6% of familial dominant PD and for 1-2% of sporadic forms with a north-south gradient of G2019S frequency in European countries and reaching frequency up to 41% in North African cases [20], while the second variation (G2385R) is common mainly in Asian populations [19, 21]. To date, apparent discrepancies between these variations have been reported, suggesting a more complicated phenotype in the G2385R mutation carriers than in *LRRK2* G2019S mutation carriers [19].

Although the evidence about LRRK2 role in inflammatory processes and in the endolysosomal system and cytoskeleton impairment has been identified [22], its involvement in PD development is still not fully defined. Interestingly, different studies highlighted that carriers of a given LRRK2 mutation show a clinical and pathological variability in the manifestation of the disorder, with nigral degeneration associated with absence and limited or wide diffusion of Lewy bodies [16, 17, 23–25]. This phenotypic and pathological variability, however, is found in nearly all monogenic causes of PD, even within nuclear families (e.g., SNCA A53T) [26].

Some variability has also been observed regarding non-motor symptoms, where LRRK2 G2019S olfactory phenotype may be less pronounced than idiopathic PD and possibly G2385R mutation, and it is not clear that all G2019S mutation carriers have olfactory impairment [19, 27–36].

Given the above reported phenotypic variability in PD olfactory dysfunction, it seems of particular interest to have a simple model to study this nonmotor symptom, particularly in a LRRK2 mutant.

The LRRK2 gene coding for unusually large protein composed of 2527 amino acids is widely expressed in the brain and other organs [37–40]. The LRRK2 roles, listed in the Berwick and Harvey review [22], include neurogenesis and neurite outgrowth, cytoskeleton assembly, endocytosis/vesicles trafficking, and autophagy coordination.

LRRK2 is a member of the ROCO protein family characterized by the presence of two conserved domains: a Roc (Ras in complex proteins) domain belonging to the Ras/GTPase superfamily and a COR domain (C-terminal of Roc). Three further conserved domains have been described: a leucine-rich repeat (LRR); a tyrosine kinase catalytic domain (MAPKKK); and finally a WD40 domain [17]. This latter is known to be crucial in several basic cell functions such as vesicle sorting during endocytosis and exocytosis of synaptic vesicles as well as vesicle-mediated transport and cytoskeleton assembly [41, 42].

Recently, De Rose et al. [43] reported that *Drosophila* LRRK2 *loss-of-function* mutant for deletion of the domain

WD40 (LRRK2^{WD40}; LRRK^{ex1} mutant, [44, 45]) showed a motor age-dependent impairment and a correlated mitochondrial impairment in the thoracic ganglia. Besides, a mitochondrial impairment was detected in the antennal lobe area, where olfactory signal from the peripheral chemoreceptors projects. Similarly, a morphological impairment was reported by Poddighe et al. [46] in another *Drosophila* mutant such as PINK1^{B9} which also showed a decrease in the olfactory detection, both in the electrophysiologically recorded olfactory signals and in the olfactory behaviour.

On this basis, the aim of this study was to estimate any possible olfactory dysfunction in the *Drosophila* LRRK2 model of PD correlated to LRRK2 mutation (LRRK^{WD40}). This model most closely approximates human LRRK2 G2385R mutations, which occur in the human WD40 domain and are a risk factor for PD. The results showed that the LRRK^{WD40} mutant presents an unexpected dramatic increase in the amplitude of electrophysiological responses, but a decrease in the olfactory discrimination, with respect to wild type flies (WT).

2. Materials and Methods

2.1. Insects. For these experiments adult wild type (WT; Canton-S) and LRRK^{WD40} mutant (LRRK^{ex1}, #34750, from Bloomington Stock Center) *Drosophila melanogaster* (Dm) males were used. Soon after emergence from pupae, WT or LRRK^{WD40} mutant males were separated from females. WT and mutant flies were reared on a standard cornmeal-yeast-agar medium in controlled environmental conditions (24-25°C; 60% relative humidity; light/dark = 12/12 hours). Flies ranging 10–15 days in age were tested according to previous experiments [43].

2.2. Electroantennograms (EAGs) Recordings. Electroantennogram (EAG) recordings were performed *in vivo* as previously described [47, 48].

By taking into account the circadian cycle in olfactory sensitivity [49], WT and mutant flies were always tested in parallel. Briefly, living 10- to 15-day-old male flies were singly inserted in a 100 μL truncated plastic pipette, with the head protruding at the tip. The preparation was fixed with dental wax on a microscope slide and positioned under the viewer of an Olympus BX51WI light microscope (Olympus, Tokyo, Japan). Glass capillaries with a silver wire were filled with a conductive 0.15 M NaCl solution. The recording glass electrode was gently placed on the tip of the antennal funiculus, whereas the reference electrode was inserted in the compound eye. The EAG signal was amplified with an AC/DC probe and then acquired with an IDAC-4 interface board (Syntech, Hilversum NL). A charcoal purified and humidified airflow was constantly blown over the antennae (speed 0.5 m/s) via a glass tube, placed approximately 1 cm from the antenna. The tip of a Pasteur pipette containing an odour-loaded filter paper (5 mm × 25 mm) was inserted into a small hole in the glass tube. Odour stimulation was administered by injecting a puff of purified air (0.5 s at 10 mL/s airflow) through the pipette using the stimulus delivery controller (Syntech).

Odour stimuli tested were dissolved in hexane and presented in series from minor to higher concentration (resp., 0.01, 0.1, 1, and 10% v/v). 1-Hexanol was chosen for its well-known stimulant activity in *Drosophila* [50–52], and 1-linalool, a terp commonly found in plants, was chosen for its capability to excite olfactory sensory neurons in different species of insects [53]. As the standard reference, 1-hexanol was administered at the 10% v/v dilution at the beginning of the experiments, to confirm the activity of the antenna. Both 1-hexanol and 1-linalool were purchased from Sigma-Aldrich (Milan, Italy).

Mean values of EAG amplitude were calculated and then analysed by comparing the results obtained in LRRK^{WD40} mutant groups with the age-matched WT control group.

The significance of differences was tested by repeated-measures ANOVA or one-way ANOVA (followed by HSD *post hoc* test) with a threshold level of statistical significance set at $P \leq 0.05$ (statistical software package). EAG results are expressed as average values + SEM and represented by histograms.

2.3. Olfactory Behaviour.

Free-walking bioassays were performed following the experimental procedures used by Dekker et al. [54]. Briefly, males of WT and LRRK^{WD40} were given the opportunity to choose between vials containing water with or without odour (1-hexanol or 1-linalool). Two 4 mL glass vials were placed symmetrically and equally spaced in a large Petri dish (the arena) and then fitted with truncated pipette tips. The vials were filled with 300 μL of water with 0.25% Triton X with or without the odorant. On the basis of the EAG response, the odour dilution chosen to trap the flies was 0.1% for both compounds. The dehydration of flies was prevented by placing a cotton ball with 3 mL of water in the arenas. Flies were starved for 9 hours prior to starting the experiments. Twelve bioassays were carried out for each experimental group of flies (15 flies per arena) and for each odour source and then replicated three times. Bioassays were performed in controlled environmental conditions and lasted 18 hours [54] that comprised the most active phase of olfactory sensitivity [49]. The attraction index (AI) was calculated as follows: $(T - C)/(T + C + NR - D)$, in which T is the number of flies in the treatment, C is the number in the control, NR is the number of living flies remaining in the arena, and D is the number of dead flies.

Data obtained were expressed as average of percentages of flies reaching the treatment vial (with 1-hexanol or 1-linalool) or the control vial (water) and statistically evaluated by means of Student's *t*-test (Statistical software package) with a 95% confidence level.

2.4. Morphological Observations.

For scanning electron microscopy (SEM), 4–6-day-old flies were anesthetized with carbon dioxide, immediately immersed in hexane, shaken for 3 minutes to remove the external wax layer, then dehydrated in a graded ethanol series for ten minutes each concentration up to absolute ethanol, subsequently air-dried, and finally glued to stubs and gold coated. At least ten specimens were prepared and observed using a FEI Quanta 200 high-vacuum SEM at the Department of Tree Science, Entomology and Plant Pathology "G. Scaramuzzi," University of Pisa. The density of antennal sensilla in both WT and LRRK^{WD40} mutant males was determined by counting the number of different types of sensilla present in a sample area enclosed by an electronic square frame (1,000 μm^2) applied to the SEM screen in the central part of the flagellum. This area of the flagellum was chosen since it was plain displayed in all samples and the arrangement of the antennal structures allowed to count easily the number of each type of sensilla included by the frame. Moreover, in this area all kinds of sensilla were present, with the exception of one type (large basiconic sensilla) located mainly in the basal part of the flagellum [53]. Sensilla were counted in the flagellar area of one antenna per specimen; differences in the number of the three types of sensilla counted in the analysed area of males of the two strains were evaluated by Student's *t*-test with a 95% confidence level (Statistica 6.0, StatSoft, Italy). Higher magnification was used to study in detail the morphology of different types of sensilla.

3. Results

3.1. LRRK^{WD40} Mutants Show Enhancement of the EAG Response to Both 1-Hexanol and 1-Linalool.

As shown in Figures 1(a) and 2(a), the olfactory stimulations of flies' antennae with both 1-hexanol and 1-linalool (0.01, 0.1, 1, and 10% v/v) consistently elicited responses with the typical EAG waveform, that is, a rapid depolarization followed by a slower recovery phase, ending with the hyperpolarized wave before complete reversal to the baseline, in both WT and in LRRK^{WD40} mutants, the repolarization phase in LRRK^{WD40} being slower than WT.

Contrary to expectations, the EAG response values elicited after stimulation with both 1-hexanol (Figure 1) and 1-linalool (Figure 2) in LRRK^{WD40} mutants were higher than those obtained in WT specimens, exhibiting a dose response for both stimuli administered, although this tendency was more evident for 1-hexanol. In detail, LRRK^{WD40} flies showed a significant increase ($P < 0.05$) in the EAG amplitudes with respect to WT after stimulation with 1-hexanol and 1-linalool for all concentrations tested, except the lowest (Figures 1 and 2).

3.2. LRRK^{WD40} Mutants Show Impairment of the Behavioural Response to Both 1-Hexanol and 1-Linalool.

As for the EAG tests, free-walking bioassays were performed on WT and LRRK^{WD40} adult males, by testing the responses to 1-hexanol or 1-linalool, both at the dilution 0.1% v/v. Contrary to electrophysiological results, LRRK^{WD40} males presented a behavioural impairment, with a significant decrease in the behavioural scores for both odours with respect to the WT control groups (Figure 3). In fact, in the trap assays with 1-hexanol, the percentage of odour-trapped insects was 37 ± 3.7% for LRRK^{WD40} compared to 71.4 ± 3.7% for WT control groups; in the case of 1-linalool, only 14.8 ± 3.3% of LRRK^{WD40} mutants were attracted in the vial with the odour as compared to 41.4 ± 3.2% of WT control groups.

(a)

(b)

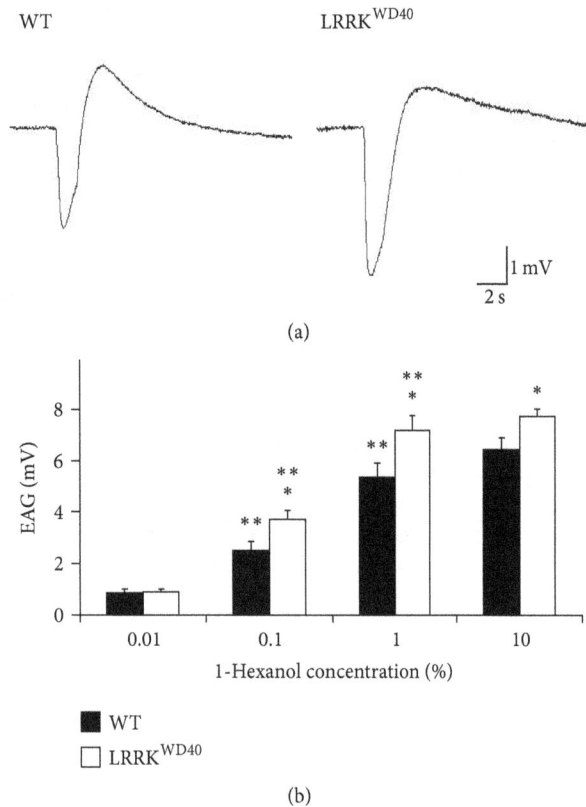

FIGURE 1: Electroantennogram (EAG) responses to 1-hexanol. Sample EAG recordings (a) and EAG amplitude values (b) elicited by stimulation with the different concentrations of 1-hexanol (0.01, 0.1, 1, and 10% v/v) in male antennae of WT and LRRK^{WD40} mutant flies. Mean values + SEM from 24–26 antennae for each stimulus concentration and insect sample. $*$ and $**$ indicate significant differences (P < 0.05; HSD *post hoc* test subsequent to one-way ANOVA or repeated-measures ANOVA) from WT and from preceding concentration of same stimulus, respectively.

(a)

(b)

FIGURE 2: Electroantennogram (EAG) responses to 1-linalool. Sample EAG recordings (a) and EAG amplitude values (b) elicited by stimulation with the different concentrations of 1-linalool (0.01, 0.1, 1, and 10% v/v) in male antennae of WT and LRRK^{WD40} mutant flies. Mean values + SEM from 24–26 antennae for each stimulus concentration and insect sample. $*$ and $**$ indicate significant differences (P < 0.05; HSD *post hoc* test subsequent to one-way ANOVA or repeated-measures ANOVA) from WT and from preceding concentration of same stimulus, respectively.

As for the water response, the numbers of trapped flies in the blank baits were higher for LRRK^{WD40} compared to WT (21.3 ± 3 and 11 ± 2.3%, resp., P < 0.05) in response to 1-hexanol, while the number of insects trapped in the blank did not differ in response to 1-linalool. Moreover, in the latter, no difference exists between mutant insects trapped by the odour with respect to the blank.

3.3. Morphological Observations. The unexpected increase in EAG response combined with the impairment of the behavioural response of mutants with respect to WT led us to investigate any possible variation in the antennal olfactory apparatus.

According to our results, no differences are found between WT and LRRK^{WD40} flies in the gross structure. As shown in Figure 4(a), antennae are located between the compound eyes in two pits separated by a prominent face. The antennae consist of three segments: scape (basal segment), pedicel, and flagellum. The pedicel is marked dorsally by a longitudinal antennal seam. The flagellum, the most relevant

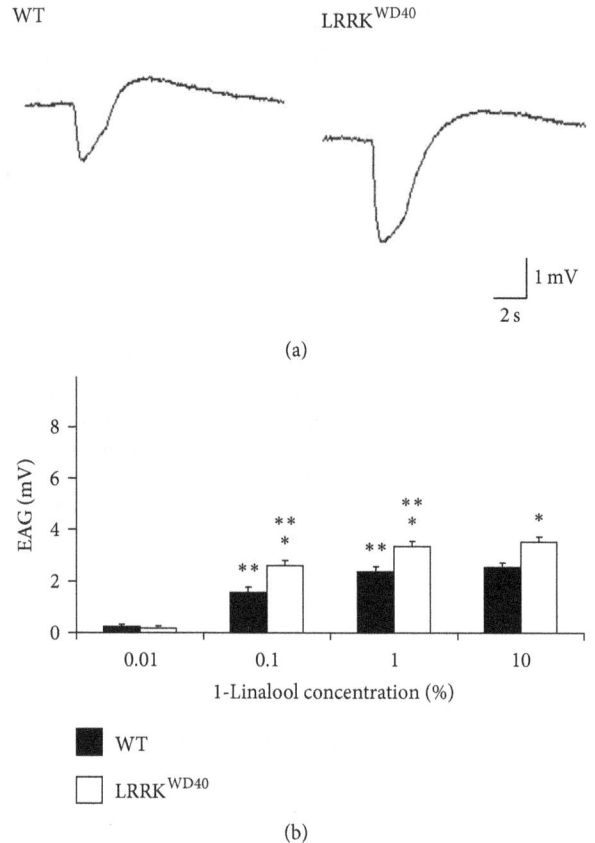

sensory area, bears different types of sensilla interspersed with cuticular setae which are in general markedly curved and furrowed. There are 4 types of sensilla: trichoid, large basiconic, small basiconic, and grooved sensilla (Figures 4(b), 4(c), and 4(d)). Trichoid sensilla are the longest, most predominant sensilla which are spread in the whole flagellum; large basiconic sensilla are present mainly in the basal part of flagellum and show a multiporous surface (Figure 4(c)), while small basiconic sensilla are present mainly in the middle and in the distal part of the flagellum. Grooved sensilla are present only in the central and in the distal part of the flagellum; they appear very small and are formed by a series of 6–8 finger-like projections (Figure 4(d)).

However, as shown in Table 1, significant differences were found in the mean number of different types of sensilla counted in the selected area of flagellum between WT and LRRK^{WD40} mutants.

In detail, as a general pattern, mutants show a higher number of all sensilla in the considered area than WT

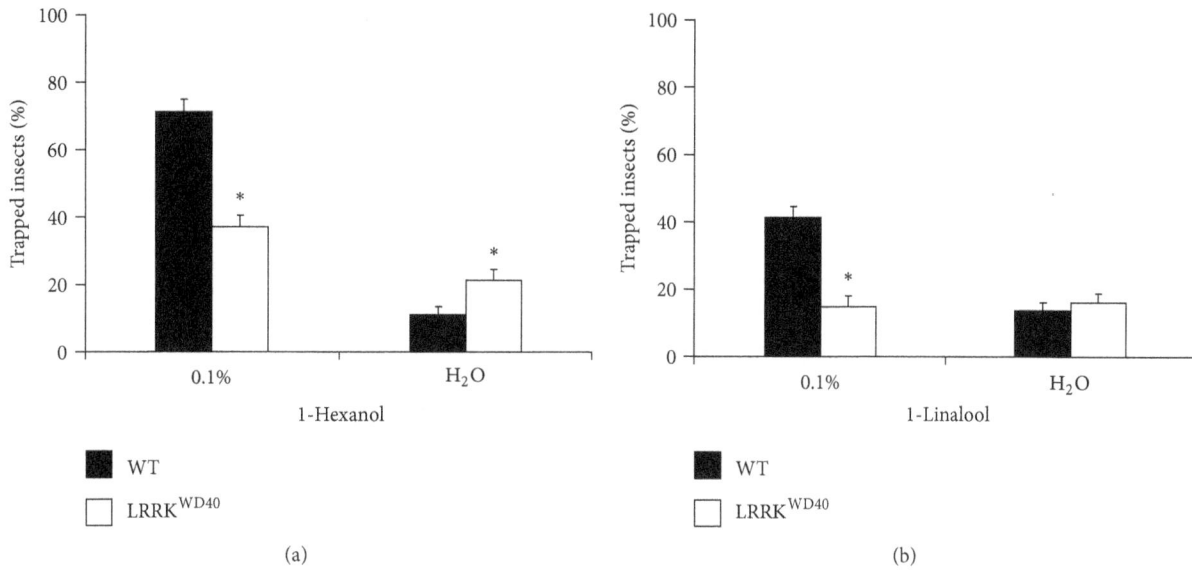

(a)

(b)

FIGURE 3: Behavioural olfactory response to 0.1% v/v 1-hexanol (a) and 0.1% v/v 1-linalool (b) in WT and LRRK^{WD40} mutant flies. Mean values of trapped males + SEM; experiments in triplicate; n = 12 bioassays for each experimental group of flies, n = 15 flies per arena. ∗ indicates significant differences ($P < 0.05$; Student's t-test) with respect to WT.

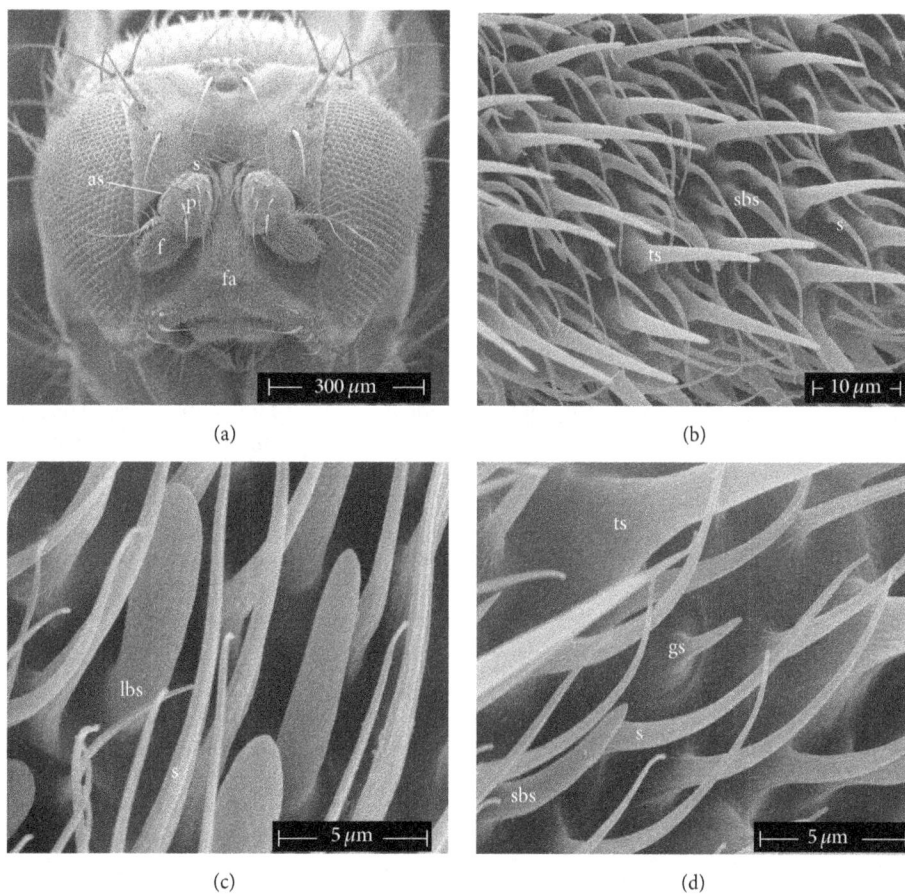

(a)

(b)

(c)

(d)

FIGURE 4: Scanning electron micrographs of $D.$ $melanogaster$ WT male. (a) Head showing the antennal pattern: scape (s), pedicel (p), antennal seam (as), flagellum (f), and face (fa). (b) Magnification of the central part of flagellum with sensilla: trichoid sensillum (ts), small basiconic sensillum (sbs), and setae (s). (c) High magnification of the basal part of the flagellum showing some large basiconic sensilla with porous wall (lbs). (d) High magnification of different types of sensilla in the central part of flagellum with a grooved sensillum (gs).

TABLE 1: Average number ($\pm$SD) of the three types of sensilla present in a sample area (1,000 μm^2) in the central part of the flagellum of *D. melanogaster* WT and LRRK^{WD40} mutants (Student's *t*-test, 95% confidence level).

Type of sensilla	Wild type ($n = 7$)	LRRK^{WD40} ($n = 8$)	P
Trichoid sensilla	8.86 ± 1.06	11.50 ± 1.07	0.00036
Small basiconic sensilla	2.00 ± 0	2.63 ± 0.74	0.04549
Grooved sensilla	0.86 ± 0.38	1.50 ± 0.53	0.02003

flies, although these differences are evident only at high magnification (Figure 5). As a matter of fact, the number of trichoid sensilla in LRRK^{WD40} mutants males exceeded the WT number with highly significant difference ($P \leq 0.001$). Similarly, also small basiconic and grooved sensilla were present in LRRK^{WD40} mutants males with a slightly higher density than in the WT males ($P \leq 0.05$).

4. Discussion

The aim of this study was to estimate in the PD translational model *Drosophila melanogaster* any possible olfactory dysfunction correlated to a specific LRRK2 mutation (LRRK^{WD40}) [43], by analogy with a previous study in a PINK1 *Drosophila* model [9, 46].

The used LRRK2 translational model most closely approximates human LRRK2 G2385R mutation, which occurs in the human WD40 domain and is a risk factor for PD, mainly in Asian populations [21].

Contrary to PINK1^{B9} [9, 46], where the EAG response was lower with respect to the WT, our results showed that the LRRK^{WD40} mutant, compared to the WT, presents an unexpected dramatic increase in the amplitude of the EAG responses and this is coupled with a higher number of olfactory sensilla.

Nevertheless, similarly to what was observed for PINK1^{B9} [46] also the LRRK^{WD40} mutants present an impairment in the behavioural response to odours.

4.1. LRRK^{WD40} Mutants Show Enhancement of the EAG Response to Both 1-Hexanol and 1-Linalool.
In detail, even if LRRK^{WD40} shows an increase in EAG response at any concentration to both tested stimuli (1-hexanol and 1-linalool), at the lowest one, no differences in threshold were found between mutants and WT. Despite the great variability in the sensilla number in different strains [55], we cannot exclude the notion that the electrophysiological response is due to the higher sensillar density found in the flagellum of LRRK^{WD40} compared to WT, mostly in consideration of the relevant number of trichoid sensilla which can cause an increased summed antennal sensitivity. Further, we cannot exclude a role of the perireceptor environment in the chemoreceptor response. In this respect, it is possible that in mutants more

odorant binding proteins could be present and/or interact with the odorants more tightly, but the presence of a diminished concentration of the odour degrading enzymes is also possible [56–58]. Accordingly, Corvol et al. [59] found in PD patients a persistent increase in an olfactory type G-protein (G$_{olf}$) that was first identified in the olfactory epithelium [60, 61] homologous to the olfactory sensilla in *Drosophila* antennae.

More recently, Yun and Park [62], analysing shape and amplitude of the EAG curve, indicated some parameters for the analysis of the EAG curve, with the peak amplitude being the most important one and therefore it is widely used for studying the odour detection. According to these authors, other parameters like the shape cannot be used for odorant concentration measurements but they can help in discriminating between different odorants. In this respect, our results show that EAGs evoked by 1-linalool are longer than those evoked by 1-hexanol. The overall lower amplitude of the EAG in response to 1-linalool with respect to 1-hexanol is also in accordance with the data in literature, according to which the former interacts with a reduced number of ORs with respect to the latter [50].

4.2. LRRK^{WD40} Mutants Show Impairment of the Behavioural Response to Both 1-Hexanol and 1-Linalool.
Looking at the behavioural response to the odours, 1-hexanol attracts a number of insects statistically higher than 1-linalool, in both WT and mutant flies, but the number of LRRK^{WD40} mutants trapped is lower than WT regardless of the stimulus tested. As for the functional significance of the two stimulants, 1-hexanol was reported to involve both the appetitive and the aversive response in flies, even if with great variability in its effects [51, 63], and it interacts with a number of olfactory receptor neurons (ORNs) distributed on the small and the large basiconic and on the trichoid sensilla [50, 53, 64]. In this respect, our behavioural data point to a prevailing appetitive response to 1-hexanol, thus making the differences with the above reported data in literature. 1-Hexanol is reported to also interact with a number of olfactory receptors (ORs) located in the trichoid ones responding to pheromones [64] that could give reason for the attractive effects we observed. In other words, we suggest possible sex-related differences, that is, male used in the present study versus male and female in a 1 : 1 ratio in the study by Knaden et al. [51]. We cannot exclude other possible methodological differences among different studies. Analogous considerations can be made for 1-linalool that was previously reported to be an aversive stimulus [51] but that may also interact with the pheromone-sensitive OR19a in the trichoid sensilla [64].

As for the response to water, in our opinion, results showing that LRRK2 mutants are trapped by water in the 1-hexanol experiments and especially the absence of difference between water and the odour in the case of 1-linalool point to an impairment in the discrimination capability of LRRK2 mutants. In fact, even if mutants present a higher electrophysiological response to both stimuli with respect to WT, the percentage of mutants which goes to the odours under a double-choice situation is about half that of WT flies. These results can be attributable to an impairment we found

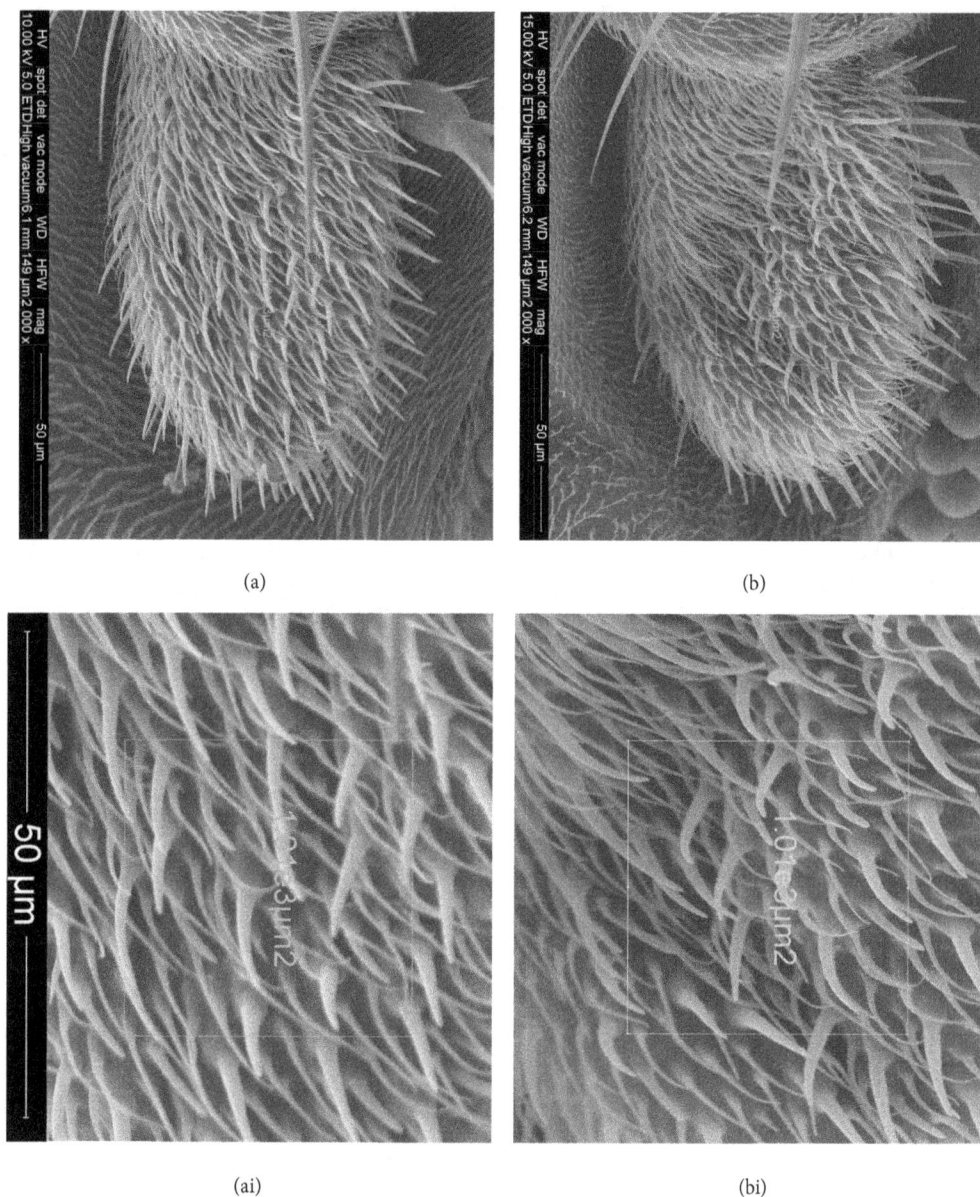

FIGURE 5: Scanning electron micrographs of flagellum of *D. melanogaster* WT (a) and LRRK^{WD40} mutant (b); (ai and bi) the respective magnifications of the central area with the frame used to count the density of sensilla.

in the mitochondrial morphology in the antennal lobes [43], where olfactory neurons project.

4.3. Morphological Observations. Our observations on antennal flagellum of *Drosophila* WT males showed the presence of four types of sensilla as previously reported [65] and mapped for this species [53]; further, the LRRK^{WD40} mutant did not display noticeable gross morphological differences with respect to the WT, but a general increase in the number of sensilla in the central part of the flagellum was highlighted. As far as we know, no data are available to correlate the number of sensilla with LRRK function; we recall that LRRK2 is known to be involved in cytoskeleton assembly [22], but how a deletion of WD40 domain can be correlated to an increase

of sensilla number is hard to hypothesize. In this respect, we recall that researches on *lozenge Drosophila* mutants showed changes at different extent in morphological features of antennal sensilla, including a reduction or an increase in the number and/or lack of some sensilla [66].

4.4. Concluding Remarks. Our functional approach to merging olfactory sensory electrophysiology with behavioural response was used to go in depth in the analysis of odour detection with the aim of considering olfaction as a diagnostic marker for PD in the LRRK^{WD40}.

Our results show that, despite the dose-response relationship and the unexpected high EAG amplitude which point to a "normal" olfactory function, the LRRK^{WD40} mutants present an impairment in the behavioural response to odours. In this respect in a pioneeristic work on human odour stimuli detection in correlating electrophysiological activity from human olfactory bulb and the subjective response to stimuli, Hughes et al. [67] stated "the significance of this type of correlation remains questionable as long as there is no indication of the total response of the organism."

In conclusion, our results suggest that olfactory behavioural impairment is a common feature for two *Drosophila* PD models such as LRRK^{WD40} and PINK1^{B9} [46] despite the two opposite electrophysiological peripheral responses and highlight the fact that *Drosophila* is a powerful model also for the LRRK2 *loss-of-function* variant.

Abbreviations

Dm:	*Drosophila melanogaster*
EAG:	Electroantennogram
LRRK2:	Leucine-rich repeat kinase 2
LRRK^{WD40}:	LRRK *loss-of-function* in the WD40 domain
PD:	Parkinson's disease
PINK1^{B9}:	PTEN-induced putative kinase 1
WT:	Wild type.

Authors' Contributions

Francescaelena De Rose, Valentina Corda, Paolo Solari, and Patrizia Sacchetti contributed equally to this work.

Acknowledgments

The authors would like to thank Dr. Ignazio Collu and Dr. Giuliana Colella (University of Cagliari) for taking care of flies.

References

[1] N. J. Strausfeld and J. G. Hildebrand, "Olfactory systems: common design, uncommon origins?" *Current Opinion in Neurobiology*, vol. 9, no. 5, pp. 634–639, 1999.

[2] D. A. Deems, R. L. Doty, R. G. Settle et al., "Smell and taste disorders, a study of 750 patients from the University of Pennsylvania Smell and Taste Center," *Archives of Otolaryngology—Head and Neck Surgery*, vol. 117, no. 5, pp. 519–528, 1991.

[3] R. S. Wilson, L. Yu, and D. A. Bennett, "Odor identification and mortality in old age," *Chemical Senses*, vol. 36, no. 1, pp. 63–67, 2011.

[4] K. A. Ansari and A. Johnson, "Olfactory function in patients with Parkinson's disease," *Journal of Chronic Diseases*, vol. 28, no. 9, pp. 493–497, 1975.

[5] R. L. Doty, D. A. Deems, and S. Stellar, "Olfactory dysfunction in parkinsonism: a general deficit unrelated to neurologic signs, disease stage, or disease duration," *Neurology*, vol. 38, no. 8, pp. 1237–1244, 1988.

[6] E. C. Wolters, C. Francot, P. Bergmans et al., "Preclinical (premotor) Parkinson's disease," *Journal of Neurology, Supplement*, vol. 247, no. 2, pp. 103–109, 2000.

[7] M. Politis, K. Wu, S. Molloy, P. G. Bain, K. R. Chaudhuri, and P. Piccini, "Parkinson's disease symptoms: the patient's perspective," *Movement Disorders*, vol. 25, no. 11, pp. 1646–1651, 2010.

[8] A. Haehner, T. Hummel, and H. Reichmann, "Olfactory loss in parkinson's disease," *Parkinson's Disease*, vol. 2011, Article ID 450939, 6 pages, 2011.

[9] S. Poddighe, K. M. Bhat, M. D. Setzu et al., "Impaired sense of smell in a *Drosophila* Parkinson's model," *PLoS ONE*, vol. 8, no. 8, Article ID e73156, 2013.

[10] K. R. Chaudhuri, D. G. Healy, and A. H. V. Schapira, "Non-motor symptoms of Parkinson's disease: diagnosis and management," *The Lancet Neurology*, vol. 5, no. 3, pp. 235–245, 2006.

[11] R. L. Doty, "Olfaction in Parkinson's disease and related disorders," *Neurobiology of Disease*, vol. 46, no. 3, pp. 527–552, 2012.

[12] W. R. G. Gibb and A. J. Lees, "The relevance of the Lewy body to the pathogenesis of idiopathic Parkinson's disease," *Journal of Neurology, Neurosurgery and Psychiatry*, vol. 51, no. 6, pp. 745–752, 1988.

[13] H. Braak, K. Del Tredici, U. Rüb, R. A. I. De Vos, E. N. H. J. Steur, and E. Braak, "Staging of brain pathology related to sporadic Parkinson's disease," *Neurobiology of Aging*, vol. 24, no. 2, pp. 197–211, 2003.

[14] A. J. Lees, J. Hardy, and T. Revesz, "Parkinson's disease," *The Lancet*, vol. 373, no. 9680, pp. 2055–2066, 2009.

[15] C. Klein and A. Westenberger, "Genetics of Parkinson's disease," *Cold Spring Harbor Perspectives in Medicine*, vol. 2, no. 1, 2012.

[16] C. Paisán-Ruíz, S. Jain, E. W. Evans et al., "Cloning of the gene containing mutations that cause PARK8–linked Parkinson's disease," *Neuron*, vol. 44, no. 4, pp. 595–600, 2004.

[17] A. Zimprich, S. Biskup, P. Leitner et al., "Mutations in LRRK2 cause autosomal-dominant parkinsonism with pleomorphic pathology," *Neuron*, vol. 44, no. 4, pp. 601–607, 2004.

[18] U. Kumari and E. K. Tan, "LRRK2 in Parkinson's disease: genetic and clinical studies from patients," *FEBS Journal*, vol. 276, no. 22, pp. 6455–6463, 2009.

[19] C. Marras, R. N. Alcalay, C. Caspell-Garcia et al., "Motor and nonmotor heterogeneity of *LRRK2*-related and idiopathic Parkinson's disease," *Movement Disorders*, vol. 31, no. 8, pp. 1192–1202, 2016.

[20] N. Change, G. Mercier, and G. Lucotte, "Genetic screening of the G2019S mutation of the LRRK2 gene in southwest European, North African, and sephardic Jewish subjects," *Genetic Testing*, vol. 12, no. 3, pp. 333–339, 2008.

[21] C.-L. Xie, J.-L. Pan, W.-W. Wang et al., "The association between the LRRK2 G2385R variant and the risk of Parkinson's disease: a meta-analysis based on 23 case-control studies," *Neurological Sciences*, vol. 35, no. 10, pp. 1495–1504, 2014.

[22] D. C. Berwick and K. Harvey, "LRRK2: an éminence grise of Wnt-mediated neurogenesis?" *Frontiers in Cellular Neuroscience*, vol. 7, pp. 1–13, 2013.

[23] Z. K. Wszolek, R. F. Pfeiffer, Y. Tsuboi et al., "Autosomal dominant parkinsonism associated with variable synuclein and tau pathology," *Neurology*, vol. 62, no. 9, pp. 1619–1622, 2004.

[24] A. Rajput, D. W. Dickson, C. A. Robinson et al., "Parkinsonism, Lrrk2 G2019S, and tau neuropathology," *Neurology*, vol. 67, no. 8, pp. 1506–1508, 2006.

[25] O. A. Ross, M. Toft, A. J. Whittle et al., "Lrrk2 and Lewy body disease," *Annals of Neurology*, vol. 59, no. 2, pp. 388–393, 2006.

[26] K. Markopoulou, D. W. Dickson, R. D. McComb et al., "Clinical, neuropathological and genotypic variability in SNCA A53T familial Parkinson's disease. Variability in familial Parkinson's disease," *Acta Neuropathologica*, vol. 116, no. 1, pp. 25–35, 2008.

[27] N. L. Khan, S. Jain, J. M. Lynch et al., "Mutations in the gene LRRK2 encoding dardarin (PARK8) cause familial Parkinson's disease: clinical, pathological, olfactory and functional imaging and genetic data," *Brain*, vol. 128, no. 12, pp. 2786–2796, 2005.

[28] J. J. Ferreira, L. C. Guedes, M. M. Rosa et al., "High prevalence of LRRK2 mutations in familial and sporadic Parkinson's disease in Portugal," *Movement Disorders*, vol. 22, no. 8, pp. 1194–1201, 2007.

[29] D. G. Healy, M. Falchi, S. S. O'Sullivan et al., "Phenotype, genotype, and worldwide genetic penetrance of LRRK2-associated Parkinson's disease: a case-control study," *The Lancet Neurology*, vol. 7, no. 7, pp. 583–590, 2008.

[30] L. Silveira-Moriyama, L. C. Guedes, A. Kingsbury et al., "Hyposmia in G2019S LRRK2-related parkinsonism: clinical and pathologic data," *Neurology*, vol. 71, no. 13, pp. 1021–1026, 2008.

[31] L. Silveira-Moriyama, R. P. Munhoz, M. D. J. Carvalho et al., "Olfactory heterogeneity in LRRK2 related Parkinsonism," *Movement Disorders*, vol. 25, no. 16, pp. 2879–2883, 2010.

[32] J. Ruiz-Martínez, A. Gorostidi, E. Goyenechea et al., "Olfactory deficits and cardiac 123I-MIBG in Parkinson's disease related to the LRRK2 R1441G and G2019S mutations," *Movement Disorders*, vol. 26, no. 11, pp. 2026–2031, 2011.

[33] R. Saunders-Pullman, K. Stanley, C. Wang et al., "Olfactory dysfunction in LRRK2 G2019S mutation carriers," *Neurology*, vol. 77, no. 4, pp. 319–324, 2011.

[34] C. Gaig, D. Vilas, J. Infante et al., "Nonmotor symptoms in LRRK2 G2019S associated Parkinson's disease," *PLoS ONE*, vol. 9, no. 10, Article ID e108982, 2014.

[35] K. K. Johansen, B. J. Warø, and J. O. Aasly, "Olfactory dysfunction in sporadic Parkinson's disease and LRRK2 carriers," *Acta Neurologica Scandinavica*, vol. 129, no. 5, pp. 300–306, 2014.

[36] R. Saunders-Pullman, A. Mirelman, C. Wang et al., "Olfactory identification in LRRK2 G2019S mutation carriers: a relevant marker?" *Annals of Clinical and Translational Neurology*, vol. 1, no. 9, pp. 670–678, 2014.

[37] S. Biskup, D. J. Moore, F. Celsi et al., "Localization of LRRK2 to membranous and vesicular structures in mammalian brain," *Annals of Neurology*, vol. 60, no. 5, pp. 557–569, 2006.

[38] S. Higashi, D. J. Moore, R. E. Colebrooke et al., "Expression and localization of Parkinson's disease-associated leucine-rich repeat kinase 2 in the mouse brain," *Journal of Neurochemistry*, vol. 100, no. 2, pp. 368–381, 2007.

[39] S. Higashi, S. Biskup, A. B. West et al., "Localization of Parkinson's disease-associated LRRK2 in normal and pathological human brain," *Brain Research*, vol. 1155, no. 1, pp. 208–219, 2007.

[40] D. Gaiter, M. Westerlund, A. Carmine, E. Lindqvist, O. Sydow, and L. Olson, "LRRK2 expression linked to dopamine-innervated areas," *Annals of Neurology*, vol. 59, no. 4, pp. 714–719, 2006.

[41] D. Li and R. Roberts, "WD-repeat proteins: structure characteristics, biological function, and their involvement in human diseases," *Cellular and Molecular Life Sciences*, vol. 58, no. 14, pp. 2085–2097, 2001.

[42] G. Piccoli, S. B. Condliffe, M. Bauer et al., "LRRK2 controls synaptic vesicle storage and mobilization within the recycling pool," *The Journal of Neuroscience*, vol. 31, no. 6, pp. 2225–2237, 2011.

[43] F. De Rose, R. Marotta, S. Poddighe et al., "Functional and morphological correlates in the *Drosophila* LRRK2 loss-of-function model of Parkinson's disease: drug effects of *Withania somnifera* (Dunal) administration," *PLoS ONE*, vol. 11, no. 1, Article ID e0146140, 2016.

[44] S. B. Lee, W. Kim, S. Lee, and J. Chung, "Loss of LRRK2/PARK8 induces degeneration of dopaminergic neurons in *Drosophila*," *Biochemical and Biophysical Research Communications*, vol. 358, no. 2, pp. 534–539, 2007.

[45] T. Li, D. Yang, S. Sushchky, Z. Liu, and W. W. Smith, "Models for LRRK2-linked parkinsonism," *Parkinson's Disease*, vol. 2011, Article ID 942412, 16 pages, 2011.

[46] S. Poddighe, F. De Rose, R. Marotta et al., "*Mucuna pruriens* (Velvet bean) rescues motor, olfactory, mitochondrial and synaptic impairment in PINK1^{B9} *Drosophila melanogaster* genetic model of Parkinson's disease," *PLoS ONE*, vol. 9, no. 10, Article ID e110802, 2014.

[47] I. Ibba, A. M. Angioy, B. S. Hansson, and T. Dekker, "Macroglomeruli for fruit odors change blend preference in *Drosophila*," *Naturwissenschaften*, vol. 97, no. 12, pp. 1059–1066, 2010.

[48] S. Poddighe, T. Dekker, A. Scala, and A. M. Angioy, "Olfaction in the female sheep botfly," *Naturwissenschaften*, vol. 97, no. 9, pp. 827–835, 2010.

[49] B. Krishnan, S. E. Dryer, and P. E. Hardin, "Circadian rhythms in olfactory responses of *Drosophila melanogaster*," *Nature*, vol. 400, no. 6742, pp. 375–378, 1999.

[50] E. A. Hallem and J. R. Carlson, "Coding of odors by a receptor repertoire," *Cell*, vol. 125, no. 1, pp. 143–160, 2006.

[51] M. Knaden, A. Strutz, J. Ahsan, S. Sachse, and B. S. Hansson, "Spatial representation of odorant valence in an insect brain," *Cell Reports*, vol. 1, pp. 392–399, 2012.

[52] E. Fishilevich and L. B. Vosshall, "Genetic and functional subdivision of the *Drosophila* antennal lobe," *Current Biology*, vol. 15, no. 17, pp. 1548–1553, 2005.

[53] M. de Bruyne, K. Foster, and J. R. Carlson, "Odor coding in the *Drosophila* antenna," *Neuron*, vol. 30, no. 2, pp. 537–552, 2001.

[54] T. Dekker, I. Ibba, K. P. Siju, M. C. Stensmyr, and B. S. Hansson, "Olfactory shifts parallel superspecialism for toxic fruit in *Drosophila melanogaster* sibling, *D. sechellia*," *Current Biology*, vol. 16, no. 1, pp. 101–109, 2006.

[55] R. F. Stocker, "*Drosophila* as a focus in olfactory research: mapping of olfactory sensilla by fine structure, odor specificity, odorant receptor expression, and central connectivity," *Microscopy Research and Technique*, vol. 55, no. 5, pp. 284–296, 2001.

[56] K. E. Kaissling, "Kinetics of olfactory receptor potentials," in *Proceedings of the 3rd International Symposium on Olfaction and Taste*, C. Pfaffmann, Ed., pp. 52–70, Rockefeller University Press, New York, NY, USA, 1969.

[57] V. G. Dethier, *The Hungry Fly: A Physiological Study of the Behavior Associated with Feeding*, Harvard University Press, London, UK, 1976.

[58] P. Solari, R. Crnjar, A. Frongia et al., "Oxaspiropentane derivatives as effective sex pheromone analogues in the gypsy moth: electrophysiological and behavioral evidence," *Chemical Senses*, vol. 32, no. 8, pp. 755–763, 2007.

[59] J.-C. Corvol, M.-P. Muriel, E. Valjent et al., "Persistent increase in olfactory type G-protein α subunit levels may underlie D_1 receptor functional hypersensitivity in Parkinson disease," *The Journal of Neuroscience*, vol. 24, no. 31, pp. 7007–7014, 2004.

[60] D. T. Jones, S. B. Masters, H. R. Bourne, and R. R. Reed, "Biochemical characterization of three stimulatory GTP-binding proteins: the large and small forms of Gs and the olfactory-specific G-protein, Golf," *Journal of Biological Chemistry*, vol. 265, no. 5, pp. 2671–2676, 1990.

[61] L. Belluscio, G. H. Gold, A. Nemes, and R. Axel, "Mice deficient in G(olf) are anosmic," *Neuron*, vol. 20, no. 1, pp. 69–81, 1998.

[62] E. S. Yun and T. H. Park, "Quantitative measurement of general odorant using electroantennogram of male silkworm moth, *Bombyx mori*," *Biotechnology and Bioprocess Engineering*, vol. 5, no. 2, pp. 150–152, 2000.

[63] M. Schwaerzel, M. Monastirioti, H. Scholz, F. Friggi-Grelin, S. Birman, and M. Heisenberg, "Dopamine and octopamine differentiate between aversive and appetitive olfactory memories in *Drosophila*," *Journal of Neuroscience*, vol. 23, no. 33, pp. 10495–10502, 2003.

[64] P. P. Laissue and L. B. Vosshall, "The olfactory sensory map in *Drosophila*," *Advances in Experimental Medicine and Biology*, vol. 628, pp. 102–114, 2008.

[65] J. R. Riesgo-Escovar, W. B. Piekos, and J. R. Carlson, "The *Drosophila* antenna: ultrastructural and physiological studies in wild-type and lozenge mutants," *Journal of Comparative Physiology A: Sensory, Neural, and Behavioral Physiology*, vol. 180, no. 2, pp. 151–160, 1997.

[66] S. E. Goulding, P. Z. Lage, and A. P. Jarman, "amos, a proneural gene for Drosophila olfactory sense organs that is regulated by lozenge," *Neuron*, vol. 25, no. 1, pp. 69–78, 2000.

[67] J. R. Hughes, D. E. Hendrix, N. Wetzel, and J. W. J. Johnston, "Correlations between electrophysiological activity from the human olfactory bulb and the subjective response to odouriferous stimuli," in *Olfaction and Taste—Proceedings of the III International Symposium*, C. Pfaffmann, Ed., pp. 172–191, The Rockfeller University Press, New York, NY, USA, 1969.

4

Accuracy of Markerless 3D Motion Capture Evaluation to Differentiate between On/Off Status in Parkinson's Disease after Deep Brain Stimulation

Hector R. Martinez, Alexis Garcia-Sarreon, Carlos Camara-Lemarroy ⓘ, Fortino Salazar, and María L. Guerrero-González ⓘ

Tecnologico de Monterrey, Escuela de Medicina y Ciencias de la Salud, Ave. Morones Prieto 3000, 64710 Monterrey, NL, Mexico

Correspondence should be addressed to María L. Guerrero-González; lucy.guerrero.gzz@gmail.com

Academic Editor: Hélio Teive

Background. Body motion evaluation (BME) by markerless systems is increasingly being considered as an alternative to traditional marker-based technology because they are faster, simpler, and less expensive. They are increasingly used in clinical settings in patients with movement disorders; however, the wide variety of systems available makes results conflicting. *Research Question*. The objective of this study was to determine whether a markerless 3D motion capture system is a useful instrument to objectively differentiate between PD patients with DBS in On and Off states and controls and its correlation with the evaluation by means of MDS-UPDRS. *Methods*. Six PD patients who underwent deep brain stimulation (DBS) bilaterally in the subthalamic nucleus were evaluated using BME and the Unified Parkinson's Disease Rating Scale (UPDRS-III) with DBS turned On and Off. BME of 16 different movements in six controls paired by age and sex was compared with that in PD patients with DBS in On and Off states. *Results*. A better performance in the BME was correlated with a lower UPDRS-III score. There was no statistically significant difference between patients in Off and On states of DBS regarding BME. However, some items such as left shoulder flexion ($p = 0.038$), right shoulder rotation ($p = 0.011$), and left trunk rotation ($p = 0.023$) were different between Off patients and healthy controls. *Significance*. Kinematic data obtained with this markerless system could contribute to discriminate between PD patients and healthy controls. This emerging technology may help to clinically evaluate PD patients more objectively.

1. Introduction

Three-dimensional (3D) markerless motion capture systems are continuously being considered as an alternative to traditional sensor-based systems in analyzing human movement kinematics and gait [1–8]. Markerless systems are being used increasingly for several reasons. First, traditional systems are time-consuming because they require the placement of several sensors as well as calibration prior to testing (which altogether can take up to 1 hour). In addition, thanks to this rapidness, technicians may scan a greater number of people per day and therefore allowing this study to be at a more reasonable price (in our hospital, the most expensive study is $80 USD while marker-based evaluation may cost around $500 USD).

Lastly, marker-based systems are susceptible to marker placement error, meaning a sensor can be accidentally placed in a different location in test-retest; therefore, reliability is low and operator dependent, which may cause conflicting results [4]. Markerless motion capture systems use light reflection from the skin or specific colored clothes to capture the patient's avatar, and they have been proven to be more consistent when the test is repeated [4, 9].

The markerless system we use in this study is called DARI (Dynamic Athletic Research Institute) (Motion Platform, version 3.2-Denali from Scientific Analytics Inc., Kansas City, KS, USA). The DARI system generates a full-body motion capture skeleton from cloud voxels, which translate to a human's volumetric silhouette that generates the parameters. Using consistent clothing, the algorithms that generate the skeleton also do it consistently. Rosengarden et al. assessed the repeatability of this system by tracking the change in skeleton segment lengths between sessions, totaling 480 sessions, and 9,120 bone segments. He found that the bone length change for a person between sessions was 1.02% with a variance of 0.002 mm and a 99% confidence interval of 0.81 mm [5]. In another study, Perrott concluded that when comparing marker-based versus markerless evaluations, they both report statistically similar ranges of change in the angle of squats in pelvis and lower limbs [9]. These findings illustrate that a 3D markerless motion capture is a highly repeatable system which can have a variety of new applications for athletic and healthcare settings [3–7, 9]. However, there is currently no gold-standard for motion capture systems and the results are not always consistent because they vary from device to device.

Also, traditional marker-based analysis of a single human motion may require days of intensive data compiling and error-correction. By the time the data is ready, the window of application has passed. Markerless systems usually process data faster; however, DARI's software is an advanced tool that consists of a powerful cloud processing software engine that takes thousands of data points comprising each motion and processes them in under a second. An interesting study conducted by Ceseracciu et al. compared markerless and marker-based motion capture technologies by recording the same movement simultaneously. They found that the markerless 3D motion capture was not as accurate as marker-based. However, because of setup compromise, they only used six cameras for the markerless system (instead of eight that the system asked for) [1].

Most of the published studies that use the DARI system and other markerless systems are applied in the field of sports medicine, for professional athletes, rehabilitation, and injury prevention [4]. However, one of the most affordable ones, the Microsoft Kinect has been used in a number of studies to analyze gait and movement disorders. Galna et al. found that the Microsoft Kinect can accurately measure timing and gross spatial characteristics of relevant PD movements, but smaller movements (e.g., hand clasping) did not have the same spatial accuracy [10]. Another study by Bovonsunthonchai examined gait initiation in patients with PD using a force distribution measurement platform and was successful in documenting specific gait characteristics in PD [11]. A similar study but with a different objective was conducted by Ferrarin et al.; they used a marker-based system to examine the effects of subthalamic stimulation on gait kinematics and kinetics in PD, and they were able to find clinical differences in the effects produced by medication (L-dopa) and DBS [12]. Although none of these studies used exactly the same system we did, they describe high accuracy rate in discriminating between PD patients in the DBS On and DBS Off states. To date, there are no published studies using DARI motion capture technology in neurological diseases, including PD. Based on the hardware and software characteristics described, we believe DARI will show even higher accuracy rate than other markerless systems previously used.

The validity and test-retest reliability in a Parkinson's disease patient are complicated to acquire due the heterogeneity of its clinical presentation. This clinical variability is not only present from patient to patient but also may even change several times a day on the same patient, even after medical or surgical treatment. For this reason, we recruited patients that had previously undergone DBS implantation, this made it possible for a single patient to become its own control in On/Off status. Also, in order to have a baseline to which we could compare the data obtained, we recruited healthy patients matched by age and gender. The objective of this study was to determine if a markerless 3D motion capture system is a useful instrument to objectively differentiate between PD patients with DBS in On and Off states and healthy control subjects.

2. Methodology

2.1. Patients.

Six patients with PD, diagnosed in accordance with the UK Parkinson's Disease Society Brain Bank Clinical Diagnostic Criteria by a certified neurologist and movement disorder specialist, were included (Table 1). This is a pilot study, and the sample size was chosen by convenience for accessibility and proximity to the researchers. Inclusion criteria: diagnosis of PD submitted to subthalamic DBS implantation a minimum of 3 months prior to the evaluation, and age limits were 40 to 80 years old. Exclusion criteria: patients with physical disability (i.e., wheelchair, cane, and assistance to daily living activities), history of stroke and physical disability, another neurological disorder other than PD, recent head and limb trauma that limits movement, and treatment with antipsychotics drug or recent botulinum toxin treatment. The patients had undergone bilateral subthalamic nucleus DBS implantation with a mean of 15 months (range, 5–46 months) prior to this evaluation due to motor fluctuations and dyskinesia after more than 3 years of good response to levodopa. The stimulation parameters were optimized to obtain the best clinical response (140–160 Hz, pulse width 60–90 μs, 2.5–3 V). Stimuli were delivered through the deepest electrode contact 0 (−) and 1 (+) in a bipolar configuration. In addition, six healthy subjects matched by age and sex were included as controls. The study was approved by our institutional research board, and the patients and controls provided written consent. In the months preceding the test, the PD patients were clinically evaluated by the same physician according to the Unified Parkinson Disease Rating Scale or motor section (UPDRS-III).

2.2. Instrument.

Actually, there are many markerless motion capture systems in the market, with a broad range of prices, as well as a broad range of reliability. However, the DARI system has been proven to be one of the best for numerous reasons. This system requires a quick calibration at the beginning of each day that the technician can complete in less than 10 minutes. It does not have to be repeated until the following day, no matter how many patients are evaluated. The system depends on a computer-based software that acquires the patient's skeleton or avatar using eighteen high-speed cameras (120 Hz) placed around the room to collect

TABLE 1: Parkinson patients at the time of evaluation.

Patient	Age	Time since diagnosis	Time since DBS implantation	PD medication	UPDRS score Off	UPDRS score On
1	67	5 years	10 months	L-dopa, rotigotine	47	22
2	65	12 years	5 months	L-dopa, rotigotine, amantadine	53	27
3	44	5 years	6 months	L-dopa, biperidone	39	29
4	76	10 years	12 months	L-dopa, rotigotine, amantadine	42	37
5	59	5 years	11 months	L-dopa, rotigotine	57	41
6	63	10 years	46 months	L-dopa, rotigotine, rasagiline	40	25

PD medication doses: L-dopa ranged from 400 to 1000 mg per day, rotigotine 4–8 mg per day, amantadine ranged from 100 to 300 mg per day, and rasagiline 1 mg per day.

whole body data and delivers kinematic analysis almost instantly using sophisticated biomechanical algorithms.

Also, traditional motion labs use cumbersome floor-mounted pressure plates to measure the forces generated by the body. These require frequent calibration and restrict the subject's movement to a limited area. The DARI's kinetic capture system does not require force plates and can measure joint torques, ground reaction forces, and other measurements without restricting the subject's natural movement [3].

Markerless 3D motion capture evaluation of kinematics in the PD patients and controls was performed in a rectangle room that measures 6 x 6 meters and 3 meters in height. The room has a green screen on the floor, and eighteen cameras are strategically placed on the walls: twelve are placed 2.6 meters high, and 6 are on a lower level at 30 centimeters from the ground. The room has ample space, which allows for broader movements to be analyzed (Figure 1).

2.3. Evaluation. PD patients were asked to arrive in the morning wearing dark close-fitting clothing, to skip their last PD medication, and with DBS in the Off state for least 180 minutes. On PD patients, UPDRS-III evaluation was done first. Then, to begin the markerless body motion evaluation (BME), patients and controls' weight and height were entered into the system to help establish the locations of joint centers. Once inside the green room, subjects first stood with feet apart and arms outstretched to the side, while the system created a 3D silhouette of each participant's form and a biometric skeleton was acquired; this took no more than three seconds. For the BME, all subjects performed 16 different movements (Table 2). This set of movements was especially designed to evaluate PD patients and contains items that are related to three major motor symptoms in this disease: rigidity, bradykinesia, and postural instability; tremor is not possible to assess. Once the BME was done, PD patients were asked to turn their DBS to the On state and wait 30 minutes before repeating both UPDRS-III and BME. Controls only performed the BME, which took no more than 20 minutes. PD patients were evaluated twice (DBS states On and Off) with a 30-minute wait in between; their evaluation altogether took approximately 1 hour. The data files were uploaded to DARI Motion Platform where the biomechanical analysis produced full-body kinematic results, and finally, these data were exported to Excel for statistical analysis.

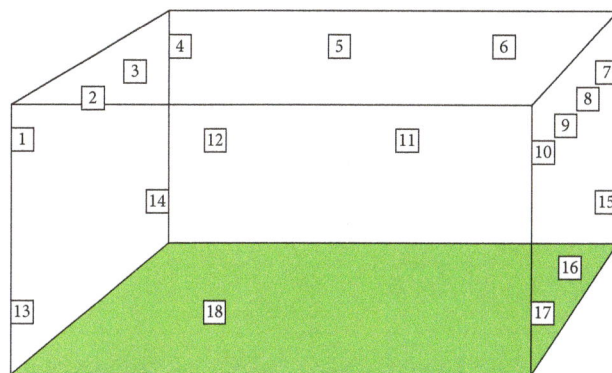

FIGURE 1: Approximate sketch of BME room, which measured $6 \times 6 \times 3$ meters. Each number represents a camera (18 in total), the different colors of the cameras represent the wall they were on. Cameras were located at two different levels: upper level cameras 1–12 were at a height of 2.6 meters and lower level cameras 13–18 at a height of 30 centimeters from the floor approximately. Distance between upper-level cameras varied but averaged 1.8 meters (range 1.4–2 meters). Distance between lower-level cameras was too variable. The floor was covered in a green screen. Subjects were able to use the entire room for evaluation.

2.4. Analysis. A paired *t*-test was used to compare mean changes in UPDRS-III between the On and Off states. Mean differences between groups were evaluated with ANOVA or Kruskal-Wallis tests depending on the distribution of the data of each independent variable. Post hoc analyses were made for pairwise comparison in statistically significant results. Bivariate correlations among evaluation modalities were examined. These correlations were examined in the On and Off states between UPDRS-III and BME items. To compare them as accurately as possible, the items on UPDRS-III and BME that were similar were correlated (e.g., rigidity in upper limbs from UPDRS-III was correlated with shoulder flexion, extension, and rotation from BME). One of the correlations was hip displacement taken from BME, which analyses balance by measuring the movement of hips when patients stand during 10 seconds with arms outstretched to the sides and eyes closed; this was correlated with the posture stability item from UPDRS-III, which is a quick pull, reactionary intervention test where patient's response is measured. Because not all UPDRS-III items were measurable by DARI, seven out of 18 were correlated; however, all BME items were correlated with the UPDRS-III global score (Table 2). IBM SPSS Statistics 21.0 software was used for data analysis. A *p* value of ≤ 0.05 was considered to

TABLE 2: Comparable items between the UPDRS-III and Body Motion Evaluation.

Functional modalities	UPDRS-III items	BME items	Description of BME items
Upper extremity	Rigidity (upper limbs 3.3)	Shoulder flexion (right and left)	All are range of motion, measured in degrees
	Body bradykinesia (3.14)	Shoulder extension (right and left) Shoulder internal/external rotation (right and left) Maximum shoulder abduction (right and left)	
Lower extremity	Rigidity (lower limbs 3.3) Gait (3.10) Body bradykinesia (3.14)	Bilateral squat depth Lunge distance (right and left)	All measured in centimeters and inches
Trunk	Rigidity (neck 3.3) Posture (3.13)	Trunk rotation (right and left) Trunk flexion Trunk extension	All measured in degrees
Balance and posture	Postural stability (3.12)	Anterior-posterior hip displacement	Patients were asked to remain for 10 seconds with arms outstretched to the sides, eyes closed, and head tilted upward
	Posture (3.13)	Medial-lateral hip displacement	Hip displacement was measured in centimeters
Gait	Arising from a chair (3.9) Gait (3.10) Freezing of gait (3.11) Posture (3.13) Body bradykinesia (3.14)	Cadence Gait speed Stride length Step length (right and left) Step width (right and left)	Strides/minute Meters/second Centimeters Centimeters Centimeters

BME, Body Motion Evaluation; UPDRS-III, Unified Parkinson's Disease Rating Scale.

indicate statistical significance, and values are given as means ± SD.

3. Results

Six patients with PD (four men and two women), with a mean age of 62.3 ± 10.6 years (range, 44–76 years), and six control subjects (four men and two women), with a mean age of 60.3 ± 10.25 years (range, 44–76 years), were included in the study.

3.1. Differences between DBS in On and Off States. The UPDRS-III motor score differed significantly between PD patients in the DBS On and Off states (30.17 vs. 46.33, $p = 0.028$). Among upper limb parameters, we found statistically significant group differences between left shoulder flexion and right shoulder rotation ($p = 0.039$ and 0.007, respectively), which in the post hoc pairwise analysis showed an important difference between Off and controls for the left shoulder flexion ($p = 0.038$) and for Off and On groups compared with controls for right shoulder rotation ($p = 0.011$ and 0.030, respectively) (Table 3).

Regarding trunk mobility, flexion/extension displacement, and right and left rotation showed significant differences between the multigroup analysis ($p = 0.046$, 0.049, 0.021, and 0.025, respectively). However, paired differences were just found between On and controls for the right

rotation of the trunk ($p = 0.024$) and between Off and controls for the left rotation ($p = 0.023$). Neither the lower limb nor gait parameters showed statistically significant difference in the multi group analysis (Table 3).

3.2. Correlation Extra Gait Items. In UPDRS-III, a higher number indicates a worse performance; in BME, a higher number usually indicates a better performance. A significant negative correlation between the BME and UPDRS-III scores for an item would mean that the item is potentially useful for evaluating patients with PD. Among PD patients in the DBS Off state, significant negative correlations were found between the global UPDRS-III motor score and right shoulder flexion ($r = -0.829$, $p = 0.042$) and maximal abduction ($r = -0.833$, $p = 0.039$). Right upper extremity rigidity also was negatively correlated with right shoulder extension ($r = -0.878$, $p = 0.021$). Negative correlations between UPDRS-III and BME were not present in PD patients in the DBS On state. With regard to the lower extremities, greater depth of bilateral squat was negatively correlated with the UPDRS-III items gait ($r = -0.926$, $p = 0.008$) and body bradykinesia ($r = -0.926$, $p = 0.008$) in the DBS Off state. This negative correlation was not present in PD patients in the DBS On state. Interestingly, when a PD patient was under stimulation, the performance of a complicated task, such as the displacement of a lunge, was correlated with lower scores for the same items (gait and

TABLE 3: Mean ± SD differences in items between patients in DBS On, DBS Off, and controls.

Items	Extra gait items			p value mean difference between groups/pos hoc pairwise comparison that showed significance
	DBS Off	DBS On	Controls	
Shoulder flexion (°)	R: 164.01 ± 13.41	R: 166.91 ± 20.82	R: 183.43 ± 14.12	NS
	L: 160.00 ± 15.23	L: 165.05 ± 16.50	**L: 183.48 ± 12.13**	0.039/**0.038**
	R: 147.33 ± 18.94	R: 152.60 ± 20.20	**R: 184.53 ± 16.91**	0.07/**0.011**
Shoulder rotation (°)*	R: 147.33 ± 18.94	**R: 152.60 ± 20.20**	**R: 184.53 ± 16.91**	0.07/**0.030**
	L: 141.41 ± 16.76	L: 142.11 ± 19.65	L: 169.93 ± 20.75	NS
Shoulder abduction (°)	R: 147.03 ± 9.56	R: 153.45 ± 13.39	R: 156.93 ± 17.12	NS
	L: 148.60 ± 13.71	L: 157.83 ± 15.94	L: 168.06 ± 22.25	NS
Trunk rotation (°)	R: 7.73 ± 2.69	**R: 6.25 ± 6.25**	**R: 16.20 ± 5.72**	0.021/**0.024**
	L: 5.36 ± 4.65	L: 9.01 ± 4.96	**L: 13.46 ± 4.01**	0.025/**0.023**
Trunk flexion/extension (°)	F: 30.11 ± 7.01	F: 32.11 ± 7.06	F: 44.78 ± 9.89	0.046
	E: 27.18 ± 7.04	E: 32.63 ± 18.91	E: 46.15 ± 7.35	0.049
Lunge distance (cm)	R: 62.11 ± 15.62	R: 70.49 ± 22.18	R: 85.11 ± 16.13	NS
	L: 58.52 ± 20.48	L: 68.52 ± 22.63	L: 83.15 ± 16.45	NS
Gait items				
Cadence (strides/min)	83.33 ± 14.21	90.38 ± 19.84	88.51 ± 4.62	NS
Stride length (cm)	97.28 ± 18.35	105.54 ± 11.66	107.07 ± 13.35	NS
Step length (cm)	R: 50.32 ± 9.65	R: 53.19 ± 7.76	R: 54.02 ± 7.80	NS
	L: 47.48 ± 8.90	L: 53.57 ± 4.49	L: 53.47 ± 5.38	NS
Step width (cm)	R: 10.01 ± 3.10	R: 10.08 ± 4.46	R: 10.13 ± 2.75	NS
	L: 8.78 ± 2.37	L: 7.76 ± 2.36	L: 8.46 ± 1.74	NS
Gait speed (m/s)	0.68 ± 0.24	0.81 ± 0.25	0.81 ± 0.09	NS

DBS, deep brain stimulation; NS, not significant; R, right; L, left; F, flexion; E, extension. *For right shoulder rotation, results are shown twice due to a double pairwise significant result.

bradykinesia) in the UPDRS-III ($r = -0.845$, $p = 0.034$ for both items).

With regard to trunk evaluation, there was a significant negative correlation when the PD patient was in the DBS On state for the global motor score in UPDRS-III and right ($r = -0.928$, $p = 0.008$) and left ($r = -0.829$, $p = 0.048$) trunk rotation in BME. Balance and posture showed no significant differences between UPDRS-III and BME (Table 4).

3.3. Correlation Gait Items. In PD patients in the DBS Off state, there was a significant negative correlation between UPDRS-III gait items and stride length ($r = -0.833$, $p = 0.039$) as well as right step length ($r = -0.926$, $p = 0.008$). In our sample, step width in the right and left feet was highly positively correlated with the gait item in UPDRS-III ($r = -0.926$, $p = 0.008$ for both feet). Interestingly, cadence, gait speed, and stride length were negatively correlated with the "rising from a chair" item of UPDRS-III ($r = -0.878$, $p = 0.021$). In PD patients in the DBS On state, posture was the only UPDRS-III item that was significantly negatively correlated with cadence and gait speed ($r = -0.926$, $p = 0.008$ for both items) and with stride length and step length on both sides ($r = -0.833$, $p = 0.039$) (Table 4).

4. Limitations

We acknowledge the limitations that may interfere with our results. The sample size was small and may not reflect the patterns of all PD patients with DBS; however, this is a pilot

study, and sample size was chosen by convenience. Items from UPDRS-III and BME are not the same and therefore, even though correlations were made based on similarity, they may not be perfectly comparable; in UPDRS-III gait, analysis is performed in 9 meters distance, while gait analysis in BME is done in a 6-meter room. However, we hypothesized that BME would have given us an objective quantification of the motor abnormalities, in contrast to the interobserver variability that may result in UPDRS-III. Also, UPDRS-III includes 18 items, and only seven of them were identifiable by the motion capture system, and the rest were not included; however, global UPDRS-III score was compared to all BME items.

5. Discussion

In the present study, we showed that a markerless 3D system correlated with UPDRS-III scores. The utility of markerless techniques in the evaluation of movement disorders in a clinical setting is controversial because analysis parameters have not been standardized yet. However, several studies have described precise acquisition of human anatomy and consistency with recommendations of biomechanical societies [1, 3, 5–7, 9, 10].

Different markerless systems have also been evaluated, including the Microsoft Kinect sensor, which accurately measures timing and gross spatial characteristics of clinically relevant movements but is much less effective for evaluating fine movements, such as tremor, hand clasping, and toe

TABLE 4: Statistically significant correlations between UPDRS-III and BME.

BME (UPDRS-III)*	DBS Off		DBS On	
	SCC	p value	SCC	p value
Right shoulder flexion (UPDRS-III score)	−0.829	0.042	−0.486	NS
Right maximal abduction (UPDRS-III score)	−0.829	0.042	−0.029	NS
Right maximal abduction (upper limb rigidity)	−0.833	0.021	−0.169	NS
Bilateral squat depth (body bradykinesia)	−0.926	0.008	−0.676	NS
Bilateral squat depth (gait)	−0.926	0.008	−0.676	NS
Stride length (gait)	−0.833	0.039	−0.338	NS
Right step length (gait)	−0.926	0.008	−0.338	NS
Right step width (gait)	0.926	0.008	0.257	NS
Left step width (gait)	0.926	0.008	−0.167	NS
Cadence (arising from a chair)	−0.878	0.021	−0.676	NS
Stride length (arising from a chair)	−0.878	0.021	NA	NS
Gait speed (arising from a chair)	−0.878	0.021	NA	NS
Right trunk rotation (UPDRS-III score)	−0.086	NS	−0.928	0.008
Left trunk rotation (UPDRS-III score)	−0.257	NS	−0.829	0.048
Lunge distance, both sides (body bradykinesia)	−0.741	NS	−0.845	0.034
Lunge distance, both sides (gait)	−0.741	NS	−0.845	0.034
Cadence (posture)	−0.516	NS	−0.926	0.008
Gait speed (posture)	−0.638	NS	−0.926	0.008
Stride length (posture)	−0.577	NS	−0.833	0.039
Right step length (posture)	−0.395	NS	−0.833	0.039
Left step length (posture)	−0.698	NS	−0.833	0.039
Right shoulder flexion (UPDRS-III score)	−0.829	0.042	−0.486	NS
Right maximal abduction (UPDRS-III score)	−0.829	0.042	−0.029	NS
Right maximal abduction (upper limb rigidity)	−0.833	0.021	−0.169	NS
Two-leg squat displacement (body bradykinesia)	−0.926	0.008	−0.676	NS
Two-leg squat displacement (gait)	−0.926	0.008	−0.676	NS
Stride length (gait)	−0.833	0.039	−0.338	NS
Right step length (gait)	−0.926	0.008	−0.338	NS
Right step width (gait)	0.926	0.008	0.257	NS
Left step width (gait)	0.926	0.008	−0.167	NS
Cadence (rising from a chair)	−0.878	0.021	−0.676	NS
Stride length (rising from a chair)	−0.878	0.021	NA	NS
Gait speed (rising from a chair)	−0.878	0.021	NA	NS
Right trunk rotation (UPDRS-III score)	−0.086	NS	−0.928	0.008
Left trunk rotation (UPDRS-III score)	−0.257	NS	−0.829	0.048
Lunge displacement, both sides (body bradykinesia)	−0.741	NS	−0.845	0.034
Lunge displacement, both sides (gait)	−0.741	NS	−0.845	0.034
Cadence (posture)	−0.516	NS	−0.926	0.008
Gait speed (posture)	−0.638	NS	−0.926	0.008
Stride length (posture)	−0.577	NS	−0.833	0.039
Right step length (posture)	−0.395	NS	−0.833	0.039
Left step length (posture)	−0.698	NS	−0.833	0.039

*Corresponding items to UPDRS-III. BME, body motion evaluation; DBS, deep brain stimulation; NA, not applicable because all data on "rising from a chair" were 0 in the On state; NS, not significant; SCC, Spearman correlation coefficient; UPDRS-III, Unified Parkinson's Disease Rating Scale.

tapping [10, 13]. Because there is a wide variety of markerless systems, it is essential to use a system that is validated and can show repeatability [14]. Even though the DARI system has not been used for neurological movement disorders, including PD, we believe that the previous publications, which acquired data from healthy subjects, confirm its validity [4].

In our study, there was a significant negative correlation between gait and stride length in the UPDRS-III and BME ($r = -0.833$, $p = 0.039$) as well as right step length ($r = -0.926$, $p = 0.008$) in the Off state. Improvement in some features in the BME was associated with positive changes in the UPDRS-III motor score. Some items showed significance on one side but not the other, this may be due to the asymmetrical clinical course that is typically observed in PD. Although our initial hypothesis of the ability of the DARI system to discriminate between Off and On states of DBS did not meet our expectations, our results suggest a potential use of the DARI system in PD. It is possible that the small sample size used in this pilot study may have reflected statistical results that are not representative. A greater sample size would contribute to establish parameters and give rise to new tools for the objective evaluation of motor disorders; this way, avoiding inter-rater variability. Validation of markerless systems for evaluating patients with PD will require further study protocols involving a greater number of patients in different clinical conditions. There is a wide area of opportunity in the evaluation of movement disorders using emerging technology. Prospective studies would also be useful to establish the clinical significance of markerless systems.

Authors' Contributions

Hector R. Martinez, MD, PhD, FACP, supervised the study; conceived the presented research idea, conception; and design; recruited patients and controls; was responsible for analysis and interpretation of data, drafting and revision of the manuscript, and critical revision and final approval of the manuscript. Alexis Garcia-Sarreon, MD, conceived the study and design, carried out evaluations on patients and controls, was responsible for acquisition of data, performed the statistical analysis and interpretation of data, and wrote the initial manuscript. Carlos Camara-Lemarroy, MD, was responsible for conception and design, verified the statistical analysis methods, contributed to the interpretation of the results, drafting, and critical revision of the manuscript. Fortino Salazar, MD, conceived the study and design, carried out the DBS implantation surgery in all patients, and was responsible for critical revision of the manuscript. María L. Guerrero-González, MD, performed analysis and interpretation of data, designed the tables, drafted and revised the manuscript, and was in charge of drafting the final version once input from all the authors was received.

Acknowledgments

We thank Instituto de Neurologia y Neurocirugia Hospital Zambrano-Hellion, Monterrey, N.L., Mexico, for being our study's headquarters. We also thank Francisco Rodriguez-Leal, MD, and Norma L. Alvarado-Franco, MD, for reviewing the clinical files and for their valuable comments on the statistical analysis of this study. We also acknowledge the unrestricted support of UCB México. Before submission, the paper was sent to Enago-Global for a substantive editing, which was funded by Tecnológico de Monterrey ITESM.

References

[1] E. Ceseracciu, Z. Sawacha, and C. Cobelli, "Comparison of markerless and marker-based motion capture technologies through simultaneous data collection during gait: proof of concept," *PLOS One*, vol. 9, no. 3, Article ID e87640, 2014.

[2] A. P. Rocha, H. Choupina, J. M. Fernandes, M. J. Rosas, R. Vaz, and J. P. Silva Cunha, "Parkinson's disease assessment based on gait analysis using an innovative RGB-D camera system," in *Proceedings of 2014 36th Annual International Conference of the IEEE Engineering in Medicine and Biology Society*, pp. 3126–3129, Chicago, Illinois, USA, August 2014.

[3] A. C. Fry, T. J. Herda, A. J. Sterczala, M. A. Cooper, and M. J. Andre, "Validation of a motion capture system for deriving accurate ground reaction forces without a force plate," *Big Data Analytics*, vol. 1, no. 1, p. 11, 2016.

[4] P. Moodie, *Validation: reviewing 3d motion capture technology types and what the gold standard should be for human movement*, Dynamic Athletic Research Institute, Lenexa, Kansas.

[5] S. Rosengarden, S. Docking, D. Wassom, and N. Moodie, "The long term repeatability of a 3D markerless motion capture system and the implications it has on healthcare," *Journal Applied Human Movement*, vol. 1, no. 1, pp. 21–25, 2015.

[6] D. Wassom, A. Fry, and N. Moodie, "Repeatability of 3D markerless motion capture and how it could affect between-session variability," *Journal Applied Human Movement*, vol. 1, no. 1, pp. 21–25, 2015.

[7] L. Mündermann, D. Anguelov, S. Corazza, A. M. Chaudhari, and T. P. Andriacchi, "Validation of a markerless motion capture system for the calculation of lower extremity kinematics," in *Proceedings of the International Society of Biomechanics XXth Congress & American Society of Biomechanics 29th Annual Meeting*, Stanford University, Cleveland, OH, USA, August 2005.

[8] S. Chen, S. Lin, L. Liao et al., "Quantification and recognition of parkinsonian gait from monocular video imaging using kernel-based principal component analysis," *BioMedical Engineering OnLine*, vol. 10, no. 1, p. 99, 2011.

[9] M. A. Perrott, T. Pizzari, J. Cook, and J. A. McClelland, "Comparison of lower limb and trunk kinematics between markerless and marker-based motion capture systems," *Gait & Posture*, vol. 52, pp. 57–61, 2017.

[10] B. Galna, G. Barry, D. Jackson, D. Mhiripiri, P. Olivier, and L. Rochester, "Accuracy of the Microsoft Kinect sensor for measuring movement in people with Parkinson's disease," *Gait & Posture*, vol. 39, no. 4, pp. 1062–1068, 2014.

[11] S. Bovonsunthonchai, R. Vachalathiti, A. Pisarnpong, F. Khobhun, and V. Hiengkaew, "Spatiotemporal gait parameters for patients with parkinson's disease compared with normal individuals," *Physiotherapy Research International*, vol. 19, no. 3, pp. 158–165, 2013.

[12] M. Ferrarin, M. Rizzone, B. Bergamasco et al., "Effects of bilateral subthalamic stimulation on gait kinematics and kinetics in Parkinson's disease," *Experimental Brain Research*, vol. 160, no. 4, pp. 517–527, 2004.

[13] D. C. Dewey, M. Svjetlana, I. Bernstein et al., "Automated gait and balance parameters diagnose and correlate with severity in Parkinson Disease," *Journal of the Neurological Sciences*, vol. 345, no. 1-2, pp. 131–138, 2014.

[14] D. D. Espy, F. Yang, T. Bhatt, and Y. C. Pai, "Independent influence of gait speed and step length on stability and fall risk," *Gait & Posture*, vol. 32, no. 3, pp. 378–382, 2010.

5

Deep Brain Stimulation Frequency of the Subthalamic Nucleus Affects Phonemic and Action Fluency in Parkinson's Disease

Valéria de Carvalho Fagundes,[1,2,3] **Carlos R. M. Rieder,**[3,4] **Aline Nunes da Cruz,**[3,5] **Bárbara Costa Beber,**[3] **and Mirna Wetters Portuguez**[1,2]

[1]*Pontifical Catholic University of Rio Grande do Sul (PUCRS), Porto Alegre, RS, Brazil*
[2]*Brain Institute of Rio Grande do Sul (InsCer), Porto Alegre, RS, Brazil*
[3]*Hospital de Clínicas de Porto Alegre (HCPA), Porto Alegre, RS, Brazil*
[4]*Federal University of Health Sciences from Porto Alegre (UFCSPA), Porto Alegre, RS, Brazil*
[5]*Federal University of Rio Grande do Sul (UFRGS), Porto Alegre, RS, Brazil*

Correspondence should be addressed to Mirna Wetters Portuguez; mirna@pucrs.br

Academic Editor: Hélio Teive

Introduction. Deep brain stimulation of the subthalamic nucleus (STN-DBS) in Parkinson's disease (PD) has been linked to a decline in verbal fluency. The decline can be attributed to surgical effects, but the relative contributions of the stimulation parameters are not well understood. This study aimed to investigate the impact of the frequency of STN-DBS on the performance of verbal fluency tasks in patients with PD. *Methods.* Twenty individuals with PD who received bilateral STN-DBS were evaluated. Their performances of verbal fluency tasks (semantic, phonemic, action, and unconstrained fluencies) upon receiving low-frequency (60 Hz) and high-frequency (130 Hz) STN-DBS were assessed. *Results.* The performances of phonemic and action fluencies were significantly different between low- and high-frequency STN-DBS. Patients showed a decrease in these verbal fluencies for high-frequency STN-DBS. *Conclusion.* Low-frequency STN-DBS may be less harmful to the verbal fluency of PD patients.

1. Introduction

Deep brain stimulation (DBS) at the subthalamic nucleus (STN) improves motor function and the quality of life of patients with advanced Parkinson's disease (PD) [1]. However, some adverse effects are well documented in the literature, such as reduced verbal fluency (VF) [2–9].

The decline in VF observed in PD patients who undergo DBS is not well understood. Studies have hypothesized that this impairment is due to a possible lesion effect from surgery and/or an effect of the neurostimulator parameters, for instance, the frequency of stimulation [1, 2, 4, 6, 8, 9]. Thus, studies assessing the impact of neurostimulation parameters, such as stimulation frequency, on VF are needed.

Low-frequency stimulation has been associated with improved motor symptoms, including freezing of gait and swallowing, in patients with STN-DBS [10, 11]. Similarly,

a study on the effects of low-frequency (10 Hz) and high-frequency (130 Hz) DBS-STN on semantic and phonemic verbal fluency found that performance on all VF tasks was significantly better for the low-frequency condition [12]. Further studies are needed to understand how frequency affects VF by analyzing additional VF tasks and the performance of various populations due to language and educational differences.

VF tasks are often used as operating measures of language and executive functions [13]. Among VF tasks are tasks that measure semantic VF (requests for words from a specific semantic group, such as animals or fruits) [13, 14], phonemic VF (requests for words that start with a certain letter) [13, 15], verb fluency or action fluency (requests for words designating things that people do) [13, 16], and unconstrained VF (requests any word without a criterion) [17].

The various VF tasks may provide different types of information regarding cognition because each VF task requires accessing specific lexical and/or semantic representations according to the criteria. The VF tasks activate overlapping areas of the frontal brain regions, but different word retrieval criteria likely activate additional distinct regions [13]. Semantic fluency is thought to be associated with temporal-lobe dysfunction, whereas phonemic fluency is associated with frontal-lobe dysfunction [18]. The action fluency deficit has been reported as a possible marker of frontostriatal impairment [16, 19]. Although both phonemic and action VF rely on frontal brain areas, evidence has indicated that action VF relies more heavily on semantic information that involves motor content (and because action VF may involve motor brain areas) [13, 19], whereas phonemic fluency relies more heavily on lexical retrieval to access words with phonemic similarities [13]. The action fluency task appears to be an important task for evaluating PD, as studies have shown that the action fluency task may be more sensitive to cognitive impairment in PD patients compared to other VF tasks [16, 19]. Currently, little is known regarding the neural and cognitive substrates of unconstrained VF because the few studies that have used this VF task only verified the influence of demographic factors on its performance [20, 21]. The absence of a retrieval criterion, as in the unconstrained VF task, may reinforce the need for inhibitory capacity, cognitive flexibility, working memory, and planning. Additionally, the unconstrained VF task may be considered as the absence of specific semantic or lexical involvement.

This study aimed to analyze the impact of low-frequency (60 Hz) and high-frequency (130 Hz) STN-DBS on VF tasks of PD patients. We hypothesized that PD patients would present VF deficits due to the frontosubcortical impairment caused by the disease. Thus, if there is an influence of the frequency of stimulation in our population, the frequency should affect the VF tasks that rely more on frontosubcortical functions, as required by the phonemic and action VFs. To test this hypothesis, not only is it important to assess phonemic and action VF tasks, but also the VF tasks that we hypothesized would not be affected by the frequency of stimulation, that is, semantic and unconstrained VFs.

2. Methods

2.1. Patients.
The present study was a randomized double-blinded experimental study. The study was conducted with outpatients from the Neurology Service of *Hospital de Clínicas de Porto Alegre* (HCPA).

The study included 20 patients with idiopathic PD diagnosed according to the criteria of the UK Parkinson's Disease Society Brain Bank [22] and aged between 30 and 75 years. All participants had a bilateral STN-DBS implanted. Only patients with DBS parameters stabilized to the best motor control were included. Also, all patients were Brazilian Portuguese native speakers.

Exclusion criteria included the abuse of illicit drugs or benzodiazepines within the last six months, the presence of auditory impairment, as evaluated by an audiometric screening performed by an audiologist, the presence of visual impairment, a clinical diagnosis of depression or the presence of important signs or symptoms of depression (measured according to the 17-item Hamilton Depression Rating Scale, with a cutoff of 23 for very severe depression) [23], a clinical diagnosis of dementia or Mini-Mental State Examination (MMSE) with scores lower than the expected for the patient's educational level (cutoff of 20 for illiterates, 25 for 1 to 4 years of education, 26.5 for 5 to 8 years, 28 for 9 to 11 years, and 29 for higher levels of education) [24], a history of psychotic symptoms, or a history of alcoholism (screening according to the CAGE questionnaire with a score ≤1) [25].

2.2. Procedures.
This study was conducted in a randomized, double-blinded manner. The order of the initial DBS conditions was defined by a medical student using the website http://www.random.com/. The order offered by the website was random but with an equal distribution of the initial DBS conditions. The low-frequency (60 Hz) and high-frequency (130 Hz) conditions were termed A-condition and B-condition, respectively. Each participant was assigned the AB order ($n = 10$) or the BA order ($n = 10$). A neurologist adjusted the frequency of stimulation, according to the randomization order, but was not allowed to participate in any rating or evaluation. The participants, the neuropsychologist who administered the VF tasks, and the neurologist who rated the Unified Parkinson's Disease Rating Scale (UPDRS-III) were blinded to the DBS condition. When the experiment was finalized, the A and B codes were revealed to compute the scores in the database.

After adjusting the frequency, the participants waited one hour to carry out the VF tasks. They then performed the following VF tasks: phonemic VF (FAS version and letter P version), semantic VF (animals), unconstrained VF, and action fluency. For the FAS version of the phonemic VF task, the participants were asked to say words beginning with the letters "F," "A," and "S" for one minute for each letter. The final score was the total number of words beginning with "F," "A," or "S" that the participants were able to say [12]. For the letter P version of the phonemic VF task, the participants were asked to say as many words as possible beginning with the letter "P" within two minutes [15, 26]. For the semantic VF task, the participants were asked to say as many animals as possible within one minute [14]. For the unconstrained VF, the participants were asked to say as many words as possible, excluding names and numbers, within 2.5 minutes while keeping their eyes closed [26]. For the action fluency task, the participants were asked to say as many actions or "things that people can do" as possible within one minute [16, 27]. The instruction of these previous VF did not allow participants to say proper names or numbers. On semantic VF, no score was given for subcategory (e.g., bird) if specific exemplars were also given (e.g., dove, canary). Additionally, sex- and age-specific names of the same animal species were considered to be the same animal (e.g., hen, rooster). On action VF, it was not allowed to use the same verb with different endings (e.g., eat, eating, eaten). Intrusions and perseverations were not scored [14–16, 28]. The UPDRS-III

TABLE 1: Baseline characteristics of the participants.

Variables	Mean ± SD or n (%)	Range
Sex, male	16 (80)	—
Age	56.65 ± 10.71	31–75
Education	10.10 ± 5.23	2–22
Time of disease, years	15.30 ± 4.71	10–29
Levodopa equivalent dose, mg/day	1165.00 ± 615.08	300–2300
Time after surgery, months	2.21 ± 1.38	0–7
MMSE	26.45 ± 2.52	21–30
Hamilton Depression Rating Scale		
Normal	14 (70)	—
Mild depression	4 (20)	—
Moderate depression	2 (10)	—
Amplitude (V), left	3.02 (0.65)	1–3.90
Amplitude (V), right	2.98 (0.60)	1.80–3.60
Pulse width (μs), left	79.50 (17.61)	60–120
Pulse width (μs), right	81.00 (17.14)	60–120
Frequency (Hz), left and right	124.00 (26.04)	60–180

SD: standard deviation; MMSE: Mini-Mental State Examination.

was used for the motor assessment [29]. After performing these evaluations, the neurologist readjusted the frequency of stimulation according to the assigned randomization to evaluate the other conditions. The participants waited one hour to repeat the VF testing and motor assessment. Upon completion of the assessments, the neurologist adjusted the parameters of the STN-DBS implanted back to the stabilized values used by each participant.

Demographic (sex, age, and education), cognitive (MMSE), and clinical (time of disease in years, time after surgery in months, Hamilton Depression Rating Scale, and the levodopa-equivalent dose (LED)) variables were considered in secondary analyses. The LED was measured as mg/day and was calculated using conversion formulae [30].

The ethics committees of out institution approved this study, and all participants gave written informed consent.

2.3. Statistical Analysis. Statistical analyses were performed using the Statistical Package for Social Sciences (SPSS version 21.0) with a significance level of 5% ($p \leq 0.05$). Continuous variables were reported as the mean (M) and standard deviation (SD). Categorical variables were described by the absolute and relative frequencies. The distribution of variables was verified using the Shapiro-Wilk test. To compare the VF performance between 60 Hz and 130 Hz frequencies, we used the generalized estimating equation (GEE) model. To verify if any demographic, clinical, or cognitive aspects influenced the effect of stimulation frequency on VF, we conducted Spearman's correlation. We used the delta value of each VF task (VF task score for the 60 Hz condition minus the VF task score for the 130 Hz condition) and of the UPDRS-III scores (UPDRS-III score for 60 Hz minus UPDRS-III score for 130 Hz) in the correlational analysis.

3. Results

3.1. Patients Characteristics. The initial study sample consisted of 25 individuals; however, 5 were excluded for not meeting the inclusion criteria. Three included patients were not able to complete some of the verbal fluency tasks in both frequency conditions. However, these participants were still included in the data analysis. All participants were on levodopa drugs, only 6 participants were on amantadine (mean dose of 283.33 mg/day), and no one was on anticholinergics or antipsychotics. The baseline characteristics of the participants are presented in Table 1. Table 2 presents sex, age, the parameters of stimulation, and the VF outcomes of the VF tasks that were significantly different between frequencies of stimulations, for each participant.

3.2. Verification of Practice Effect. The first and second sets of VF tasks were compared to determine if there was a practice/learning effect due to the repetition of the tasks. The results showed that there was no significant difference between the two sets of tasks for any of the VF tasks (Table 3).

3.3. Verification of the Effect of Stimulation Frequency. Table 4 shows that, after 60 Hz stimulation, the performances of the phonemic (FAS and P version) and action fluency tasks were significantly better than those after 130 Hz stimulation.

The performances for the VF tasks according to the STN-DBS frequency are shown in Figure 1(a). Despite the significant difference between stimulation conditions for phonemic and action fluencies, the individual performances for each of the VF tasks presented in Figures 1(b), 1(c), and 1(d) indicate that the participants did not exhibit the same outcome pattern. In addition to the comparison analyses, we assessed the distribution of patients who improved or

TABLE 2: Stimulation parameters at the moment of inclusion and verbal fluency outcomes of each subject.

Subject	Sex	Age	Frequency (Hz)	Stimulation contacts (all cases +)		Amplitude (V)		Pulse width (μs)		Verbal fluency outcomes (at 60 Hz)		
				L	R	L	R	L	R	Action	Phonemic (P)	Phonemic (FAS)
1	M	49	90	3-	11-	3.0	3.0	60	60	—	↑	↑
2	F	66	110	3-	10-	3.6	1.8	90	90	↓	↑	ND
3	M	75	130	0-, 1-	8-, 9-	3.3	3.3	60	60	ND	↑	↓
4	M	65	130	2-, 3-	11-	3.0	3.6	60	90	↓	↓	ND
5	F	62	110	2-	11-	2.8	2.6	90	60	ND	↑	↓
6	M	53	180	1-	9-, 10-	2.6	2.7	90	90	↑	↑	↑
7	M	31	140	2-, 3-	8-, 9-	3.6	3.6	90	120	↑	ND	↑
8	M	50	60	0-	8-, 9-	2.5	3.0	90	90	↑	↑	↑
9	M	70	130	1-, 2-	9-, 10-	3.0	3.2	90	90	↓	↑	↑
10	M	47	110	0-	11-	2.8	2.8	60	60	↑	↑	↑
11	M	46	140	0-	9-	2.6	3.0	90	90	ND	↑	↑
12	M	70	110	3-	11-	3.6	3.6	90	90	↑	↑	↑
13	M	59	160	2-	8-	3.5	3.5	120	90	ND	—	ND
14	M	47	110	1-	9-	1.0	2.0	60	90	—	↑	↑
15	M	61	120	2-	11-	3.4	3.4	60	60	↓	ND	ND
16	M	66	160	2-	9-	3.2	3.6	90	90	↑	↑	↑
17	F	59	120	2-	5-	3.2	3.2	90	90	↑	↑	↑
18	F	48	130	3-	8-	3.9	2.2	60	60	—	—	ND
19	M	51	110	2-	10-	3.6	3.6	90	90	↑	↑	↑
20	M	58	130	0-	8-	2.2	2.0	90	60	—	↓	↓

F: female; L: left; M: male; R: right; ↑: improvement; ↓: worsening; ND: no difference; "-": cathode/negative electrode contact.

TABLE 3: Comparisons of verbal fluency tasks between moments of administration.

Verbal fluency task	Moment 1 Mean ± SD	Moment 2 Mean ± SD	Difference	CI 95%	p
Phonemic, P	14.53 ± 1.61	14.47 ± 1.89	0.05	−2.96–3.07	0.973
Phonemic, FAS	25.26 ± 2.88	25.39 ± 15.33	−0.11	−3.36–3.15	0.949
Semantic, animals	13.26 ± 1.07	13.42 ± 1.22	−0.16	−1.86–1.54	0.856
Unconstrained	29.63 ± 2.50	27.58 ± 3.00	2.05	−1.76–5.87	0.292
Action	8.39 ± 1.00	9.11 ± 1.30	−0.72	−2.65–1.21	0.463

SD: standard deviation; CI: confidence interval.

TABLE 4: Comparisons of the verbal fluency tasks and UPDRS-III between the different frequencies of SNT-DBS.

Variables	60 Hz Mean ± SE	130 Hz Mean ± SE	Difference	CI 95%	p
UPDRS III, total	34.33 ± 4.74	35.44 ± 4.30	−1.11	−9.38–7.15	0.792
UPDRS III, tremor	2.72 ± 1.20	2.00 ± 1.09	0.72	−2.19–3.63	0.627
UPDRS III, gait	1.28 ± 0.26	1.61 ± 0.33	−0.33	−0.80–0.13	0.157
UPDRS III, pull test	1.28 ± 0.29	1.83 ± 0.34	−0.56	−1.12–0.00	0.052
Phonemic VF, P	16.53 ± 1.82	12.47 ± 1.56	4.05	1.65–6.45	0.001*
Phonemic VF, FAS	26.84 ± 3.36	23.79 ± 2.79	3.05	0.10–6.00	0.042*
Semantic VF, animals	13.70 ± 1.20	12.89 ± 1.08	0.89	−0.76–2.55	0.290
Unconstrained VF	29.63 ± 2.92	27.58 ± 2.59	1.95	−1.76–5.87	0.292
Action VF	9.94 ± 1.22	7.56 ± 1.94	2.39	0.77–4.00	0.004*

CI: confidence interval; SE: standard error; UPDRS: Unified Parkinson's Disease Rating Scale; VF: verbal fluency; $^*p \leq 0.05$.

worsened for 60 Hz stimulation in the phonemic and action fluency tasks. The differences (delta values) in the outcomes of the VF tasks between the frequency conditions (60 Hz minus 130 Hz conditions) were classified as "improvement at 60 Hz" (positive delta values), "worsening at 60 Hz" (negative values of delta), or "no difference" (zero values of delta) (Table 5). The individual description of the VF outcomes is also shown in Table 2.

3.4. Correlational Analysis. In the correlational analysis, we included the delta values of the VF task outcomes that showed significant differences between the frequency conditions (P and FAS versions of the phonemic fluency tasks and the action fluency task) to determine if the difference was correlated with additional variables (including the delta values of UPDRS-III). The delta value of the FAS version of the phonemic VF task was negatively associated with age ($r = -0.0473$; $p = 0.041$). The delta value of the P version of the phonemic VF task was negatively associated with UPDRS-III ($r = -0.686$; $p = 0.002$) (Table 6).

4. Discussion

The present study aimed to investigate the impact of modulating the frequency of STN-DBS on the performance of VF tasks in patients with PD. We assessed the effect of low-frequency stimulation of 60 Hz compared to high-frequency stimulation of 130 Hz in patients who had undergone bilateral STN-DBS in the medication-on state. We found that low-frequency stimulation had a positive impact on phonemic

and action fluency, and this effect was not due to practice. Furthermore, we observed different outcome patterns for the VF tasks based on the frequency conditions, which could not be explained by the demographic, cognitive, and clinical variables that were studied here.

Previous studies have pointed to a decline in VF after STN-DBS surgery in PD patients, although the reason behind this decline is not well understood. There are many methodological differences among such studies, such as evaluations performed while stimulation is "on" or "off," at pre- and postsurgical time points, and with or without a control group [2–9].

Greater declines in VF over time in STN-DBS patients compared to nonsurgical PD patients have been reported, which suggests that VF impairment is related to the DBS intervention [3]. VF may decline as a consequence of microsurgical injuries, which affect the cortical-basal circuits involved in the recovery process of words [31–33]. The number of microelectrode recordings required during surgery for lead placement does not adversely affect VF [4], although this finding does not exclude the possibility of an effect due to the lesions caused by the macroelectrode, suggesting that other factors in addition to microlesions may be involved in VF impairment after surgery.

The frequency of stimulation for treatment of PD has been studied in other clinical situations regarding STN-DBS. For example, 60 Hz stimulation, compared with the routine 130 Hz, improved swallowing function and freezing of gait in patients with PD who underwent bilateral STN-DBS [10, 11]. A previous study that evaluated semantic and

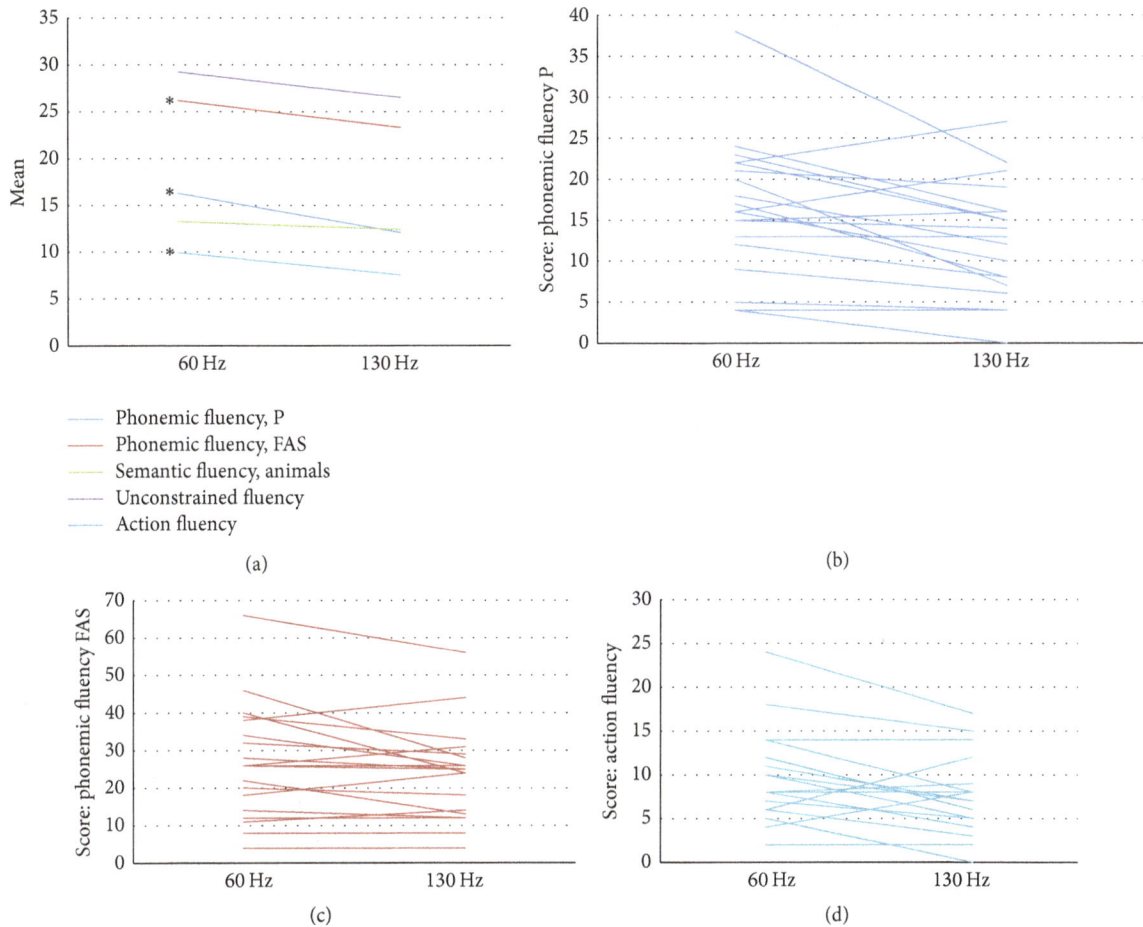

FIGURE 1: Patients' performances on VF tasks at low and high stimulation frequencies. (a) Performance of the entire sample for each VF task. * denotes the significant difference between frequency conditions for the respective task. (b) Phonemic fluency performance (P version) by the patient. (c) Phonemic fluency performance (FAS version) by the patient. (d) Action fluency performance by the patient.

TABLE 5: Distribution of delta values for phonemic and action fluency tasks.

	Phonemic VF P version	Phonemic VF FAS version	Action VF
Delta value, mean ± SD	4.05 (5.50)	3.05 (6.73)	2.40 (3.60)
Delta classification, n (%)			
Improvement at 60 Hz	14 (70)	11 (55)	10 (50)
Worsening at 60 Hz	2 (10)	3 (15)	3 (15)
No difference	2 (10)	4 (20)	3 (15)

SD: standard deviation; VF: verbal fluency.

phonemic VF for 10 Hz and 130 Hz stimulation reported greater performances in both VF tasks for low-frequency stimulation [12]. Our results also showed that low-frequency stimulation was associated with better scores of phonemic VF but no improvement was found for semantic VF. Wojtecki et al. [12] did not exclude participants with dementia or lower scores in their cognitive screening, and they did not describe the global cognitive status of the participants. It is known that patients with dementia may also present deficits in semantic VF [16]. Furthermore, differences in language and education may contribute to differences among populations.

When we compared the VF scores and the motor performances between the low-frequency (60 Hz) and high-frequency (130 Hz) stimulation trials, we found that phonemic and action fluency significantly declined for 130 Hz stimulation. However, no significant difference was found between stimulation frequencies for the semantic and unconstrained VF tasks. Our findings indicate that the influence of the stimulation frequency relies more heavily on specific frontosubcortical pathways involved in lexical-word and action-semantic processes, as there was an influence of frequency on phonemic and action VF tasks but not

TABLE 6: Correlational analysis between VF tasks (phonemic and action), demographic, cognitive, and clinical measures.

	Phonemic - P		Phonemic - FAS		Action	
	r	p	r	p	r	p
Age	−0.207	0.382	−0.473	0.041[*]	−0.352	0.152
Education	−0.192	0.416	0.300	0.212	−0.021	0.935
MMSE	−0.014	0.953	0.215	0.377	0.108	0.669
Time of disease, years	0.400	0.081	0.358	0.132	−0.036	0.887
Time after surgery, months	0.288	0.218	0.440	0.060	0.284	0.253
Levodopa equivalent dose	0.351	0.140	0.131	0.592	−0.003	0.992
HDRS, total score	0.011	0.964	0.078	0.757	−0.138	0.599
UPDRS, total	−0.686	0.002[*]	−0.342	0.165	−0.058	0.825
UPDRS, tremor	−0.200	0.426	−0.133	0.600	0.020	0.939
UPDRS, gait	−0.378	0.122	0.004	0.986	0.003	0.990
UPDRS, pull test	−0.312	0.207	−0.479	0.068	−0.321	0.209

HDRS: Hamilton Depression Rating Scale; MMSE: Mini-Mental State Examination; UPDRS: Unified Parkinson's Disease Rating Scale; [*] $p \leq 0.05$.

on semantic and unconstrained VF tasks. As we expected, the frequency affected the VF tasks that rely more heavily on frontosubcortical functions, which are impaired in PD, supporting our *a priori* hypothesis.

Phonemic and action fluency, which were hampered by high-frequency neurostimulation, are both tasks that involve frontal circuits and that rely more heavily on executive functions. Semantic VF depends on lexical-semantic processes and temporal circuits [13, 34]. Unconstrained VF is used to assess clinical conditions due to right or left hemisphere lesions, although there are no studies regarding its construct validity and the brain areas involved in adults [17]. One hypothesis regarding the cognitive processing of verbs, based on the theory of embodied cognition, states that the same brain areas involved in planning and motor execution participate in accessing lexical and semantic processes of verbs. This theory, though still controversial, helps to explain the deficits in verb production that have been observed in different clinical groups with Parkinsonian syndromes [35, 36]. STN-DBS could affect lexical-semantic processing of actions, such as those involved in the action fluency task; in the same way, it affects neural motor circuitry. The mechanism whereby the stimulus frequency may affect different circuitries remains unknown.

In the present study, no significant difference was found in the motor performance of the patients in relation to the stimulation frequency. One hypothesis for this finding is that the patients were under the effect of dopaminergic medication during the evaluation. If there was no effect of the medication, the low-frequency stimulation (60 Hz) would be expected to correspond to worse motor symptoms, whereas an improvement in motor performance for the high-frequency stimulation would be expected [10].

The comparison analyses revealed that most patients performed better in phonemic and action VF tasks for the low-frequency condition. However, a few of the participants presented an opposite pattern (worse VF scores for low-frequency stimulation) or no difference between the conditions. In an attempt to elucidate the cause of these different patterns, correlational analyses were conducted with the delta values of the phonemic and action VF scores. The scores from the FAS version of the phonemic VF task were negatively correlated with age, indicating a possible effect of age on the benefit of low-frequency stimulation; that is, older participants may exhibit lower improvements in performance for low-frequency stimulation compared to younger patients. The scores from the P version of the phonemic VF task were negatively correlated with UPDRS-III total score, indicating that increased improvements in motor performance were associated with smaller improvements in this phonemic VF task for low-frequency stimulation. This latter finding indicates that motor performance and phonemic VF scores (P version) are characterized by opposite outcomes at low-frequency stimulation. Future studies should seek identifying the factors that explain the different VF improvement profiles for varying frequency stimulation conditions by studying larger samples of PD patients with STN-DBS.

Our study is the first one that called attention to different outcomes of verbal fluency when frequency conditions were compared. Many aspects may influence the modulation of frequency on verbal fluency. Because the STN is thought to have separate functional subregions [37], we hypothesize that the volume and locus of activated STN tissue may interact with the effect of DBS frequency. Besides that, there are studies suggesting that DBS leads to neural plasticity in motor cortex and in modulating corticobasal circuits [38, 39]. Then, it is possible that frequency of stimulation may also interact with the effect of neural plasticity leading to different outcomes on verbal fluency. These possibilities of interactions may be further investigated in future studies.

Our results should be interpreted in light of some limitations. First, the improvement in the VF task for the low-frequency condition could be due to an improvement in other cognitive functions, such as attention. However, this study did not evaluate other cognitive functions. We chose to utilize a less-extensive assessment because some patients do not tolerate adjustments in stimulation frequency for long periods of time. Second, the participants were not evaluated in the DBS-off condition so that they were not exposed to unpleasant symptoms for long periods of time, and this study did not include a control group. The lack of information for the DBS-off condition and the lack of a control group do not allow surgical effects to be assessed. Third, the administration order of the VF tasks was the same in both conditions. There is the possibility of an order effect, but based on a previous study, we do not believe an order effect occurred, at least pertaining to the action VF task [27].

5. Conclusion

In summary, the results of the present study led to two important conclusions. First, the frequency of STN-DBS affects phonemic and action fluency in PD patients. Second, low-frequency (60 Hz) stimulation is associated with less negative side effects on VF than high-frequency (130 Hz) stimulation. Therefore, whenever possible, low-frequency stimulation should be the first choice for PD patients, especially for patients who present any cognitive impairments, such as reduced VF, in their daily activities. Future studies utilizing larger sample populations and those incorporating longer study periods should be performed to investigate stimulation effects on VF with regard to electrode position in the STN and other stimulation parameters (amplitude and pulse width).

Acknowledgments

The authors would like to thank the patients for their participation, the *Coordenação de Aperfeiçoamento de Pessoal de Nível Superior* (CAPES) for scholarships, and the *Fundo de Incentivo à Pesquisa e Eventos* (FIPE) from *Hospital de Clínicas de Porto Alegre* (HCPA) for financial support.

References

[1] A.-S. Moldovan, S. J. Groiss, S. Elben, M. Südmeyer, A. Schnitzler, and L. Wojtecki, "The treatment of Parkinson's disease with deep brain stimulation: current issues," *Neural Regeneration Research*, vol. 10, no. 7, pp. 1018–1022, 2015.

[2] K. Witt, O. Granert, C. Daniels et al., "Relation of lead trajectory and electrode position to neuropsychological outcomes of subthalamic neurostimulation in Parkinson's disease: results from a randomized trial," *Brain*, vol. 136, part 7, pp. 2109–2119, 2013.

[3] D. F. Marshall, A. M. Strutt, A. E. Williams, R. K. Simpson, J. Jankovic, and M. K. York, "Alternating verbal fluency performance following bilateral subthalamic nucleus deep brain stimulation for Parkinson's disease," *European Journal of Neurology*, vol. 19, no. 12, pp. 1525–1531, 2012.

[4] K. M. Smith, M. O'Connor, E. Papavassiliou, D. Tarsy, and L. C. Shih, "Phonemic verbal fluency decline after subthalamic nucleus deep brain stimulation does not depend on number of microelectrode recordings or lead tip placement," *Parkinsonism and Related Disorders*, vol. 20, no. 4, pp. 400–404, 2014.

[5] A. Borden, D. Wallon, R. Lefaucheur et al., "Does early verbal fluency decline after STN implantation predict long-term cognitive outcome after STN-DBS in Parkinson's disease?" *Journal of the Neurological Sciences*, vol. 346, no. 1-2, pp. 299–302, 2014.

[6] F. Ehlen, L. K. Krugel, I. Vonberg, T. Schoenecker, A. A. Kühn, and F. Klostermann, "Intact lexicon running slowly—prolonged response latencies in patients with subthalamic DBS and verbal fluency deficits," *PLoS ONE*, vol. 8, no. 11, Article ID e79247, 2013.

[7] A. Merola, L. Rizzi, M. Zibetti et al., "Medical therapy and subthalamic deep brain stimulation in advanced Parkinson's disease: a different long-term outcome?" *Journal of Neurology, Neurosurgery & Psychiatry*, vol. 85, no. 5, pp. 552–559, 2014.

[8] A. Harati and T. Müller, "Neuropsychological effects of deep brain stimulation for Parkinson's disease," *Surgical Neurology International*, vol. 4, supplement 6, pp. S443–S447, 2013.

[9] R. Cilia, C. Siri, G. Marotta et al., "Brain networks underlining verbal fluency decline during STN-DBS in Parkinson's disease: an ECD-SPECT study," *Parkinsonism and Related Disorders*, vol. 13, no. 5, pp. 290–294, 2007.

[10] T. Xie, J. Vigil, E. MacCracken et al., "Low-frequency stimulation of STN-DBS reduces aspiration and freezing of gait in patients with PD," *Neurology*, vol. 84, no. 4, pp. 415–420, 2015.

[11] T. Xie, U. J. Kang, and P. Warnke, "Effect of stimulation frequency on immediate freezing of gait in newly activated STN DBS in Parkinson's disease," *Journal of Neurology, Neurosurgery and Psychiatry*, vol. 83, no. 10, pp. 1015–1017, 2012.

[12] L. Wojtecki, L. Timmermann, S. Jörgens et al., "Frequency-dependent reciprocal modulation of verbal fluency and motor functions in subthalamic deep brain stimulation," *Archives of Neurology*, vol. 63, no. 9, pp. 1273–1276, 2006.

[13] S. Pekkala, "Verbal fluency tasks and the neuropsychology of language," in *The Handbook of the Neuropsychology of Language*, pp. 619–634, Blackwell, Oxford, UK, 2012.

[14] S. M. D. Brucki, S. M. Fleury Malheiros, I. H. Okamoto, and P. H. F. Bertolucci, "Dados normativos para o teste de fluência verbal categoria animais em nosso meio," *Arquivos de Neuro-Psiquiatria*, vol. 55, no. 1, pp. 56–61, 1997.

[15] T. H. Machado, H. C. Fichman, E. L. Santos et al., "Normative data for healthy elderly on the phonemic verbal fluency task—FAS," *Dementia e Neuropsychologia*, vol. 3, no. 1, pp. 55–60, 2009.

[16] A. L. Piatt, J. A. Fields, A. M. Paolo, W. C. Koller, and A. I. Tröster, "Lexical, semantic, and action verbal fluency in Parkinson's disease with and without dementia," *Journal of Clinical and Experimental Neuropsychology*, vol. 21, no. 4, pp. 435–443, 1999.

[17] B. Le Blanc and Y. Joanette, "Unconstrained oral naming in left- and right-hemisphere-damaged patients: an analysis for naturalistic semantic strategies," *Brain and Language*, vol. 55, pp. 42–45, 1996.

[18] S. Schwartz, J. Baldo, R. E. Graves, and P. Brugger, "Pervasive influence of semantics in letter and category fluency: a multidimensional approach," *Brain and Language*, vol. 87, no. 3, pp. 400–411, 2003.

[19] B. C. Beber and M. L. F. Chaves, "The basis and applications of the action fluency and action naming tasks," *Dementia e Neuropsychologia*, vol. 8, no. 1, pp. 47–57, 2014.

[20] N. Zimmermann, M. A. de Mattos Pimenta Parente, Y. Joanette, and R. P. Fonseca, "Unconstrained, phonemic and semantic verbal fluency: age and education effects, norms and discrepancies," *Psicologia: Reflexao e Critica*, vol. 27, no. 1, pp. 55–63, 2014.

[21] D. M. Jacobsen, *Funções executivas na infância: impacto de idade, sexo, tipo de escola, escolaridade parental e sintomas de desatenção/hiperatividade [M.S. thesis]*, Programa de Pós-Graduação em Psicologia da Pontifícia Universidade Católica do Rio Grande do Sul, Porto Alegre, Brazil, 2016.

[22] A. J. Hughes, S. E. Daniel, L. Kilford, and A. J. Lees, "Accuracy of clinical diagnosis of idiopathic Parkinson's disease: a clinico-pathological study of 100 cases," *Journal of Neurology, Neurosurgery & Psychiatry*, vol. 55, no. 3, pp. 181–184, 1992.

[23] C. L. Hooper and D. Bakish, "An examination of the sensitivity of the six-item Hamilton Rating Scale for Depression in a sample of patients suffering from major depressive disorder," *Journal of Psychiatry and Neuroscience*, vol. 25, no. 2, pp. 178–184, 2000.

[24] S. M. D. Brucki, R. Nitrin, P. Caramelli, P. H. F. Bertolucci, and I. H. Okamoto, "Suggestions for utilization of the mini-mental state examination in Brazil," *Arquivos de Neuro-Psiquiatria*, vol. 61, no. 3, pp. 777–781, 2003.

[25] R. A. do Amaral and A. Malbergiera, "Evaluation of a screening test for alcohol-related problems (CAGE) among employees of the Campus of the University of São Paulo," *Revista Brasileira de Psiquiatria*, vol. 26, no. 3, pp. 156–163, 2004.

[26] R. P. Fonseca, M. A. D. M. P. Parente, H. Cote, B. Ska, and Y. Joanette, *Bateria MAC—Bateria Montreal de Avaliação da Comunicação*, Pró-Fono, 2008.

[27] B. C. Beber and M. L. F. Chaves, "Does previous presentation of verbal fluency tasks affect verb fluency performance?" *Dementia & Neuropsychologia*, vol. 10, no. 1, pp. 31–36, 2016.

[28] S. M. D. Brucki and M. S. G. Rocha, "Category fluency test: effects of age, gender and education on total scores, clustering and switching in Brazilian Portuguese-speaking subjects," *Brazilian Journal of Medical and Biological Research*, vol. 37, no. 12, pp. 1771–1777, 2004.

[29] S. Fahn, C. Marsden, D. Calne, and M. Goldstein, "Fahn S, Elton RL. and members of the UPDRS Development Committee. Unified Parkinson's disease rating scale," in *Recent Developments in Parkinson's Disease*, pp. 153–163, Macmillan Healthcare Information, Florham Park, NJ, USA, 1987.

[30] C. L. Tomlinson, R. Stowe, S. Patel, C. Rick, R. Gray, and C. E. Clarke, "Systematic review of levodopa dose equivalency reporting in Parkinson's disease," *Movement Disorders*, vol. 25, no. 15, pp. 2649–2653, 2010.

[31] A. I. Troster, "Neuropsychology of deep brain stimulation in neurology and psychiatry," *Frontiers in Bioscience*, vol. 14, no. 5, pp. 1857–1879, 2009.

[32] A. I. Tröster, S. P. Woods, and J. A. Fields, "Verbal fluency declines after pallidotomy: an interaction between task and lesion laterality," *Applied Neuropsychology*, vol. 10, no. 2, pp. 69–75, 2003.

[33] A. I. Tröster, J. A. Fields, J. A. Testa et al., "Cortical and subcortical influences on clustering and switching in the performance of verbal fluency tasks," *Neuropsychologia*, vol. 36, no. 4, pp. 295–304, 1998.

[34] M. Pihlajamäki, H. Tanila, T. Hänninen et al., "Verbal fluency activates the left medial temporal lobe: a functional magnetic resonance imaging study," *Annals of Neurology*, vol. 47, no. 4, pp. 470–476, 2000.

[35] G. Vigliocco, D. P. Vinson, J. Druks, H. Barber, and S. F. Cappa, "Nouns and verbs in the brain: a review of behavioural, electrophysiological, neuropsychological and imaging studies," *Neuroscience and Biobehavioral Reviews*, vol. 35, no. 3, pp. 407–426, 2011.

[36] T. H. Bak, "The neuroscience of action semantics in neurodegenerative brain diseases," *Current Opinion in Neurology*, vol. 26, no. 6, pp. 671–677, 2013.

[37] A. Mikos, D. Bowers, A. M. Noecker et al., "Patient-specific analysis of the relationship between the volume of tissue activated during DBS and verbal fluency," *NeuroImage*, vol. 54, supplement 1, pp. S238–S246, 2011.

[38] S. J. Kim, K. Udupa, Z. Ni et al., "Effects of subthalamic nucleus stimulation on motor cortex plasticity in Parkinson disease," *Neurology*, vol. 85, no. 5, pp. 425–432, 2015.

[39] X.-H. Li, J.-Y. Wang, G. Gao, J.-Y. Chang, D. J. Woodward, and F. Luo, "High-frequency stimulation of the subthalamic nucleus restores neural and behavioral functions during reaction time task in a rat model of Parkinson's disease," *Journal of Neuroscience Research*, vol. 88, no. 7, pp. 1510–1521, 2010.

6

Alpha-Synuclein in Parkinson's Disease: From Pathogenetic Dysfunction to Potential Clinical Application

Lingjia Xu and Jiali Pu

Department of Neurology, 2nd Affiliated Hospital, School of Medicine, Zhejiang University, Hangzhou, Zhejiang 310009, China

Correspondence should be addressed to Jiali Pu; carrie_1105@163.com

Academic Editor: Shu Wen

Parkinson's disease is a neurodegenerative disease/synucleinopathy that develops slowly; however, there is no efficient method of early diagnosis, nor is there a cure. Progressive dopaminergic neuronal cell loss in the substantia nigra pars compacta and widespread aggregation of the α-synuclein protein (encoded by the *SNCA* gene) in the form of Lewy bodies and Lewy neurites are the neuropathological hallmarks of Parkinson's disease. The *SNCA* gene has undergone gene duplications, triplications, and point mutations. However, the specific mechanism of α-synuclein in Parkinson's disease remains obscure. Recent research showed that various α-synuclein oligomers, pathological aggregation, and propagation appear to be harmful in certain areas in Parkinson's disease patients. This review summarizes our current knowledge of the pathogenetic dysfunction of α-synuclein associated with Parkinson's disease and highlights current approaches that seek to develop this protein as a possible diagnostic biomarker and therapeutic target.

1. Introduction

Parkinson's disease (PD) is the second most common neurodegenerative disorder [1] and is defined as one of the synucleinopathies, which include other disorders featuring Lewy bodies [2]. It is characterized by the relatively selective loss of dopaminergic neuronal cells in the substantia nigra pars compacta (SNpc) and the presence of Lewy bodies and Lewy neurites in surviving affected neurons [3]. As the main component of the Lewy bodies and Lewy neurites, α-synuclein is the product of the first gene identified as associated with PD: *SNAC*, which was reported in 1997 by Polymeropoulos et al. [4]. Mutations in *SNCA* (duplications, triplications, or point mutation) cause autosomal dominant forms of PD and are the basis of the risk of developing sporadic PD [5]. Recent studies [6–8] suggested that the misfolding of α-synuclein causes it to aggregate and spread in certain sites, where the inflammation induced by it is intimately involved in the pathogenetic dysfunction underlying PD. All this indicates that α-synuclein plays a central role in the pathogenesis of PD.

Currently, the main treatment for PD is replacement therapy using levodopa, which may be effective in the early stage of the disease [9]. However, as the disease progresses, levodopa has less effect, and a series of side effects, such as movement complications, occur. Therefore, other therapeutic strategies, such as deep brain stimulation (DBS), have also been attempted for advanced patients; however, it is only an alleviative treatment. Consequently, biomarkers for early diagnosis and neuroprotective therapy are urgently required for this chronic disorder. Alpha-synuclein is the distinctive hallmark of PD; therefore, it has a potential application in the clinical diagnosis and treatment of PD [10].

To fully understand the pathogenetic dysfunction of α-synuclein associated with PD, in this review, we summarize the current knowledge of the physiology and pathology of α-synuclein, including its structure, physiological function, degradation, spread, and toxicity. We also highlight current approaches that seek to develop this protein as a potential diagnostic biomarker and therapeutic target.

2. Alpha-Synuclein Structure and Physiological Function

In humans, α-synuclein is a member of a three-protein family: α-synuclein, β-synuclein, and γ-synuclein [11]. Alpha-synuclein is a small protein comprising 140 amino acids with three domains: an N-terminal domain (aa 1–65), a non-amyloid-β component of plaques (NAC) domain (aa 66–95), and a C-terminal domain (aa 96–140) [12]. Rare point mutations in the N-terminal domain of α-synuclein, such as Ala53Thr, Ala30Pro, Glu46Lys, and the recently described His50Gln, Gly51Asp, and Ala53Glu, result in autosomal dominant familial PD and PD-like syndromes, presumably caused by misfolding and/or aggregation of the mutant α-synuclein protein [4, 13–17]. All known clinical mutations are present in this N-terminal region [10], emphasizing the importance of this domain in the pathological dysfunction of α-synuclein. The NAC domain, which is unique to α-synuclein [18], has a stretch of 12 amino acid residues that are responsible for the aggregation properties of α-synuclein via inhibition of its degradation and promotion of its fibrillation [19]. Nowadays, most studies focus on the N-terminal peptide; however, future studies should also consider the C-terminal peptide, because this is where truncation more typically occurs [20]. The truncations discovered to date include Tyr39T, Tyr125T, Tyr133T, and Tyr136T [10]. To date, very few studies have investigated the effects of the smallest peptide produced by truncation. Research on this peptide might give us a new and distinct view of the potential application of this protein.

Concerning the native state of α-synuclein, there are two hypotheses: one is the monomeric conformation, and the other one is the α-helically folded tetramer. Early studies of α-synuclein isolated from bacterial expression systems or mouse tissues indicated that it is monomeric, with a limited secondary structure [21]; however, Bartels et al. [22] identified the state of endogenous α-synuclein in living human cells by examining freshly collected human red blood cells and showed that natively, endogenous cellular α-synuclein exists largely as an α-helically folded, 58 kDa tetramer. They hypothesized that the contrasting results might have resulted from the different materials and protocols applied in this research, namely, denaturing detergents. The tetramer circulates in plasma and can become destabilized which promotes α-synuclein aggregation from monomers to oligomers. Further studies by Burré et al. [23], using similar methods in the mouse brain, indicated that the predominant native conformation of α-synuclein might be an unstructured monomer, exhibiting a random coil structure in solution, and it can aggregate age-dependently, while the α-helical structure was only adopted upon membrane binding [24].

However, the normal physiological structure and function of α-synuclein still remain unclear.

Recent studies showed that the normal physiological function of α-synuclein involves roles in compartmentalization, storage, and recycling of neurotransmitters [25]. In addition, α-synuclein is associated with the physiological regulation of certain enzymes and is thought to increase the number of dopamine transporter molecules [26]. Neurotransmitter release [27] and interaction with the synaptic SNARE- (soluble N-ethylmaleimide-sensitive factor attachment protein receptors) complex are partly mediated by its role as molecular chaperone [23]. Cycling between SNARE-complex assembly and disassembly is required, with continuous generation of reactive SNARE-protein intermediates. Cysteine string protein α (CSPα) is a chaperone that is essential for synaptic health, whose deletion in mice led to a decrease in the SNARE-complex, nerve terminal degeneration, motor impairment, and cell death [28]. In CSPα knockout mice, α-synuclein could rescue this degenerative phenotype and restore levels of SNARE-complexes in synaptic terminals. Moreover, mice lacking both α-synuclein and CSPα exhibited nerve terminal dysfunction and cell death [29]. These findings suggested that α-synuclein is able to complement the activity of CSPα as a molecular chaperone. This interaction was documented in further research in which α-synuclein was demonstrated to directly bind to the SNARE-protein synaptobrevin-2 and promote SNARE-complex via binding of its C-terminal 44 residues to the N-terminal 28 residues from synaptobrevin-2 [30].

3. Alpha-Synuclein Aggregation, Degradation, and Spread

Alpha-synuclein exists in various conformations in a dynamic equilibrium, modulated by many factors, comprising internal and external factors that either accelerate or inhibit fibrillation [31–33]. As mentioned before, disease-related mutations affect the aggregation of α-synuclein (Figure 1). All known mutations associated with familial PD (Ala53Thr, Ala30Pro, Glu46Lys, His50Gln, Gly51Asp, and Ala53Glu) are found in the N-terminal domain [10]. The mutations Glu46Lys, His50Gln, and Ala53Glu [14, 15, 17] can promote α-synuclein to form insoluble aggregates and produce oligomers. However, how these mutations accelerate aggregation has not been completely clarified. Based on Burré et al.'s later study [30], it is likely to be due to the destabilization of the native N-terminal conformation. The NAC domain plays a central role in α-synuclein's self-propagation [19]. Recently, Rodriguez et al. [34] resolved the crystal structures of residues 68–78 (termed NACore) and residues 47–56 (PreNAC) using microelectron diffraction, which revealed that, in certain regions, these strands transferring into β-sheets are typical of amyloid assemblies. Lastly, the C-terminal domain was identified to be necessary to maintain the solubility of α-synuclein. The presence of residues consisting of five prolines suggested that this region lacks secondary structure [35]. In addition, C-terminally truncated forms of α-synuclein appeared to aggregate faster than the full-length protein [36, 37]. In addition, the C-terminus appears to be important for the interaction of α-synuclein with other proteins in the nervous system and with some small molecules [23]. These findings indicated that all three domains play a role in aggregation and that they might influence each other, either promoting or inhibiting its pathological fibrillation and oligomerization.

Phosphorylation of α-synuclein is essential and sufficient in the process of degradation in neurodegenerative diseases. Mass methodologies revealed that α-synuclein extracted from human Lewy bodies was phosphorylated at S129 [38]. Some data indicated that polo-like kinase (PLK) 2-mediated phosphorylation of S129 increased autophagy-mediated degradation of α-synuclein, suggesting that phosphorylation might be a neuroprotective mechanism to accelerate the clearance of aggregated protein [39]. Chemical

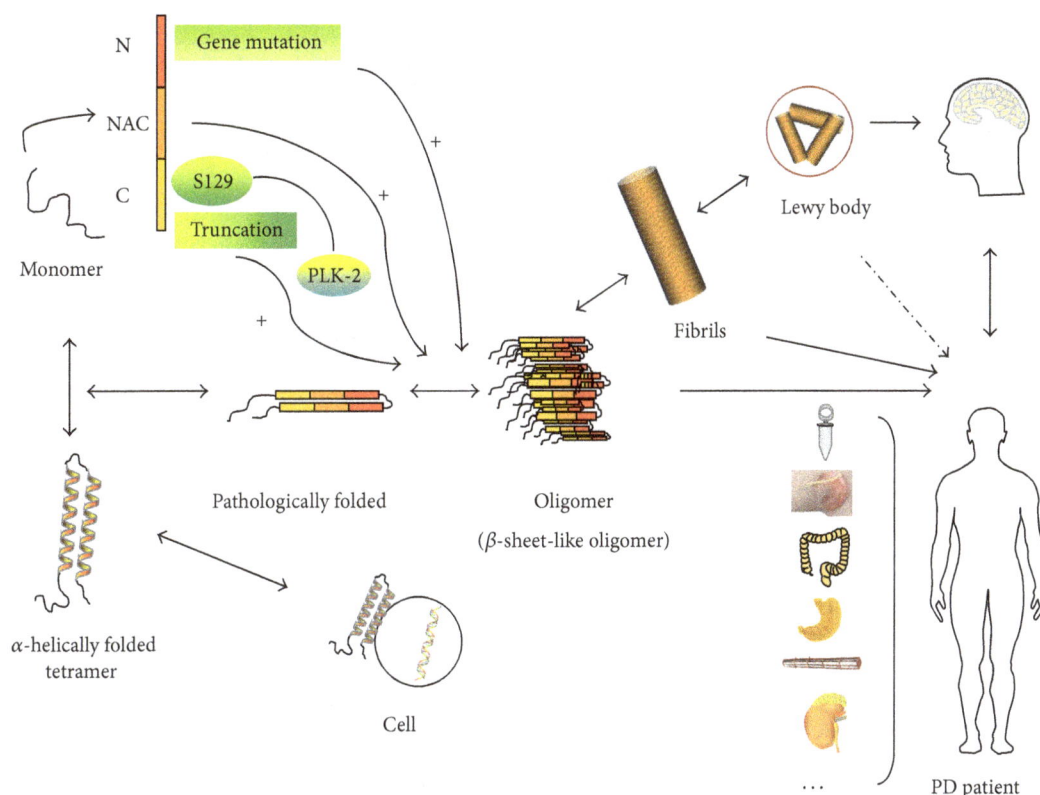

FIGURE 1: Alpha-synuclein's aggregation pathway and role as a diagnostic biomarker in PD. Alpha-synuclein is a small protein comprising 140 amino acids with three domains that exist in dynamic states. The α-helically folded tetramer is thought to be only adopted upon membrane binding. The three domains each have a role in aggregation, as shown in the figure. All known gene mutations are found in the N-terminal domain, and some have been proven to accelerate aggregation. The NAC domain has a stretch of 12 amino acid residues that are unique and typical in the formation of oligomers and fibrils. C-terminally truncated α-synuclein appears to aggregate faster. In addition, the phosphorylation of amino acid 129, located in C-terminal domain, plays a central role in the pathway and is promoted by PLK2. Alpha-synuclein leads to toxicity when aggregated into pathological oligomers, fibrils, and Lewy bodies. In the search for a diagnostic biomarker in PD, α-synuclein from the CSF, plasma, the submandibular gland, saliva, colonic and gastric mucosa samples, and peripheral nerve fibers has been tested.

nitration of α-synuclein resulted in the formation of both tyrosine-nitrated monomers and nitrated dimers [40], which also affected the degradation of α-synuclein, and immunoelectron microscopy confirmed that nitrated monomers and dimers are incorporated into amyloid fibrils. Purified nitrated α-synuclein monomer by itself was unable to form fibrils, whereas the nitrated dimer accelerated the aggregation of unmodified α-synuclein [41]. Additionally, nitration of certain residues in the N-terminal domain decreased binding to synthetic vesicles and prevented the protein from adopting the α-helical conformation to the membrane [41]. The structure has been identified by Snead and Eliezer [42], clarifying the physiological function of α-synuclein binding to the membrane. Using the synthetic nitrated α-synuclein, the results showed that nitration did not interfere with phosphorylation of S129 by PLK3 and reaffirmed that intermolecular interactions between the N- and C-terminal domains of α-synuclein are critical to direct nitration-induced oligomerization of α-synuclein [30].

Alpha-synuclein is degraded by the ubiquitin-proteasome system (UPS) and the autophagy-lysosomal pathway [43]. Ebrahimi-Fakhari et al. [44] provided *in vivo*

evidence that normal soluble α-synuclein is degraded mainly by the UPS, whereas more complex conformations, including aggregates, are degraded by the autophagy-lysosomal pathway. The finding that α-synuclein in both the monomeric and oligomeric states can be detected in human plasma, cerebrospinal fluid, and other peripheral tissues [45, 46] suggested the idea that α-synuclein is secreted. Although the exact mechanism of α-synuclein's release has not been fully demonstrated, it seems that α-synuclein might be released by exosomes in a calcium-dependent manner and be further degraded after lysosomal inhibition [47]. Lööv et al. [48] found that insoluble conformations of α-synuclein do not themselves appear to have significant neurotoxic effects, despite being misfolded and even aggregated in certain areas. By contrast, various α-synuclein oligomers are harmful, and structures termed extracellular vesicles (EVs) might mediate the propagation of toxic α-synuclein between neurons [48]. In one study, recombinant α-synuclein monomers produced together with EV fractions from cultured neuroblastoma cells accelerated the formation of toxic oligomers compared with monomeric α-synuclein produced alone [49]. EVs are mediators of cellular information; thus, genetic information can be carried from one cell to another and consequently can aggravate the toxicity [50]. In conclusion, propagation and spreading are key to the pathogenetic dysfunction in PD. Recent *in vivo* and *in vitro* studies [26] confirmed that transfer and interaction through the membranes by α-synuclein might contribute to the pathogenetic dysfunction in PD and thus progress the disease. These results suggest that α-synuclein propagation is a major factor in the progression of PD pathology.

Moreover, numerous data have suggested that α-synuclein self-propagates [7]. Normally, small numbers of aggregates are disposed of by the protein degradation pathways; however, if, over time, the aggregates accumulate above a certain threshold, they could self-propagate, contributing to the progression of PD. Lewy bodies and neurites, a histopathological signature of PD, found in grafted fetal dopaminergic neurons in the SNpc of PD patients, are of significant importance [51]. These observations led to the development of the "prion-like hypothesis" [51]. Several *in vitro* and *in vivo* studies suggested that α-synuclein can spread from cell to cell and from region to region, which dramatically promotes PD pathogenesis and progression [52–58]. Recently, one of these studies focused on the postmortem analyses of brains from patients with PD who received fetal mesencephalic transplants and demonstrated that α-synuclein-containing Lewy bodies gradually appeared in the grafted neurons [53]. Subsequently, The authors in [53] seeded α-synuclein aggregates in recipient neurons to explore whether intercellular transfer of α-synuclein could occur from the host to the graft. Ultimately, they demonstrated that α-synuclein could transfer between host cells and grafted dopaminergic neurons. In summary, intercellularly transferred α-synuclein can propagate its pathology by interacting with cytoplasmic α-synuclein. However, whether the pathological conversion of endogenous α-synuclein is triggered by material derived from patients with PD or from recombinant α-synuclein remains to be discussed. In addition, whether preformed fibrils might occur directly through a seeding prion process or occur indirectly as a general response to cellular stress remains unknown.

4. Alpha-Synuclein Toxicity in PD

The precise mechanism whereby α-synuclein leads to toxicity and cell death remains obscure. It is likely that aggregation of α-synuclein results either from an increased release of α-synuclein and increased cell-to-cell transfer or via accumulated cellular levels of the protein [38]. Here, we discuss the latest research in this area.

Alpha-synuclein's toxicity is interconnected with its physiological function, and to better understand its toxicity, animal models, including wild-type ones and those with genetic mutations, are needed. One of the most important physiological functions that α-synuclein regulates, synaptic activity, was tested directly in mice lacking α-synuclein. Originally, α-synuclein null mice develop normal brain architecture and contacts and do not exhibit gross behavioral phenotypes [59]. Upon repeated stimulation, dopaminergic synapses from α-synuclein null mice showed highly elevated

dopamine release [59]. In α/β-synuclein double knockout mice, synaptic plasticity appears unaltered relative to α-synuclein single knockouts, although the dopamine levels in the striatum were reduced [60]. Meanwhile, in the $\alpha/\beta/\gamma$-synuclein triple knockout mice, the synucleins were proved to be very important, because of the decreased life span and age-dependently synaptic dysfunction compared with wild-type mice [23]. Collectively, these reports emphasized the important role of the synucleins in long-term synaptic maintenance and flexibility. Kokhan et al. [61] carried out behavioral evaluations in α-synuclein knockout mice, and the results showed that α-synuclein knockout mice had worse learning ability in tests requiring both working and spatial memory. For the first time, they demonstrated that α-synuclein is necessary for these types of learning and explained this phenomenon by discussing neurotransmitters involved in the pathology of cognitive dysfunction, like monoamine, glutamate, and acetylcholine-mediated neurotransmission [61]. The physiological function and pathological dysfunction of α-synuclein are both involved in synaptic neuronal transmitters, which prompts the question as to what triggers this protein's toxicity.

The neuronal toxicities of α-synuclein caused by genetic mutations or epigenetic mechanisms appear to involve many pathways and cellular functions, including endocytosis, Golgi homeostasis, ER-to-Golgi transport, presynaptic trafficking, UPS, autophagy, ER, and oxidative and nitration stress [62–64]. Alpha-synuclein oligomers are thought to be the toxic species and the cause of the neurodegenerative process. These oligomers would spread throughout the brain and other parts of body and induce α-synuclein pathology in interconnected structures [48].

There are several pathological factors that contribute to the toxicity of α-synuclein. Firstly, dysfunction of autophagy and UPS, the two main ways to clear toxic α-synuclein [65, 66], might lead to neuronal toxicities; secondly, both nitration and oxidation decrease the propensity of α-synuclein to form stable conformations, which might contribute to the progression of PD; in addition, truncated α-synuclein species have also been reported in Lewy bodies [20]. Truncation, typically occurring in the C-terminal domain of the protein, is associated with an increased propensity of α-synuclein to form fibrils and with increased toxicity in fly and rat models of PD [67, 68]. Currently, inflammation is a hot topic in studies of the pathogenesis in PD. Glial cells are the culprit in the mechanism of neuroinflammation, and this makes sense considering the prion-like hypothesis of α-synuclein's spread throughout the brain. The direct transfer of α-synuclein from neurons to astrocytes was demonstrated *in vivo* using transgenic mice overexpressing human α-synuclein under a neuronal promoter by Lee et al. [69]. In these transgenic mice, accumulation of human α-synuclein was observed not only in neurons, but also in glial cells [69]; the authors also found that the secretion of α-synuclein by neurons induced toxicity not only inside the cytoplasm of neighboring cells, but also in the extracellular space. The results clarified what activates glial cells and induces chronic inflammation, thereby contributing to the progression of the pathology throughout the brain. In other reports, the preferential binding of iron, copper, and other metals, including Cu(II), Mn(II), Co(II), and Ni(II), to the C-terminus of α-synuclein at residues D121, N122, and E123 [70, 71] has been shown to influence α-synuclein's function and aggregation and to promote the disease.

The spread of α-synuclein suggests that its toxicity would affect both the nervous system and other systems throughout the human body. This prompted us to consider the relationship between α-synuclein and the nonmotor symptoms in PD, such as the deficit of the olfactory sensation and astriction, which are nonspecific and always appear before the motor symptoms. Olfactory filaments are the only nerves directly exposed to the exterior environment [10, 56]. Transgenic animals expressing human α-synuclein under the control of the tyrosine hydroxylase promoter (ensuring catecholaminergic neuron-specific expression) presented olfactory impairments compared with wild-type animals during the olfaction test, and the olfactory deficits appeared long before the motor alterations in that study [52]. This brain region is of particular interest, because Lewy neurites and bodies are present in this area in the very early stages of PD [52]. This also provided a new insight into the toxicity of α-synuclein and its potential as a biomarker. However, it remains to be determined whether the misfolding of α-synuclein occurs randomly, where and when it first appears, and how self-propagation is initiated.

5. Alpha-Synuclein as a Diagnostic Biomarker in PD

To date, the diagnosis of PD still relies mostly on clinical features, because neuropathological confirmation is only possible with autopsy examination in postmortem studies [72]. Early diagnosis is required urgently, since PET-CT (Positron Emission Computed Tomography) or functional MRI (Magnetic Resonance Imaging) scans are not specific enough for this disease. Alpha-synuclein, with its unique characteristics in the occurrence and development of synucleinopathies, exists widely, not only in the central nervous system, but also in the peripheral nervous system, submandibular gland, skin, and saliva gland [72], making it a good candidate as a diagnostic biomarker, especially at the early stage of the disease.

About five years ago, studies provided evidence that α-synuclein was present in the CSF from PD patients [73]; however, the role of α-synuclein species in PD prognosis remains unclear [74]. Subsequently, some studies tested the level of α-synuclein in plasma after controlling several major variables; however, unlike CSF, there were no obvious differences between PD patients and controls. Recently, the submandibular gland was shown to be involved in synucleinopathy in the early stages of PD [75]. Consequently, Devic et al. [76] investigated human saliva, and the results seemed positive, suggesting that saliva α-synuclein is another potential biomarker for PD's diagnosis and progression. Recently, the presence of α-synuclein reactive antibodies in the serum of PD patients has become a hot topic [77].

New evidence has emerged indicating that CNS-derived EVs in plasma could serve as diagnostic biomarkers [48]. In addition, other studies have shown that urine harbors EVs; therefore, if the EVs could be isolated successfully, urine

would be another example of an easily accessible biofluid [78]. Hypothetically, in addition to testing for α-synuclein itself, the whole structure that generated, transported, and even cleared α-synuclein could be detected. Zange et al. [79] tested skin from 10 patients with multiple system atrophy and 10 with PD together with six control subjects suffering from essential tremor; the phosphorylated α-synuclein in the specimens was examined by immunohistochemistry, and both phosphorylated α-synuclein deposits in skin sympathetic nerve fibers and dermal nerve fiber density were assessed. Their results showed that all patients with PD expressed phosphorylated α-synuclein in sympathetic skin nerve fibers, correlating with age-independent denervation of autonomic skin elements. In contrast, no phosphorylated α-synuclein was found in patients with multiple system atrophy or in the essential tremor-control subjects. These findings supported the view that phosphorylated α-synuclein deposition may cause nerve fiber degeneration in PD. Although the peripheral synuclein tissue is a closer step to diagnosis of PD, Tolosa and Vilas [80] pointed out that Miki et al. [81] and Navarro-Otano et al. [82] made efforts to find abnormal α-synuclein deposition in the gastrointestinal tract and failed. Afterwards, several studies have identified phosphorylated α-synuclein in gastric and colonic specimens, as well as in the salivary glands. However, there are still some important methodological issues that need to be discussed. Firstly, the optimal site of α-synuclein deposits in skin has not yet been identified and current evidence suggests it might occur in skin tissue obtained from the cervical region [83]. Secondly, the number of biopsies needed to obtain a convincing result is also unclear. Thus, further studies are needed to determine the sensitivity and specificity of α-synuclein as a diagnostic biomarker for PD. Eventually, studies targeting testing phosphorylated α-synuclein in the peripheral nervous system in PD are still desperately needed [80]. Studies that aimed to achieve pathological confirmation of PD by biopsying these accessible tissues or chemical examinations evaluating the levels of α-synuclein are summarized in Table 1 [45, 46, 73–77, 83–91]. Currently, the nonmotor symptoms are becoming more and more important in the diagnosis of PD; however, they are always nonspecific and easily ignored by the patients. If physicians could find successfully a way to identify the close relationship between synucleins and the pathology of PD, great progress in the early and differential diagnosis of PD would be made. In addition, there have been few studies targeting synuclein using magnetic resonance or PET; therefore, more research effort is required.

6. Alpha-Synuclein as a Therapeutic Target in PD

There are four common ways to combat the toxicity produced by α-synuclein: decrease α-synuclein aggregation, control its propagation, increase its clearance, and stabilize its existing circumstances. A correct protein balance has a central role in cellular homeostasis of the nervous system [92].

Many mediators participate in the neurotoxicity induced by α-synuclein in synucleinopathies. For example, the

TABLE 1: Selected studies targeting α-synuclein as biomarker for the diagnosis of PD.

Ref	Materials	Analytical/measuring methods	Results in PD patients compared to controls
Lebouvier et al., 2008 [84]	Colonic tissue	Biopsy and immunohistochemical studies	TH-IR (tyrosine-hydroxylase immunoreactive) neurons were not a marker but phospho-α-synuclein-IR neurities were found in PD patients
Beach et al., 2010 [75]	Lower esophagus and submandibular tissue	Biopsy and a sensitive immunohistochemical method for phosphorylated α-synuclein	A rostrocaudal gradient of decreasing phosphorylated α-synuclein histopathology frequency and density
Shi et al., 2010 [45]	Alpha-synuclein in plasma	Blood component separation and analysis	No statistical difference was observed
Cersósimo et al., 2011 [85]	Salivary gland	Biopsy and immunohistochemical studies	The presence of α-synuclein inclusions in the submandibular glands
Devic et al., 2011 [76]	Saliva	Immunoblotting with a rabbit anti-human α-synuclein antibody ASY-1	The level of α-synuclein decreased
Yanamandra et al., 2011 [77]	Alpha-synuclein reactive antibodies in blood *sera*	ELISA, western blot, and Biacore surface plasmon resonance	Higher antibody levels towards monomeric α-synuclein
Shannon et al., 2012 [86]	Colonic submucosa	Biopsy and immunohistochemical studies	Staining for α-synuclein in nerve fibers in colonic submucosa
Alexoudi et al., 2013 [87]	Submandibular gland	Topic discussion	Positive
Schmid et al., 2013 [88]	Alpha-synuclein posttranslational modifications (PTMs)	A new chemical synthesis scheme	Relevant PTMs associated with disease progression and severity
Adler et al., 2014 [89]	Submandibular gland	Biopsy and immunohistochemical studies	Microscopic evidence of the tissue was positive for Lewy type α-synucleinopathy
Gao et al., 2015 [46]	CSF	Meta-analysis	The mean CSF α-synuclein concentration was significantly lower
Sanchez-Ferro et al., 2015 [90]	Gastric mucosa samples	Biopsy and immunohistochemical studies	Positive fibers for the α-synuclein protein were observed
Zhou et al., 2015 [73]	CSF	Meta-analysis	Mean concentration of CSF α-synuclein was slightly decreased; mean concentration of CSF α-synuclein oligomers was significantly higher
Adler et al., 2016 [91]	Submandibular gland	Biopsy and immunohistochemical studies	Positive staining
Donadio et al., 2016 [83]	Skin nerve	Skin biopsy	Only 49% of samples with a higher positivity rate for abnormal α-synuclein deposits at the proximal site in IPD
Parnetti et al., 2016 [74]	CSF	Review of 32 selected articles	The role of α-synuclein species in PD prognosis remained unsatisfactory

inflammatory protease caspase-1 mediates the C-terminal truncation and was implicated in the mechanism in promoting aggregation of α-synuclein *in vitro* and *in vivo* [20]. Interestingly, a caspase-1 inhibitor could provide neuroprotective effects on PD by reducing α-synuclein cleavage, hence limiting its ability to form aggregates. Preventing aggregation could also be achieved using passive or active immunization approaches, such as gene-silence technologies or active protein immunization. There are already some transgenic mouse models of PD reported [93] that have reached the clinical investigation stage.

Dehay et al. aimed to prevent either direct α-synuclein's seeds' toxicity or cell-to-cell transmission and have developed some *in vitro* screens for compounds targeting these phenomena [94]. Models with human Lewy body-derived α-synuclein assemblies can also be used to prevent cell-to-cell transmission. As discussed above, the spread of α-synuclein includes neuron to neuron, neuron to glia, glia to neuron, and glia to glia [69]. A combination of these methods would allow the identification of potential therapeutics.

The two major degradation systems are autophagy and the UPS. The UPS is thought to be responsible for the degradation of misfolded proteins [95]. A study aimed at this system indicated that downregulation of the UPS might contribute to the pathogenesis of PD [66]. Moreover, considering neurodegenerative diseases, aging is the most significant risk factor for the development of such diseases and is associated with progressive decline of the UPS and accumulation of oxidized proteins [96]. This suggests that targeting these two systems to increase the clearance of α-synuclein might be an efficient treatment for PD in the future.

Many studies have reported the development of powerful tools and models targeting α-synuclein. In addition, much attention is now being paid to the proteotoxic mechanisms and inflammation induced by α-synuclein and how to block them using strategies such as enhancing cellular clearance through innate and adaptive immunization [25]. The accumulation of C-terminal domain truncated α-synuclein can be inhibited by immunotherapy [8]. In addition, improvements in axonal and motor deficits can be achieved by protecting C-terminal domain truncated α-synuclein from C-terminal cleavage [68]. Furthermore, the antibodies that inhibit C-terminal truncation could, theoretically, reduce cell-to-cell propagation of α-synuclein. Immunization with antibodies targeting the C-terminal truncation sites of α-synuclein, the oxidation and nitration of α-synuclein, or even those promoting increased clearance might have therapeutic potential, not only as agents to reduce the amount of α-synuclein itself, but also as inhibitors of its pathological oligomerization and propagation. Several important questions concerning the antibodies remain, the most fundamental one being how antibodies could reach the brain compartment at sufficient levels and how they could recognize their intracellular targeting protein and promote its intracellular toxicity.

Small molecules that stabilize α-synuclein's physiological tetramer could reduce its pathogenicity. The JAK/STAT (Janus kinase/signal transducer and activator of transcription) pathway is known to function in cell proliferation, differentiation, and apoptosis and in immune regulation and hematopoietic cells generation and plays a variety of biological functions in tumorigenesis and neural development. Cytokines such as interleukin, interferon, and epidermal growth factor can contribute to the protection of the nervous system through this pathway, which also provided new insights into the future therapy of PD [97].

7. Conclusion

Alpha-synuclein is a major component of Lewy bodies and Lewy neurites, which are the neuropathological hallmarks of Parkinson's disease. Currently, gene-targeting therapy and biotherapy are hot topics in research into neurodegenerative disorders such as Parkinson's disease, Alzheimer's disease,

and Huntington's disease. Here, we summarized recent progress targeting this unique protein. However, further research effort is required and several questions remain: What is the specific mechanism of this protein in PD? Do other, as yet undiscovered, gene mutations or duplications or triplications lead to the production of the toxic version of this protein? Did the gene mutations initiate its dysfunction? How can we control the toxic effects of this protein if we aim to limit the accumulation of misfolded proteins without disturbing its physiological function? In conclusion, we still lack critical knowledge necessary to develop α-synuclein as a diagnostic biomarker and therapeutic target.

Acknowledgments

This work was supported by the National Natural Science Foundation of China (81400933) and the Zhejiang Medical Science and Technology Plan Project (2016KYB119).

References

[1] W. G. Meissner, M. Frasier, T. Gasser et al., "Priorities in Parkinson's disease research," Nature Reviews Drug Discovery, vol. 10, no. 5, pp. 377–393, 2011.

[2] W. Peelaerts, L. Bousset, A. Van der Perren et al., "α-synuclein strains cause distinct synucleinopathies after local and systemic administration," Nature, vol. 522, no. 7556, pp. 340–344, 2015.

[3] K. Wakabayashi, K. Tanji, S. Odagiri, Y. Miki, F. Mori, and H. Takahashi, "The Lewy body in Parkinson's disease and related neurodegenerative disorders," Molecular Neurobiology, vol. 47, no. 2, pp. 495–508, 2013.

[4] M. H. Polymeropoulos, C. Lavedan, E. Leroy et al., "Mutation in the α-synuclein gene identified in families with Parkinson's disease," Science, vol. 276, no. 5321, pp. 2045–2047, 1997.

[5] E.-K. Tan, V. R. Chandran, S. Fook-Chong et al., "Alpha-synuclein mRNA expression in sporadic Parkinson's disease," Movement Disorders, vol. 20, no. 5, pp. 620–623, 2005.

[6] E. Angot, J. A. Steiner, C. M. Tomé et al., "Alpha-synuclein cell-to-cell transfer and seeding in grafted dopaminergic neurons in vivo," PLoS ONE, vol. 7, no. 6, Article ID e39465, 2012.

[7] A. Recasens and B. Dehay, "Alpha-synuclein spreading in Parkinson's disease," Frontiers in Neuroanatomy, vol. 8, article 159, 2014.

[8] H. T. Tran, C.-Y. Chung, M. Iba et al., "α-synuclein immunotherapy blocks uptake and templated propagation of misfolded α-synuclein and neurodegeneration," Cell Reports, vol. 7, no. 6, pp. 2054–2065, 2014.

[9] B. S. Connolly and A. E. Lang, "Pharmacological treatment of Parkinson disease: a review," The Journal of the American Medical Association, vol. 311, no. 16, pp. 1670–1683, 2014.

[10] B. Dehay, M. Bourdenx, P. Gorry et al., "Targeting α-synuclein for treatment of Parkinson's disease: mechanistic and therapeutic considerations,," The Lancet Neurology, vol. 14, no. 8, pp. 855–866, 2015.

[11] H. A. Lashuel, C. R. Overk, A. Oueslati, and E. Masliah, "The many faces of α-synuclein: from structure and toxicity to therapeutic target," *Nature Reviews Neuroscience*, vol. 14, no. 1, pp. 38–48, 2013.

[12] R. Jakes, M. G. Spillantini, and M. Goedert, "Identification of two distinct synucleins from human brain," *FEBS Letters*, vol. 345, no. 1, pp. 27–32, 1994.

[13] R. Krüger, W. Kuhn, T. Müller et al., "Ala30Pro mutation in the gene encoding α-synuclein in Parkinson's disease," *Nature Genetics*, vol. 18, no. 2, pp. 106–108, 1998.

[14] J. J. Zarranz, J. Alegre, J. C. Gómez-Esteban et al., "The new mutation, E46K, of α-synuclein causes parkinson and lewy body dementia," *Annals of Neurology*, vol. 55, no. 2, pp. 164–173, 2004.

[15] S. Appel-Cresswell, C. Vilarino-Guell, M. Encarnacion et al., "Alpha-synuclein p.H50Q, a novel pathogenic mutation for Parkinson's disease," *Movement Disorders*, vol. 28, no. 6, pp. 811–813, 2013.

[16] S. Lesage, M. Anheim, F. Letournel et al., "G51D α-synuclein mutation causes a novel Parkinsonian-pyramidal syndrome," *Annals of Neurology*, vol. 73, no. 4, pp. 459–471, 2013.

[17] P. Pasanen, L. Myllykangas, M. Siitonen et al., "A novel α-synuclein mutation A53E associated with atypical multiple system atrophy and Parkinson's disease-type pathology," *Neurobiology of Aging*, vol. 35, no. 9, pp. 2180.e1–2180.e5, 2014.

[18] J. M. George, "The synucleins," *Genome Biology*, vol. 3, Article ID REVIEWS3002, 2002.

[19] B. I. Giasson, I. V. J. Murray, J. Q. Trojanowski, and V. M.-Y. Lee, "A hydrophobic stretch of 12 amino acid residues in the middle of α-synuclein is essential for filament assembly," *The Journal of Biological Chemistry*, vol. 276, no. 4, pp. 2380–2386, 2001.

[20] D. Games, E. Valera, B. Spencer et al., "Reducing C-terminal-truncated alpha-synuclein by immunotherapy attenuates neurodegeneration and propagation in Parkinson's disease-like models," *Journal of Neuroscience*, vol. 34, no. 28, pp. 9441–9454, 2014.

[21] D. E. Mor, S. E. Ugras, M. J. Daniels, and H. Ischiropoulos, "Dynamic structural flexibility of α-synuclein," *Neurobiology of Disease*, vol. 88, pp. 66–74, 2016.

[22] T. Bartels, J. G. Choi, and D. J. Selkoe, "α-Synuclein occurs physiologically as a helically folded tetramer that resists aggregation," *Nature*, vol. 477, no. 7362, pp. 107–110, 2011.

[23] J. Burré, M. Sharma, T. Tsetsenis, V. Buchman, M. R. Etherton, and T. C. Südhof, "α-Synuclein promotes SNARE-complex assembly in vivo and in vitro," *Science*, vol. 329, no. 5999, pp. 1663–1667, 2010.

[24] J. Burré, S. Vivona, J. Diao, M. Sharma, A. T. Brunger, and T. C. Südhof, "Properties of native brain α-synuclein," *Nature*, vol. 498, no. 7453, pp. E4–E6, 2013.

[25] H. E. A. Reish and D. G. Standaert, "Role of α-synuclein in inducing innate and adaptive immunity in Parkinson disease," *Journal of Parkinson's Disease*, vol. 5, no. 1, pp. 1–19, 2015.

[26] D. Lee, S.-Y. Lee, E.-N. Lee, C.-S. Chang, and S. R. Paik, "α-synuclein exhibits competitive interaction between calmodulin and synthetic membranes," *Journal of Neurochemistry*, vol. 82, no. 5, pp. 1007–1017, 2002.

[27] V. M. Nemani, W. Lu, V. Berge et al., "Increased expression of α-synuclein reduces neurotransmitter release by inhibiting synaptic vesicle reclustering after endocytosis," *Neuron*, vol. 65, no. 1, pp. 66–79, 2010.

[28] N. M. Bonini and B. I. Giasson, "Snaring the function of α-synuclein," *Cell*, vol. 123, no. 3, pp. 359–361, 2005.

[29] S. Chandra, G. Gallardo, R. Fernández-Chacón, O. M. Schlüter, and T. C. Südhof, "α-Synuclein cooperates with CSPα in preventing neurodegeneration," *Cell*, vol. 123, no. 3, pp. 383–396, 2005.

[30] J. Burré, M. Sharma, and T. C. Südhof, "Definition of a molecular pathway mediating α-synuclein neurotoxicity," *Journal of Neuroscience*, vol. 35, no. 13, pp. 5221–5232, 2015.

[31] K. A. Conway, J. D. Harper, and P. T. Lansbury, "Accelerated in vitro fibril formation by a mutant α-synuclein linked to early-onset Parkinson disease," *Nature Medicine*, vol. 4, no. 11, pp. 1318–1320, 1998.

[32] K. A. Conway, S.-J. Lee, J.-C. Rochet, T. T. Ding, R. E. Williamson, and P. T. Lansbury Jr., "Acceleration of oligomerization, not fibrillization, is a shared property of both α-synuclein mutations linked to early-onset Parkinson's disease: implications for pathogenesis and therapy," *Proceedings of the National Academy of Sciences of the United States of America*, vol. 97, no. 2, pp. 571–576, 2000.

[33] D. P. Karpinar, M. B. G. Balija, S. Kügler et al., "Pre-fibrillar α-synuclein variants with impaired B-structure increase neurotoxicity in parkinson's disease models," *The EMBO Journal*, vol. 28, no. 20, pp. 3256–3268, 2009.

[34] J. A. Rodriguez, M. I. Ivanova, M. R. Sawaya et al., "Structure of the toxic core of α-synuclein from invisible crystals," *Nature*, vol. 525, no. 7570, pp. 486–490, 2015.

[35] T. S. Ulmer, A. Bax, N. B. Cole, and R. L. Nussbaum, "Structure and dynamics of micelle-bound human α-synuclein," *The Journal of Biological Chemistry*, vol. 280, no. 10, pp. 9595–9603, 2005.

[36] W. Hoyer, D. Cherny, V. Subramaniam, and T. M. Jovin, "Impact of the acidic C-terminal region comprising amino acids 109-140 on α-synuclein aggregation in vitro," *Biochemistry*, vol. 43, no. 51, pp. 16233–16242, 2004.

[37] W. Li, N. West, E. Colla et al., "Aggregation promoting C-terminal truncation of α-synuclein is a normal cellular process and is enhanced by the familial Parkinson's disease-linked mutations," *Proceedings of the National Academy of Sciences of the United States of America*, vol. 102, no. 6, pp. 2162–2167, 2005.

[38] F. Samuel, W. P. Flavin, S. Iqbal et al., "Effects of serine 129 phosphorylation on alpha-synuclein aggregation, membrane association, and internalization," *Journal of Biological Chemistry*, vol. 291, no. 9, pp. 4374–4385, 2016.

[39] K. J. Inglis, D. Chereau, E. F. Brigham et al., "Polo-like kinase 2 (PLK2) phosphorylates α-synuclein at serine 129 in central nervous system," *The Journal of Biological Chemistry*, vol. 284, no. 5, pp. 2598–2602, 2009.

[40] J. M. Souza, B. I. Giasson, Q. Chen, V. M.-Y. Lee, and H. Ischiropoulos, "Dityrosine cross-linking promotes formation of stable α-synuclein polymers: implication of nitrative and oxidative stress in the pathogenesis of neurodegenerative synucleinopathies," *The Journal of Biological Chemistry*, vol. 275, no. 24, pp. 18344–18349, 2000.

[41] R. Hodara, E. H. Norris, B. I. Giasson et al., "Functional consequences of α-synuclein tyrosine nitration: diminished binding to lipid vesicles and increased fibril formation," *The Journal of Biological Chemistry*, vol. 279, no. 46, pp. 47746–47753, 2004.

[42] D. Snead and D. Eliezer, "Alpha-synuclein function and dysfunction on cellular membranes," *Experimental Neurobiology*, vol. 23, no. 4, pp. 292–313, 2014.

[43] J. L. Webb, B. Ravikumar, J. Atkins, J. N. Skepper, and D. C. Rubinsztein, "α-Synuclein is degraded by both autophagy and the proteasome," *Journal of Biological Chemistry*, vol. 278, no. 27, pp. 25009–25013, 2003.

[44] D. Ebrahimi-Fakhari, I. Cantuti-Castelvetri, Z. Fan et al., "Distinct roles in vivo for the ubiquitin-proteasome system and the autophagy-lysosomal pathway in the degradation of α-synuclein," *The Journal of Neuroscience*, vol. 31, no. 41, pp. 14508–14520, 2011.

[45] M. Shi, C. P. Zabetian, A. M. Hancock et al., "Significance and confounders of peripheral DJ-1 and alpha-synuclein in Parkinson's disease," *Neuroscience Letters*, vol. 480, no. 1, pp. 78–82, 2010.

[46] L. Gao, H. Tang, K. Nie et al., "Cerebrospinal fluid alpha-synuclein as a biomarker for Parkinson's disease diagnosis: a systematic review and meta-analysis," *International Journal of Neuroscience*, vol. 125, no. 9, pp. 645–654, 2015.

[47] E. Emmanouilidou, K. Melachroinou, T. Roumeliotis et al., "Cell-produced α-synuclein is secreted in a calcium-dependent manner by exosomes and impacts neuronal survival," *Journal of Neuroscience*, vol. 30, no. 20, pp. 6838–6851, 2010.

[48] C. Lööv, C. R. Scherzer, B. T. Hyman, X. O. Breakefield, and M. Ingelsson, "α-Synuclein in extracellular vesicles: functional implications and diagnostic opportunities," *Cellular and Molecular Neurobiology*, vol. 36, no. 3, pp. 437–448, 2016.

[49] M. Grey, C. J. Dunning, R. Gaspar et al., "Acceleration of alpha-synuclein aggregation by exosomes," *Journal of Biological Chemistry*, vol. 290, no. 5, pp. 2969–2982, 2015.

[50] C. P. Lai, E. Y. Kim, C. E. Badr et al., "Visualization and tracking of tumour extracellular vesicle delivery and RNA translation using multiplexed reporters," *Nature Communications*, vol. 6, article 7029, 2015.

[51] S. B. Prusiner, "A unifying role for prions in neurodegenerative diseases," *Science*, vol. 336, no. 6088, pp. 1511–1513, 2012.

[52] P. Desplats, H.-J. Lee, E.-J. Bae et al., "Inclusion formation and neuronal cell death through neuron-to-neuron transmission of α-synuclein," *Proceedings of the National Academy of Sciences of the United States of America*, vol. 106, no. 31, pp. 13010–13015, 2009.

[53] C. Hansen, E. Angot, A.-L. Bergström et al., "α-Synuclein propagates from mouse brain to grafted dopaminergic neurons and seeds aggregation in cultured human cells," *The Journal of Clinical Investigation*, vol. 121, no. 2, pp. 715–725, 2011.

[54] K. C. Luk, V. Kehm, J. Carroll et al., "Pathological α-synuclein transmission initiates Parkinson-like neurodegeneration in nontransgenic mice," *Science*, vol. 338, no. 6109, pp. 949–953, 2012.

[55] K. C. Luk, V. M. Kehm, B. Zhang, P. O'Brien, J. Q. Trojanowski, and V. M. Y. Lee, "Intracerebral inoculation of pathological α-synuclein initiates a rapidly progressive neurodegenerative α-synucleinopathy in mice," *The Journal of Experimental Medicine*, vol. 209, no. 5, pp. 975–986, 2012.

[56] F. Lelan, L. Lescaudron, C. Boyer et al., "Effects of human alpha-synuclein A53T-A30P mutations on SVZ and local olfactory bulb cell proliferation in a transgenic rat model of Parkinson disease," *Parkinson's Disease*, vol. 2011, Article ID 987084, 11 pages, 2011.

[57] S. Aulić, T. T. N. Le, F. Moda et al., "Defined α-synuclein prion-like molecular assemblies spreading in cell culture," *BMC Neuroscience*, vol. 15, article 69, 2014.

[58] A. Ulusoy, R. E. Musgrove, R. Rusconi et al., "Neuron-to-neuron α-synuclein propagation in vivo is independent of neuronal

injury," *Acta Neuropathologica Communications*, vol. 3, article 13, 2015.

[59] A. Abeliovich, Y. Schmitz, I. Fariñas et al., "Mice lacking α-synuclein display functional deficits in the nigrostriatal dopamine system," *Neuron*, vol. 25, no. 1, pp. 239–252, 2000.

[60] S. Chandra, F. Fornai, H.-B. Kwon et al., "Double-knockout mice for α- and β-synucleins: effect on synaptic functions," *Proceedings of the National Academy of Sciences of the United States of America*, vol. 101, no. 41, pp. 14966–14971, 2004.

[61] V. S. Kokhan, M. A. Afanasyeva, and G. I. Van'kin, "α-Synuclein knockout mice have cognitive impairments," *Behavioural Brain Research*, vol. 231, no. 1, pp. 226–230, 2012.

[62] T. Wang and J. C. Hay, "Alpha-synuclein toxicity in the early secretory pathway: how it drives neurodegeneration in Parkinsons disease," *Frontiers in Neuroscience*, vol. 9, article 433, 2015.

[63] E. H. Norris, B. I. Giasson, H. Ischiropoulos, and V. M.-Y. Lee, "Effects of oxidative and nitrative challenges on α-synuclein fibrillogenesis involve distinct mechanisms of protein modifications," *The Journal of Biological Chemistry*, vol. 278, no. 29, pp. 27230–27240, 2003.

[64] G. Yamin, V. N. Uversky, and A. L. Fink, "Nitration inhibits fibrillation of human α-synuclein in vitro by formation of soluble oligomers," *FEBS Letters*, vol. 542, no. 1–3, pp. 147–152, 2003.

[65] M. Martinez-Vicente, "Autophagy in neurodegenerative diseases: from pathogenic dysfunction to therapeutic modulation," *Seminars in Cell and Developmental Biology*, vol. 40, pp. 115–126, 2015.

[66] F. J. A. Dennissen, N. Kholod, and F. W. van Leeuwen, "The ubiquitin proteasome system in neurodegenerative diseases: culprit, accomplice or victim?" *Progress in Neurobiology*, vol. 96, no. 2, pp. 190–207, 2012.

[67] M. Periquet, T. Fulga, L. Myllykangas, M. G. Schlossmacher, and M. B. Feany, "Aggregated α-synuclein mediates dopaminergic neurotoxicity in vivo," *The Journal of Neuroscience*, vol. 27, no. 12, pp. 3338–3346, 2007.

[68] A. Ulusoy, F. Febbraro, P. H. Jensen, D. Kirik, and M. Romero-Ramos, "Co-expression of C-terminal truncated alpha-synuclein enhances full-length alpha-synuclein-induced pathology," *European Journal of Neuroscience*, vol. 32, no. 3, pp. 409–422, 2010.

[69] H.-J. Lee, J.-E. Suk, C. Patrick et al., "Direct transfer of α-synuclein from neuron to astroglia causes inflammatory responses in synucleinopathies," *The Journal of Biological Chemistry*, vol. 285, no. 12, pp. 9262–9272, 2010.

[70] R. M. Rasia, C. W. Bertoncini, D. Marsh et al., "Structural characterization of copper(II) binding to α-synuclein: insights into the bioinorganic chemistry of Parkinson's disease," *Proceedings of the National Academy of Sciences of the United States of America*, vol. 102, no. 12, pp. 4294–4299, 2005.

[71] A. Binolfi, R. M. Rasia, C. W. Bertoncini et al., "Interaction of α-synuclein with divalent metal ions reveals key differences: a link between structure, binding specificity and fibrillation enhancement," *Journal of the American Chemical Society*, vol. 128, no. 30, pp. 9893–9901, 2006.

[72] M. G. Cersosimo, "Gastrointestinal biopsies for the diagnosis of alpha-synuclein pathology in Parkinson's disease," *Gastroenterology Research and Practice*, vol. 2015, Article ID 476041, 6 pages, 2015.

[73] B. Zhou, M. Wen, W.-F. Yu, C.-L. Zhang, and L. Jiao, "The diagnostic and differential diagnosis utility of cerebrospinal

fluid α-synuclein levels in Parkinson's disease: a meta-analysis," *Parkinson's Disease*, vol. 2015, Article ID 567386, 11 pages, 2015.

[74] L. Parnetti, C. Cicognola, P. Eusebi, and D. Chiasserini, "Value of cerebrospinal fluid α-synuclein species as biomarker in Parkinson's diagnosis and prognosis," *Biomarkers in Medicine*, vol. 10, no. 1, pp. 35–49, 2016.

[75] T. G. Beach, C. H. Adler, L. I. Sue et al., "Multi-organ distribution of phosphorylated α-synuclein histopathology in subjects with Lewy body disorders," *Acta Neuropathologica*, vol. 119, no. 6, pp. 689–702, 2010.

[76] I. Devic, H. Hwang, J. S. Edgar et al., "Salivary α-synuclein and DJ-1: potential biomarkers for Parkinson's disease," *Brain*, vol. 134, no. 7, article e178, 2011.

[77] K. Yanamandra, M. A. Gruden, V. Casaite, R. Meskys, L. Forsgren, and L. A. Morozova-Roche, "α-synuclein reactive antibodies as diagnostic biomarkers in blood sera of parkinson's disease patients," *PLoS ONE*, vol. 6, no. 4, Article ID e18513, 2011.

[78] A. Gámez-Valero, S. I. Lozano-Ramos, I. Bancu, R. Lauzurica-Valdemoros, and F. E. Borràs, "Urinary extracellular vesicles as source of biomarkers in kidney diseases," *Frontiers in Immunology*, vol. 6, article 6, 2015.

[79] L. Zange, C. Noack, K. Hahn, W. Stenzel, and A. Lipp, "Phosphorylated α-synuclein in skin nerve fibres differentiates Parkinson's disease from multiple system atrophy," *Brain*, vol. 138, no. 8, pp. 2310–2321, 2015.

[80] E. Tolosa and D. Vilas, "Peripheral synuclein tissue markers: a step closer to Parkinson's disease diagnosis," *Brain*, vol. 138, no. 8, pp. 2120–2122, 2015.

[81] Y. Miki, M. Tomiyama, T. Ueno et al., "Clinical availability of skin biopsy in the diagnosis of Parkinson's disease," *Neuroscience Letters*, vol. 469, no. 3, pp. 357–359, 2010.

[82] J. Navarro-Otano, J. Casanova-Mollà, M. Morales, J. Valls-Solé, and E. Tolosa, "Cutaneous autonomic denervation in Parkinson's disease," *Journal of Neural Transmission*, vol. 122, no. 8, pp. 1149–1155, 2015.

[83] V. Donadio, A. Incensi, C. Piccinini et al., "Skin nerve misfolded α-synuclein in pure autonomic failure and Parkinson disease," *Annals of Neurology*, vol. 79, no. 2, pp. 306–316, 2016.

[84] T. Lebouvier, T. Chaumette, P. Damier et al., "Pathological lesions in colonic biopsies during Parkinson's disease," *Gut*, vol. 57, no. 12, pp. 1741–1743, 2008.

[85] M. G. Cersósimo, C. Perandones, F. E. Micheli et al., "Alpha-synuclein immunoreactivity in minor salivary gland biopsies of Parkinson's disease patients," *Movement Disorders*, vol. 26, no. 1, pp. 188–190, 2011.

[86] K. M. Shannon, A. Keshavarzian, E. Mutlu et al., "Alpha-synuclein in colonic submucosa in early untreated Parkinson's disease," *Movement Disorders*, vol. 27, no. 6, pp. 709–715, 2012.

[87] A. Alexoudi, S. A. Schneider, and G. Deuschl, "Submandibular gland biopsy for the diagnosis of Parkinson's disease," *Movement Disorders*, vol. 28, no. 6, p. 734, 2013.

[88] A. W. Schmid, B. Fauvet, M. Moniatte, and H. A. Lashuel, "Alpha-synuclein post-translational modifications as potential biomarkers for parkinson disease and other synucleinopathies," *Molecular & Cellular Proteomics*, vol. 12, no. 12, pp. 3543–3558, 2013.

[89] C. H. Adler, B. N. Dugger, M. L. Hinni et al., "Submandibular gland needle biopsy for the diagnosis of Parkinson disease," *Neurology*, vol. 82, no. 10, pp. 858–864, 2014.

[90] A. Sanchez-Ferro, A. Rabano, M. J. Catalan et al., "In vivo gastric detection of alpha-synuclein inclusions in Parkinson's disease," *Movement Disorders*, vol. 30, no. 4, pp. 517–524, 2015.

[91] C. H. Adler, B. N. Dugger, J. G. Hentz et al., "Peripheral synucleinopathy in early Parkinson's disease: submandibular gland needle biopsy findings," *Movement Disorders*, vol. 31, no. 2, pp. 250–256, 2016.

[92] P. Rivero-Ríos, J. Madero-Pérez,, B. Fernández, and S. Hilfiker, "Targeting the autophagy/lysosomal degradation pathway in Parkinson's disease," *Current Neuropharmacology*, vol. 14, no. 3, pp. 238–249, 2016.

[93] M. Mandler, E. Valera, E. Rockenstein et al., "Next-generation active immunization approach for synucleinopathies: implications for Parkinson's disease clinical trials," *Acta Neuropathologica*, vol. 127, no. 6, pp. 861–879, 2014.

[94] B. Dehay, M. Decressac, M. Bourdenx et al., "Targeting alpha-synuclein: therapeutic options," *Movement Disorders*, vol. 31, no. 6, pp. 882–888, 2016.

[95] A. Ciechanover and Y. T. Kwon, "Degradation of misfolded proteins in neurodegenerative diseases: therapeutic targets and strategies," *Experimental & Molecular Medicine*, vol. 47, no. 3, article e147, 2015.

[96] C. McKinnon and S. J. Tabrizi, "The ubiquitin-proteasome system in neurodegeneration," *Antioxidants and Redox Signaling*, vol. 21, no. 17, pp. 2302–2321, 2014.

[97] E. Himpe and R. Kooijman, "Insulin-like growth factor-I receptor signal transduction and the Janus Kinase/Signal Transducer and Activator of Transcription (JAK-STAT) pathway," *BioFactors*, vol. 35, no. 1, pp. 76–81, 2009.

7

Theatre is a Valid Add-On Therapeutic Intervention for Emotional Rehabilitation of Parkinson's Disease Patients

Giovanni Mirabella,[1,2] Paolo De Vita,[3] Michele Fragola,[1] Silvia Rampelli,[3] Francesco Lena,[1] Fulvia Dilettuso,[3] Marta Iacopini,[3] Raffaella d'Avella,[3] Maria Concetta Borgese,[3] Silvia Mazzotta,[3] Deborah Lanni,[1] Marco Grano,[1] Sara Lubrani,[3] and Nicola Modugno[1]

[1]Istituto Neurologico Mediterraneo "Neuromed", Pozzilli, Italy
[2]Department of Anatomy, Histology, Forensic Medicine & Orthopedics, Sapienza University of Rome, Rome, Italy
[3]PARKIN-ZONE onlus, Roma, Italy

Correspondence should be addressed to Giovanni Mirabella; giovanni.mirabella@uniroma1.it

Academic Editor: Hélio Teive

Conventional medical treatments of Parkinson's disease (PD) are effective on motor disturbances but may have little impact on nonmotor symptoms, especially psychiatric ones. Thus, even when motor symptomatology improves, patients might experience deterioration in their quality of life. We have shown that 3 years of active theatre is a valid complementary intervention for PD as it significantly improves the well-being of patients in comparison to patients undergoing conventional physiotherapy. Our aim was to replicate these findings while improving the efficacy of the treatment. We ran a single-blinded pilot study lasting 15 months on 24 subjects with moderate idiopathic PD. 12 were assigned to a theatre program in which patients underwent "emotional" training. The other 12 underwent group physiotherapy. Patients were evaluated at the beginning and at the end of their treatments, using a battery of eight clinical and five neuropsychological scales. We found that the emotional theatre training improved the emotional well-being of patients, whereas physiotherapy did not. Interestingly, neither of the groups showed improvements in either motor symptoms or cognitive abilities tested by the neuropsychological battery. We confirmed that theatre therapy might be helpful in improving emotional well-being in PD.

1. Introduction

Parkinson's disease is a progressive neurodegenerative disease that causes motor disturbances (e.g., slowness, rigidity, tremor, and disorders of gait and balance) and nonmotor disturbances such as neuropsychiatric symptoms (e.g., depression, anxiety, obsessive-compulsive disorders, and cognitive impairments) and autonomic dysfunction (e.g., decreased control of urinary bladder and sexual dysfunctions) [1]. Consequently, the general health and the social lives of patients can be deeply impaired [2].

Standard medical treatments based on the administration of dopaminergic drugs [3, 4] allow optimal control of the motor symptoms, especially in the initial stages of PD; however, with chronic treatment, motor and behavioral complications partly unmasked by dopaminergic medications

may develop [5]. Moreover, dopaminergic drugs are not often fully effective in controlling the full clinical spectrum of nonmotor symptoms. Often physiotherapy is used as an additional therapy [6], but even though it has been shown to be effective [7, 8], benefits tend to disappear as soon as the treatment is over [9] and there is no clear evidence of its efficacy on nonmotor symptoms.

Thus, as PD progresses, the increasing difficulties in its management may lead to social isolation as patients start to feel embarrassed by the disease, with a consequent deterioration in their quality of life (QoL; [10]). That said, there is a gap between the effects of the best available medical treatment and patients' expectations. In some instances, a paradoxical discrepancy between an objectively good control of motor disturbances and an increasing negative feeling of well-being reported by patients may occur.

Given that PD has worldwide prevalence of approximately 10 million people and that this number is expected to double by 2050 because of increasing longevity [11], management and treatment of this disease will be a very important public health problem. Accordingly, the demand for the development of appropriate complementary strategies aimed at improving personal and social life of patients and caregivers is rapidly increasing. Activities such as tai chi [12], dancing tango [13], and Irish dance [14] have been shown to produce positive effects mainly on balance and frequency of falls. However, improvements in nonmotor cognitive and affective symptoms were absent or very limited. An exception is given in a study [15] that demonstrated that 3 months of active music therapy improved both motor abilities and the emotional status of PD patients. Nevertheless, these effects disappeared 2 months after the end of therapy. Some preliminary evidence indicates that group psychotherapy [16] and occupational therapies [17, 18] might be a useful treatment for emotional disorders such as depression and/or anxiety, but samples are usually very small, measurements are too few, and control groups are not always present. Therefore, more systematic research is necessary to quantify the effects of those approaches.

Recently, we have shown that active theatre, in which patients are directly involved in the representations, is a valid add-on therapeutic intervention for PD [19]. Compared to patients undergoing physiotherapy, only PD patients performing theatre had progressive improvements in most nonmotor clinical scales (especially those tapping into the affective domains) and, to a lesser extent, in those assessing motor symptoms. In particular, patients performing theatre showed remarkable improvements in their level of depression, in their self-esteem, and in the quality of sleep. However, most of these beneficial effects emerged only after a training of 3 years and this evidence casts doubts on the transferability of the theatre therapy program. In addition, our sample was relatively small (20 subjects). Finally, as only five clinical scales were used, they might not be enough to fully appreciate the effects of the interventions. The present study was designed to both (i) replicate and extend our previous results, by collecting data on more clinical and neuropsychological scales, and (ii) develop a form of theatre therapy which would speed up the emergence of benefits in order to improve its transferability. Because in the previous study PD patients showed a significant improvement in most of clinical scales evaluating the emotional sphere, we hypothesized that a way to make theatre training more efficient would have been to train patients to represent emotional events on the stage. The effects of such "emotional" theatre were compared with those induced by physiotherapy in other groups of PD patients.

2. Materials and Methods

2.1. Study Participants. Forty-five patients were recruited from the outpatients of several hospitals in Rome ($n = 25$) and from IRCCS Neuromed Hospital, Italy ($n = 20$), by means of referrals from neurologists and of advertising through local PD associations. Eligibility criteria for including PD patients were (i) a diagnosis of idiopathic PD with a

moderate disease severity (Hoehn-Yahr stage 2-3), (ii) a stable treatment with levodopa (L-dopa) and dopamine agonists, (iii) absence of cognitive impairment (MMSE score ≥ 24), (iv) absence of severe sensory deficits, (v) absence of severe motor disability so that they could stand and walk unaided, and (vi) not being involved in other rehabilitation studies.

We allowed patients recruited from Rome hospitals to be assigned to the theatre rehabilitation program *(theatre group)*, while patients from Neuromed Hospital were allowed to enter in the physiotherapy rehabilitation therapy *(control group)*. Two main motivations produced this choice: (1) actors were only available in Rome; (2) the two groups of patients would not be in contact (Neuromed Hospital is about 200 km from Rome), avoiding possible complaints about being assigned to a given group.

After the initial screening, patients who met inclusion criteria underwent a one-to-one interview (sometimes by telephone) led by one member of the staff who explained the type of study in which they were taking part. Ten patients refused to participate in the theatre group and five in the physiotherapy group. Motivations were mainly related to the programmed length of the study or to logistic problems. Of the remaining 30 patients, six (three from each group) did not conclude the study because (a) two moved to another town; (b) three experienced physical problems; and (c) one had lack of motivation (1). We ended up having 24 patients, 12 per group, who took part in more than 75% of the study sessions. Throughout the entire course of the study, patients were allowed to continue taking their dopaminergic therapy, which was optimized whenever necessary according to the patient's needs. The use of antidepressant and hypnotic agents was equally distributed between the two groups during the entire course of the study.

All subjects gave their informed consent and were free to withdraw from the study at any time. The procedures were approved by the local Institutional Ethics Committee and were in accordance with the ethical standards laid down in the Declaration of Helsinki of 1964.

2.2. Clinical Assessment. All patients underwent a clinical evaluation at the beginning ($T0$) of the training period and after 15 months ($T1$). A neurologist and a psychologist, blinded to the study groups, evaluated PD patients on clinical and neuropsychological scales, respectively. We employed eight clinical scales: (i) the Unified Parkinson's Disease Rating Scale (UPDRS), which rates patients' mood and cognition (UPDRS I), activities of daily living (UPDRS II), motor symptoms (UPDRS III), and complications of therapy (UPDRS IV); (ii) the Gait and Falls Questionnaire, which measures gait disturbances; (iii) the Parkinson's Disease Quality of Life Scale (PDQ39), which measures the QoL by summing the scores of its eight subscales (mobility, activities of daily living, emotional well-being, stigma, social support, cognition, communication, and bodily discomfort); (iv) the Beck Depression Inventory, which measures the level of depression; (v) the Apathy Evaluation Scale, which measures the level of apathy (lack of feelings, emotions, interests, or concerns); (vi) the Hamilton Anxiety Rating Scale, which measures the level of anxiety; (vii) the Parkinson's Disease Sleep Scale

(PDSS), which measures sleep and nocturnal disability in PD; and (viii) the Schwab and England Scale, which assesses the degree of functional independence in daily living. In addition, we assessed some cognitive functions exploiting five neuropsychological tests: (i) the Raven test, which measures general intelligence; (ii) the Stroop test, which measures attention and/or inhibitory functions; (iii) the Rey test, which measures verbal memory; (iv) the digit span task, which measures working memory's capacity for numbers; and (v) the phonological fluency test, which measures the ability of participants to generate words that begin with a given letter.

The rating of all scales was carried out in their best ON medication state calculated after the first morning dose which normally allowed the patient to attain the best control of symptoms. As a result, patients were rated 45–60 minutes after the administration of an L-dopa dose ranging from 100 to 200 mg.

2.3. Emotional Theatre Workshop. The theatrical workshop consisted of 3-hour daily session, once a week, giving a total of ~12 h/month for 15 months. Each session was led by two professionals, an actor and in turn a dancer or a singer. Approximately 50 minutes were spent performing either movement or voice training, while the following 50 minutes were spent in theatrical training (see Table 1 and Movies 1 and 2 in Supplementary Material available online at https://doi.org/10.1155/2017/7436725). All exercises were organized according to a theme (e.g., the experience and expression of anger). All the remaining time (~80 minutes) was focused on performing theatre scenes or theatrical tasks that required the representation of the chosen theme. The whole program was divided into three phases: (i) welcome, self-confidence, and group foundation (~4 months); (ii) emotional stress work focusing on six different emotional moods: anger, fear, happiness, sadness, surprise, and sensuality (~8 months); and (iii) free organization, interpretation, and representation of emotional states by each patient using either texts or improvisations and/or body movements (~3 months).

2.4. Physiotherapy. Physiotherapy consisted of 1.5-hour group sessions, 2 days a week, giving a total of ~12 h/month for 15 months. Each session was led by a physiotherapist. The physical therapy program was designed to increase strength, power, endurance, and aerobic capacity and to improve motor functions, postural control, balance, and gait according to the European Physiotherapy Guideline for Parkinson's Disease (for more details, see Table 2).

2.5. Statistics. Using the Shapiro-Wilk test, we verified that, in the vast majority of instances, the assumption of normality was verified (108/112 or 96.4%; see Table 3), with the exception of data recorded with the Schwab and England Scale. Thus, in the latter case, we used the Wilcoxon signed-rank test for comparisons within a group and the Mann–Whitney U test for comparisons between groups, lowering the alpha value according to the number of comparisons (alpha: 0.05/4 = 0.0125). For all the other scales, a two-way mixed-design ANOVA [between-subjects factor: GROUP (theatre; controls); within-subjects factor: TIME ($T0, T1$)] was employed

for assessing changes in the scores across the experimental conditions. Bonferroni corrections were applied to all post hoc tests (pairwise comparisons). In order to provide a measure of the "effect size," we computed the partial eta-squared (η_p^2) for each ANOVA, with values of 0.139, 0.058, and 0.01 indicating large, medium, and small effects, respectively, and Cohen's d as the effect size for t-tests, with values of 0.2, 0.5, and 0.8 indicating large, medium, and small effects [20]. As η_p^2 and Cohen's d allow comparison between the effects of a given manipulation regardless of other factors that have been manipulated, they allow comparison of our results with those of future studies.

3. Results

As shown in Table 4, at time $T0$, demographic and clinical data did not differ between the two groups. The levels of instruction were similar, preventing a possible criticism that people from a great metropolis, such as Rome, may be more educated than those coming from more rural areas.

A two-way mixed-design ANOVA on the amount of L-dopa equivalent daily dose (LEDD) (mg) administered did not show a main effect of group (M_{diff} = 117; SD = 123) ($F(1, 22)$ = 0.91; p = 0.35; η_p^2 = 0.04; 95% CI [−137; 373]) or a main effect of time (M_{diff} = 15; SD = 39) ($F(1, 22)$ = 0.15; p = 0.69; η_p^2 = 0.07; 95% CI [−65; 95]) or an interaction ($F(1, 22)$ = 2.22; p = 0.15; η_p^2 = 0.09). However, theatre-group patients on average had a small decrease in dopaminergic drug therapy during the course of the study (LEDD = 34.1 mg), while control patients needed on average an increase in dopaminergic drug therapy (LEDD = 73.8 mg).

All the other effects of theatrical training are reported in Tables 5, 6, and 7. None of the clinical scales measuring motor symptoms (UPDRS III, GFQ, and PDQ39-mobility), daily activities (UPDRS II, Schwab and England Scale (The Wilcoxon signed-rank test did not show any significant difference between $T0$ and $T1$ either in theatre patients (p = 0.65) or in controls (p = 1). The Mann–Whitney U test did not show differences between theatre patients and controls either at $T0$ (p = 0.89) or at $T1$ (p = 0.55).), and PDQ39-activities of daily living), or physical problems (UPDRS IV and PDQ39-bodily discomfort) showed significant differences either within or between the two groups. The same applied to cognitive functions measured either by the UPDRS I or by the neuropsychological tests, with the exception of the reading time of the Stroop test. Here, the main effect of time indicates that, overall, patients increased the speed of reading over the 15 months. This effect was qualified by the interaction group * time, which showed that only theatre patients improved their reading time (Tables 5, 6, and 7 and Figure 1).

While motor symptoms and cognitive functions were not affected by either treatment, four scales addressing the emotional/affective domains, that is, those measuring depression, apathy, stigma, and emotional well-being, showed significant improvements from $T0$ to $T1$ in the theatre group but not in the control group (Tables 5, 6, and 7 and Figure 1). In all these cases, the main effect of the factor time was

TABLE 1: Exercises included in a typical emotional theatre training session. It must be remarked that some but not all exercises were performed in each session.

Movement training	
Proprioception	Visualization; self-awareness; breath exercises; postural exercises
Basic motor skills practice	Breathing exercises; spinal column exercises; head exercises; limb exercises; foot exercises; hand exercises; muscle exercises; joint exercises; stretching; strength and flexibility; coordination; dissociation; active/passive motion; balance; memory; sequences; meaningful actions; nonfunctional, expressive movement
Space	Body space; personal space; proximal space; medial and distal space; imaging space; spatial cues
Time	Internal time; external time; temporal cues; rhythm
Relationship	Sound; solo work; couple work; group work; contact
Voice training	
Proprioception	Visualization; self-awareness; postural exercises
Basic motor skills practice	Spinal column exercises; head/neck exercises; limb exercises; foot exercises; hand exercises; pelvic exercises; shoulder exercises
Breathing	Diaphragmatic breathing; movements of abdominal muscles; pelvis exercises; emission of breath for increasing time/with puffs; vocal emission of the consonant "S," "SH," and "TS" for increasing time/with puffs
Resonators	Vocal emission of the "M" consonant, with closed mouth and rhythmic movements, from low to high pitches
Vowels emission	Individual emission of vowels following different orders with a single breath, from low to high pitches, from low to high volume
Articulation	Mouth and tongue exercises; facial muscles exercises; articulation of single consonants; exasperated articulations of words; rhythmic articulation of lyrics
Musicianship	Performing scales and arpeggios with different syllables/with two-syllable words from low to high pitches in different rhythms, from low to high volume
Singing	Improvisation (solo work, couple work, and choral work); learning and performing a song (choral work)
Theatre training	
Vocal technique	Breathing; diaphragmatic breathing; vocal exercise; articulation of consonant; syllables and word exercises; increasing and decreasing voice
Improvisation and experimentation	Improvisation linked on a given idea; timing and rhythm; variations about the story; including all the partners on stage in a common happening; self-collocate in a drama; fixing the acme; exit the situation; totally enter again in the drama; use of the text; apperceive a personal feeling; communicate it to audience; use of the stage like a chessboard; any step is an emotional stage; Performing with one, two, or three partners; create a story, interpreting and closing it with a comic end. Control and experience the emotional states associated with the story and, finally, reinterpret it with expressing the opposite emotion; exercises of theatrical strategies to be useful for partners; increase and decrease scenic rhythms; deconstruction of a drama, linked to bodily and vocal reps; positive training to prepare to facing audience
Dramaturgy	Comedy of Arts techniques; techniques of pantomime; use of the body to create a feature; kind of walking to fix it; study of classic text; dramaturgical analysis; methods to memorize the learned techniques of the Comedy of Arts

explained by the interaction group * time, which showed a significant improvement in theatre patients and no changes in the controls over the period of treatment. The levels of anxiety and the social support (PDQ39-social support) had a very similar tendency, but the decrease in anxiety in the theatre group did not reach significance. In addition, the theatre training led to an improvement in the quality of sleep (PDSS), the cognition measured by the subscale of the PDQ39

and, more marginally, the ability to communicate (PDQ39-communication).

4. Discussion

The present study successfully replicates our previous results by confirming the efficacy of theatre therapy as an add-on rehabilitative tool for PD patients [19]. The novel finding is

TABLE 2: Exercises included in the physiotherapy rehabilitation program. Depending on the single patient's motor and functional status, the physiotherapist could include exercises other than those indicated as basic exercises.

Activities	Basic exercises
Supine position (15 minutes)	Diaphragmatic, segmental, and deep breathing exercises; movements to the fullest range of motion of hip, knee, ankle, shoulder, elbow, and wrist; postural changes to lateral and prone position
Seated position (15 minutes)	Muscle-stretching of scapular, hip flexor, hamstring, and gastrocnemius; active flexion, extensions, and rotation of upper and lower limbs
Standing position (15 minutes)	Standing wall push-up; pelvic mobility (anterior and posterior tilts); side to side tilts; pelvic clock exercise and ball exercise to facilitate sitting control; sit to stand transfer
Overground gait training (20 minutes)	Overground gait training (forwards, backwards, and lateral); walking on the spot
Balance training (15 minutes)	Weight shifts in both sitting and standing; sitting and standing activities on gymnastic ball

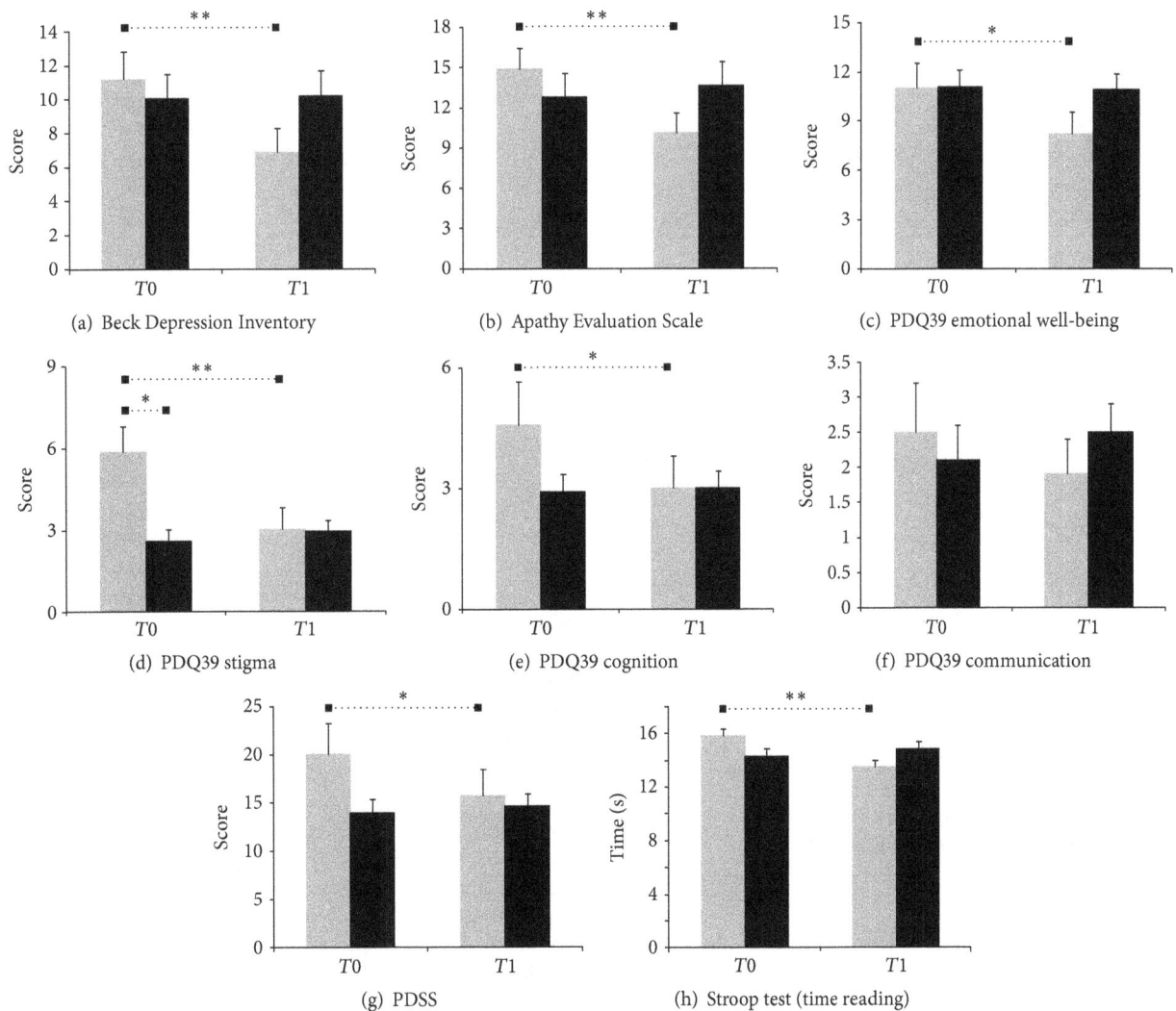

FIGURE 1: Mean scores and standard error of the means at the two time points for the theatre (gray bars) and control group (black bars) in the scales or subscales showing a significant effect at the mixed-design ANOVAs (see text and Table 5 for more details). Bars indicate significant differences after post hoc analyses, the single * indicates values of $p < 0.01$, and the double * indicates values of $p < 0.001$. PDQ39: Parkinson's Disease Quality of Life Scale; PDSS: Parkinson's Disease Sleep Scale.

TABLE 3: *p* values obtained from the Shapiro-Wilk test of normality for the two groups of PD patients (theatre group and control group) in all clinical scales and subscales at the beginning (*T*0) and the end (*T*1) of the rehabilitation treatments. *p* values less than 0.05 indicate that the data are not from a normally distributed population and are indicated in bold. UPDRS: Unified Parkinson's Disease Rating Scale; GFQ: Gait and Falls Questionnaire; PDQ39: Parkinson's Disease Quality of Life Scale; PDSS: Parkinson's Disease Sleep Scale.

	Theatre		Controls	
	*T*0	*T*1	*T*0	*T*1
UPDRS I	0.147	0.563	0.109	0.370
UPDRS II	0.18	0.38	0.579	**0.047**
UPDRS III	0.666	0.638	0.596	0.375
UPDRS IV	0.303	0.091	0.175	0.762
Schwab and England Scale	**0.020**	**0.012**	0.051	**0.004**
GFQ	0.148	0.302	0.599	0.684
PDQ39 (*total score*)	0.240	0.542	0.062	0.784
PDQ39 (*mobility*)	0.834	0.526	0.247	0.667
PDQ39 (*activities of daily living*)	0.559	0.703	0.733	0.088
PDQ39 (*Emotional well-being*)	0.303	0.956	0.137	0.825
PDQ39 (*stigma*)	0.133	**0.008**	0.071	0.412
PDQ39 (*social support*)	0.144	0.083	0.333	0.598
PDQ39 (*cognition*)	0.201	0.109	0.143	0.135
PDQ39 (*communication*)	0.071	0.095	0.135	0.174
PDQ39 (*bodily discomfort*)	0.745	0.360	0.916	0.813
Beck Depression Inventory	0.126	0.324	0.103	**0.013**
Apathy Evaluation Scale	0.252	0.291	0.071	0.144
Hamilton Anxiety Rating Scale	0.338	0.286	0.440	0.366
PDSS	0.702	0.341	0.343	0.479
Raven test	0.099	0.051	0.623	0.256
Stroop (word reading time)	0.448	0.659	0.393	0.189
Stroop (color reading time)	0.080	0.262	0.542	**0.025**
Stroop (interference reading time)	0.321	0.080	0.278	0.365
Rey immediate recall	0.778	0.757	0.128	0.088
Rey delayed recall	0.551	0.923	0.086	0.062
Forward digit span	0.197	0.543	0.432	0.354
Backward digit span	0.069	0.123	0.433	0.187
Phonological fluency test	0.382	0.216	0.450	0.416

that theatre training based on the representation of emotions speeds up the appearance of benefits in the affective domain. We will discuss why theatre might represent a very effective form of cognitive rehabilitation.

4.1. Why Is Theatre Training Effective? Even though motor disturbances are mandatory to make the diagnosis of PD, there is now a consensus around the idea that this is not a pure motor disorder but a multifaceted one. Several factors contribute to its severity. Nonmotor symptoms have been shown to play a more important role than motor symptoms in reducing the health-related and perceived QoL in PD [21, 22]. In particular, depression seems to deeply affect the feelings

about the disease perception and its future consequences [21, 23].

Recent findings have started to shed light on the link between the depletion of dopaminergic neurons occurring in PD and the genesis of neuropsychiatric nonmotor symptoms. The disruption of the dopaminergic system seems to affect the decision-making processes underlying the genesis of motor acts (see [24]) because of a wrong evaluation of the costs of movements [25, 26], making this cost too high [26]. The wrong value assignment decreases the motivation to act, inducing either bradykinesia or akinesia and even apathy. Other evidence indicates that, in healthy subjects, L-dopa not only plays a role during decision-making under risky choices but also has a critical role in generating a subjective feeling of happiness which follows the receipt of reward [27]. Therefore, the loss of dopamine is likely to affect both the planning of actions and the pleasant feelings normally associated with rewarding events possibly leading to anhedonia, a core symptom of major depression. Overall, it is not surprising that an objectively good control of motor symptoms might not be coupled with a positive feeling of well-being experienced by patients. This evidence has prompted the need for developing auxiliary approaches to medical therapy. However, the effectiveness of these approaches had rarely been explored with proper randomized controlled trials (for a review, see [28, 29]). Most studies suffer from having small and/or heterogeneous samples, and sometimes methodologies are not rigorous enough (see [12] for a remarkable exception). In addition, the effects of most interventions do not last more than a few months, a span of time that is very likely too short to promote the so-called brain plasticity, that is, the neural mechanism underlying behavioral changes (e.g., [30, 31]). Moreover, another factor has to be considered to evaluate the effectiveness of a therapy, that is, the different degrees to which it affects motor, emotional, and interpersonal components. For instance, art therapies based on drawing, painting, sculpting, or music playing allow patients to express themselves spontaneously, but they tend to lack the intersubjective interactions normally occurring in real life, and their impact on body motor control is rather limited. Dance and martial arts require physical involvement but they do not reproduce the intersubjective interactions of real life. The opposite holds true for occupational therapies. In contrast, theatre training allows a more holistic approach as, to successfully impersonate a character, an actor needs to control his body, reproduce the character's emotions and way of thinking, and identify himself with his social role. To some extent, an actor needs to learn a way to become another person on the stage and to behave accordingly. This is potentially a successful exercise through which PD patients could develop new strategies for carefully controlling their bodies and minds within a protected environment, that is, in a place where they do not feel judged by others. In addition, both during and outside the performance, patients have to continuously interact and thus they are forced to socialize. These unique features make theatre an ideal playground for deeply motivating patients, allowing them to reacquire the control of their social, psychological, and emotional life and to transfer these abilities to everyday life situations.

TABLE 4: Clinical data of PD patients of theatre (TH) and control (CT) groups. For each patient, sex, age, years of education, side of disease onset (L = left; R = right), years since diagnosis, mini-mental state examination (MMSE) scores, Hoehn and Yahr scores (H&Y) in ON and OFF state (see text for definitions), and L-dopa equivalent daily dose (LEDD) (mg) at time $T0$ are given. At the bottom of the table, the t values, the corresponding degrees of freedom, the p values, and Cohen's d values for the comparisons between the two groups are reported. *Equal variances were not assumed. §This patient had a deep brain stimulator.

	Sex		Age		Years of education		Side of onset		Years since diagnosis		MMSE		H&Y		LEDD (mg)	
	TH	CT	TH	CT	TH	CT	TH	CT	TH	CT	TH	CT	TH	CT	TH	CT
1	M	M	72	57	18	13	L	R	17	8	29	29	3	3	1260	936
2	F	F	57	65	13	5	R	R	7	7	29	30	2	3	505	700
3	M	F	66	64	18	13	R	L	7	6	30	30	3	3	1584	500
4	M	F	67	55	18	13	R	L	8	8	29	29	3	3	728	300
5	M	F	61	68	13	18	R	L	12	8	27	28	3	3	480	630
6	F	F	62	57	13	13	R	R	18	10	29	28	2	3	1073	850
7	F	F	60	47	5	8	L	R	11	4	29	27	2	2	739	453
8	F	F	60	50	18	13	R	R	3	9	30	27	1	2	153	500
9§	F	M	42	65	12	13	L	L	10	5	25	30	2	3	480	353
10	F	M	56	63	10	13	L	R	4	5	25	29	2	2	327	400
11	M	M	39	72	18	8	R	R	7	18	28	30	3	3	1051	605
12	F	M	64	62	11	13	L	L	8	6	28	30	2	2	200	250
Mean			58.8	60.3	13.9	11.9			9.3	7.8	28.2	28.9	2.4	2.7	715	539.8
SD			9.6	7.6	4.2	3.4			4.2	3.7	1.7	1.2	0.2	0.5	445.2	212.7
t-test			$t(22) = 0.4$		$t(22) = -1.3$				$t(22) = 0.9$		$t(22) = -1.3$		$t(22) = -1.0$		$t(15.8) = 1.2$	
			p = 0.67		**p = 0.21**				**p = 0.38**		**p = 0.22**		**p = 0.31**		**p = 0.24***	
			Cohen's		Cohen's				Cohen's		Cohen's		Cohen's		Cohen's	
			d = 0.18		**d = 0.54**				**d = 0.39**		**d = 0.5**		**d = 0.82**		**d = 0.52**	

TABLE 5: Mean scores and standard deviations obtained by the two groups of PD patients (theatre group and control group) in all clinical scales and subscales at the beginning (T0) and the end (T1) of the rehabilitation treatments.

	Theatre		Controls	
	T0	T1	T0	T1
UPDRS I	2.9 ± 1.9	3 ± 1.9	2.8 ± 1.7	3.1 ± 1.4
UPDRS II	8.1 ± 4.9	7.8 ± 4.9	6.6 ± 3.8	7.6 ± 4.9
UPDRS III	21.4 ± 9.3	24.2 ± 9.9	21.2 ± 5	22 ± 4.9
UPDRS IV	4.4 ± 3.9	3.2 ± 3.2	3.9 ± 2.2	4.1 ± 1.7
Schwab and England Scale	90 ± 7.4	89.2 ± 6.7	90 ± 9.5	90 ± 10.4
GFQ	20.1 ± 15.8	20.7 ± 15.7	10.5 ± 6.2	10.9 ± 6.4
PDQ39 (total score)	58.1 ± 27.1	50.3 ± 22.6	47.3 ± 14	52.2 ± 16.9
PDQ39 (mobility)	15.4 ± 9.2	16.8 ± 9.3	12.8 ± 5.7	15.8 ± 5.5
PDQ39 (activities of daily living)	9.3 ± 5.3	9.1 ± 4.1	8 ± 2.9	9.7 ± 4.2
PDQ39 (Emotional well-being)	11 ± 5.5	8.2 ± 4.9	11.1 ± 3.6	10.9 ± 3.3
PDQ39 (stigma)	6.8 ± 3.9	3.5 ± 3.3	3 ± 1.8	3.4 ± 1.7
PDQ39 (social support)	2.4 ± 2.1	1.9 ± 1.4	1.9 ± 1.4	1.9 ± 1.1
PDQ39 (cognition)	4.6 ± 3.7	3 ± 2.8	2.9 ± 1.5	3 ± 1.5
PDQ39 (communication)	2.5 ± 2.3	1.9 ± 1.6	2.1 ± 1.6	2.5 ± 1.3
PDQ39 (bodily discomfort)	6.1 ± 2.1	5.9 ± 2.4	5.5 ± 2	5 ± 2.1
Beck Depression Inventory	11.4 ± 5.9	7 ± 5	10.3 ± 5.2	10.4 ± 5.3
Apathy Evaluation Scale	14.9 ± 5.6	10.1 ± 5.3	12.8 ± 6.1	13.7 ± 6.2
Hamilton Anxiety Rating Scale	13.4 ± 5.6	10.2 ± 6.1	13.8 ± 7.2	14.3 ± 6.8
PDSS	20.1 ± 11.1	15.8 ± 9.5	13.9 ± 5.4	14.7 ± 4.3
Raven test	29.1 ± 5.1	29.4 ± 5.5	28.9 ± 3.8	29.2 ± 3.1
Stroop (word reading time)	15.8 ± 1.7	13.5 ± 1.9	14.3 ± 1.9	14.8 ± 2.2
Stroop (color reading time)	22.3 ± 4.4	21.3 ± 4.6	19.8 ± 3	20 ± 2.7
Stroop (interference reading time)	39.5 ± 10.6	38.5 ± 11.8	42.8 ± 8	43.2 ± 6.8
Rey immediate recall	47.8 ± 8.4	48.4 ± 9.3	43.3 ± 9.3	43.9 ± 7.3
Rey delayed recall	9.3 ± 2.2	9.5 ± 2.5	9.3 ± 3	9.8 ± 2.6
Forward digit span	6.8 ± 1.5	6.9 ± 1.6	6.9 ± 1.2	7 ± 1.3
Backward digit span	4.3 ± 1.1	4.2 ± 0.9	4.1 ± 1.2	4.5 ± 1
Phonological fluency test	45.3 ± 15.4	46.1 ± 13.4	38.2 ± 9.8	39 ± 9.1

4.2. The Effectiveness of Emotional Theatre. A novel finding of the current work is that the emotional theatre training boosts the improvements in the emotional sphere, allowing the emergence of significant ameliorations in more clinical scales tapping the affective domain than in our previous study [19]. After 15 months, there were no improvements in any of the clinical scales measuring either motor symptoms, daily activities, or physical problems. Nevertheless, even though patients still suffered from physical discomforts, their feelings about the disease and about its evolution were so positive that they declared they could not stop their theatrical activities (Movies 3 and 4). The improvements in the quality of sleep are likely to be associated with the increased psychological well-being. This is in keeping with the idea that improvements in mood bring about an improved perception of the disease [21, 22, 32]. It must be remarked that performing this type of theatre training is not an enjoyable activity by definition. Patients experienced some form of distress when playing emotionally negative events (e.g., the feeling of being powerless in front of someone else; see Movie 2), and some of them reexperienced, directly or indirectly, painful situations

(e.g., the loss of some beloved person). Therefore, our results could not be simply explained by the fact that patients were attending an enjoyable social activity: the training was a complex pathway into an emotional world, leading the patients to regain the ability to manage their emotions much better than patients who were having physiotherapy (i.e., the most common treatment associated with medical therapy). In our opinion, these elements could explain the different outcomes of other types of complementary therapies, for example, dance [13, 14] or martial arts [12].

4.3. Limitations of the Study. We are aware of some methodological limitations of our study. First, this is not a randomized study and in Materials and Methods we have explained why we exploited this experimental design. However, we measured several clinical parameters (diagnosis, age, years of disease, onset of disease, education, H&Y, LEDD, and MMSE) and we demonstrated that they were not different across theatre and control groups. In addition, the two groups were scored by blind raters, thus avoiding bias during the evaluations. Obviously, as in similar studies, it was impossible

TABLE 6: Results of the two-way mixed-design ANOVA with GROUP (theatre; controls) as between subjects' factor and TIME ($T0, T1$) as within subjects' factor, comparing scores of clinical scales (or subscales, top part of the table) and of neuropsychological tests (lower part of the table). Asterisk ($*$) indicates subscales of Parkinson's Disease Quality of Life Scale (PDQ39). η_p^2 represents the partial eta-squared; values higher than 0.14 indicate strong effect sizes (see Section 2.5 for further details). p values less than 0.05 as well as the corresponding F and η_p^2 values are indicated in bold. Unified UPDRS: Parkinson's Disease Rating Scale; GFQ: Gait and Falls Questionnaire; PDSS: Parkinson's Disease Sleep Scale; TR: time for reading words; TC: time for naming color; TI: time for naming color during interference.

	TIME			GROUP			TIME × GROUP		
	$F(1, 22)$	p value	η_p^2	$F(1, 22)$	p value	η_p^2	$F(1, 22)$	p value	η_p^2
UPDRS I	0.83	0.37	0.04	0.004	0.95	<0.001	0.29	0.59	0.01
UPDRS II	0.26	0.62	0.01	0.22	0.64	0.01	1.03	0.32	0.04
UPDRS III	1.55	0.23	0.07	0.19	0.67	0.01	0.44	0.51	0.02
UPDRS IV	1.16	0.29	0.05	0.04	0.85	0.002	1.98	0.17	0.08
GFQ	0.26	0.62	0.01	4.06	0.06	0.16	0.01	0.93	<0.001
PDQ39	0.47	0.49	0.02	0.26	0.61	0.01	3.92	0.06	0.15
Mobility*	3.09	0.09	0.12	0.41	0.53	0.02	0.37	0.55	0.02
Activities of daily living*	0.57	0.46	0.02	0.06	0.81	0.003	0.86	0.36	0.04
Emotional well-being*	**5.4**	**0.03**	**0.19**	0.71	0.41	0.03	**4.2**	**0.05**	**0.16**
Stigma*	**14.1**	**0.001**	**0.39**	3.24	0.08	0.13	**23.3**	**<0.001**	**0.51**
Social support*	1.44	0.24	0.61	0.12	0.73	0.005	2.82	0.11	0.11
Cognition*	**5.13**	**0.03**	**0.19**	0.72	0.41	0.03	**6.3**	**0.02**	**0.22**
Communication*	0.14	0.71	0.006	0.01	0.9	0.001	**5.11**	**0.03**	**0.19**
Bodily discomfort*	1.26	0.27	0.05	0.82	0.38	0.04	0.31	0.58	0.01
Beck Depression Inventory	**29.6**	**<0.001**	**0.57**	0.27	0.6	0.12	**34.4**	**<0.001**	**0.61**
Apathy Evaluation Scale	**8.78**	**0.007**	**0.28**	0.09	0.76	0.004	**18.93**	**<0.001**	**0.46**
Hamilton Anxiety Rating Scale	1.47	0.24	0.06	0.85	0.37	0.04	2.73	0.11	0.11
PDSS	**4.34**	**0.049**	**0.16**	0.13	0.27	0.06	**8.7**	**0.007**	**0.28**
Raven test	0.65	0.43	0.03	0.13	0.91	0.001	0.13	0.9	0.001
Stroop test (TR)	**6.81**	**0.016**	**0.24**	0.14	0.91	0.001	**14.4**	**0.001**	**0.4**
Stroop test (TC)	0.82	0.37	0.04	1.59	0.22	0.07	2.28	0.14	0.09
Stroop test (TI)	0.06	0.81	0.003	1.15	0.29	0.05	0.35	0.56	0.016
Rey test (immediate recall)	0.24	0.63	0.01	1.84	0.19	0.08	<0.001	1	<0.001
Rey test (delayed recall)	0.94	0.34	0.04	0.04	0.84	0.002	0.1	0.75	0.005
Digit span test (forward)	0.08	0.77	0.004	0.03	0.87	0.001	<0.001	1	<0.001
Digit span test (backward)	0.37	0.55	0.02	0.07	0.8	0.003	0.83	0.37	0.04
Phonological fluency test	0.6	0.44	0.03	2.12	0.16	0.09	<0.001	1	<0.001

TABLE 7: Post hoc analyses of significant interactions obtained in two-way mixed-design ANOVAs [between subjects' factor: GROUP (theatre; controls); within subjects' factor: TIME ($T0, T1$), see Table 5]. Data are reported just for those post hoc tests which survived the Bonferroni correction. Asterisk ($*$) indicates subscales of Parkinson's Disease Quality of Life Scale. M_{diff}: differences between the means; SD_{diff}: standard deviation of M_{diff}, CI_{diff}: confidence interval of M_{diff}. Other abbreviations are as in Table 6.

	Theatre $T0$ versus theatre $T1$					Theatre $T0$ versus controls $T0$				
	M_{diff}	SD_{diff}	CI_{diff}	Cohen's d	p value	M_{diff}	SD_{diff}	CI_{diff}	Cohen's d	p value
Emotional well-being*	2.8	0.9	[0.9, 4.7]	0.72	0.005	—	—	—	—	—
Stigma*	3.3	0.5	[2.2, 4.5]	1.2	<0.001	3.8	1.2	[1.3, 6.4]	1.5	0.005
Cognition*	1.6	0.5	[0.6, 2.5]	0.63	0.003	—	—	—	—	—
Beck Depression Inventory	4.4	0.5	[3.3, 5.6]	1.07	<0.001	—	—	—	—	—
Apathy Evaluation Scale	4.8	0.9	[2.9, 6.8]	1.18	<0.001	—	—	—	—	—
PDSS	4.3	1.2	[1.8, 6.8]	0.55	0.002	—	—	—	—	—
Stroop test (TR)	2.2	0.5	[1.2, 3.3]	1.71	<0.001	—	—	—	—	—

to make patients blind to the treatment condition. Overall, we believe that the limitation of this experimental approach is more theoretical than practical, as it must be supposed that unpredictable and hidden factors systematically affected a certain group.

Second, our sample is relatively small (but similar to those of most studies in this field (e.g., [13–15])). To address this problem, we performed very stringent statistical analyses providing parameters that allow estimation of the effect size and facilitate the interpretation of the substantive as well as the statistical significance of the results [20]. In all instances, we had strong or very strong effect sizes, indicating the consistency of our findings.

Third, we had a relatively high drop-out rate, mainly at the recruitment stage, which was principally due to the length of the treatment. Patients at the beginning of the study were requested to give their availability for 15 months, that is, a very long period of time especially for people affected by a neurodegenerative disorder. Indeed, we are not aware of other studies able to keep patients for such a long period of time.

Fourth, as in the previous study, we included patients with a moderate form of PD because they are likely to fully enjoy the theatrical experience. However, whether this treatment could also be effective on patients with more severe forms of PD, maybe implementing a virtual reality training (e.g., [33]) for those who could not walk, needs to be tested.

Fifth, as clinical scales are self-reported measures, they require the conscious participation of the person, which can alter the final outcomes. Thus, there is a need to collect data such as psychophysiological measurements which can be used to monitor the emotional state of patients independently of their conscious reporting to assess how theatre training changes the processing of affective states of PD patients during the therapy.

5. Conclusions

In conclusion, even though this work suffers from some weaknesses and must be viewed as a pilot study, it confirms that theatre represents a valid add-on therapy for PD and it provides some evidence that emotional training improves the patients' mood and thus patients' QoL.

Disclosure

An earlier version of this work was presented as a poster at the 21st World Congress on Parkinson's Disease and Related Disorders, 2016 (http://www.prd-journal.com/article/S1353-8020(15)00966-9/fulltext).

Acknowledgments

The authors thank all patients for their participation in the study. Giovanni Mirabella wishes to acknowledge the Fondazione Neurone (http://www.fondazioneneurone.it/) and PARKIN-ZONE onlus for their financial support.

References

[1] K. R. Chaudhuri and A. H. Schapira, "Non-motor symptoms of Parkinson's disease: dopaminergic pathophysiology and treatment," *The Lancet Neurology*, vol. 8, no. 5, pp. 464–474, 2009.

[2] R. B. Postuma and J. Montplaisir, "Predicting Parkinson's disease—why, when, and how?" *Parkinsonism & Related Disorders*, vol. 15, supplement 3, pp. S105–S109, 2009.

[3] G. C. Cotzias, P. S. Papavasiliou, and R. Gellene, "L-dopa in parkinson's syndrome," *The New England Journal of Medicine*, vol. 281, no. 15, p. 272, 1969.

[4] S. Fahn, "The history of dopamine and levodopa in the treatment of Parkinson's disease," *Movement Disorders*, vol. 23, supplement 3, pp. S497–S508, 2008.

[5] A. E. Lang and A. M. Lozano, "Parkinson's disease. First of two parts," *The New England Journal of Medicine*, vol. 339, no. 15, pp. 1044–1053, 1998.

[6] R. W. Bohannon, "Physical rehabilitation in neurologic diseases," *Current Opinion in Neurology*, vol. 6, no. 5, pp. 765–772, 1993.

[7] L. Tickle-Degnen, T. Ellis, M. H. Saint-Hilaire, C. A. Thomas, and R. C. Wagenaar, "Self-management rehabilitation and health-related quality of life in Parkinson's disease: a randomized controlled trial," *Movement Disorders*, vol. 25, no. 2, pp. 194–204, 2010.

[8] C. L. Tomlinson, S. Patel, C. Meek et al., "Physiotherapy versus placebo or no intervention in Parkinson's disease," *Cochrane Database of Systematic Reviews*, vol. 8, Article ID CD002817, 2012.

[9] W. Carne, D. X. Cifu, P. Marcinko et al., "Efficacy of multidisciplinary treatment program on long-term outcomes of individuals with Parkinson's disease," *Journal of Rehabilitation Research and Development*, vol. 42, no. 6, pp. 779–786, 2005.

[10] C. W. Olanow, M. B. Stern, and K. Sethi, "The scientific and clinical basis for the treatment of Parkinson disease," *Neurology*, vol. 72, no. 21, pp. S1–S136, 2009.

[11] J.-P. Bach, U. Ziegler, G. Deuschl, R. Dodel, and G. Doblhammer-Reiter, "Projected numbers of people with movement disorders in the years 2030 and 2050," *Movement Disorders*, vol. 26, no. 12, pp. 2286–2290, 2011.

[12] F. Li, P. Harmer, K. Fitzgerald et al., "Tai chi and postural stability in patients with Parkinson's disease," *The New England Journal of Medicine*, vol. 366, no. 6, pp. 511–519, 2012.

[13] M. E. Hackney and G. M. Earhart, "Effects of dance on movement control in Parkinson's disease: a comparison of Argentine tango and American ballroom," *Journal of Rehabilitation Medicine*, vol. 41, no. 6, pp. 475–481, 2009.

[14] D. Volpe, M. Signorini, A. Marchetto, T. Lynch, and M. E. Morris, "A comparison of Irish set dancing and exercises for people with Parkinson's disease: a phase II feasibility study," *BMC Geriatrics*, vol. 13, no. 1, article 54, 2013.

[15] C. Pacchetti, F. Mancini, R. Aglieri, C. Fundaró, E. Martignoni, and G. Nappi, "Active music therapy in Parkinson's disease: an integrative method for motor and emotional rehabilitation," *Psychosomatic Medicine*, vol. 62, no. 3, pp. 386–393, 2000.

[16] E. Sproesser, M. A. Viana, E. M. A. B. Quagliato, and E. A. P. de Souza, "The effect of psychotherapy in patients with PD: a

controlled study," *Parkinsonism & Related Disorders*, vol. 16, no. 4, pp. 298–300, 2010.

[17] M. E. A. Armento, M. A. Stanley, L. Marsh et al., "Cognitive behavioral therapy for depression and anxiety in Parkinson's disease: a clinical review," *Journal of Parkinson's Disease*, vol. 2, no. 2, pp. 135–151, 2012.

[18] E. R. Foster, M. Bedekar, and L. Tickle-Degnen, "Systematic review of the effectiveness of occupational therapy-related interventions for people with Parkinson's disease," *The American Journal of Occupational Therapy*, vol. 68, no. 1, pp. 39–49, 2014.

[19] N. Modugno, S. Iaconelli, M. Fiorilli, F. Lena, I. Kusch, and G. Mirabella, "Active theater as a complementary therapy for Parkinson's disease rehabilitation: a pilot study," *The Scientific World Journal*, vol. 10, pp. 2301–2313, 2010.

[20] D. Lakens, "Calculating and reporting effect sizes to facilitate cumulative science: a practical primer for t-tests and ANOVAs," *Frontiers in Psychology*, vol. 4, article 863, 2013.

[21] B. Müller, J. Assmus, K. Herlofson, J. P. Larsen, and O.-B. Tysnes, "Importance of motor vs. non-motor symptoms for health-related quality of life in early Parkinson's disease," *Parkinsonism & Related Disorders*, vol. 19, no. 11, pp. 1027–1032, 2013.

[22] D. Santos-García and R. de la Fuente-Fernández, "Impact of non-motor symptoms on health-related and perceived quality of life in Parkinson's disease," *Journal of the Neurological Sciences*, vol. 332, no. 1-2, pp. 136–140, 2013.

[23] E. B. Forsaa, J. P. Larsen, T. Wentzel-Larsen, K. Herlofson, and G. Alves, "Predictors and course of health-related quality of life in Parkinson's disease," *Movement Disorders*, vol. 23, no. 10, pp. 1420–1427, 2008.

[24] G. Mirabella, "Should I stay or should I go? Conceptual underpinnings of goal-directed actions," *Frontiers in Systems Neuroscience*, vol. 8, no. 206, 2014.

[25] P. Mazzoni, A. Hristova, and J. W. Krakauer, "Why don't we move faster? Parkinson's disease, movement vigor, and implicit motivation," *The Journal of Neuroscience*, vol. 27, no. 27, pp. 7105–7116, 2007.

[26] S. Tinaz, A. S. Pillai, and M. Hallett, "Sequence effect in Parkinson's disease is related to motor energetic cost," *Frontiers in Neurology*, vol. 7, no. 83, 2016.

[27] R. B. Rutledge, N. Skandali, P. Dayan, and R. J. Dolan, "Dopaminergic modulation of decision making and subjective well-being," *The Journal of Neuroscience*, vol. 35, no. 27, pp. 9811–9822, 2015.

[28] D. Bega, P. Gonzalez-Latapi, C. Zadikoff, and T. Simuni, "A review of the clinical evidence for complementary and alternative therapies in parkinson's disease," *Current Treatment Options in Neurology*, vol. 16, no. 10, article 314, 2014.

[29] G. Mirabella, "Is art therapy a reliable tool for rehabilitating people suffering from brain/mental diseases?" *The Journal of Alternative and Complementary Medicine*, vol. 21, no. 4, pp. 196–199, 2015.

[30] T. Elbert, C. Pantev, C. Wienbruch, B. Rockstroh, and E. Taub, "Increased cortical representation of the fingers of the left hand in string players," *Science*, vol. 270, no. 5234, pp. 305–307, 1995.

[31] M. A. Lebedev, G. Mirabella, I. Erchova, and M. E. Diamond, "Experience-dependent plasticity of rat barrel cortex: redistribution of activity across barrel-columns," *Cerebral Cortex*, vol. 10, no. 1, pp. 23–31, 2000.

[32] C. S. Hurt, J. Weinman, R. Lee, and R. G. Brown, "The relationship of depression and disease stage to patient perceptions of Parkinson's disease," *Journal of Health Psychology*, vol. 17, no. 7, pp. 1076–1088, 2012.

[33] A. Gorini, A. Gaggioli, C. Vigna, and G. Riva, "A second life for eHealth: prospects for the use of 3-D virtual worlds in clinical psychology," *Journal of Medical Internet Research*, vol. 10, no. 3, article e21, 2008.

8

Resting State fMRI: A Valuable Tool for Studying Cognitive Dysfunction in PD

Kai Li,[1,2] **Wen Su,**[1] **Shu-Hua Li,**[1] **Ying Jin,**[1] **and Hai-Bo Chen** ⓘ[1]

[1]*Department of Neurology, Beijing Hospital, National Center of Gerontology, No. 1 Dahua Road, Dong Dan,*
 Beijing 100730, China
[2]*Department of Geriatric Medicine, Beijing Hospital, National Center of Gerontology, No. 1 Dahua Road, Dong Dan,*
 Beijing 100730, China

Correspondence should be addressed to Hai-Bo Chen; chenhbneuro@263.net

Academic Editor: Jan Aasly

Cognitive impairment is a common disabling symptom in PD. Unlike motor symptoms, the mechanism underlying cognitive dysfunction in Parkinson's disease (PD) remains unclear and may involve multiple pathophysiological processes. Resting state functional magnetic resonance imaging (rs-fMRI) is a fast-developing research field, and its application in cognitive impairments in PD is rapidly growing. In this review, we summarize rs-fMRI studies on cognitive function in PD and discuss the strong potential of rs-fMRI in this area. rs-fMRI can help reveal the pathophysiology of cognitive symptoms in PD, facilitate early identification of PD patients with cognitive impairment, distinguish PD dementia from dementia with Lewy bodies, and monitor and guide treatment for cognitive impairment in PD. In particular, ongoing and future longitudinal studies would enhance the ability of rs-fMRI in predicting PD dementia. In combination with other modalities such as positron emission tomography, rs-fMRI could give us more information on the underlying mechanism of cognitive deficits in PD.

1. Introduction

Parkinson's disease (PD) is one of the most common neurodegenerative diseases. Traditionally, it has been regarded as a movement disorder characterized by the motor symptoms, such as bradykinesia, resting tremor, and rigidity. Up to now, it is well known that cognitive impairment is a common nonmotor symptom in patients with PD, even in the early stages or before motor symptom onset [1]. Furthermore, about 40% of the PD patients suffer from PD dementia (PDD) in cross-sectional studies [2]. In a longitudinal study, 83% of the PD patients developed dementia during the 20-year follow-up [3]. Despite the heavy burden caused by cognitive impairments in PD, we still lack effective treatments for cognitive symptoms in PD. Although acetylcholinesterase inhibitors could provide modest help, the progression of cognitive decline is inevitable [4].

The underlying mechanism of motor symptoms of PD is depleted dopaminergic cells in the substantia nigra [5].

In contrast, the pathophysiological basis of cognitive impairments in PD remains uncertain. Disrupted frontal-subcortical circuits due to dopaminergic neuron damage and wide deposition of α-synuclein, β-amyloid, and tau proteins might play a role [6, 7]. Various neurotransmitters including dopamine, acetylcholine, serotonin, and noradrenaline are involved [7]. A better understanding of the pathophysiology of cognitive impairments in PD can facilitate early identification and improved intervention for cognitive symptoms.

Functional MRI (fMRI) measures the blood-oxygen-level dependent (BOLD) signal in the brain, which is determined by the amount of oxyhemoglobin and deoxyhemoglobin and reflects neuronal activity. Resting state fMRI (rs-fMRI) estimates the brain BOLD signal while the subjects are awake without performing any specific task [8]. MRI is widely equipped by hospitals and research institutions; rs-fMRI is easy to perform and has an excellent safety profile compared to other imaging modalities such as computed tomography (CT), positron emission tomography (PET), and single photon emission computed tomography (SPECT). Therefore, the application of rs-fMRI in neurological and psychiatric disorders has been rapidly increasing in the recent two decades. There are many approaches that can analyze the rs-fMRI data, including amplitude of low-frequency fluctuations (ALFF) and regional homogeneity (ReHo) which reflect local activity of individual regions or voxels, as well as seed-based functional connectivity (FC), independent component analysis (ICA), effective connectivity, machine learning, and graph theory-based analyses which measure the connectivity characteristics of different regions [8, 9]. rs-fMRI has been applied to investigate the pathophysiology of motor and nonmotor symptoms in PD, help early and differential diagnosis, predict disease progression, and guide treatment. In this review, we summarize recent developments of rs-fMRI studies on cognitive impairments in PD.

2. Uncovering the Pathophysiology of Cognitive Impairment in PD Using rs-fMRI

2.1. rs-fMRI Studies on PD Patients with Mild Cognitive Impairment (MCI) or Dementia. Cognitive activities rely on the coordination of various brain regions. Several networks have been established by rs-fMRI: the default mode network (DMN), the visual network, the sensorimotor network, the executive control network, and the frontoparietal network [10]. rs-fMRI is useful for improving our understanding of the mechanism of cognitive impairment in PD. Gorges et al. performed seed-based analyses on rs-fMRI in PD patients with and without MCI and healthy controls. Compared with the controls, PD patients without cognitive impairment had increased FC in multiple regions, while PD-MCI patients had decreased FC mainly within the DMN. The increased FC in PD patients without cognitive impairment might be a compensatory mechanism preceding PD-MCI [11]. Hou et al. conducted a study on drug-naïve PD patients with and without MCI and found FC reduction in both PD groups. In addition, compared with PD patients without cognitive impairment, PD-MCI patients had significantly reduced FC between DMN and the middle frontal and middle temporal gyri; within the DMN, PD-MCI patients had reduced FC between the anterior temporal lobe and inferior frontal gyrus. The FC alterations in the PD group were associated with attention/working memory and memory function [12]. Chen et al. studied the FC between posterior cingulate cortex and other regions of the bran in PD patients with and without MCI. They found decreased FC between the posterior cingulate cortex and the right temporal gyrus and increased FC between the posterior cingulate cortex and multiple brain regions in PD patients without cognitive impairment compared with healthy controls and reduced FC between the posterior cingulate cortex and several areas including bilateral prefrontal cortex, the left parietal-occipital junction, and the right temporal gyrus in PD-MCI patients compared with PD patients without cognitive impairment. The FC of the posterior cingulate cortex with other brain areas was associated with MoCA and MMSE scores in the PD patients [13]. Baggio et al. performed ICA and seed-based rs-fMRI analyses in PD patients without cognitive impairment, PD-MCI patients, and healthy controls. They found that PD-MCI patients had decreased connectivity between the dorsal attention network and the right frontoinsular regions, and this alteration was associated with attention/executive function. The DMN showed increased connectivity with medial and lateral occipito-parietal regions in PD-MCI patients, which was correlated with worse visuospatial/visuoperceptual abilities [14]. In another study by Baggio et al., graph theory-based analysis showed that PD-MCI patients had reduced long-range connections and increased local interconnectedness including higher measures of clustering, small-worldness, and modularity. The local interconnectedness was associated with visuospatial/visuoperceptual and memory functions in the PD patients [15]. Peraza et al. compared the intra- and inter-network changes in PD patients with and without MCI and found that PD-MCI patients had intranetwork impairments in the attention, executive function, and motor control networks compared with PD patients with normal cognitive function, as well as internetwork alterations in the visual perception together with the three above-mentioned networks [16]. Amboni et al. assessed the brain networks using ICA analysis in PD patients with and without MCI. Both PD groups showed impaired DMN connectivity, while the PD-MCI group showed impaired FC in the frontoparietal network. In addition, the decreased prefrontal cortex connectivity was associated with memory, visuospatial, and executive function [17]. Shin et al. compared the FC of PD-MCI patients with shorter and longer periods of motor symptoms before cognitive impairment using seed-based analyses and found that these two groups showed different characteristics of decreased FC in the DMN. Their findings implied that these two types might have different mechanisms and might help predict cognitive decline in future studies [18]. Lopes et al. investigated the brain network features of PD patients with different levels of cognitive function using the graph theory and network-based statistics. They showed that the functional organization decreased in accordance with the degree of cognitive impairment, and PD patients with cognitive impairment had reduced FC in the basal ganglia, ventral prefrontal, parietal, temporal, and occipital cortices [19]. The above studies confirmed the commonly impaired cognitive domains in PD, executive, attention, visuospatial function, and memory [7], and uncovered the impaired brain regions.

2.2. rs-fMRI Study on PD Patients without Cognitive Impairment. rs-fMRI is a sensitive imaging modality that can reveal dysfunction in cognition-related brain regions in PD patients with only subtle cognitive changes or even without cognitive symptoms. This property makes rs-fMRI a promising tool for the early identification of patients with a high risk for PDD. Lucas-Jimenez et al. used a seed-based FC analysis and showed reduced DMN FC in nondemented PD patients, and this FC change was correlated with lower verbal and visual memory and visual abilities in PD [20].

Manza et al. also used a seed-based approach to investigate the striatum FC in PD patients, the results showed that the stronger FC between the dorsal caudate and the rostral anterior cingulate cortex was associated with cognitive dysfunction (especially memory and visuospatial function) [21]. Muller-Oehring utilized a seed-based rs-fMRI and task fMRI and demonstrated that stronger putamen-medial parietal and pallidum-occipital FC than controls was associated with executive function and motor symptoms [22]. Tessitore et al. assessed the brain FC of cognitively unimpaired PD patients using the ICA analysis and found decreased FC within the DMN, and the FC changes correlated with memory, visuospatial, and attention/executive function [23]. Madhyastha et al. showed impaired brain network dynamic connectivity at rest in PD patients without cognitive impairment using factor analysis of overlapping sliding windows, and the factors in the dorsal attention network and frontoparietal task control network were correlated with patients' performance in attention examinations [24]. Luo et al. performed a graph theory-based analysis in drug-naive PD patients and found disrupted network organization in the PD patients at global, nodal, and connectional levels. Node centralities and connectivity strength were reduced mainly in the temporal-occipital and sensorimotor regions. Furthermore, the changed global network properties were associated with cognitive function [25]. In a group of rigidity-dominant drug-naive PD patients without cognitive impairment using a seed-based approach, Hou et al. found a decreased FC in DMN (especially the posterior DMN) and an increased FC in the anterior DMN in the PD patients, and increased FC of the anterior and ventral parts were negatively correlated with Hopkins verbal learning test-revised scores [26]. In a 3-year longitudinal study by Olde Dubbelink et al., the multivariate exploratory linear optimized decomposition into independent components analysis showed widespread reduction of FC in the PD patients compared with the controls. After 3 years, the FC in the PD patients decreased further on, and the FC changes were most prominent for posterior parts of the brain. The FC change over time was correlated with the alteration of global cognitive function, as well as perception, praxis and the spatial span subscores [27]. It is noteworthy that some patients in their study had dementia, and the cognitive performance of the PD patients was inferior to the controls at baseline [7]. In a study by Huang et al., left onset PD patients had worse performance in feedback-based associative learning than the right onset PD patients and the controls. In the left onset PD patients, the impaired cognitive function was associated with the ReHo in the right dorsal rostral putamen [28]. These studies showed that rs-fMRI was a sensitive tool detecting brain network abnormalities in PD patients without obvious cognitive impairment, and some motor symptom features implied higher risk for cognitive dysfunction in PD.

3. Combining rs-fMRI with Other Modalities

Until now, various methods have been applied in investigating neurological disorders, and each has its advantage

and disadvantage. PET and SPECT using different radio ligands can display abnormalities of neurotransmitters in the brain and deposition of aggregated proteins such as α-synuclein, β-amyloid, and tau proteins in neurological disorders [29]. EEG has a very high temporal resolution. CSF laboratory examinations are able to detect the culprit protein and the degree of neurodegeneration [30]. Combining rs-fMRI and other modalities can deepen our understanding of the pathophysiology of cognitive dysfunction in PD. Madhyastha et al. used the "network kernel analysis" in PD patients and found widespread alterations in the correlations of network kernels in the PD patients, and the degree of network disturbance was associated with lower cerebrospinal fluid α-synuclein and amyloid-β_{42} levels. In addition, increased correlation of the insula with the DMN was associated with worse attentional function. Therefore, both α-synuclein and amyloid-β_{42} might play a role in disrupting cognitive-related brain regions [30]. Lebedev et al. combined a graph theory-based rs-fMRI analysis with ^{123}I-FP-CIT SPECT imaging. In their study, executive function was associated with dorsal frontoparietal cortical processing and sensory involvement, as well as the striatal dopamine transporter binding ratios. Memory performance was correlated with prefrontolimbic processing but not associated with nigrostriatal dopaminergic function. Their study confirmed that distinct from executive dysfunction, memory deficits in PD was not induced by dopaminergic insufficiency [31]. In future studies, integration of more CSF laboratory examinations, EEG/fMRI, and PET imaging utilizing more radio ligands including for other transmitters (cholinergic, serotonergic, norepinephrinergic systems, etc.) and abnormal proteins (such as α-synuclein, β-amyloid, and tau proteins) and laboratory examinations using other body fluids can promote our recognition of the underlying mechanism of cognitive impairment in PD.

4. rs-fMRI as a Diagnostic Tool

So far, most of the rs-fMRI studies in PD enrolled small numbers of patients. However, we can obtain preliminary consistent conclusions on the networks disrupted in PD and their relationship with cognitive dysfunction. We still need more evidence to apply rs-fMRI as a diagnostic tool in clinical practice. Abos et al. used a support vector machine method to distinguish PD patients with and without MCI with an accuracy of 80%, and the connectivity of the selected edges was correlated with memory and executive function in the PD patients [32]. Peraza et al. compared the brain network between patients with dementia with Lewy bodies and PDD using seed-based analyses. Their results implied that there might be subtle differences in attention and motor-related networks between these two disorders [33]. Borroni et al. performed rs-fMRI in patients with PD, PDD, and DLB using ReHo. PD and PDD patients had decreased ReHo in the frontal regions, while DLB patients had lower ReHo in the posterior regions [34]. Future studies enrolling large samples would pave the road for clinical diagnostic applications in PD.

5. Prediction of Cognitive Impairment in PD

Disease-modifying therapies targeting α-synuclein, β-amyloid, and tau proteins are under active investigation and are hopeful to be available in clinical practice in the near future. Early identification of PD patients with a high risk for dementia is critical for potential disease-modifying therapies. As far as we know, most of the studies using rs-fMRI for cognitive function in PD are cross-sectional. Only two studies explored the progression of cognitive impairment and brain network changes in a longitudinal design. However, they only enrolled small numbers of patients and had a short time of follow-up (1 and 3 years, resp.) [21, 27]. Ongoing prospective studies such as the Parkinson's Progression Markers Initiative (PPMI) would help answer the question of PDD prediction.

6. Evaluating and Assisting Intervention

rs-fMRI has been applied in the assessment of the effects of levodopa and cognitive rehabilitation in PD cognition. Simioni et al. tested the effect of levodopa on brain networks and cognitive function using seed-based and ICA analyses. Levodopa increased resting state FC between caudate and right parietal cortex (within the frontoparietal attentional network), and this effect was associated with improvement in working memory performance [35]. Diez-Cirarda employed a seed-based rs-fMRI analysis in a randomized controlled trial of cognitive rehabilitation in PD and showed increased FC between the left inferior temporal lobe and the bilateral dorsolateral prefrontal cortex in the rehabilitation group than the control group. Moreover, the increased FC was correlated with executive function in the treatment group [36]. Eighteen months later, they performed a follow-up examination of 15 patients in the rehabilitation group and found preserved effect of rehabilitation on both cognitive function and brain FC even after 18 months [37]. Cerasa et al. also evaluated the effect of cognitive rehabilitation using rs-fMRI. They employed ICA and SPM and showed improved attention/executive function together with the attention and central executive neural networks [38]. There are other studies evaluating the effect of varied interventions on the resting brain networks, but the associations with cognitive function has been less investigated [39–45]. In the future, rs-fMRI can play a more important role in evaluating treatment effects as well as guiding neuromodulation therapies.

In summary, rs-fMRI might be a useful tool for the exploration of underlying mechanism of cognitive dysfunction in PD and can help diagnose cognitive dysfunction in PD and assist treatments. More longitudinal studies using rs-fMRI and the combination of rs-fMRI with other modalities are needed.

Authors' Contributions

Kai Li and Wen Su contributed equally to this work.

References

[1] S. Fengler, I. Liepelt-Scarfone, K. Brockmann, E. Schäffer, D. Berg, and E. Kalbe, "Cognitive changes in prodromal Parkinson's disease: a review," *Movement Disorders*, vol. 32, no. 12, pp. 1655–1666, 2017.

[2] M. Emre, D. Aarsland, R. Brown et al., "Clinical diagnostic criteria for dementia associated with Parkinson's disease," *Movement Disorders*, vol. 22, no. 12, pp. 1689–1707, 2007.

[3] M. A. Hely, W. G. J. Reid, M. A. Adena, G. M. Halliday, and J. G. L. Morris, "The Sydney multicenter study of Parkinson's disease: the inevitability of dementia at 20 years," *Movement Disorders*, vol. 23, no. 6, pp. 837–844, 2008.

[4] K. Seppi, D. Weintraub, M. Coelho et al., "The movement disorder society evidence-based medicine review update: treatments for the non-motor symptoms of Parkinson's disease," *Movement Disorders*, vol. 26, no. 3, pp. S42–S80, 2011.

[5] L. V. Kalia and A. E. Lang, "Parkinson's disease," *The Lancet*, vol. 386, no. 9996, pp. 896–912, 2015.

[6] S. Tekin and J. L. Cummings, "Frontal-subcortical neuronal circuits and clinical neuropsychiatry: an update," *Journal of Psychosomatic Research*, vol. 53, no. 2, pp. 647–654, 2002.

[7] D. Aarsland, B. Creese, M. Politis et al., "Cognitive decline in Parkinson disease," *Nature Reviews Neurology*, vol. 13, no. 4, pp. 217–231, 2017.

[8] A. K. Azeez and B. B. Biswal, "A review of resting-state analysis methods," *Neuroimaging Clinics of North America*, vol. 27, no. 4, pp. 581–592, 2017.

[9] M. Tahmasian, L. M. Bettray, T. van Eimeren et al., "A systematic review on the applications of resting-state fMRI in Parkinson's disease: does dopamine replacement therapy play a role?," *Cortex*, vol. 73, pp. 80–105, 2015.

[10] S. M. Smith, P. T. Fox, K. L. Miller et al., "Correspondence of the brain's functional architecture during activation and rest," *Proceedings of the National Academy of Sciences*, vol. 106, no. 31, pp. 13040–13045, 2009.

[11] M. Gorges, H.-P. Müller, D. Lulé, E. H. Pinkhardt, A. C. Ludolph, and J. Kassubek, "To rise and to fall: functional connectivity in cognitively normal and cognitively impaired patients with Parkinson's disease," *Neurobiology of Aging*, vol. 36, no. 4, pp. 1727–1735, 2015.

[12] Y. Hou, J. Yang, C. Luo et al., "Dysfunction of the default mode network in drug-naive Parkinson's disease with mild cognitive impairments: a resting-state fMRI study," *Frontiers in Aging Neuroscience*, vol. 8, p. 247, 2016.

[13] B. Chen, S. Wang, W. Sun et al., "Functional and structural changes in gray matter of Parkinson's disease patients with mild cognitive impairment," *European Journal of Radiology*, vol. 93, pp. 16–23, 2017.

[14] H. C. Baggio, B. Segura, R. Sala-Llonch et al., "Cognitive impairment and resting-state network connectivity in Parkinson's disease," *Human Brain Mapping*, vol. 36, no. 1, pp. 199–212, 2015.

[15] H. C. Baggio, R. Sala-Llonch, B. Segura et al., "Functional brain networks and cognitive deficits in Parkinson's disease," *Human Brain Mapping*, vol. 35, no. 9, pp. 4620–4634, 2014.

[16] L. R. Peraza, D. Nesbitt, R. A. Lawson et al., "Intra- and inter-network functional alterations in Parkinson's disease with mild cognitive impairment," *Human Brain Mapping*, vol. 38, no. 3, pp. 1702–1715, 2017.

[17] M. Amboni, A. Tessitore, F. Esposito et al., "Resting-state functional connectivity associated with mild cognitive impairment in Parkinson's disease," *Journal of Neurology*, vol. 262, no. 2, pp. 425–434, 2015.

[18] N. Y. Shin, Y. S. Shin, P. H. Lee et al., "Different functional and microstructural changes depending on duration of mild cognitive impairment in Parkinson disease," *American Journal of Neuroradiology*, vol. 37, no. 5, pp. 897–903, 2016.

[19] R. Lopes, C. Delmaire, L. Defebvre et al., "Cognitive phenotypes in Parkinson's disease differ in terms of brain-network organization and connectivity," *Human Brain Mapping*, vol. 38, no. 3, pp. 1604–1621, 2017.

[20] O. Lucas-Jimenez, N. Ojeda, J. Peña et al., "Altered functional connectivity in the default mode network is associated with cognitive impairment and brain anatomical changes in Parkinson's disease," *Parkinsonism & Related Disorders*, vol. 33, pp. 58–64, 2016.

[21] P. Manza, S. Zhang, C.-S. R. Li, and H.-C. Leung, "Resting-state functional connectivity of the striatum in early-stage Parkinson's disease: cognitive decline and motor symptomatology," *Human Brain Mapping*, vol. 37, no. 2, pp. 648–662, 2016.

[22] E. M. Muller-Oehring, E. V. Sullivan, A. Pfefferbaum et al., "Task-rest modulation of basal ganglia connectivity in mild to moderate Parkinson's disease," *Brain Imaging and Behavior*, vol. 9, no. 3, pp. 619–638, 2015.

[23] A. Tessitore, F. Esposito, C. Vitale et al., "Default-mode network connectivity in cognitively unimpaired patients with Parkinson disease," *Neurology*, vol. 79, no. 23, pp. 2226–2232, 2012.

[24] T. M. Madhyastha, M. K. Askren, P. Boord, and T. J. Grabowski, "Dynamic connectivity at rest predicts attention task performance," *Brain Connectivity*, vol. 5, no. 1, pp. 45–59, 2015.

[25] C. Y. Luo, X. Y. Guo, W. Song et al., "Functional connectome assessed using graph theory in drug-naive Parkinson's disease," *Journal of Neurology*, vol. 262, no. 6, pp. 1557–1567, 2015.

[26] Y. Hou, C. Luo, J. Yang et al., "Default-mode network connectivity in cognitively unimpaired drug-naive patients with rigidity-dominant Parkinson's disease," *Journal of Neurology*, vol. 264, no. 1, pp. 152–160, 2017.

[27] K. T. Olde Dubbelink, M. M. Schoonheim, J. B. Deijen, J. W. R. Twisk, F. Barkhof, and H. W. Berendse, "Functional connectivity and cognitive decline over 3 years in Parkinson disease," *Neurology*, vol. 83, no. 22, pp. 2046–2053, 2014.

[28] P. Huang, Y.-Y. Tan, D. Qiang et al., "Motor-symptom laterality affects acquisition in Parkinson's disease: a cognitive and functional magnetic resonance imaging study," *Movement Disorders*, vol. 32, no. 7, pp. 1047–1055, 2017.

[29] J. Jankovic and E. Tolosa, *Parkinson's Disease and Movement Disorders*, Lippincott Williams & Wilkins, Philadelphia, PA, USA, 2015.

[30] T. M. Madhyastha, M. K. Askren, J. Zhang et al., "Group comparison of spatiotemporal dynamics of intrinsic networks in Parkinson's disease," *Brain*, vol. 138, no. 9, pp. 2672–2686, 2015.

[31] A. V. Lebedev, E. Westman, A. Simmons et al., "Large-scale resting state network correlates of cognitive impairment in Parkinson's disease and related dopaminergic deficits," *Frontiers in Systems Neuroscience*, vol. 8, p. 45, 2014.

[32] A. Abos, H. C. Baggio, B. Segura et al., "Discriminating cognitive status in Parkinson's disease through functional connectomics and machine learning," *Scientific Reports*, vol. 7, p. 45347, 2017.

[33] L. R. Peraza, S. J. Colloby, M. J. Firbank et al., "Resting state in Parkinson's disease dementia and dementia with Lewy bodies: commonalities and differences," *International Journal of Geriatric Psychiatry*, vol. 30, no. 11, pp. 1135–1146, 2015.

[34] B. Borroni, E. Premi, A. Formenti et al., "Structural and functional imaging study in dementia with Lewy bodies and Parkinson's disease dementia," *Parkinsonism & Related Disorders*, vol. 21, no. 9, pp. 1049–1055, 2015.

[35] A. C. Simioni, A. Dagher, and L. K. Fellows, "Effects of levodopa on corticostriatal circuits supporting working memory in Parkinson's disease," *Cortex*, vol. 93, pp. 193–205, 2017.

[36] M. Diez-Cirarda, N. Ojeda, J. Peña et al., "Increased brain connectivity and activation after cognitive rehabilitation in Parkinson's disease: a randomized controlled trial," *Brain Imaging and Behavior*, vol. 11, no. 6, pp. 1640–1651, 2016.

[37] M. Diez-Cirarda, N. Ojeda, J. Peña et al., "Long-term effects of cognitive rehabilitation on brain, functional outcome and cognition in Parkinson's disease," *European Journal of Neurology*, vol. 25, no. 1, pp. 5–12, 2017.

[38] A. Cerasa, M. Cecilia Gioia, M. Salsone et al., "Neurofunctional correlates of attention rehabilitation in Parkinson's disease: an explorative study," *Neurological Sciences*, vol. 35, no. 8, pp. 1173–1180, 2014.

[39] C. C. Quattrocchi, M. F. de Pandis, C. Piervincenzi et al., "Acute modulation of brain connectivity in Parkinson disease after automatic mechanical peripheral stimulation: a pilot study," *PLoS One*, vol. 10, no 10, article e0137977, 2015.

[40] Z. Wen, J. Zhang, J. Li, J. Dai, F. Lin, and G. Wu, "Altered activation in cerebellum contralateral to unilateral thalamotomy may mediate tremor suppression in Parkinsons disease: a short-term regional homogeneity fMRI study," *PLoS One*, vol. 11, no 6, article e0157562, 2016.

[41] W. Yang, B. Liu, B. Huang et al., "Altered resting-state functional connectivity of the striatum in Parkinson's disease after levodopa administration," *PLoS One*, vol. 11, no 9, article e0161935, 2016.

[42] B. Ng, G. Varoquaux, J. Baptiste et al., "Distinct alterations in Parkinson's medication-state and disease-state connectivity," *NeuroImage: Clinical*, vol. 16, pp. 575–585, 2017.

[43] M. F. Dirkx, H. E. M. den Ouden, E. Aarts et al., "Dopamine controls Parkinson's tremor by inhibiting the cerebellar thalamus," *Brain*, vol. 140, no. 3, pp. 721–734, 2017.

[44] Z. Ye, A. Hammer, and T. F. Munte, "Pramipexole modulates interregional connectivity within the sensorimotor network," *Brain Connectivity*, vol. 7, no. 4, pp. 258–263, 2017.

[45] J. Kahan, M. Urner, R. Moran et al., "Resting state functional MRI in Parkinson's disease: the impact of deep brain stimulation on 'effective' connectivity," *Brain*, vol. 137, no. 4, pp. 1130–1144, 2014.

9

Ex Vivo and In Vivo Characterization of Interpolymeric Blend/Nanoenabled Gastroretentive Levodopa Delivery Systems

Ndidi C. Ngwuluka,[1] Yahya E. Choonara,[1] Girish Modi,[2] Lisa C. du Toit,[1] Pradeep Kumar,[1] Leith Meyer,[3] Tracy Snyman,[4] and Viness Pillay[1]

[1] Wits Advanced Drug Delivery Platform Research Unit, Department of Pharmacy and Pharmacology, School of Therapeutic Sciences, Faculty of Health Sciences, University of the Witwatersrand, Johannesburg, 7 York Road, Parktown 2193, South Africa

[2] Department of Neurology, Faculty of Health Sciences, University of the Witwatersrand, Johannesburg, 7 York Road, Parktown 2193, South Africa

[3] Department of Paraclinical Sciences, Faculty of Veterinary Science, University of Pretoria, Pretoria, South Africa

[4] National Laboratory Services, Faculty of Health Sciences, University of the Witwatersrand, Johannesburg, 7 York Road, Parktown 2193, South Africa

Correspondence should be addressed to Viness Pillay; viness.pillay@wits.ac.za

Academic Editor: Wei-dong Le

One approach for delivery of narrow absorption window drugs is to formulate gastroretentive drug delivery systems. This study was undertaken to provide insight into in vivo performances of two gastroretentive systems (*PXLNET* and IPB matrices) in comparison to Madopar® HBS capsules. The pig model was used to assess gastric residence time and pharmacokinetic parameters using blood, cerebrospinal fluid (CSF), and urine samples. Histopathology and cytotoxicity testing were also undertaken. The pharmacokinetic parameters indicated that levodopa was liberated from the drug delivery systems, absorbed, widely distributed, metabolized, and excreted. C_{max} were 372.37, 257.02, and 461.28 ng/mL and MRT were 15.36, 14.98, and 13.30 for Madopar HBS capsules, *PXLNET*, and IPB, respectively. In addition, X-ray imaging indicated that the gastroretentive systems have the potential to reside in the stomach for 7 hours. There was strong in vitro-in vivo correlation for all formulations with r^2 values of 0.906, 0.935, and 0.945 for Madopar HBS capsules, *PXLNET*, and IPB, respectively. Consequently, *PXLNET* and IPB matrices have pertinent potential as gastroretentive systems for narrow absorption window drugs (e.g., L-dopa) and, in this application specifically, enhanced the central nervous system and/or systemic bioavailability of such drugs.

1. Introduction

Although a number of in vitro drug delivery studies are undertaken, the ultimate goal in developing and evaluating a drug delivery device is to achieve the desired drug delivery outcomes in vivo. Despite attempts at simulating in vivo environment, in vitro studies still do not exactly replicate the operation and impact of an in vivo environment on drug delivery devices. Hence, after development and in vitro analyses, there is still the need to assess the device in vivo (within a living organism) before it is commercialized for administration to the end-user consumer for complete description of the pharmacodynamics and pharmacokinetics data of the drug delivery device. The degree of absorption of a drug in the gastrointestinal tract is based on certain events which include drug release, drug in solution at absorptive sites, drug absorption into systemic circulation, liver and gut metabolism, decomposition, and transit [1]. Absorption and subsequent bioavailability of a drug are not only determined by the properties of the drug, such as solubility, which in turn is based on its crystallinity and lipophilicity, but are also affected by the gastrointestinal environment which is determined by its pH and presence of food and certain substances such as surfactants in gastric juice or bile as well as enzymes. Other factors include viscosity of luminal contents, motility patterns and flow rate, secretions and coadministered fluids [2]. Hence, oral drug delivery devices are developed to accommodate a number of these factors and at the same time ensure the absorption and subsequent bioavailability of the incorporated drug.

Optimized interpolymeric blend/nanoenabled levodopa- (L-dopa-) loaded delivery systems have been developed to be gastroretentive and release levodopa at a constant rate in order to maintain a constant concentration over a prolonged period for potential in vivo attainment of enhanced bioavailability of the narrow absorption window L-dopa. Hence, it was necessary to assess in vivo the gastric residence time and drug release properties, as well as the degree of toxicity of the device. The pig model was chosen because of the close resemblance of its gastrointestinal tract to that of humans, consequently, being best suited for in vivo studies of oral drug delivery. The anatomy and physiology of each section of the pig's gastrointestinal tract are comparable to that of humans [3, 4]. The pig model has also been employed to model brain disorders. This is due to the similarities of the pig's brain to that of a human in extent of peak brain growth at the time of birth, the gross anatomy, and the growth patterns [5, 6]. The catecholaminergic neurons in the pig brain are similar to those in other vertebrates [6]. Furthermore, a study by Minuzzi and coworkers indicated that the saturation binding parameters (B_{max} and K_d) of ligands specific for dopamine D_1 and D_2 receptors in pig brain cryostat sections are similar to the human receptors [7] implicated in the pathophysiology of Parkinson's disease [8]. Consequently, the choice of a pig model was deemed appropriate to assess the in vivo performance of L-dopa-loaded gastroretentive delivery systems.

2. Materials and Methods

2.1. Materials. The following materials were sourced for cell and animal studies: heparin sodium 1000 i.u./mL (Bodene (PTY) Limited as Intramed, Port Elizabeth, South Africa), normal saline (Adcock Ingram, Midrand, South Africa), two-lumen central venous catheterization set with ARROWgard Blue (Arrow International, Inc., Reading, PA, USA), CaCo 2 adhesion cells, CytoTox-Glo™ Kit (Promega Corporation, Madison, WI, USA) fetal bovine serum, penicillin and streptomycin, Dulbecco's modified Eagle's medium (DMEM) (Sigma-Aldrich Chemie, GmbH, Steinheim, Germany), acid washed alumina, TRIS buffer, phosphoric acid (Bio-Rad Laboratories, Hercules, CA, USA), Oasis® HLB cartridges (3cc, Waters Corporation, Milford, MA, USA), silicone Foley catheters (two-way French size 10, Supra Latex, Kempton Park, Gauteng, South Africa), clinical speculum and veterinary laryngoscope, levodopa, dopamine, methyldopa, benserazide, and carbidopa (Sigma-Aldrich Chemie, GmbH, Steinheim, Germany). Materials used for formulation of the tablet matrices were methacrylate copolymer (Eudragit E100, Evonik Röhm GmbH & Co. KG, Darmstadt, Germany), sodium carboxymethylcellulose (NaCMC, Fluka Biochemika, Sigma-Aldrich Chemie, GmbH, Buchs, Switzerland), locust bean from *Ceratonia siliqua* seeds (Sigma-Aldrich, Inc., Steinheim, Germany), barium sulphate, pullulan from *Aureobasidium pullulans* (Sigma-Aldrich, Inc.,

Steinheim, Germany), silica, magnesium stearate (Merck Chemicals (Pty), Ltd., Gauteng, South Africa), chitosan (Wellable Group, Fujian, China), sodium tripolyphosphate (TPP) (Sigma-Aldrich, Germany), and lecithin from egg yolk (Lipoid E PC S, Lipoid AG, Ludwigshafen, Germany).

2.2. Preparation of Gastroretentive Formulations. The formulations *Poly-x-Lipo Nanoenabled Tablets (PXLNET)* and interpolymeric blend (IPB) matrices were prepared as previously described, where the IPB had L-dopa and the decarboxylase inhibitor, benserazide, directly compressed into the matrix, whereas the *PXLNET* L-dopa and benserazide were incorporated into the IPB matrix within poly-lipo-nanoparticles [9, 10]. However, the *PXLNET* was modified in this study for easy administration to the pigs. A tablet of not more than 1000 mg in total was permitted due to the method of administration. Consequently, the quantity of IPB was reduced to 224.22 mg, while the quantity of levodopa-loaded nanoparticles was 375.78 mg. Madopar HBS, a controlled release as well as a gastroretentive dosage form, was employed to analyze the performance of IPB and *PXLNET* gastroretentive drug delivery systems.

2.3. Arrival of Pigs and Habituation. The animal ethics clearance (2009/01/05) was obtained from the animal ethics screening committee of University of the Witwatersrand, Johannesburg, South Africa. Five White Large pigs (four females and a male) weighing 32.55 ± 4.38 kg were used for the study. The pigs were housed in cages with access to food and water under a controlled temperature (20–24°C) and a 12-hour light/dark cycle. Habituation was ensured before the pigs were subjected to surgery and dosing.

2.4. Venous Catheterization of the Pigs for Blood Sampling. Approximately ten days after arrival, surgery was undertaken under aseptic conditions to insert a catheter in the internal jugular veins of the pigs for easy withdrawal of blood samples during dosing. Briefly, each pig was anesthetized with ketamine (11 mg/kg) and midazolam (0.3 mg/kg) intramuscularly and maintained by intubation with 2% isoflurane in 100% oxygen. Analgesia was provided by intramuscular administration of buprenorphine (0.05 mg/kg) and carprofen (4 mg/kg). An incision was made on the lateral side of the neck to expose the jugular vein, which was isolated and a two-lumen central venous catheter was inserted into the lumen of the vein. The remainder of the catheter was tunneled subcutaneously with the aid of a trocar to an exit point cranial to the dorsal aspect of the scapular. To avoid untimely removal of the catheter by the movements of the pig, the external sampling ports were sutured to the skin of the pig. The catheter was tested and cleaned by withdrawal of blood and flushing with heparinized saline (5000 i.u./L of 0.9% saline). The pigs were monitored after surgery to ensure full recovery from anesthesia and allowed more than seven days to recover before the commencement of gastric dosing and sampling.

2.5. Flushing and Bleeding of Pigs. In order to keep the catheters open throughout the period of the study, the

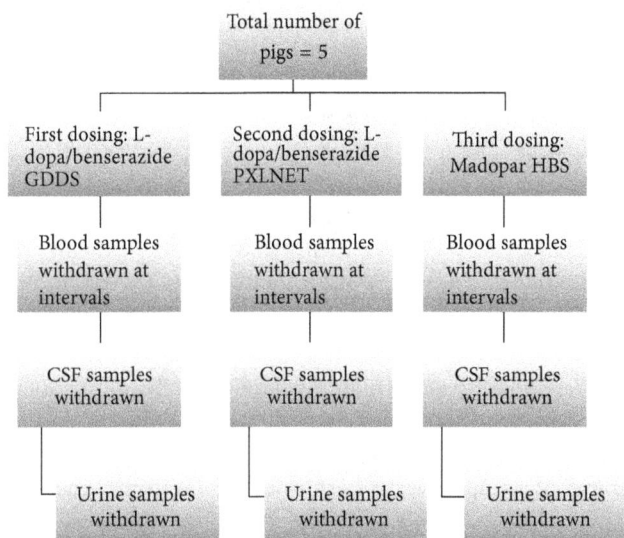

FIGURE 1: Flow diagram detailing in vivo animal studies for three drug delivery systems.

catheters had to be flushed twice a day with heparinized saline. Bleeding was also undertaken at intervals to ensure flow of blood through the catheters as well as to obtain blank plasma. In addition, the ports of the catheters had to be sprayed with antiseptic before and after flushing to avoid infection.

2.6. Gastric Dosing and Blood Sampling of the Pigs. The pigs were fasted overnight before dosing. The formulations *PXLNET* and IPB matrices as well as Madopar HBS were administered via intragastric tubes. However, before dosing, baseline blood samples were withdrawn for control analysis. The procedures for flushing and bleeding were utilized to withdraw the baseline blood samples and subsequent blood samples from the pigs after dosing. The pigs were anesthetized as described earlier and subsequently each pig was raised in an upright position and, with the aid of an intragastric tube, the drug was administered via the tube and flushed down into the stomach with about 20–50 mL of water. The pigs are taken back to their cages and monitored until they recovered from anesthesia. The study was a crossover study with two-day wash-out period, whereby the same pigs were employed for the different dosage forms. Blood samples were withdrawn from the chronically implanted venous catheters at specific time intervals (2, 4, 6, 8, 10, 12, 16, 20, and 24 hours) and collected in EDTA vacutainers (BD Vacutainers®, Franklin Lakes, NJ, USA) to avoid coagulation. The blood samples were centrifuged at 5000 rpm for 15 mins to obtain plasma samples. Into 2 mL of each plasma sample, 30 uL of 10% sodium metabisulphite was added and the plasma samples were stored in a −80°C freezer until analysis. Figure 1 explicates the crossover design and the dosage forms administered.

2.7. Cerebrospinal Fluid Collection from Pigs. Cerebrospinal fluid (CSF) was obtained from an anaesthetized pig by

puncturing the cisterna magna. The cistern magna can be accessed through the foramen magnum. The pig's neck was leaned on the table to flex the neck by an assistant. The caudal end of the occipital bone and the nuchal tubercles were palpated. A 20-gauge spinal needle was passed slightly caudal to this area at an angle approximately 60° towards the oral cavity to enter the foramen magnum cranial to the body of the axis. CSF was withdrawn with a 2 mL syringe and transferred into a collection tube containing 10% sodium metabisulphite. The CSF sample was then stored at −80°C until analysis. CSF was collected at the 2nd and 4th hour after dosing. CSF sampling was not carried out over the day because the pigs could only be anaesthetized a limited number of times in a day and puncturing of the cisterna magna was also limited.

2.8. Urine Collection from Pigs. The pigs were anaesthetized and placed on their abdomens. A lubricated speculum with a long blade was inserted into the urogenital opening to open the vaginal wall. To visualize the external urethral orifice, a veterinary laryngoscope with straight blade was inserted. The female urethral opening is located on the floor of the vagina, about a third or half the distance to the cervix. A Foley catheter French size 10 with a stylet was controlled with a blunt tip forceps and inserted into the bladder. As the catheter got into the bladder, the stylet was removed and urine was allowed to flow into the collection tube. Urine was collected at the 2nd and 4th hour after dosing. More time point urine sampling was limited due to the same reasons for CSF collection. This study adhered to the scope of approval by the animal ethics committee.

2.9. In Vivo Measurement of the IPB GDDS and PXLNET Residence Times in a Large White Pig Model. Measurement of the gastric residence time of a drug delivery system at the application site is to provide information on the gastroretentive ability of the drug delivery system. X-ray imaging was employed as a noninvasive method of determining the residence time without affecting gastrointestinal (GIT) motility. A radio-opaque marker, barium sulphate, was incorporated into the GDDS and *PXLNET* formulations to determine the extent of gastroretention. Two of the Large White pigs were fasted overnight and a radiolabeled GDDS and *PXLNET* was administered to them on different occasions. The animals were anaesthetized twice: first, it was during drug delivery system administration and, second, at the 7th hour after administration, to undergo X-ray imaging each time point.

2.10. Histopathological Evaluation in Control and Dosed Pigs. The stomach of a euthanized pig was cut open and the area the PXLNET was located, was excised, as well as the posterior and anterior section, and was fixed in neutral buffered formalin. The same sections were excised from the control pig and fixed in neutral buffered formalin in order to preserve the tissues. The tissue samples were embedded on labeled cassettes and sectioned into blocks. An automated processor was used for fixation, dehydration, and paraffin embedding. Routine histological methodology was undertaken which involved Mayer's hematoxylin and eosin staining procedure.

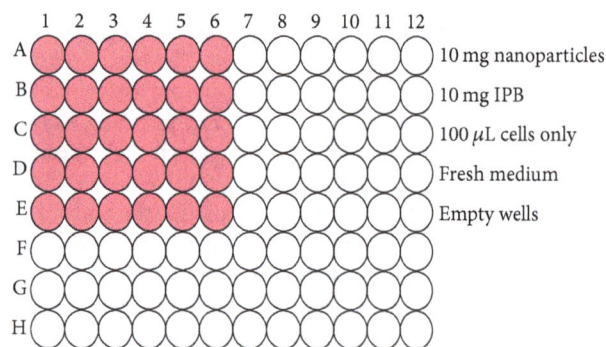

FIGURE 2: Schematic diagram of a 96-well plate depicting the arrangement of the samples, no-cell background and cells only.

TABLE 1: Multiple reaction monitoring parameters.

	Parent (m/z)	Daughter (m/z)
Dopamine	154.30	137.40
Levodopa	198.50	152.10
Methyldopa	212.90	165.90
Methyldopa	212.90	194.60
Carbidopa	226.40	181.1
Benserazide	258.70	139.10
Benserazide	294.70	258.70

Coverslipping was undertaken to prevent the tissue from being scratched and to provide better optical quality during microscopic viewing. Descriptions of the microscopic features were made and a final microscopic diagnosis was reported.

2.11. Cytotoxicity Testing of the IPB and Nanoparticles.

CaCo-2 adhesion cells were cultured in 10 mL cocktail media comprising 10% fetal bovine serum (5 mL), 0.1% v/v of penicillin (100 IU/mL) and streptomycin (100 μg/mL), and Dulbecco's modified Eagle's medium (DMEM). The cells were maintained in a humidified atmospheric incubator (RS Biotech Galaxy, Irvine, UK) with 5% CO_2 at 37°C. The cells were cultured under aseptic conditions to avoid contamination and death. After growing the cells for two weeks, the medium was decanted and the adherent cells were rinsed with DMEM. Thereafter, the adherent cells were harvested by trypsinization (100 μL trypsin was added and incubated for 5 minutes). The cells were washed with fresh medium (DMEM) to remove residual trypsin and resuspended in fresh medium. The suspended cells (100 μL each) were placed in a 96-well plate as shown in Figure 2 and 10 μL of samples (0.1 mg/μL) was added to each of the wells containing cells. The colored wells as shown in Figure 2 contain cells and samples tested. The 96-well plate was incubated for 24 hours.

After 24 hours of incubation, the cytotoxicity assay was performed employing CytoTox-Glo Kit (Promega Corporation, Madison, WI, USA). CytoTox-Glo cytotoxicity assay is a homogenous luminescent assay which enables the number of dead cells in a well to be counted. The assay has two steps: first is the addition of the luminogenic peptide substrate which enables the measurement of dead-cell protease activity released from cells that have lost membrane integrity, and the second step requires the addition of the lysis reagent to deliver a luminescent signal associated with the total numbers of cells in each well. The number of dead cells was measured at each step after 15 mins incubation at ambient temperature by a multilabel reader (PerkinElmer 2030 Victor™, Turku, Finland).

2.12. Ultraperformance Liquid Chromatographic Analysis of Samples

2.12.1. Quantitative Analyses of Samples.
Quantitative assays of samples were performed on Waters Acquity™ UPLC/MS/MS system (Waters Corporation, Milford, MA, USA). The column used was an Acquity UPLC® BEH shield RP18 1.7 μm, 2.1 × 100 mm. Carbidopa was used as internal standard and a gradient method was employed using mobile phase, 2 mmol/L ammonium acetate and 0.1% formic acid in deionized water as solvent A and acetonitrile as solvent B. The ratio of the mobile phase gradient started at 30% A for 0.5 min and increased linearly to 100% B for 1 minute, returning to the original settings over the following 0.5 min at a flow rate of 0.3 mL/min. The injection volume was 10 μL, run time was 2 min, and sample temperature was maintained at 4°C. The data was captured with Waters MassLynx™ software. Standards and analytes were detected using a triple quadrupole mass spectrometer fitted with electrospray ionization probe (ES+) and multiple reaction monitoring scan; parameters are as shown in Table 1.

2.12.2. Standard Preparation of Actives.
Stock solutions of L-dopa, dopamine, methyldopa, benserazide, and carbidopa were prepared by dissolving 100 mg of each drug in 100 mL of 0.1 N hydrochloric acid individually. From the stock solutions, a series of working standards was prepared in blank plasma to give 4000, 2000, 1000, 500, 250, and 125 ng/mL each of L-dopa, dopamine, methyldopa, and benserazide combined in each working standard, while carbidopa added to the standards was 2000 ng/mL to provide a standard curve required for quantitation. Extraction from plasma was undertaken before injection and a standard curve was obtained from the peak ratio of drug/internal standard versus the concentrations of standards. The curve type is linear with a weighting factor of 1/concentration.

2.12.3. Extraction of Drugs and Metabolites from Plasma and CSF Samples.
Frozen plasma and CSF samples were thawed and 2 mL of each sample was transferred into separate extraction tubes. A designated measuring spoon was used to add one level spoonful of alumina into each tube. Thereafter, 2000 μL of the internal standard, carbidopa, was added, followed by 1 mL of TRIS Buffer. The tubes were capped and agitated using a mechanical shaker for 5 min. The tubes were centrifuged at 2500 rpm for 2 min. A disposable pipette was used to remove as much liquid as possible from each tube without disturbing the alumina. To wash the alumina, 1 mL Milli-Q water was added to each tube; the tubes

vortexed for 15 secs and centrifuged for 2 min at 2500 rpm. Water was removed using disposable pipettes. The washing procedure was repeated and 200 μL of 0.1% phosphoric acid was added to the tubes and vortexed for 30 secs. The tubes were centrifuged for 2 min at 2500 rpm and the supernatant was transferred into sample vials for subsequent injection into the column.

2.12.4. Extraction of Drug and Metabolites from Urine. Solvent-phase extraction was employed to isolate metabolites from urine. Briefly, 2 mL of methanol was used to condition each of the Oasis HLB cartridges and 2 mL of deionized water was used for washing. Thereafter, 2 mL of urine sample was loaded onto each cartridge, followed by 2 mL of 5% methanol in water. The metabolites were then eluted with 500 μL methanol and acetonitrile in the ratio of 1:1. The eluates were then transferred into sample vials for subsequent injection into the column.

2.13. Pharmacokinetic Modelling and Analysis. PKSolver, an add-in program for Microsoft Excel written in visual basic for application (VBA) for decoding problems in pharmacokinetic and pharmacodynamic data analysis, was used to model and estimate the pharmacokinetic parameters. Analysis of variance (ANOVA) was used to determine the statistical significance of the differences between the data.

3. Results and Discussion

Venous catheterization was successful. The pigs healed as anticipated without infection and dosing commenced. There was successful blood sampling at time intervals as well as CSF withdrawals. Urine collection was not as successful in all pigs on all days of dosing and sampling. One of the pigs had a skewed urethra and three attempts on different days proved abortive. In another, the urogenital canal began to bleed during the process and urine was not sampled from the pig.

3.1. In Vivo Measurement of the GDDS and PXLNET Residence Times in a Large White Pig Model. Two pigs were utilized for the in vivo gastroretentive study and the radiographic images were captured at the lateral and anterior-posterior positions as shown in Figure 3. The images in Figure 3(a) are the anterior-posterior position of the pig showing the presence of the device in the stomach immediately after dosing and at the 7th hour indicating that the IPB GDDS is able to be retained in the stomach for at least 7 hours. The position of the GDDS can be found within the red circles on the images. The radiographic images at the 7th hour showed that GDDS retained its three-dimensional network. However, the presence of the GDDS could not be seen in the second pig. It is envisaged that GDDS could have been obscured by food as the pigs were allowed to eat after administration and recovery from anesthesia or it could have been emptied from the stomach which may be an indication of intersubject variability.

However, as observed during in vitro drug release studies, PXLNET lost its three-dimensional network due to more rapid erosion in the presence of fluid [9] and may be showing as dispersed particles faintly seen in Figure 3(c) within the red circle. Furthermore, when a dosed pig was euthanized to harvest the stomach for histopathological testing 4-5 hours after administration, PXLNET was found adhering to the wall of the stomach perhaps kept in place by the presence of food but it had lost its shape. This is indicative that PXLNET may be able to withstand peristalsis up to 5 hours.

3.2. Histopathological Findings in Dosed and Control Pigs. Histopathological findings for the dosed (either with IPB or PXLNET) and control pigs are shown in Figure 4.

3.2.1. Dosed Animal. The mucosal epithelium was multifocally lost, likely due to autolytic changes of an early degree. The gastric glands appeared normal. Few normal appearing lymphoid follicles were visible in some sections, within the muscularis mucosa. The submucosa in few areas appeared mildly edematous. Very few lymphoplasmacytic aggregates were present in the lamina propria interstitium, mostly in one of the biopsy specimens from the pyloric area of the stomach wall.

3.2.2. Control. The stomach mucosal epithelium was multifocally lost, likely due to early autolytic changes. Where intact, the mucosal epithelium appeared normal with mucus accumulation together with intact desquamated epithelium cells on the surface. The underlying lamina propria multifocally showed mild lymphocytic infiltrates. These infiltrates extended to the muscularis mucosa but not beyond that. The gastric glands appeared within normal limits. Samples from both the fundus and pyloric portions of the stomach wall were available for examination. One section from the pylorus revealed moderate interstitial inflammation in which lymphocytes, plasma cells, and eosinophils were all present in a mixed reaction. The submucosa appeared mildly edematous.

The control sample yielded more inflammatory changes in the stomach lamina propria than the dosed sample. Mild inflammation was, however, present in dosed and control pigs and changes can therefore not be related directly to the polymeric drug delivery system used in the dosed pig. Mild gastric inflammation is a nonspecific lesion in many production animals and may be related to intestinal flora, intestinal pathogens, and presence of worms.

3.3. Cytotoxicity Testing of the IPB and Nanoparticles. The results obtained from the cytotoxicity testing are shown in Tables 2–5. Table 5 shows the percentage cytotoxicity for all samples. The luminescent signals observed for fresh medium and empty wells were used to correct those obtained for the samples and the percentage cytotoxicity was calculated thereafter. The cytotoxicity data obtained indicated that the drug delivery devices were not cytotoxic. This is not unexpected as the polymer utilized such as sodium carboxymethylcellulose [11–13] and chitosan [14–16] have been found to be cytoprotective. While studies on the cytoprotective nature of locust bean could not be obtained, it is generally regarded as safe (GRAS). Figure 5 shows confocal microscopy images of the cells viewed during culturing.

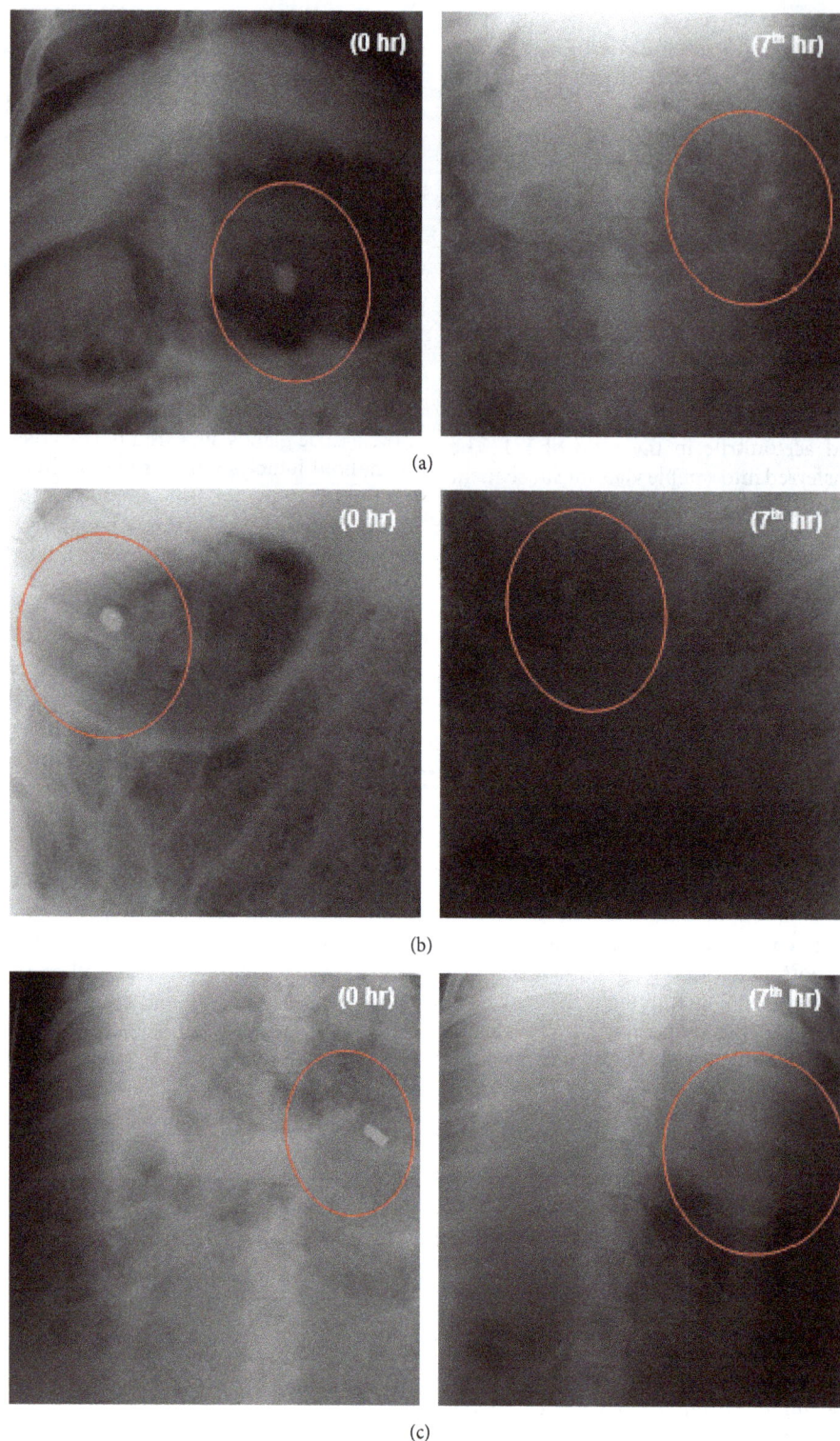

(a)

(b)

(c)

FIGURE 3: Radiographic images of (a) GDDS with the pig in the anterior-posterior position; (b) GDDS with the pig in the lateral position; and (c) PXLNET with the pig in the anterior-posterior position.

3.4. UPLC/MS/MS Method Validation: Recovery, Linearity, and Limit of Detection. Efforts have been made to optimize the quantitation of L-dopa, benserazide, and the metabolites. However, catecholamines are in the submicroanalysis range, a few parts per billion in the plasma; further, they are to be extracted from complex biological systems such as plasma, which usually poses a challenge of obtaining sufficient yields [17]. The recovery of the drugs was assessed by comparing

(a)

(b)

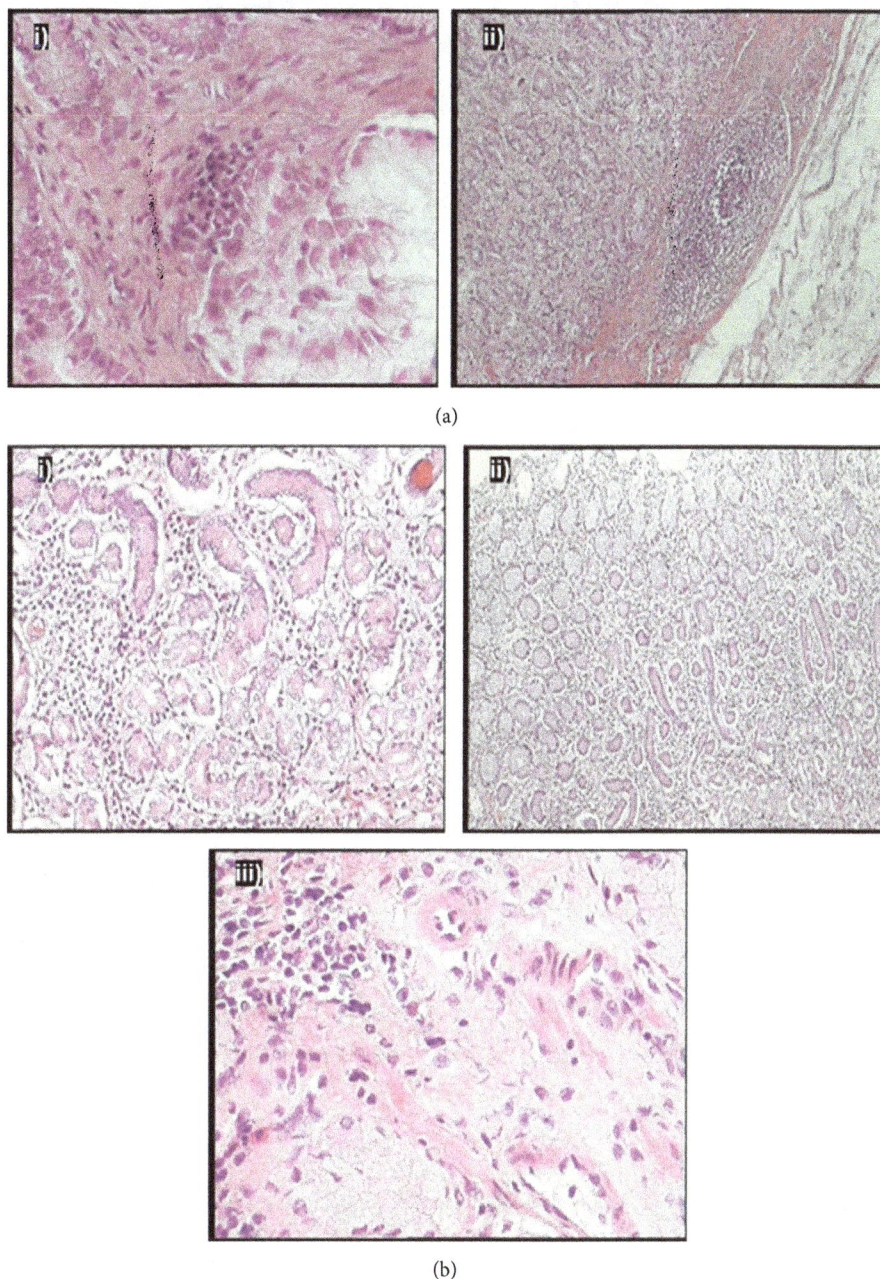

FIGURE 4: (a) Images from dosed pigs' stomach showing (i) mild lymphocytic aggregate in lamina propria interstitium and (ii) lymphoid follicle in deep lamina propria and submucosal edema. (b) Images from control tissue: (i) moderate lymphoplasmacytic interstitial lamina propria infiltration, higher magnification (×20); (ii) moderate lymphoplasmacytic interstitial lamina propria infiltration, lower magnification (×10); (iii) mild lymphoplasmacytic interstitial aggregated in the lamina propria.

TABLE 2: Measurement of dead cells (step 1).

Samples	Well 1	Well 2	Well 3	Well 4	Well 5	Well 6
10 mg nanoparticles	684	772	716	732	656	576
10 mg IPB	1474	1558	1428	1484	1466	1590
Cells only	970	1066	1014	1076	1228	960
Fresh medium	142	66	80	80	64	142
Empty wells	64	58	64	58	68	54

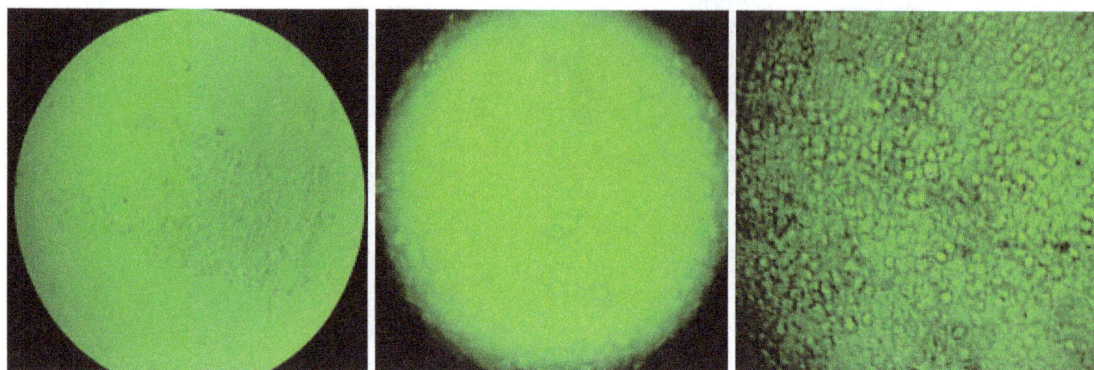

FIGURE 5: Microscopic images of CaCo-2 adhesion cells.

TABLE 3: Measurement of total cytotoxicity (step 2).

Samples	Well 1	Well 2	Well 3	Well 4	Well 5	Well 6
10 mg nanoparticles	778	744	834	924	832	868
10 mg IPB	1676	1662	1576	1414	1628	1836
Cells only	2784	2344	2810	2404	2576	2810
Fresh medium	118	108	102	92	80	118
Empty wells	150	164	148	172	144	116

TABLE 4: Signal from viable cells (step 2 − step 1).

Samples	Well 1	Well 2	Well 3	Well 4	Well 5	Well 6
10 mg nanoparticles	94	−28	118	192	176	292
10 mg IPB	202	104	148	−70	162	246
Cells only	1814	1278	1796	1328	1348	1850
Fresh medium	−24	42	22	12	16	−24
Empty wells	86	106	84	114	76	62

TABLE 5: Percentage cytotoxicity.

Samples	Well 1	Well 2	Well 3	Well 4	Well 5	Well 6
10 mg nanoparticles	5.18	−2.19	6.57	14.46	13.06	15.78
10 mg IPB	11.14	8.14	8.24	−5.27	12.02	13.30
Cells only	—	—	—	—	—	—
Fresh medium	—	—	—	—	—	—
Empty wells	—	—	—	—	—	—

the area under the curves and peak heights of the standards extracted from the plasma to those in aqueous solutions and of the same concentrations. Percentage recovery ranged from 82 to 122% for methyldopa, 89 to 125% for dopamine, and 81 to 114% for L-dopa at concentration ranges from 125 to 8000 ng/mL. The limit of detection is described as the concentration of the analyte that produces a signal equal to three times the standard deviation of the signal from the blank. The error limit of detection is calculated as 3 times the standard deviation obtained from the blank or as 3 times the height of the baseline of the blank. The limit of detection was 40.60 ng/mL, 85.69 ng/mL, and 54.94 ng/mL for methyldopa, dopamine, and L-dopa, respectively. Specificity is derived from the mass selectivity and multiple reaction monitoring transitions, while linearity is related to correlation coefficients ranging from 94 to 99% for methyldopa, 86 to 97% for dopamine, and 96–99% for L-dopa.

3.5. Pharmacokinetic Data Analysis. Pharmacokinetic analysis is crucial in order to assess the in vivo performance of a drug delivery system. Before a drug is orally absorbed, it has to be liberated from its carrier. The factors that influence the

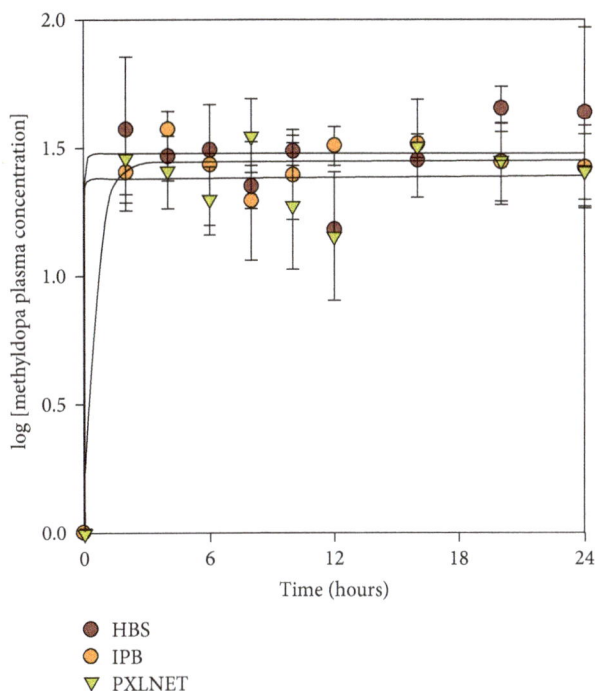

FIGURE 6: Mean methyldopa plasma concentration after administration of Madopar HBS capsules and *PXLNET* and IPB matrices.

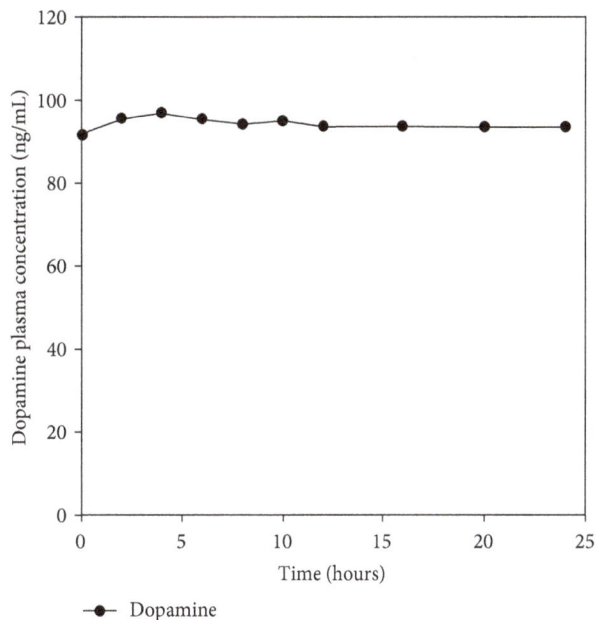

FIGURE 7: A typical mean dopamine plasma concentration observed for all formulations.

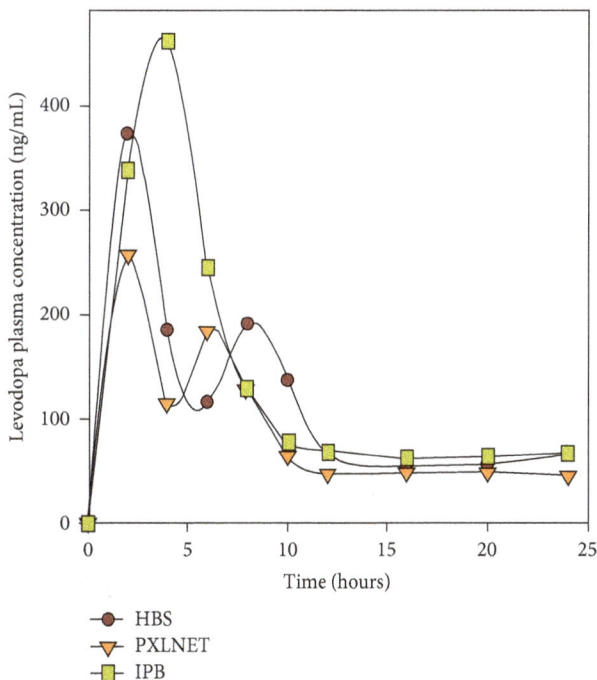

FIGURE 8: Comparative L-dopa pharmacokinetic curve of Madopar HBS capsules and *PXLNET* and IPB matrices after single dose administration.

oral absorption are broadly categorized as biological factors, physiochemical properties of the drug, and formulation factors. These factors influence the pharmacokinetic phase of drug administration and so determine the drug level in the systemic circulation, site of action, and subsequently the therapeutic effect of the drug administered.

The pigs fared well after administration of drug and recovery from anesthesia, though two pigs took a longer time to recover from the effect of anesthesia and puncturing of the cisterna magna. On visual observation, they did not seem to exhibit any side effects associated with administration of L-dopa. The metabolites and L-dopa plasma concentrations are presented in Figures 6, 7, and 8, while CSF and urine concentrations are shown in Tables 6 and 7, respectively; and the pharmacokinetic parameters are presented in Table 8. Benserazide was not detected in the samples. Benserazide, as observed during the study and confirmed in the literature, is highly chemically unstable, making its analytical quantitation challenging. It is rapidly metabolized to its main metabolite trihydroxybenzylhydrazine, a highly potent decarboxylase inhibitor [18]. Jorga and coworkers [18] also could not measure benserazide in some of the patients used in their study. They observed an increase in benserazide levels in patients given a 50 mg dose. In this study, 25 mg of benserazide was administered to the pigs. Furthermore, Jorga and coworkers [18] observed that the metabolite trihydroxybenzylhydrazine was rapidly formed after the administration of benserazide and its concentration exceeded that of benserazide. Although benserazide was metabolized, the presence of its metabolite, trihydroxybenzylhydrazine, ensured continued carboxylase inhibition leading to the presence of unchanged L-dopa in the

urine and no significant difference in the level of dopamine plasma concentration.

The plasma concentration of methyldopa was observed to vary between 8 and 50 ng/mL in the three formulations (Figure 6) and there was no marked increase over the period of sampling. Nutt and coworkers also observed that each dose

TABLE 6: Mean cerebrospinal fluid concentration after oral administration of Madopar HBS capsules, *PXLNET*, and IPB matrices.

Time (h)	Mean CSF concentration (ng/mL)								
	Madopar HBS			*PXLNET*			IPB		
	M-D	D-M	L-D	M-D	D-M	L-D	M-D	D-M	L-D
2.00	36.47	—	88.69	35.63	83.01	70.48	3.27	—	71.96
4.00	28.31	—	224.12	27.86	82.94	87.79	30.44	—	97.15

M-D, methyldopa; D-M, dopamine; and L-D, levodopa.

TABLE 7: Mean urine concentration after oral administration of Madopar HBS capsules, *PXLNET*, and IPB matrices.

Time (h)	Mean urine concentration (ng/mL)								
	Madopar HBS			*PXLNET*			IPB		
	M-D	D-M	L-D	M-D	D-M	L-D	M-D	D-M	L-D
2.00	604.6	5888	196.8	1532.7	4449	784.8	459.4	111.2	425.5
4.00	853.3	21938	755.1	—	—	—	1221.8	4571.1	1328

M-D, methyldopa; D-M, dopamine; and L-D, levodopa.

TABLE 8: Levodopa noncompartmental pharmacokinetic parameters following oral administration of Madopar HBS capsules, *PXLNET*, and IPB matrices.

Pharmacokinetic parameter	Madopar HBS	*PXLNET*	IPB
T_{max} (h)	2	2	4
C_{max} (ng/mL)	372.37	257.02	461.28
AUC_{0-t} (ng/mL*h)	2816.47	2121.43	3347.45
AUC_{0-inf} (ng/mL*h)	3685.03	2722.42	4147.16
$AUMC_{0-inf}$ (ng/mL*(h)^2)	56590.17	40775.35	55147.93
MRT (h)	15.36	14.98	13.30
Vz/F [mg/(ng/mL)]	0.3598	0.4847	0.2874
Cl/F [mg/(ng/mL)/h]	0.0271	0.0367	0.0241

T_{max}, time for maximum concentration of drug; C_{max}, maximum drug concentration; AUC_{0-t}, area under the concentration-time curve; AUC_{0-inf}, area under the concentration-time curve from time 0 to infinity; $AUMC_{0-inf}$, area under the first moment of concentration-time curve from time 0 to infinity; MRT, mean residence time. Cl/F is apparent clearance and Vz/F is apparent volume of distribution.

of L-dopa probably made a small contribution to the plasma concentration of methyldopa [19]. They deduced that methyldopa fluctuations observed in the plasma concentrations may be due to redistribution within the tissues. Furthermore, the concentrations of methyldopa in the plasma in comparison to other large neutral amino acids suggest that it is not a major competitor with L-dopa for transport to the brain; and, hence, at the concentrations detected during L-dopa dosing, it is not an important determinant of clinical response [20]. In the absence of a carboxylase inhibitor, more than 90% of L-dopa is converted to dopamine [21]. In this study, dopamine was essentially constant in all the formulations and confirms the effective carboxylase inhibition by benserazide/its active metabolite. A typical dopamine plasma concentration-time curve is shown in Figure 7. Dopamine was not detected in most of the CSF samples (Table 6). However, there is a noted dopamine concentration in the CSF for the PXLNET system. This is possibly due to enhanced targeted delivery of both L-dopa and benserazide attained by the nanoenabled system due to intact nanoparticles potentially achieving more site-specific conversion of L-dopa to dopamine. Olanow and coworkers also could not detect free dopamine in CSF [22]. Furthermore, the large presence of dopamine in the urine (Table 7) did not stem mainly from L-dopa dosing. The bulk

of the urinary dopamine may be from renal production and uptake of dopamine and decarboxylation of circulating dihydroxyphenylalanine (dopa), [23, 24] which is in turn from hydrolysis of tyrosine. However, the rationale for the large concentration of dopamine at the 4th hour for Madopar HBS in comparison to *PXLNET* and IPB matrices is uncertain. It is known that urinary dopamine is increased by feeding [25] and stress [26] amongst other factors.

A comparative display of L-dopa concentration-time curves for the three formulations is provided in Figure 8. The pharmacokinetic curves and parameters obtained for each formulation are dependent on the rate of release of L-dopa from the formulation and biological factors such as health/disposition of GIT, gastric emptying rate, rate of absorption, rate of metabolism, transporters, and extent of distribution, amongst other factors. These factors are expected to vary from pig to pig (intersubject variation) and it is also possible to vary within a pig over time (intrasubject variation). Furthermore, a protein-loaded diet is known to decrease the oral absorption of L-dopa. This is due to competitive absorption in the presence of proteins as L-dopa uses the same transport system as large amino acids. However, it is also been found that food effects vary with formulations [21].

In addition, double peaks observed in the pharmacokinetic curves of Madopar HBS capsules and *PXLNET* matrices may be attributed to the effect of L-dopa on gastric emptying time. Studies have shown that L-dopa produces intermittent delays in gastric emptying time [27–29]. In the studies undertaken by Robertson and coworkers, the double peaks were shown to correspond to the two distinct phases of gastric emptying separated by a period of negligible or no significant emptying. They employed paracetamol which is a biomarker for gastric emptying with radiolabeled diethylenetriamine-pentaacetic acid (^{99}Tc-DTPA) and gamma-camera imaging to explore the impact of L-dopa on gastric emptying [28]. The mechanisms postulated by which L-dopa delays gastric emptying were stimulations of dopamine and osmoreceptors [27]. It is also envisaged that it could also be a metabolite that may be responsible for delayed gastric emptying [27]; however, whichever it is, it affects both the absorption of L-dopa and its metabolite as this may also explicate the multiple peaks of methyldopa as well. Although the mean pharmacokinetic curve of IPB matrices has a single peak, some of individual pigs had double peaks and this may also explain the mean T_{max} of IPB matrices being at the 4th hour. Furthermore, the variability of gastric emptying is high and, apart from the presence of L-dopa, is an outcome of a complex interaction between the structure and function of the stomach and its nutrient content, which affects gastric emptying by meal volume and nutrient density. Gastric emptying is also affected by the physical and chemical properties of the meal, body movement, and position during emptying [30].

PKSolver, an add-in program for Microsoft Excel with user-friendly interface, predefined menus, and forms for easy recall [31], was used for computation. It is a visual basic for application (VBA) program which can run a range of applications for PK/PD data analysis including noncompartmental and compartmental analyses and modelling of pharmacodynamic data; and also embedded are 20 frequently used pharmacokinetic functions that can be executed on an open spreadsheet. PKSolver was validated by comparing its results with those of WinNonlin (Pharsight, Mountain View, USA) and Scientist (Micromath, Saint Louis, USA) employing two sample data sets obtained from a published book [31]. The parameters generated with PKSolver were similar to those obtained from WinNonlin and Scientist [31]. In fact, the results were identical to Scientist in all parameters to two decimal points and to WinNonlin to one or two decimal points. Consequently, PKSolver is not only flexible and user-friendly but also robust and reliable.

A noncompartmental pharmacokinetic model was chosen to decode the parameters for L-dopa plasma concentration-time curve as it best describes the data obtained (Table 8). The IPB matrices are characterized by higher C_{max}, T_{max}, AUC_{0-t}, AUC_{0-inf} and less apparent volume of distribution and clearance in comparison to Madopar HBS capsules and *PXLNET*, indicating a potential enhancement in the systemic bioavailability of L-dopa. The mean T_{max} of 4 hours for IPB matrices is attributed to the variations in individual pigs attaining peak plasma concentrations at different times. However, its mean residence time was decoded to be less than those of Madopar HBS capsules and *PXLNET*.

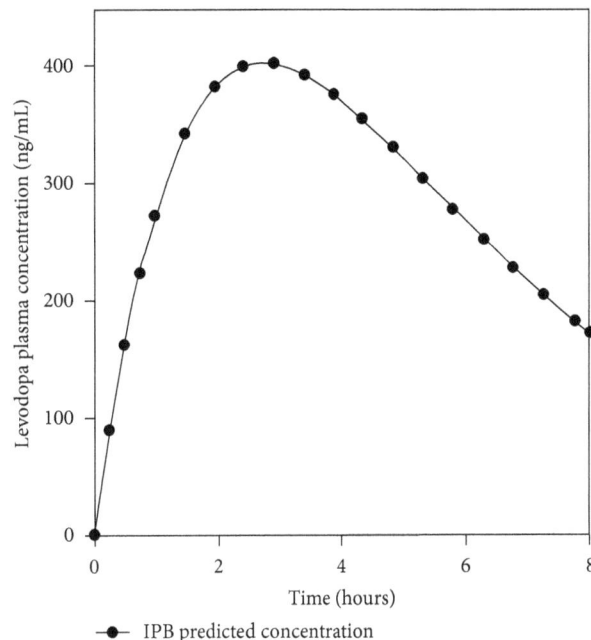

FIGURE 9: Predicted L-dopa plasma concentrations from 0.24 to 8 hours.

On application of ANOVA, the pharmacokinetic curves of the three formulations were found not to be statistically different ($p = 0.49$) at significance level of 0.05. C_{max} was also not statistically different ($p = 0.44$). Furthermore, when Madopar HBS capsules were compared with either IPB or PXLNET, there was no difference. However, statistical equivalence does not imply pharmaceutical equivalence or therapeutic equivalence. As modelled using the similarity factor, f_2, the in vitro drug release profiles of IPB and *PXLNET* matrices were not bioequivalent to that of Madopar HBS capsules.

L-dopa is known to distribute widely into the body tissues while small amounts are found in the central nervous system. This is replicated and affirmed in this study by the large apparent volume of distribution for the three formulations and the small concentrations found in CSF. The volume of distribution when quantified per kilogram was 8.94, 15.09, and 11.20 L/kg for the IPB, *PXLNET*, and Madopar HBS, respectively. Furthermore, the large apparent volume of distribution may also clarify the low concentration of L-dopa in the plasma and appreciable concentration in urine when compared with plasma concentration. There was no urine data for *PXLNET* at the 4th hour as urine collection at that period proved abortive.

Based on the impracticality of continuous blood sampling throughout the day, from the observed values, the plasma concentrations for the time points samples that were not collected can be predicted. Figure 9 is a predicted pharmacokinetic curve for IPB matrices for 8 hours showing the possible concentration of L-dopa for the times that samples were not collected. Obtaining predicted values is crucial in clinical situations as limited samples are collected after a dose to measure drug concentrations.

(a)

(b)

(c)

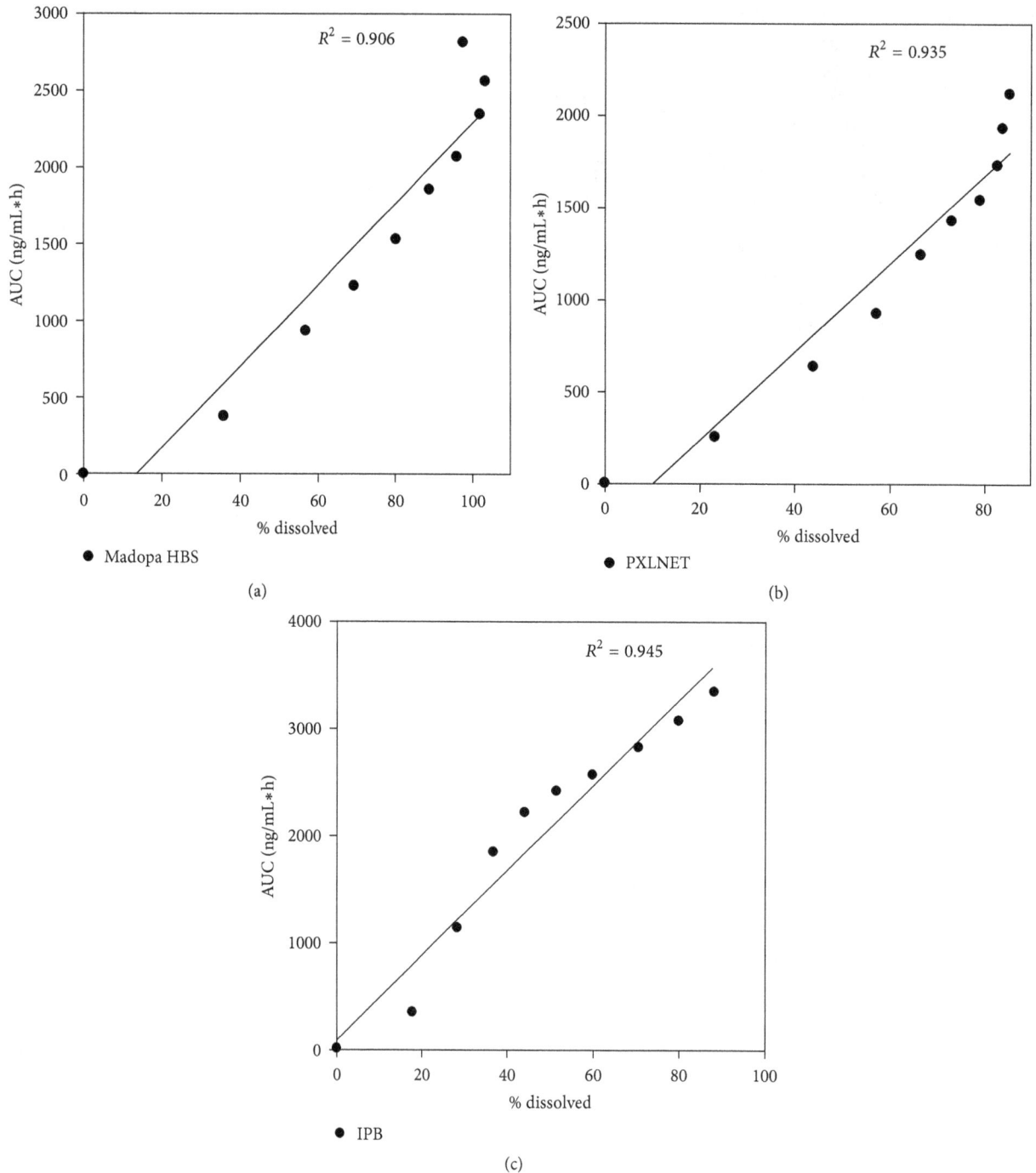

FIGURE 10: Linear regression multiple-level C IVIVC correlation models for (a) Madopar HBS capsules; (b) *PXLNET* matrices; and (c) IPB matrices.

3.6. *In Vitro-In Vivo Correlation of Dissolution and Pharmacokinetic Parameters.* In vitro-in vivo correlation describes the relationship between in vitro and in vivo outcomes. Various parameters can be used to assess correlations-dissolution time points such as $T_{50\%}$, $T_{90\%}$, MDT, and % dissolved for in vitro parameters and AUC, C_{max}, and MRT for in vivo parameters. Of the five correlation levels, multiple-level C correlation was employed in this study. Multiple-level C correlation relates one or more pharmacokinetic parameters

to the amount of drug dissolved (in vitro) at different time points of the dissolution profile [32]. In this study, a pharmacokinetic parameter, AUC was used to demonstrate a relationship with in vitro dissolution profile (% dissolved). A correlation is declared strong if it is greater than 0.8 and weak if it is less than 0.5. Linear regression multiple-level C IVIVC correlation models were constructed for Madopar HBS capsules, *PXLNET*, and IPB matrices and are shown in Figure 10. The correlation models had r^2 values of 0.906,

0.935, and 0.945 for Madopar HBS capsules, *PXLNET*, and IPB matrices, respectively.

4. Conclusions

The IPB and PXLNET formulation has been proven in vivo to be gastroretentive and nontoxic to the tissues and cells. The pharmacokinetic parameters elucidated that L-dopa was liberated from the drug delivery systems, absorbed, widely distributed, metabolized and excreted as both unchanged and metabolites (such as methyldopa). The in vitro and in vivo data correlated strongly implying that quality gastroretentive drug delivery systems were developed which performs identically in vitro and in vivo. Therefore, IPB and *PXLNET* matrices designed and formulated show promise as gastroretentive drug delivery systems for delivery of L-dopa. Furthermore, the IPB GDDS potentially enhanced the systemic bioavailability of L-dopa compared to the market comparator, whereas the PXLNET achieved comparatively more notable CSF dopamine levels.

Acknowledgments

This work was funded by the National Research Foundation (NRF) of South Africa.

References

[1] J. B. Dressman and C. Reppas, "In vitro-in vivo correlations for lipophilic, poorly water-soluble drugs," *European Journal of Pharmaceutical Sciences*, vol. 11, no. 2, pp. S73–S80, 2000.

[2] E. Lipka and G. L. Amidon, "Setting bioequivalence requirements for drug development based on preclinical data: Optimizing oral drug delivery systems," *Journal of Controlled Release*, vol. 62, no. 1-2, pp. 41–49, 1999.

[3] S. S. Davis, L. Illum, and M. Hinchcliffe, "Gastrointestinal transit of dosage forms in the pig," *Journal of Pharmacy and Pharmacology*, vol. 53, no. 1, pp. 33–39, 2001.

[4] K. D. Rainsford, P. I. Stetsko, S. P. Sirko, and S. Debski, "Gastrointestinal mucosal injury following repeated daily oral administration of conventional formulations of indometacin and other non-steroidal anti-inflammatory drugs to pigs: A model for human gastrointestinal disease," *Journal of Pharmacy and Pharmacology*, vol. 55, no. 5, pp. 661–668, 2003.

[5] J. Jelsing, R. Nielsen, A. K. Olsen, N. Grand, R. Hemmingsen, and B. Pakkenberg, "The postnatal development of neocortical neurons and glial cells in the Göttingen minipig and the domestic pig brain," *Journal of Experimental Biology*, vol. 209, no. 8, pp. 1454–1462, 2006.

[6] N. M. Lind, A. Moustgaard, J. Jelsing, G. Vajta, P. Cumming, and A. K. Hansen, "The use of pigs in neuroscience: modeling brain disorders," *Neuroscience and Biobehavioral Reviews*, vol. 31, no. 5, pp. 728–751, 2007.

[7] L. Minuzzi, A. K. Olsen, D. Bender et al., "Quantitative autoradiography of ligands for dopamine receptors and transporters in brain of Göttingen Minipig: comparison with results in vivo," *Synapse*, vol. 59, no. 4, pp. 211–219, 2006.

[8] P. Rosa-Neto, D. J. Doudet, and P. Cumming, "Gradients of dopamine D1- and D2/3-binding sites in the basal ganglia of pig and monkey measured by PET," *NeuroImage*, vol. 22, no. 3, pp. 1076–1083, 2004.

[9] N. C. Ngwuluka, V. Pillay, Y. E. Choonara et al., "Fabrication, modeling and characterization of multi-crosslinked methacrylate copolymeric nanoparticles for oral drug delivery," *International Journal of Molecular Sciences*, vol. 12, no. 9, pp. 6194–6225, 2011.

[10] N. C. Ngwuluka, Y. E. Choonara, G. Modi et al., "Design of an interpolyelectrolyte gastroretentive matrix for the site-specific zero-order delivery of levodopa in Parkinson's disease," *AAPS PharmSciTech*, vol. 14, no. 2, pp. 605–619, 2013.

[11] Q. Garrett, P. A. Simmons, S. Xu et al., "Carboxymethylcellulose binds to human corneal epithelial cells and is a modulator of corneal epithelial wound healing," *Investigative Ophthalmology and Visual Science*, vol. 48, no. 4, pp. 1559–1567, 2007.

[12] L. C. Huang, D. Jean, and A. M. McDermott, "Effect of preservative-free artificial tears on the antimicrobial activity of human β-defensin-2 and cathelicidin LL-37 in vitro," *Eye and Contact Lens*, vol. 31, no. 1, pp. 34–38, 2005.

[13] J. G. Vehige, P. A. Simmons, C. Anger, R. Graham, L. Tran, and N. Brady, "Cytoprotective properties of carboxymethyl cellulose (CMC) when used prior to wearing contact lenses treated with cationic disinfecting agents," *Eye and Contact Lens*, vol. 29, no. 3, pp. 177–180, 2003.

[14] M. Ito, A. Ban, and M. Ishihara, "Anti-ulcer effects of chitin and chitosan, healthy foods, in rats," *The Japanese Journal of Pharmacology*, vol. 82, no. 3, pp. 218–225, 2000.

[15] F. Khodagholi, B. Eftekharzadeh, N. Maghsoudi, and P. F. Rezaei, "Chitosan prevents oxidative stress-induced amyloid β formation and cytotoxicity in NT2 neurons: involvement of transcription factors Nrf2 and NF-κB," *Molecular and Cellular Biochemistry*, vol. 337, no. 1-2, pp. 39–51, 2010.

[16] M. Susan, I. Baldea, S. Senila et al., "Photodamaging effects of porphyrins and chitosan on primary human keratinocytes and carcinoma cell cultures," *International Journal of Dermatology*, vol. 50, no. 3, pp. 280–286, 2011.

[17] N. Unceta, E. Rodriguez, Z. G. De Balugera et al., "Determination of catecholamines and their metabolites in human plasma using liquid chromatography with coulometric multi-electrode cell-design detection," *Analytica Chimica Acta*, vol. 444, no. 2, pp. 211–221, 2001.

[18] K. M. Jorga, J. P. Larsen, A. Beiske et al., "The effect of tolcapone on the pharmacokinetics of benserazide," *European Journal of Neurology*, vol. 6, no. 2, pp. 211–219, 1999.

[19] J. G. Nutt, W. R. Woodward, S. T. Gancher, and D. Merrick, "3-O-Methyldopa and the response to levodopa in Parkinson's disease," *Annals of Neurology*, vol. 21, no. 6, pp. 584–588, 1987.

[20] J. G. Nutt, J. H. Carter, E. S. Lea, and W. R. Woodward, "Motor fluctuations during continuous levodopa infusions in patients with Parkinson's disease," *Movement Disorders*, vol. 12, no. 3, pp. 285–292, 1997.

[21] S.-P. Khor and A. Hsu, "The pharmacokinetics and pharmacodynamics of Levodopa in the treatment of Parkinson's disease," *Current Clinical Pharmacology*, vol. 2, no. 3, pp. 234–243, 2007.

[22] C. W. Olanow, L. L. Gauger, and J. M. Cedarbaum, "Temporal relationships between plasma and cerebrospinal fluid pharmacokinetics of levodopa and clinical effect in Parkinson's disease," *Annals of Neurology*, vol. 29, no. 5, pp. 556–559, 1991.

[23] J. R. Gill Jr., E. Grossman, and D. S. Goldstein, "High urinary dopa and low urinary dopamine-to-dopa ratio in salt-sensitive hypertension," *Hypertension*, vol. 18, no. 5, pp. 614–621, 1991.

[24] E. Grossman, D. S. Goldstein, A. Hoffman, I. R. Wacks, and M. Epstein, "Effects of water immersion on sympathoadrenal and dopa-dopamine systems in humans," *American Journal of Physiology—Regulatory Integrative and Comparative Physiology*, vol. 262, no. 6, pp. R993–R999, 1992.

[25] B. Mühlbauer and H. Osswald, "Feeding but not salt loading is the dominant factor controlling urinary dopamine excretion in conscious rats," *Naunyn-Schmiedeberg's Archives of Pharmacology*, vol. 346, no. 4, pp. 469–471, 1992.

[26] W. Fibiger and G. Singer, "Urinary dopamine in physical and mental effort," *European Journal of Applied Physiology and Occupational Physiology*, vol. 52, no. 4, pp. 437–440, 1984.

[27] D. Robertson, A. Renwick, N. Wood et al., "The influence of levodopa on gastric emptying in man.," *British Journal of Clinical Pharmacology*, vol. 29, no. 1, pp. 47–53, 1990.

[28] D. Waller, C. Roseveare, A. Renwick, B. Macklin, and C. George, "Gastric emptying in healthy volunteers after multiple doses of levodopa," *British Journal of Clinical Pharmacology*, vol. 32, no. 6, pp. 691–695, 1991.

[29] D. R. C. Robertson, A. G. Renwick, B. Macklin et al., "The influence of levodopa on gastric emptying in healthy elderly volunteers," *European Journal of Clinical Pharmacology*, vol. 42, no. 4, pp. 409–412, 1992.

[30] T. Müller, C. Erdmann, D. Bremen et al., "Impact of gastric emptying on levodopa pharmacokinetics in Parkinson disease patients," *Clinical Neuropharmacology*, vol. 29, no. 2, pp. 61–67, 2006.

[31] Y. Zhang, M. Huo, J. Zhou, and S. Xie, "PKSolver: An add-in program for pharmacokinetic and pharmacodynamic data analysis in Microsoft Excel," *Computer Methods and Programs in Biomedicine*, vol. 99, no. 3, pp. 306–314, 2010.

[32] J. Emami, "In vitro-in vivo correlation: from theory to applications," *Journal of Pharmacy and Pharmaceutical Sciences*, vol. 9, pp. 169–189, 2006.

10

Abdominal Massage for the Relief of Constipation in People with Parkinson's

D. McClurg,[1] **K. Walker,**[1] **P. Aitchison,**[1] **K. Jamieson,**[1] **L. Dickinson,**[2] **L. Paul,**[3] **S. Hagen,**[1] **and A.-L. Cunnington**[4]

[1]*Nursing, Midwifery, and Allied Health Professions, Research Unit, Glasgow Caledonian University, Glasgow G4 0BA, UK*
[2]*Nursing, Midwifery and Allied Health Professions, Research Unit, Stirling University, Stirling, UK*
[3]*School of Medicine, Dentistry & Nursing, Nursing & Health Care School, 59 Oakfield Avenue,
  Gilmorehill Campus, Glasgow University, Glasgow, UK*
[4]*Care of Elderly Department, Glasgow Royal Infirmary, 84 Castle Street, Glasgow G4 0SF, UK*

Correspondence should be addressed to D. McClurg; doreen.mcclurg@gcu.ac.uk

Academic Editor: Peter Hagell

Objectives. To explore the experiences of people with Parkinson's (PwP) who suffer from constipation, the impact this has on their lives, and the effect of using lifestyle changes and abdominal massage as a form of constipation management. *Method.* Fourteen semistructured interviews were completed (8 males and 6 females; mean age 72.2 years) at the end of a care programme, which consisted of either lifestyle advice and abdominal massage (intervention group; $n = 7$) or lifestyle advice only (control group; $n = 7$). Data were analysed using constant-comparison techniques and Framework methods. Themes and key quotes were identified to depict major findings. *Findings.* Four key themes were identified: (i) the adverse impact of bowel problems on quality of life; (ii) positive experience of behaviour adjustments: experimentation; (iii) abdominal massage as a dynamic and relaxing tool: experiential learning (intervention group only); (iv) abdominal massage as a contingency plan: hesitation (control group only). Constipation was reported as having a significant impact on quality of life. Participants in both groups perceived lifestyle advice to relieve symptoms. Specific improvements were described in those who also received the abdominal massage. *Conclusions.* Both lifestyle advice and abdominal massage were perceived to be beneficial in relieving symptoms of constipation for PwP.

1. Introduction

Constipation is a common nonmotor symptom of neurological conditions [1] including Parkinson's [2, 3]. Constipation is the most common gastrointestinal complaint reported in people with Parkinson's (PwP) and is estimated to impact 27–67% of all sufferers [4, 5]. Furthermore, constipation in Parkinson's has been shown to occur to varying degrees at any time point during disease progression, with epidemiological data indicating that bowel dysfunction can even precede typical Parkinsonian motor symptoms by as much as 20 years [6, 7].

Constipation in Parkinson's is caused by deterioration of the neurological pathways that promote the peristaltic reflex. Reduced peristalsis often exacerbates a slow colonic transit time, resulting in defecatory dysfunction and decreased bowel movement frequency [7]. Lifestyle and individual factors such as poor diet, decreased mobility, general weakness and fatigue, and medication side-effects are also thought to exacerbate bowel dysfunction symptoms [8]. Recommendations for constipation management in Parkinson's therefore include pharmacological treatment, increased physical activity, and dietary modifications such as increased intake of fluids (6–8 glasses water per day), and a high fibre diet [9, 10]. As Parkinson's progresses many patients complain of dysphagia and experience worsening mobility leading to poor diet and difficulty with maintaining levels of activity. Instead, these individuals rely on medicines such as osmotic or stimulant laxatives and stool softeners to help relieve gastrointestinal distress. Though at times effective, laxatives can cause side-effects such as abdominal cramps and diarrhoea, which may lead to faecal incontinence [11].

People with Parkinson's have reported the experience of constipation as distressing, painful, and often debilitating [7]. A UK based National Audit (2015) identified that 80% of patients had been asked about their bladder and bowel symptoms at a routine clinical appointment; however it has also been found that that there is a lack of follow-up and appropriate management with consultations typically focusing on the more visually apparent motor characteristics of the disease [12]. Study of the experience of constipation in PwP is therefore warranted to produce helpful therapeutic approaches, management strategies, and education for PwP who suffer from constipation.

A growing body of research has shown that abdominal massage can reduce the severity of gastrointestinal symptoms, including those who experience chronic constipation [13–15]. Stimulating the parasympathetic division of the autonomic nervous system through a variety of pressured movements is thought to encourage rectal loading by increasing the motility of the muscles and relaxing the sphincters in the gastrointestinal canal. The resulting increase in intra-abdominal pressure promotes peristalsis and bowel sensation [16]. Using abdominal massage as a form of constipation management has also been proposed to reduce laxative use (and thus also their side-effects) [17, 18], improve health related quality of life (QoL) [19, 20], and ease the substantial cost of constipation-related-medicines to primary care [21].

Abdominal massage has been shown to be a safe, effective, and noninvasive form of bowel management in the general population [14, 22, 23], as well as people with multiple sclerosis and stroke [5, 13, 24–26]. It is therefore plausible that PwP who suffer from constipation may also benefit from using abdominal massage as a form of constipation management and this was explored in our feasibility studies [27, 28].

However the experience of living with constipation is inadequately described in the literature and particularly within neurological populations. In one of the few qualitative studies identified, McClurg and colleagues explored the impact of constipation on the QoL of people with multiple sclerosis (MS) [29]. Using phenomenological methodology, the authors highlighted that constipation had a significant impact on the QoL of some people with MS, with themes of decreased self-esteem, loss of control, and reluctance to talk about bowel problems, which was often linked to social isolation.

This study was a cohort study of a prospective two-group (intervention = abdominal massage and advice; control = advice only) single blind randomised controlled feasibility study that aimed to explore the effects of lifestyle advice and abdominal massage on constipation in PwP [27]. The study period was 10 weeks, with base-line outcome assessment (Week 0), 6 weeks of intervention with assessment (Week 6), and final outcome assessment 4 weeks later (Week 10).

Intervention Group. The intervention group were asked to self-administer or have a carer administer a 10-minute abdominal massage. The abdominal massage was demonstrated to the patient and/or their carer in their own home and a research nurse visited the patient weekly to offer support on the massage and on the suggested lifestyle changes. Step-by-step written instructions for the abdominal massage were provided with an accompanying DVD. Lifestyle advice, incorporated in a leaflet, included increasing awareness of the importance of fluid intake, fruit and vegetable consumption, physical activity levels, and varying one's position on the toilet.

Control Group. Those in the control group were also visited weekly for the 6-week intervention period by the research nurse to offer support around the suggested lifestyle changes as described above. This group was also offered a brief abdominal massage training session and given the DVD at the 10-week follow-up visit following completion of the final outcome measures [27].

It was concluded from the quantitative analysis that abdominal massage as an adjunct to treatment of constipation offers a potentially beneficial intervention to PwP.

This is the first study to explore the views and experiences of PwP in terms of abdominal massage and constipation and aims to explore the experiences of PwP and constipation, as well as the impact that this has on their lives and the effect of using lifestyle advice and abdominal massage as a form of constipation management. As a feasibility study this information is important in going on to design a fully powered randomised controlled study and implementation should be proved effective.

2. Methods

2.1. Study Design and Sample. An exploratory, qualitative research design was adopted to align with the aims of this study.

2.2. Ethical Approval. The study received ethical approval from the West of Scotland Research Ethics 10/S1001/11 and management approval from NHS Greater Glasgow & Clyde R&D GN10GE070. All participants received both oral and written information about the qualitative strand of the study during the initial consultation for the feasibility trial [27]. Informed consent was obtained for participants who wished to take part and the voluntary nature of the study was continually declared. Confidentiality and anonymity were assured. Raw data were stored in a locked filing cabinet and password-protected computer and the study investigators had sole access to data.

2.3. Data Collection. Participants in both the intervention and control groups were invited for interview at the end of the pilot study to gain an appreciation of their experiences of being constipated, how it impacted on their QoL and their views on taking part in the study. A number of participants included a family member in their medication management (some of whom also applied the massage to the participant if necessary), and in these scenarios both the patients and their carer/family member were present at interview. A research assistant (PA) who had not been involved in the intervention delivery undertook the interviews by telephone. The topics explored were description of Parkinson's symptoms and their impact on life, impact of constipation on life, management of symptoms, experience of taking part in the study and their perceptions of the effect of the lifestyle advice, and/or abdominal massage on their constipation (see Appendix A.). Interviews ranged from 11 to 31 minutes, were digitally recorded, and were then transcribed verbatim. PA checked transcripts for accuracy before coding and analysis.

2.4. Data Analysis. Throughout the data collection process, data were analysed using the constant-comparative technique [30]. DM and PA reviewed and compared interview transcripts regularly, which enabled the identification of emergent themes for exploration in subsequent interviews. Further data management and analysis was approached using the "Framework" method [31]. Familiarisation with data enabled construction of a first level coding framework and was informed by (1) *a priori* research questions underpinning the qualitative element of the study, (2) topics and issues introduced by researchers during the interviews, and (3) recurring themes emerging from interviews with participants. PA conducted this process for each transcript. Initial "indexing" was reviewed by KW, who identified a number of additional emergent codes or themes reflecting patients' experiences of constipation, abdominal massage and bowel management advice. The KW and PA contributed to descriptive analysis, interpretation of indexed data and manuscript preparation with the aid of thematic charts to compare themes within and across the intervention and control groups. In order to ensure validity of interpretation, a sample of indexed data was selected and reviewed by the first author (DM). Key themes and quotes were identified to depict major findings.

3. Results

Thirty-two PWP took part in the study from which 14 completed semistructured interviews, 2–4 weeks after completing Week-10 outcome assessments (intervention group $n = 7$; control group $n = 7$). The sample interviewed included 8 males and 6 females with a mean age of 72.2 years. Interviews were conducted either face-to-face (8 interviews) or by telephone (4 interviews). The interview sample was purposively selected to provide a broad range of demographics and equal numbers from the intervention and control group.

This study aimed to explore the experience of constipation in PwP and the feasibility and impact of lifestyle advice and abdominal massage as an intervention within this population. Four main themes emerged from the analysis: (i) *the adverse impact of bowel problems on participants' quality of life;* (ii) *positive experience of behaviour adjustments: experimentation;* (iii) *abdominal massage as a dynamic and relaxing tool: experiential learning (intervention group only);* (iv) *abdominal massage as a contingency plan: hesitation (control group only)* (see Appendix B). The themes discussed are narrated by direct quotations from participants, with an exemplar given for each theme. Numerical values have been assigned to each participant to protect their identities.

3.1. The Adverse Impact of Bowel Problems on Participants' Lives

3.1.1. The Nature and Burden of Constipation: Psychological Distress. All participants in both the intervention and control groups stated that constipation was the main bowel problem they experienced (other specific bowel problems mentioned were IBS and diverticulitis). The duration of constipation ranged from two months to five years. Three participants recalled that their constipation began around the time of their Parkinson's diagnosis, while two participants perceived an association between their constipation and their Parkinson's medication. Symptoms associated with constipation included flatulence, bloating, nausea, and lethargy and were reported as extremely bothersome. As one participant described:

> *Well you don't feel 100% because you're sluggish and I have to strain a lot to get movement. Participant 14, Male, Intervention*

Feeling constipated resulted in participants going to the toilet more frequently and for longer periods, but often without achieving a bowel movement until days later. Stools were often described as being like small pellets which involved straining, pain, and discomfort with some using digital stimulation to encourage a bowel movement.

> *The stools are very very hard like round balls . . . it's very very painful to try and go to the toilet. Participant 6, Male, Intervention*

Participants emphasised that the overall experience of constipation was time consuming and detracted from their ability to perform daily activities. Furthermore, the perception of having "no control" over their bowel movements caused concern for a number of individuals who curtailed social activity specifically due to the burden of constipation. This included going out shopping or taking part in occasions with family and friends. The constant need to be close to a toilet and the corresponding fear of not finding one close by, especially after taking laxatives, required either careful forward planning or deciding simply not to go out at all.

> *This is going to sound daft, but you don't go out so often. I'm frightened to go out in case I need to go . . . you don't know when you're going to need to go to the toilet. That's the big thing. Participant 5, Male, Control*

In summary, the burden of constipation was expressed through a range of emotional, psychological, and social outlets and was continually linked to a perceived negative impact on quality of life. A number of participants felt embarrassed because they had flatulence or had to take laxatives or were generally unhappy about having recurring constipation. One participant described how the discomfort from constipation affected his concentration during meetings at work. Another participant expressed the worry she had about her constipation because this contrasted with previous, very regular bowel movements. While for some participants, coping with the effects of constipation lowered their day-to-day mood, for a participant in the control group it had the effect of affecting him in a deeper way:

> You get depressed. A wee bit of depression set in ... even going out for a walk, I've virtually got to make sure that I'm empty before I go out because I don't want to get caught short. Participant 11, Male, Control

3.1.2. Balancing Solutions with Unpredictable Side-Effects. The psychological burden of constipation was strongly associated with the unpredictable nature of medical aids specific to easing constipation. Most participants in both the intervention and control groups relied on laxatives to contend with their constipation, though some did not use them every day and others reported that they did not always have the desired result of initiating a bowel movement. The unpredictable effect of laxatives was also a concern for many, who described a balancing act between taking laxatives to relieve temporary constipation, against managing the consequences of taking them, for example, experiencing loose stools or diarrhoea. One participant admitted that she was fearful that the physiological influence of laxatives might interfere with the effectiveness of her Parkinson's medications and would use them as a last resort depending on the severity of constipation and stability of Parkinson's combined:

> You're trying to achieve this balance, you're saying, well, on the one hand I'm getting a bit of discomfort in terms of my stomach, my bowels, but in terms of Parkinson's I'm feeling a lot better. So you're trying to do as little as you can to disrupt that. Participant 4, Female, Control

Implementing dietary changes was mentioned as an alternative approach to dealing with constipation. Examples of dietary changes that participants made included drinking prune juice and eating more fruit, vegetables, and roughage, for example, brown bread and Weetabix. In some instances, participants first implemented dietary changes before deciding to take laxatives or continued to combine the two approaches.

3.1.3. Meeting Educational Needs. The participant group was divided almost equally between those who had received information or advice about bowel problems from specialist healthcare staff and those who had not. In the former group, without exception, participants stated that their bowel problems had been discussed with Parkinson's nurses during clinic appointments. Emerging from participants' accounts was a sense that these discussions were typically quite brief and often initiated by participants themselves. As Participant 13 describes:

> I found that if you bring something up then they [specialist staff] were working things out for you, but I wouldn't say that they told me about them [bowel problems]. Participant 13, Male, Control

The input from specialist staff often made minimal difference to these individuals who instead preferred to cope with their bowel problems themselves, sometimes with the help of other information sources such as the Internet. Participants also highlighted that discussing bowel problems was not always considered an acceptable thing to do in everyday life and often felt embarrassed at initiating conversations on the subject. For a few participants, this was exacerbated by the lack of someone to share such difficulties with. These individuals reported to value the opportunity to discuss their otherwise "taboo" bowel problems with the study researcher who reduced their anxiety and encouraged them to be honest about their experiences with constipation.

Those who had not received specialist advice reflected that bowel problems were perhaps not a priority for discussion with healthcare staff, including GPs, because the focus was more on how they were coping with the general development of their Parkinson's:

> When you go to see the doctor about [husband's] Parkinson's ... they don't have the time. He's more interested in what [husband] can do with his hand and how he's able to stand up, but they never mentioned bowel to me once. Wife of Participant 5, Male, Control

3.2. Positive Experience of Behaviour Adjustments: Experimentation. All participants in the study received lifestyle advice over the 6-week study duration that aimed to help reduce their constipation. Topics included diet, fluid intake, and sitting position, and participants were recommended to monitor their bowel movements with the use of a bowel diary. In general, participants described experiences of increased self-awareness specific to their bowel problems upon implementing the lifestyle advice and often reported direct improvements to the severity of their constipation. This was achieved through a process of experimentation and determination which enabled participants to identify individualised triggers and sensitivities.

3.2.1. Bowel Diaries. All participants stated that they had kept a bowel diary during the study period, with the majority claiming that it was a useful tool to document their bowel habits. Particular reference was made to the fact that participants could easily monitor changes in stool type over time and objectively check if remedial action was needed to improve fluid levels or make dietary changes. This increase in awareness allowed participants to reflect on how their daily behaviours and established routines may impact or relate to their bowel problems. As one participant highlighted:

> ... it's not till you start writing things down you realise how many times you go to the toilet, how you do the toilet, what positions you're in. All of a sudden you're challenged to think, well, you've always done it that way, but why? [Participant 13, Male, Control]

3.2.2. *Dietary Advice.* Within the study, members of both the intervention and control groups had the opportunity to discuss their current diet with the researcher and, if appropriate, to explore ways in which dietary changes might help to alleviate their constipation. Participants' accounts of their discussions about diet were of two types: those who recounted that they were "already doing the right things" and those who were recommended to make changes. Advice included regularly eating more fruit, vegetables and high fibre foods, adding foods such as yoghurts to lunches, and increasing the frequency of snacks in between meals.

Those participants who did make changes to their diet found them to have a positive impact on their bowel movements and indicated that they had continued with the changes. Participants highlighted the role of partners and family members in encouraging them to incorporate and maintain these dietary modifications.

3.2.3. *Fluid Intake.* As an integral aspect of exploring dietary behaviour during the study, participants' levels of fluid intake were also explored and encouraged. Some individuals explained that gaining an understanding about the potential relationship between lack of fluid intake and constipation proved enlightening for them. As one participant's wife described:

> I didn't realise it was the liquid that [E] needed to take; it didn't matter so much what I was feeding him up, it was lying in the bowel because there wasn't enough liquid. [Wife of Participant 5, Male, Control]

A range of approaches were adopted to help maintain higher fluid intake such as filling bottles with water or juice and using these throughout the day, taking water regularly with their medication, or drinking alternatives to water (e.g., soda water, juices, or tea). Two-thirds of participants who had initially increased their fluid intake said that they had maintained this behaviour after participating in the study and reported that this continued to ease their symptoms of constipation. There was a variety of reasons why some participants had not been able to maintain higher fluid levels, including travelling and forgetfulness. However two participants explained that after increasing their fluid intake they had perceived no effect on their constipation and had therefore reverted back to previous levels.

3.2.4. *Sitting Position.* Those who followed advice about trying to adopt an improved sitting position to facilitate bowel movements found it generally helpful in achieving bowel movements. Specifically, some participants said that it helped reduce straining, prompted mindfulness about sitting up straighter on the toilet, and made sitting on the toilet more comfortable. Over half of the participants reported that they were continuing to use the sitting technique after the 6-week study period [4 intervention; 4 control], and one female participant recounted that her husband had even made her a small wooden stool so that she could elevate her feet when she went to the toilet. Two participants in the control group

had not continued to use the technique: one because he did not perceive it to have any effect for him and the other reported difficulty doing so due to mobility aids installed in her bathroom following a recent hip replacement operation.

3.3. *Abdominal Massage as a Dynamic and Relaxing Tool: Experiential Learning (Intervention Group Only).* Participants in the intervention group were taught abdominal massage and given a DVD at the start of the study and were visited once a week over the 6 weeks to discuss their diet, lifestyle, and how they (or their carer) were getting on with the massage. Generally, as a way of gauging the effect of the massage intervention, participants compared their bowel problems before and after intervention.

Performing abdominal massage produced a variety of effects for participants. Four individuals in the intervention group reported an improvement in their bowel problems during the study period and three saw minimal or no change. For those who reported immediate improvements (sometimes occurring after the very first massage), experiences included reduced or no constipation, more regular bowel movements, less straining, less bloating, and an increased sense of when a bowel movement was going to occur. Changes in stool type and less total time spent on the toilet were also described:

> I don't sit on the toilet for so long. I come out after ten minutes whereas before it was thirty-five minutes. Participant 8, Female, Intervention

Participants also described that they felt relaxed, comfortable, and generally at ease when receiving abdominal massage. One participant reported: "I felt like falling asleep." Additionally, a male participant [Participant 3] reflected on how the massage intervention had helped him to deal with his Parkinson's in a wider sense and increase his motivation to engage more fully and positively in managing his symptoms. Further, having the ability to apply the self-massage technique and experience its positive effect reduced the negative impact of constipation and gave him one less thing to deal with on a daily basis:

> It's getting me focused again, I'm a bit more relaxed ... in dealing with symptoms as well ... I think it's like giving you a tool ... [The massage] is a big help. It's something less you're dealing with, you know, because Parkinson's is enough to deal with. Participant 3, Male, Intervention

Those who reported a continued improvement to their bowel problems were also those who had continued to practice abdominal massage regularly, either by self-massage or given by their husband or wife. Three participants perceived continued improvements to their bowel problems following the "very good" and "very useful" intervention and felt that their bowel habits were "easier" and "more regular" as a result. For two participants this was accompanied by a reduction in laxative use, which resulted in an increase in motivation to reengage with social activities.

Three participants perceived minimal or no changes to their bowel problems even if improvements had been perceived initially. In other words, any improvements that were observed were not maintained, despite continuing to use the massage for the 6-week study duration. Symptoms of constipation remained an issue for these participants, and each continued to take daily laxatives. As Participant 9 describes:

> I'd say at the moment [my constipation] is as bad as it has ever been. Participant 9, Male, Intervention

Of those who reported little or no improvement to their bowel problems, no one had continued to carry out regular abdominal massage beyond the study period of 6 weeks. However one participant in this group did self-massage if his constipation lasted more than two or three days. Reasons given for ceasing massage were lack of perceived improvement in constipation severity, lack of physical strength in hands and arms (either self or of partner), and changes in daily routine affected by travel.

3.4. Abdominal Massage as a Contingency Plan: Hesitation (Control Group Only). Participants in the control group received advice about their diet and lifestyle once a week over the 6-week study duration. If they wanted, they were also advised and instructed on the abdominal massage by the study researcher *after* the 6-week intervention period was completed at the 10-week assessment session. Thus the control group received less training and no support to implement the abdominal massage. Participants in the control group reported mixed results of performing abdominal massage. One female participant did not practice abdominal massage after being shown, expressing that she felt "guilty" about not doing so [CP12, Female, Control]. Reasons for not continuing were her husband's reticence about applying the technique, using other ways to control constipation and experiencing other health problems. One participant stopping after approximately two weeks due to experiencing pain in his lower abdomen when his wife applied the massage techniques. The experience of abdominal massage was also reported as uncomfortable and awkward for two participants, with minimal perceived impact on constipation. This lack of immediate positive experience or impact of abdominal massage on severity of constipation caused participants to feel hesitant towards using it as a tool to alleviate their bowel problems. One individual further stated that he preferred to focus on the dietary and lifestyle advice he had received (such as increased roughage and varying his position on the toilet), as these changes incurred a reduction in his constipation severity:

> [The massage] was a lot of work, for not a lot of change. I've been concentrating more on the initial comments and remedies [that were] suggested. And they definitely helped, not 100% but maybe 95%. Participant 11, Male, Control

Of those who gave data, two participants from the control group were still continuing to use the technique at the time of interview. A female participant commented that she continued to use the self-massage technique, despite finding it quite difficult to do and anticipated continued improvement in her technique with practice. Another participant's wife explained that she continued to use massage on her husband if he experienced constipation for three to four days, because she found that this helped to initiate a bowel movement.

4. Discussion

The findings of this research confirm previous evidence that PwP can suffer from constipation, which often presents as a frequent and emotionally troublesome nonmotor feature of the disease [2, 7, 32]. The themes from the narratives also align with Kaye et al. (2006) such that many participants felt concerned at the severity of their constipation symptoms and often relied on laxatives to help ease their constipation.

Research has shown that experiencing emotional stress, anxiety, and cognitive impairment may contribute to constipation by overstimulating the sympathetic nervous system, which can result in decreased digestive motility [33, 34]. The majority of participants in this study perceived constipation to have a negative impact on their QoL, experiencing general low mood and fear regarding the consequences of laxative use, which curtailed social activity. Depression in Parkinson's has been well documented in the literature [8, 35] and the present results highlight both the physical and psychological strain of constipation within this population.

Participants described discrepancies and inconsistencies in consultation experiences such that some were alerted to associations between Parkinson's and constipation and others were not. In the latter circumstance, it seemed that emphasis was placed on the motor symptoms of Parkinson's, such as motor complications and motor disability, to the detriment of nonmotor symptoms. Those who had not received direct advice from their Parkinson's nurse (or equivalent) sought out strategies of self-management from alternate sources including the Internet; however the information gathered from these methods is not always as reliable as that from health care professionals. Helping patients realise the likelihood of developing constipation may help them feel more at ease about talking through similar nonmotor symptoms and provides an opportunity to learn simple yet effective strategies such as abdominal massage, which may have significant impact on QoL.

The topic of constipation is often reported as a "taboo" subject within clinical settings, resulting in many PwP feeling embarrassed to talk to health care professionals about their bowel movements [36]. Participants in the present study recalled similar feelings of embarrassment when discussing their constipation with healthcare professionals and thus welcomed the opportunity to openly discuss their bowel movements with the researcher. Indeed, many participants reported feelings of relief at the chance to talk freely about their experiences with constipation. This may in turn reduce stress and anxiety and enable the digestive system to work more effectively [34]. This perspective is likely to reflect both the topical nature of the study-specific conversations and the researcher's encouragement of discussing a potentially sensitive subject.

A number of study-specific tools were also believed to be helpful in relieving the impact of constipation on daily life through means of increasing one's self-awareness of the condition and its exacerbations. For example, using a bowel diary to record bowel movements allowed participants to note the nature of their constipation (e.g., stool frequency, consistency, size, and degree of straining), observe patterns in their preceding nutritional choices, and gain a deeper understanding of their overall Parkinson's health status. Other studies have affirmed diary use as a positive bowel management strategy in the alleviation of constipation and associated symptoms [26]. Increased consumption of liquids was also perceived to reduce severity of constipation. These findings provide support for HCPs to encourage the use of bowel diaries and increased fluid intake as potential constipation aids for PwP, while taking individual preference and lifestyle into consideration.

Abdominal massage was reported as a pleasant and relaxing experience which aligns with previous work [20, 22]. Most participants in the intervention group reported positive impacts both physically (including improved bowel function, reduction in time spent defecating, less straining and bloating, increased completeness of evacuation, and reduced dependence on laxatives) and emotionally, for example, feeling empowered to self-manage their symptoms. This combination of positive visual *and* kinaesthetic feedback may help to explain why the abdominal massage was perceived to be an effective treatment for constipation for these specific participants, as the evidential change in outcomes motivated them to continue.

However some participants did not perceive any improvements in their bowel movements from the abdominal massage over the study period and thus discontinued with abdominal massage sessions. A number of these individuals preferred to rely on the lifestyle advice to ease their constipation and use abdominal massage as a contingency plan if their constipation was particularly bothersome. This reiterates that abdominal massage may not be effective for all individuals who experience constipation and further work is needed to define those in whom it may work or may pose beneficial. Nonetheless, the findings from the present study suggest that abdominal massage may offer an additional treatment option for PwP who have constipation which is noninvasive and few side-effects. This may be an important perception for PwP who do not want to take additional medication to alleviate their constipation.

4.1. Limitations. Only a small number of interviews were conducted from the original cohort, which means that the findings presented here must be viewed as one possible description of experiences of individuals who live with Parkinson's and constipation. Furthermore, the participants may represent a biased sample towards those who were not only happy to talk about their treatment but had also perceived benefits from the lifestyle advice and abdominal massage specifically. Further research is therefore required with diverse samples of PwP to extend understanding of the experience of constipation and its treatments in this specific population.

5. Conclusion

This study has provided insight into the experiences of PwP who suffer with constipation taking part in a six-week lifestyle advice and abdominal massage programme as an intervention for constipation management. Many participants perceived lifestyle advice and abdominal massage to relieve symptoms and severity of constipation and increase their QoL. Lifestyle advice and abdominal massage (both in combination and separately) may therefore provide effective strategies for constipation management in those who live with Parkinson's and particularly in those who may not wish to rely on multiple medications to alleviate their symptoms of bowel dysfunction. This has implications for clinicians who wish to understand and alleviate the burden of constipation in PwP and also for further research that aims to identify and explore potential interventions for constipation.

This study also highlighted that people who live with Parkinson's and constipation warrant improved education and explanation from HCPs about the nonmotor symptoms of Parkinson's in the goal of holistic and person-centred care. In light of the results presented, HCPs may therefore wish to include lifestyle advice and abdominal massage specifically in their advice to PwP, to potentially relieve the impact and severity of constipation on daily life and increase QoL. However individual tolerability and preference must be considered before any recommendations are made.

Appendix

A. Interview Schedule

Study of the Relief of Constipation Using Abdominal Massage for Patients with Parkinson's Disease

(1) Can you describe your PD symptoms?

Probes:

(i) Would you suffer from constipation as a result of PD?

(ii) Would you suffer from any other bowel problems as a result of PD?

(iii) Have you ever suffered from faecal incontinence?

(2) What impact has PD had on your life?

(3) What impact has the constipation and/or bowel problems had?

Probes:

(i) Impact on family life

(ii) Impact on social life

(iii) Impact on self-perception

(iv) Impact on ability to work

(v) Impact on everyday tasks for example, house-work

(4) How do you manage your symptoms of PD?

Probe:

(i) How do you manage the bowel problems?
(ii) Have you used laxatives?

(5) What information had you received about PD and bowel problems/constipation?

Probes:

(i) Information about the causes of bowel problems
(ii) What symptoms to expect
(iii) How to alleviate symptoms
(iv) Sources of information (e.g. GP, PD nurses, Consultant; voluntary groups)

(6) How have you found the massage technique?

Probe:

(i) How long have you been doing it yourself?
(ii) What do you think of the technique?

(7) When do you tend to do the massage?

Probes:

(i) In bed/on toilet/night time

(8) Who does the massage?

Probe:

(i) Self massage and/or carer and/or partner
(ii) How do you feel about this?

(9) Do you think a physio or someone trained in massage would be more effective?

Probe:

(i) Positives and negatives of physio/outside person doing massage

(10) How did you find using the diary?

Probe:

(i) Was the diary useful? Why?

(11) What did you think of the DVD?

Probe:

(i) How did you use the DVD?
(ii) Was the DVD useful? Why?

(12) What did you think of the weekly visits?

(13) Was the programme long enough?

(14) Do you think that the massage helped with your constipation and/or bowel problems?

Probe:

(i) How did it help?
(ii) Did it affect your use of laxatives (if applicable?)
(iii) Has it stabilised your constipation?
(iv) Has it had any impact on overflow inconti-nence?
(v) Has it affected any bladder problems you might have had?

(15) Has the massage helped with any other problems associated with PD?

(16) Can you think of any other way the massage pro-gramme could be improved for other PD patients?

Probes:

(i) Would you use a hand-held massager? Why?
(ii) Would you like to know of any other exercises that might help your symptoms?
(iii) Would you attend a group forum or group exercise class showing how to alleviate PD symptoms?

(17) Is there anything else you want to add about the programme?

B. Themes and Subthemes from Interview Data

(3.1) The adverse impact of bowel problems on partici-pants' quality of life

(3.1.1) The nature and burden of constipation: psycho-logical distress

(3.1.2) Balancing solutions with unpredictable side-effects

(3.1.3) Meeting educational needs

(3.2) Positive experience of behaviour adjustments: exper-imentation

(3.3) Abdominal massage as a dynamic and relaxing tool: experiential learning (Intervention group only)

(3.4) Abdominal massage as a contingency plan: hesitation (Control Group only)

Acknowledgments

The authors would like to thank all of the individuals who took part in the study. This work was supported by Parkinson's UK Grant no. K-0908.

References

[1] K. Krogh, P. Christensen, and S. Laurberg, "Colorectal symptoms in patients with neurological diseases," *Acta Neurologica Scandinavica*, vol. 103, no. 6, pp. 335–343, 2001.

[2] P. Martinez-Martin, A. H. V. Schapira, F. Stocchi et al., "Prevalence of nonmotor symptoms in Parkinson's disease in an international setting; study using nonmotor symptoms questionnaire in 545 patients," *Movement Disorders*, vol. 22, no. 11, pp. 1623–1629, 2007.

[3] H. Y. Sung, M.-G. Choi, Y.-I. Kim, K.-S. Lee, and J.-S. Kim, "Anorectal manometric dysfunctions in newly diagnosed, early-stage parkinson's disease," *Journal of Clinical Neurology*, vol. 8, no. 3, pp. 184–189, 2012.

[4] R. Sakakibara, H. Shinotoh, T. Uchiyama et al., "Questionnaire-based assessment of pelvic organ dysfunction in Parkinson's disease," *Autonomic Neuroscience: Basic and Clinical*, vol. 92, no. 1-2, pp. 76–85, 2001.

[5] J. Kaye, H. Gage, A. Kimber, L. Storey, and P. Trend, "Excess burden of constipation in Parkinson's disease: a pilot study," *Movement Disorders*, vol. 21, no. 8, pp. 1270–1273, 2006.

[6] R. Savica, W. A. Rocca, and J. E. Ahlskog, "When does Parkinson's disease start?" *Archives of Neurology*, vol. 67, no. 7, pp. 798–801, 2010.

[7] M. Rossi, M. Merello, and S. Perez-Lloret, "Management of constipation in Parkinson's disease," *Expert Opinion on Pharmacotherapy*, vol. 16, no. 4, pp. 547–557, 2015.

[8] M. Pandya, C. S. Kubu, and M. L. Giroux, "Parkinson disease: not just a movement disorder," *Cleveland Clinic Journal of Medicine*, vol. 75, no. 12, pp. 856–863, 2008.

[9] P. Paré, R. Bridges, M. C. Champion et al., "Recommendations on chronic constipation (including constipation associated with irrtable bowel syndrome) treatment," *Canadian Journal of Gastroenterology*, vol. 21, pp. 3B–22B, 2007.

[10] H. J. Song, "Constipation in community-dwelling elders," *Journal of Wound, Ostomy & Continence Nursing*, vol. 39, no. 6, pp. 640–645, 2012.

[11] A. C. Ford and N. C. Suares, "Effect of laxatives and pharmacological therapies in chronic idiopathic constipation: systematic review and meta-analysis," *Gut*, vol. 60, no. 2, pp. 209–218, 2011.

[12] D. A. Gallagher, A. J. Lees, and A. Schrag, "What are the most important nonmotor symptoms in patients with Parkinson's disease and are we missing them?" *Movement Disorders*, vol. 25, no. 15, pp. 2493–2500, 2010.

[13] Ş. Ayaş, B. Leblebici, S. Sözay, M. Bayramoğlu, and E. A. Niron, "The effect of abdominal massage on bowel function in patients with spinal cord injury," *American Journal of Physical Medicine and Rehabilitation*, vol. 85, no. 12, pp. 951–955, 2006.

[14] K. Lämås, L. Lindholm, H. Stenlund, B. Engström, and C. Jacobsson, "Effects of abdominal massage in management of constipation: a randomized controlled trial," *International Journal of Nursing Studies*, vol. 46, no. 6, pp. 759–767, 2009.

[15] J. Preece, "Introducing abdominal massage in palliative care for the relief of constipation," *Complementary Therapies in Nursing and Midwifery*, vol. 8, no. 2, pp. 101–105, 2002.

[16] Z. Liu, R. Sakakibara, T. Odaka et al., "Mechanism of abdominal massage for difficult defecation in a patient with myelopathy (HAM/TSP)," *Journal of Neurology*, vol. 252, no. 10, pp. 1280–1282, 2005.

[17] D. Bromley, "Abdominal massage in the management of chronic constipation for children with disability," *Community Practitioner*, vol. 87, no. 12, pp. 25–29, 2014.

[18] M. Emly, "Abdominal massage for adults with learning disabilities," *Nursing Times*, vol. 97, no. 30, pp. 61–62, 2001.

[19] K. Lämås, L. Lindholm, B. Engström, and C. Jacobsson, "Abdominal massage for people with constipation: a cost utility analysis," *Journal of Advanced Nursing*, vol. 66, no. 8, pp. 1719–1729, 2010.

[20] L. Moss, M. Smith, S. Wharton, and A. Hames, "Abdominal massage for the treatment of idiopathic constipation in children with profound learning disabilities: a single case study design," *British Journal of Learning Disabilities*, vol. 36, no. 2, pp. 102–108, 2008.

[21] Department of Health, *Prescription Cost Analysis: Laxatives*, Department of Health, London, UK, 2001.

[22] K. Lämås, U. H. Graneheim, and C. Jacobsson, "Experiences of abdominal massage for constipation," *Journal of Clinical Nursing*, vol. 21, no. 5-6, pp. 757–765, 2012.

[23] N. Turan and T. A. Asti, "The effect of abdominal massage on constipation and quality of life," *Gastroenterology Nursing*, vol. 39, no. 1, pp. 48–59, 2016.

[24] B. Albers, H. Cramer, A. Fischer, A. Meissner, A. Schürenberg, and S. Bartholomeyczik, "Abdominal massage as intervention for patients with paraplegia caused by spinal cord injury—A Pilot Study," *Pflege Zeitschrift*, vol. 59, no. 3, pp. 2–8, 2006.

[25] C. Hu, M. Ye, and Q. Huang, "Effects of manual therapy on bowel function of patients with spinal cord injury," *Journal of Physical Therapy Science*, vol. 25, no. 6, pp. 687–688, 2013.

[26] D. McClurg, S. Hagen, S. Hawkins, and A. Lowe-Strong, "Abdominal massage for the alleviation of constipation symptoms in people with multiple sclerosis: a randomized controlled feasibility study," *Multiple Sclerosis*, vol. 17, no. 2, pp. 223–233, 2011.

[27] D. McClurg, S. Hagen, K. Jamieson, L. Dickinson, L. Paul, and A. Cunnington, "Abdominal massage for the alleviation of symptoms of constipation in people with Parkinson's: a randomised controlled pilot study," *Age and Ageing*, vol. 45, no. 2, pp. 299–303, 2016.

[28] D. McClurg, S. Hagen, A. L. Cunnington et al., "A qualitative study on the effect of constipation in patients with Parkinson's," *Nerourology and Urodynamics*, vol. 34, no. 3, pp. S1–S461, 2015.

[29] D. McClurg, K. Beattie, A. Lowe-Strong, and S. Hagen, "The elephant in the room: the impact of bowel dysfunction on people with multiple sclerosis," *Journal of the Association of Chartered Physiotherapists in Women's Health*, no. 111, pp. 13–21, 2012.

[30] D. Silverman, *Doing Qualitative Research: A Practical Handbook*, SAGE, London, UK, 2000.

[31] J. Ritchie and J. Lewis, *Qualitative Research Practice: A Guide for Social Science Students and Researchers*, SAGE, London, UK, 2003.

[32] M. F. Siddiqui, S. Rast, M. J. Lynn, A. P. Auchus, and R. F. Pfeiffer, "Autonomic dysfunction in Parkinson's disease: a comprehensive symptom survey," *Parkinsonism and Related Disorders*, vol. 8, no. 4, pp. 277–284, 2002.

[33] M. Petticrew, M. Rodgers, and A. Booth, "Effectiveness of laxatives in adults," *Quality in Health Care: QHC*, vol. 10, no. 4, pp. 268–273, 2001.

[34] M. Sinclair, "The use of abdominal massage to treat chronic constipation," *Journal of Bodywork and Movement Therapies*, vol. 15, no. 4, pp. 436–445, 2011.

[35] F. Kanda, O. Kenichi, S. Kenji et al., "Characteristics of depression in Parkinson's disease: evaluating with Zung's self'rating depression scale," *Parkinsonism and Related Disorders*, vol. 14, no. 1, pp. 19–23, 2008.

[36] K. R. Chaudhuri, C. Prieto-Jurcynska, Y. Naidu et al., "The nondeclaration of nonmotor symptoms of Parkinson's disease to health care professionals: an international study using the nonmotor symptoms questionnaire," *Movement Disorders*, vol. 25, no. 6, pp. 704–709, 2010.

11

Microarray Analysis of the Molecular Mechanism Involved in Parkinson's Disease

Cheng Tan, Xiaoyang Liu, and Jiajun Chen ⓘD

Department of Neurology, China-Japan Union Hospital of Jilin University, Changchun, Jilin 130033, China

Correspondence should be addressed to Jiajun Chen; cjj@jlu.edu.cn

Academic Editor: Amnon Sintov

Purpose. This study aimed to investigate the underlying molecular mechanisms of Parkinson's disease (PD) by bioinformatics. *Methods*. Using the microarray dataset GSE72267 from the Gene Expression Omnibus database, which included 40 blood samples from PD patients and 19 matched controls, differentially expressed genes (DEGs) were identified after data preprocessing, followed by Gene Ontology (GO) and Kyoto Encyclopedia of Genes and Genomes (KEGG) pathway enrichment analyses. Protein-protein interaction (PPI) network, microRNA- (miRNA-) target regulatory network, and transcription factor- (TF-) target regulatory networks were constructed. *Results*. Of 819 DEGs obtained, 359 were upregulated and 460 were downregulated. Two GO terms, "rRNA processing" and "cytoplasm," and two KEGG pathways, "metabolic pathways" and "TNF signaling pathway," played roles in PD development. Intercellular adhesion molecule 1 (*ICAM1*) was the hub node in the PPI network; hsa-miR-7-5p, hsa-miR-433-3p, and hsa-miR-133b participated in PD pathogenesis. Six TFs, including zinc finger and BTB domain-containing 7A, ovo-like transcriptional repressor 1, GATA-binding protein 3, transcription factor dp-1, SMAD family member 1, and quiescin sulfhydryl oxidase 1, were related to PD. *Conclusions*. "rRNA processing," "cytoplasm," "metabolic pathways," and "TNF signaling pathway" were key pathways involved in PD. *ICAM1*, hsa-miR-7-5p, hsa-miR-433-3p, hsa-miR-133b, and the abovementioned six TFs might play important roles in PD development.

1. Introduction

Parkinson's disease (PD) is one of the most common age-related neurodegenerative diseases [1]. The age at PD onset is approximately 55 years, and the incidence in the population aged > 65 years is approximately 1% [1–3]. PD mainly occurs because of the death of dopaminergic neurons in the substantia nigra [4]. Patients with PD present with symptoms such as bradykinesia, resting tremor, rigidity, and postural instability [5]. The current therapy for PD is targeted at its symptoms rather than at dopaminergic neuron degeneration [1]. The diagnosis of PD at the early stage is challenging, and successfully managing PD is difficult at its later stages [4]. To date, the cause of PD remains unknown; however, it appears to involve the intricate interplay of environmental and genetic factors [1, 4].

Much effort has been spent in investigating PD pathogenesis, and the misfolding, aggregation, and aberrance of proteins are considered to be some of the main causes

[1, 4, 5]. Some key genes such as hydrogen sulfide, chromobox 5 (*CBX5*), and transcription factor 3 (*TCF3*) are related to PD [6, 7]. Several pathways have also been identified to be related to PD. Activation of the protein kinase B (Akt)/glycogen synthase kinase 3 beta/(GSK3β) pathway by urate reportedly protects dopaminergic neurons in a rat model of PD [8]. In addition, the E2-related factor 2 (Nrf2)/antioxidant response element pathway reportedly counteracts mitochondrial dysfunction, which is a prominent PD feature [9]. The ubiquitin, lipid, nigrostriatal, autophagy-lysosome, and endosomal pathways are also involved in PD [10–15]. Furthermore, a recent study revealed several microRNAs (miRNAs) associated with PD; miR-205 suppresses LRRK2 expression and miR-205 expression levels in the brains of patients with PD decreases [16]. Furthermore, miR-34b and miR-34c are downregulated in the brains of patients with PD, which is related to the reduction in the expression of *DJ-1* and *PARKIN* [17], and miR-133 and miR-7 are also associated with PD [18–20]. Numerous

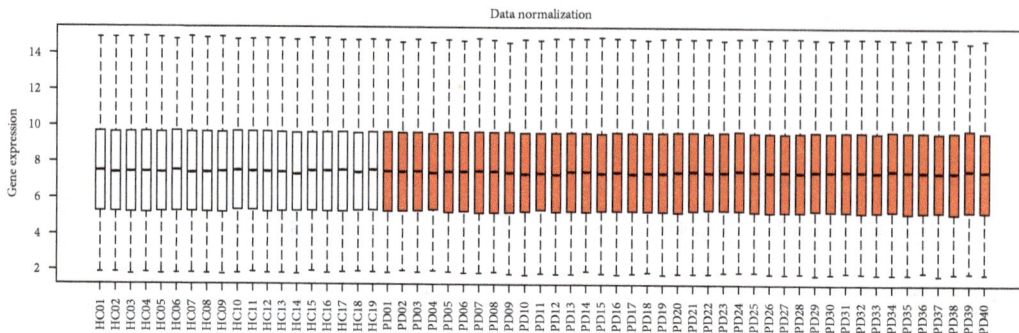

FIGURE 1: Boxplots for normalized gene expression data. Red represents the blood samples of patients with Parkinson's disease, and white represents the healthy matched control samples.

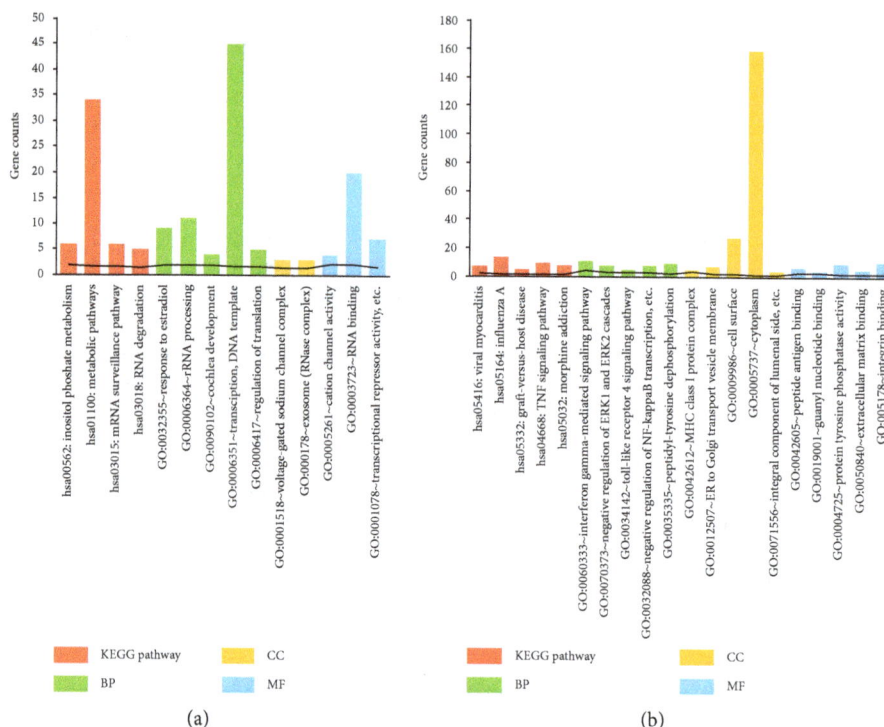

FIGURE 2: Functional enrichment analyses of differentially expressed genes (DEGs). (a) Gene Ontology (GO) terms and the Kyoto Encyclopedia of Genes and Genomes (KEGG) pathways of upregulated DEGs and (b) GO terms and KEGG pathways of downregulated DEGs. The numbers on the x-axis were the ID of pathways or GO terms. The numbers on the y-axis were gene counts.

reports that have described the roles of transcription factors (TFs) in PD have also been published. The TF paired-like homeodomain 3 has roles in developing and maintaining dopaminergic neurons [21, 22], and engrailed 1, which is downregulated in the rat models, plays a role in the apoptosis of dopaminergic neurons and the symptoms of PD [23]. Moreover, Nrf2, nuclear factor kappa B (NF-κB), GATA2, and PHD finger protein 10 are TFs involved in PD [24–27]. However, understanding the key mechanisms underlying the development of PD remains unclear.

In a previous study, the microarray dataset GSE72267 generated by Calligaris et al. [7] was used to identify key differentially expressed genes (DEGs) such as *CBX5*, *TCF3*,

dedicator of cytokinesis 10, and mannosidase alpha class 1C in the blood of patients with PD compared with those of healthy controls. Moreover, crucial pathways related to chromatin remodeling and methylation were revealed. In the current study, we downloaded this microarray dataset to comprehensively analyze DEGs in patients with PD compared with those in matched controls by bioinformatics approaches and to describe their functional annotations. Compared with the previous analysis conducted by Calligaris et al. [7], we performed additional analyses, including those for the protein-protein interaction (PPI), miRNA-target regulatory, and TF-target regulatory networks, to further elucidate the key mechanisms underlying PD. Our

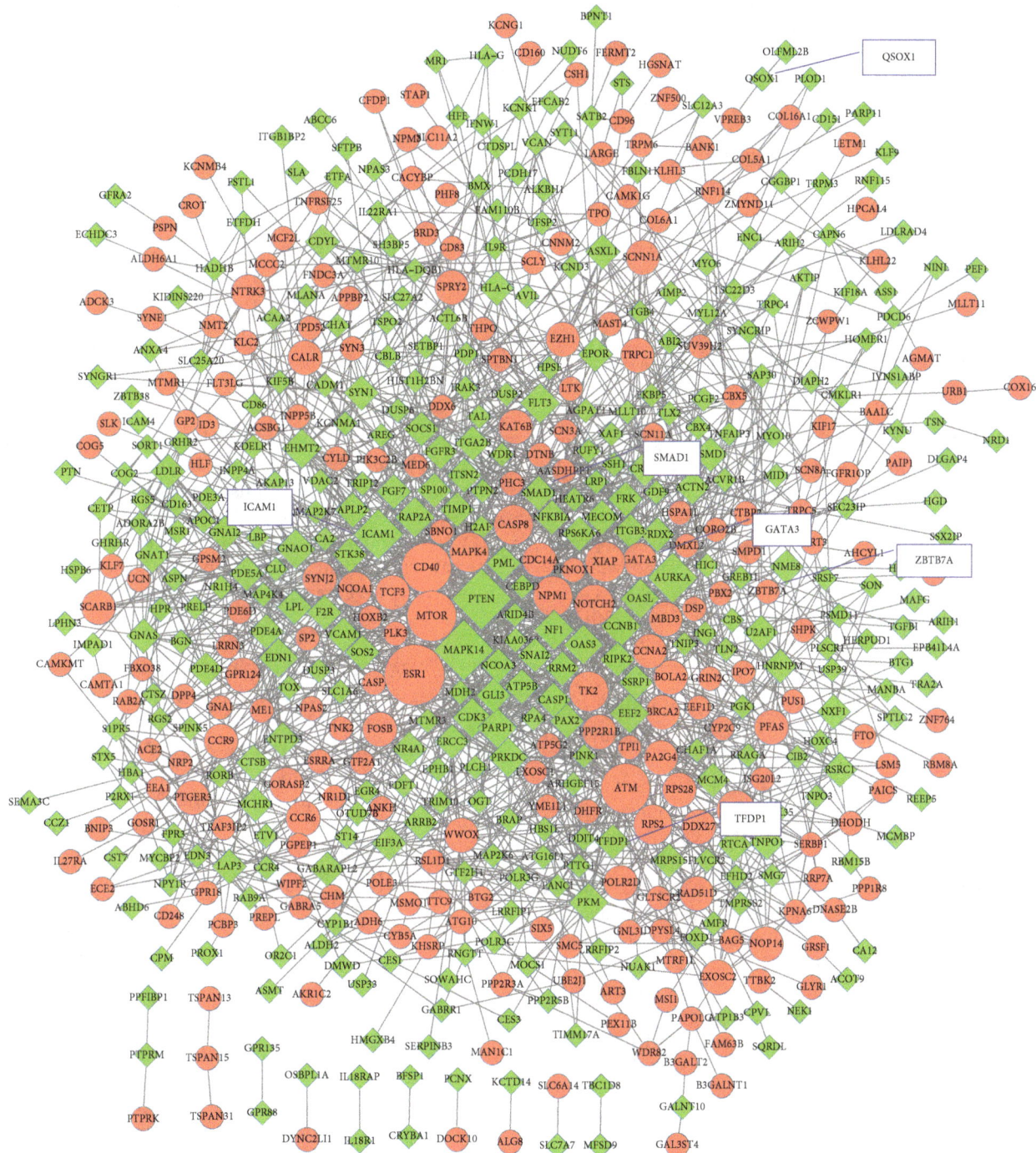

Figure 3: The protein-protein interaction (PPI) network of differentially expressed genes (DEGs). Red circles represent upregulated DEGs, and green diamonds represent downregulated DEGs.

results may provide useful data for diagnosing and treating PD.

2. Materials and Methods

2.1. Affymetrix Microarray Data. Gene expression profile data GSE72267 was extracted from the Gene Expression Omnibus database (https://www.ncbi.nlm.nih.gov/geo/) [28]. The GSE72267 dataset was deposited by Calligaris et al. [7], including blood samples from 40 PD patients and 19 healthy matched controls and was based on the platform of the GPL571 (HG-U133A-2) Affymetrix Human Genome U133A 2.0 Array (Affymetrix Inc., Santa Clara, California, USA). This dataset was downloaded and analyzed on October 2016.

2.2. Data Preprocessing and DEG Screening. The downloaded data in CEL files were preprocessed using the Affy package

TABLE 1: List of top 10 differentially expressed genes with higher degrees in protein-protein interaction network.

Gene	Full name	Description	Degree
MAPK14	Mitogen-activated protein kinase 14	Down	68
ESR1	Estrogen receptor 1	Up	54
PTEN	Phosphatase and tensin homolog	Down	52
MTOR	Mechanistic target of rapamycin	Up	40
ATM	ATM serine/threonine kinase	Up	35
ICAM1	Intercellular adhesion molecule 1	Down	33
CD40	CD40 molecule	Up	32
AURKA	Aurora kinase A	Down	31
PRKDC	Protein kinase, DNA-activated, catalytic polypeptide	Down	29
TK2	Thymidine kinase 2, mitochondrial	Up	29

Degree was used for describing the importance of protein nodes in network. The higher the degree was, the more important the nodes were in network.

(version 1.50.0) [29] in R language, including background correction, normalization, and expression calculation. Annotations to the probes were performed, and probes that were not matched to the gene symbol were excluded. The average expression values were taken if different probes mapped to the same gene. DEGs in patients with PD compared with those in healthy matched controls were analyzed using the limma package (version 3.10.3) [30] in R language. The cutoff threshold was set to a p value of <0.05.

2.3. Pathway Enrichment Analysis.

Gene ontology (GO) (http://www.geneontology.org/) analysis is commonly used for functional studies of large-scale genomic or transcriptomic data and classifies functions with respect to three aspects: molecular function (MF), cellular component (CC), and biological process (BP) [31, 32]. The Kyoto Encyclopedia of Genes and Genomes (KEGG; http://www.kegg.jp/) pathway database [33] is widely used for systematic analysis of gene functions, linking genomic data with higher order functional data. The database for annotation, visualization, and integrated discovery (DAVID) is an integrated biological knowledgebase with analytical tools used for systematic and integrative analysis of large gene lists [34]. In this study, GO terms and KEGG pathway enrichment analyses for up- and downregulated DEGs were performed using DAVID (version 6.8). The cutoff thresholds were as follows: an enrichment gene number count of ≥2 and a super geometry inspection significance threshold p value of <0.05.

2.4. PPI Network Analysis.

Search Tool for the Retrieval of Interacting Genes/Proteins (STRING; http://www.string-db.org/) [35] is an online database that assesses and integrates PPIs. In this study, DEGs were mapped into the STRING database for PPI analysis, with a PPI score of 0.4 as the parameter setting. The PPI network established by DEGs was constructed using the Cytoscape software (version 3.2.0) [36], and the topology scores of the nodes, including node degree in the PPI network, were analyzed using the CytoNCA plugin (version 2.1.6; http://apps.cytoscape.org/apps/cytonca) [37] (parameter setting: without weight). Degree was used for describing importance of

protein nodes in network. The higher the degree was, the more important the nodes were in network. In addition, subnetworks were identified using the MCODE plugin [38] in the Cytoscape software, and subnetworks with a score of >5 were identified as key subnetworks. Finally, KEGG pathway enrichment analyses for the genes in the key subnetworks were performed.

2.5. miRNA-Target Regulatory Network Analysis.

The miR2disease (http://www.mir2disease.org/) database [39] is a manually curated database that provides a comprehensive resource of miRNA deregulation in various human diseases. miRWalk2.0 (http://zmf.umm.uni-heidelberg.de/apps/zmf/mirwalk2/) [40] is a comprehensive database that presents predicted and validated data, regarding miRNA targets in human, mouse, and rats. In this study, miRNAs related to PD were extracted from the miR2disease database, and experimentally verified miRNA-gene regulatory pairs were obtained by searching miRWalk2.0. Finally, a miRNA-target regulatory network was constructed by comparing DEGs with obtained miRNA-gene regulatory pairs using the Cytoscape software.

2.6. TF-Target Regulatory Network Analysis.

The genes in the PPI network described above were further analyzed to identify TF-target interaction pairs that were then used to construct a TF-target regulatory network. The iRegulon plugin (version 1.3; http://apps.cytoscape.org/apps/iRegulon) [41] in the Cytoscape software collects multiple human TF-target interaction databases such as Transfac, Jaspar, and Encode using two computational methods: Motif and Track. In this study, we analyzed the TF-target pairs using the iRegulon plugin and compared them with TFs with DEGs in the PPI network, followed by a TF-target regulatory network construction. The parameter settings were as follows: minimum identity between orthologous genes, 0.05 and maximum false discovery rate on motif similarity, 0.001. The normalized enrichment score (NES) indicates the reliability of the results, and the cutoff threshold was NES of >3.

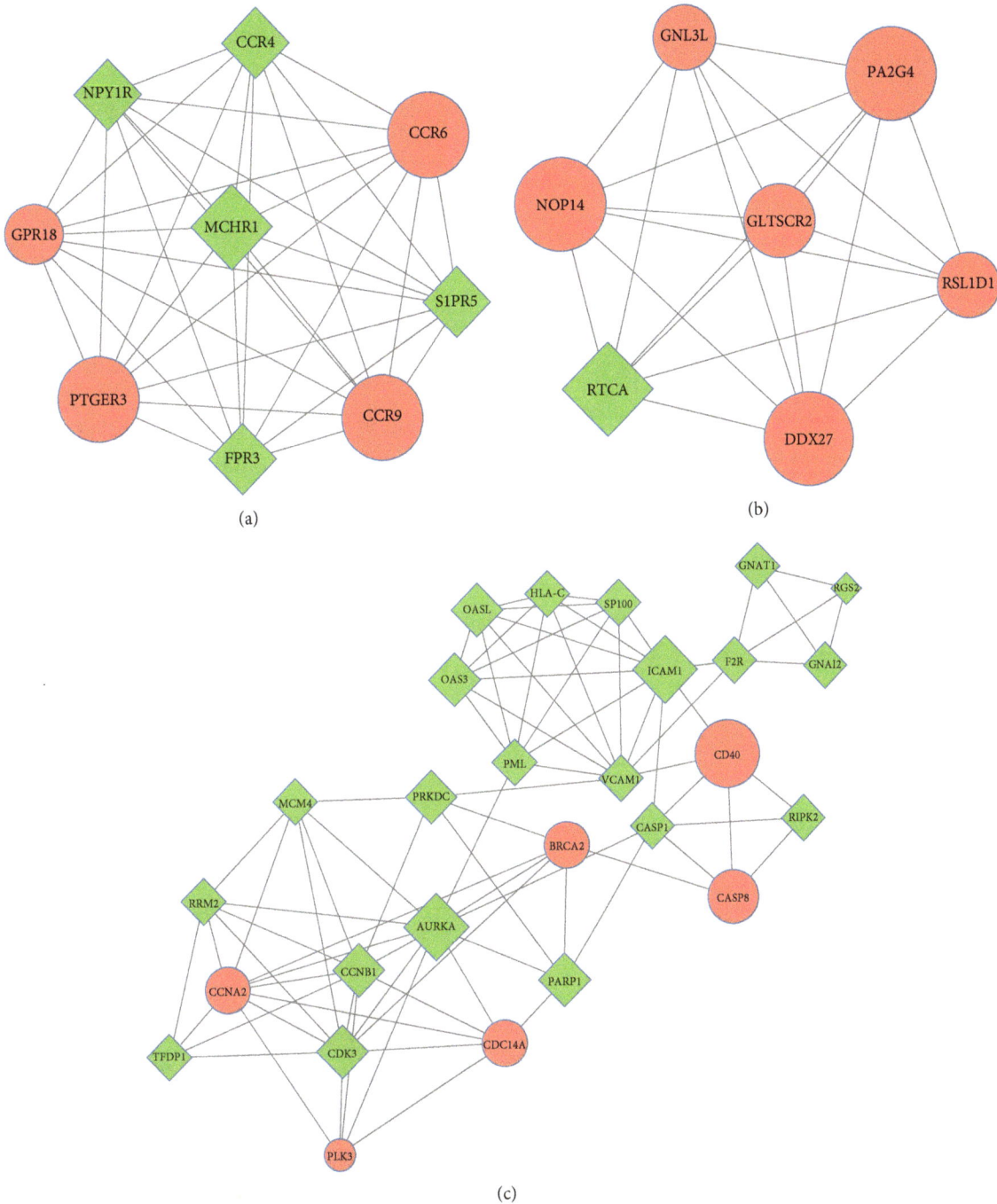

FIGURE 4: Subnetworks of differentially expressed genes (DEGs). (a) Subnetwork a; (b) subnetwork b; (c) subnetwork c. Red circles represent upregulated DEGs, and green diamonds represent downregulated DEGs.

3. Results

3.1. Analysis of DEGs.
The boxplot of the preprocessed data indicated good normalization (Figure 1). In total, 22,277 probes were obtained, among which 971 probes were differentially expressed. After annotation, 819 DEGs in patients with PD compared with those in healthy matched controls were identified (Supplementary Table 1), including 359 upregulated DEGs and 460 downregulated DEGs.

3.2. Pathway Enrichment Analysis.
GO and KEGG pathway enrichment analyses for the up- and downregulated DEGs were performed (Supplementary Table 2). The significant GO terms and KEGG pathways are shown in Figure 2. The upregulated DEGs were significantly enriched in four KEGG pathways, namely, metabolic pathways, inositol phosphate metabolism, mRNA surveillance pathway, and RNA degradation, and GO terms such as transcription, DNA-template processing, and rRNA processing (Figure 2(a)).

TABLE 2: List of KEGG pathways of subnetworks.

Subnetwork	Pathway ID	Pathway name	Count	p value	Genes
Subnetwork a	hsa04080	Neuroactive ligand-receptor interaction	5	1.40E−04	MCHR1, PTGER3, S1PR5, FPR3, NPY1R
	hsa04062	Chemokine signaling pathway	3	1.80E−02	CCR9, CCR6, CCR4
	hsa04060	Cytokine-cytokine receptor interaction	3	2.74E−02	CCR9, CCR6, CCR4
Subnetwork c	hsa04110	Cell cycle	6	1.31E−04	CCNB1, CDC14A, PRKDC, CCNA2, MCM4, TFDP1
	hsa05416	Viral myocarditis	4	1.62E−03	ICAM1, CASP8, HLA-C, CD40
	hsa05168	Herpes simplex infection	5	6.03E−03	SP100, CASP8, OAS3, PML, HLA-C
	hsa04514	Cell adhesion molecules	4	1.70E−02	VCAM1, ICAM1, HLA-C, CD40
	hsa05144	Malaria	3	1.78E−02	VCAM1, ICAM1, CD40
	hsa04621	NOD-like receptor signaling pathway	3	2.00E−02	CASP8, RIPK2, CASP1
	hsa04115	p53 signaling pathway	3	2.93E−02	CCNB1, RRM2, CASP8
	hsa05164	Influenza A	4	3.32E−02	ICAM1, OAS3, PML, CASP1
	hsa04914	Progesterone-mediated oocyte maturation	3	4.30E−02	CCNB1, GNAI2, CCNA2
	hsa05169	Epstein–Barr virus infection	4	4.42E−02	ICAM1, HLA-C, CD40, CCNA2
	hsa05203	Viral carcinogenesis	4	4.60E−02	SP100, CASP8, HLA-C, CCNA2
	hsa04064	NF-kappa B signaling pathway	3	4.84E−02	VCAM1, ICAM1, CD40

KEGG, Kyoto Encyclopedia of Genes and Genomes.

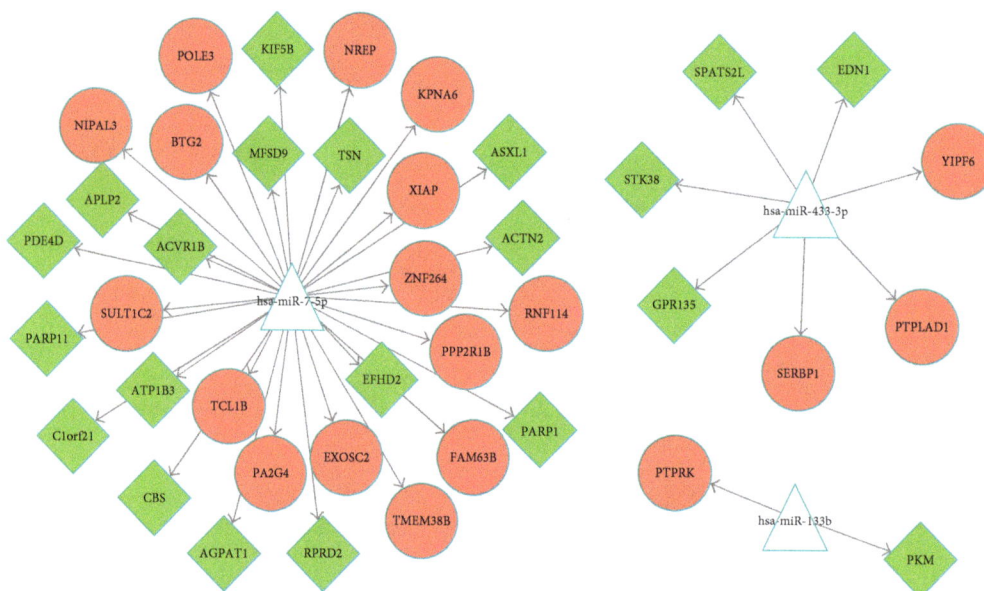

FIGURE 5: MicroRNA- (miRNA-) target regulatory networks of differentially expressed genes (DEGs). Triangles represent miRNAs, red circles represent upregulated DEGs, and green diamonds represent downregulated DEGs.

The downregulated DEGs were enriched in pathways such as those of influenza A, viral myocarditis, and TNF signaling and GO terms such as cytoplasm, cell surface, and interferon gamma-mediated signaling pathway (Figure 2(b)).

3.3. PPI Network Analysis. The PPI network, including 605 nodes and 1937 PPI pairs, is shown in Figure 3. The top 10 DEGs with the highest degree included five upregulated DEGs such as estrogen receptor 1 (*ESR1*), mechanistic target of rapamycin (*MTOR*), ATM serine/threonine kinase (*ATM*), CD40 molecule (*CD40*) and thymidine kinase 2, mitochondrial (*TK2*), and five downregulated DEGs such as mitogen-activated protein kinase 14 (*MAPK14*), phosphatase

and tensin homolog (*PTEN*), intercellular adhesion molecule 1 (*ICAM1*), aurora kinase A (*AURKA*), and protein kinase, DNA-activated, catalytic polypeptide (*PRKDC*) (Table 1). Three subnetworks were identified (subnetworks a–c). Subnetwork a (Figure 4(a)) included nine nodes and 36 PPI pairs, and these genes were significantly enriched in three KEGG pathways (Table 2), including neuroactive ligand-receptor interaction, chemokine signaling pathway, and cytokine-cytokine receptor interaction. Subnetwork b (Figure 4(b)) included seven nodes and 21 PPI pairs, and these genes were not enriched in any KEGG pathway. Subnetwork c (Figure 4(c)) included 27 nodes and 81 PPI pairs, and these genes were enriched in 12 KEGG pathways (Table 2), such as cell cycle, herpes simplex infection, and NF-κB signaling pathways.

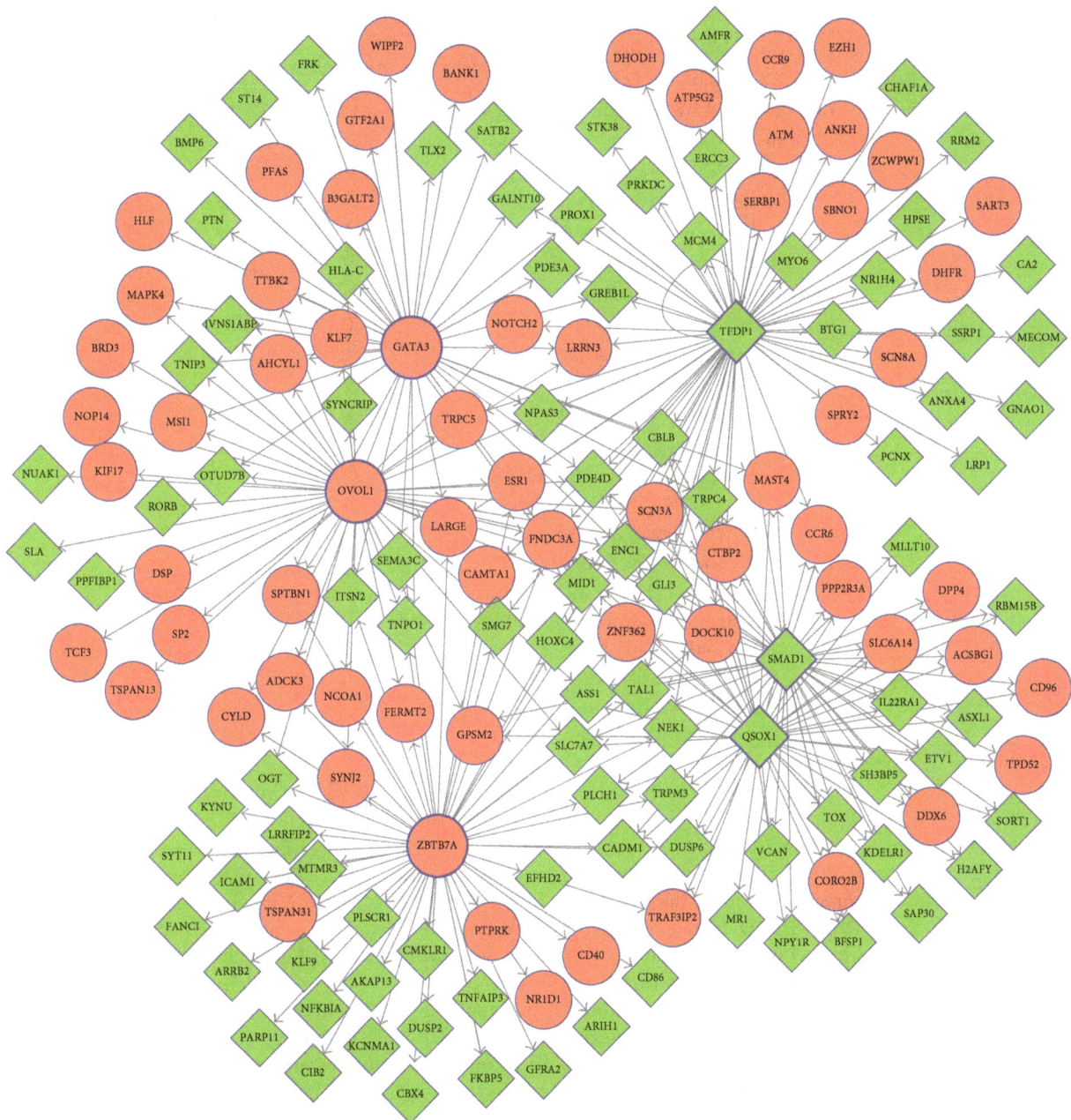

FIGURE 6: The TF-target regulatory network of differentially expressed genes (DEGs). Blue boxed figures represent TFs, red circles represent upregulated genes, and green diamonds represent downregulated genes. TF, transcription factor.

In addition, *ICAM1* was involved in six KEGG pathways of subnetwork c, such as viral myocarditis, cell adhesion molecules (CAMs), and NF-κB signaling pathways (Table 2). The detailed information existed in PPI network, and three subnetworks are shown in Supplementary Table 3.

3.4. miRNA-Target Regulatory Network Analysis. According to the data from the miR2disease database, six miRNAs were identified to be associated with PD and 698 miRNA-gene pairs were obtained by searching miRWalk2.0. A total of 40 miRNA-target interaction pairs were obtained by comparing miRNA-gene pairs with DEGs, and subsequently, the

miRNA-target regulatory network was constructed. The network (Figure 5) contained 40 miRNA-target interaction pairs and 43 nodes (Supplementary Table 4), among which three miRNAs (hsa-miR-7-5p, hsa-miR-433-3p, and hsa-miR-133b) were included.

3.5. TF-Target Regulatory Network Analysis. According the information of TF-target interaction databases such as Transfac, Jaspar, and Encode in the Cytoscape software, a total of 83 TFs were identified from the PPI network, forming 5371 TF-gene pairs. Among the 83 TFs, six were differentially expressed: three upregulated ones, that is, zinc

TABLE 3: List of top 20 nodes with higher degree in transcription factor-target regulatory network.

Gene	Full name	Description	Degree
TFDP1*	Transcription factor Dp-1	Down	62
ZBTB7A*	Zinc finger and BTB domain-containing 7A	Up	55
OVOL1*	Ovo-like transcriptional repressor 1	Up	46
SMAD1*	SMAD family member 1	Down	45
QSOX1*	Quiescin sulfhydryl oxidase 1	Down	44
GATA3*	GATA-binding protein 3	Up	38
ENC1	Ectodermal-neural cortex 1	Down	6
FNDC3A	Fibronectin type III domain-containing 3A	Up	6
MID1	Midline 1	Down	6
PDE4D	Phosphodiesterase 4D	Down	5
ZNF362	Zinc finger protein 362	Up	5
CBLB	Cbl proto-oncogene B	Down	4
LARGE	LARGE xylosyl- and glucuronyltransferase	Up	4
TRPC4	Transient receptor potential cation channel subfamily C member 4	Down	4
CTBP2	C-terminal binding protein 2	Up	4
GLI3	GLI family zinc finger 3	Down	4
SCN3A	Sodium voltage-gated channel alpha subunit 3	Up	4
TAL1	TAL BHLH transcription factor 1, erythroid differentiation factor	Down	4
LRRN3	Leucine rich repeat neuronal 3	Up	3
MAST4	Microtubule-associated serine/threonine kinase family member 4	Up	3

*Transcription factor.

finger and BTB domain-containing 7A (*ZBTB7A*), ovo-like transcriptional repressor 1 (*OVOL1*), and GATA-binding protein 3, and three downregulated ones, that is, transcription factor dp-1 (*TFDP1*), SMAD family member 1 (*SMAD1*), and quiescin sulfhydryl oxidase 1 (*QSOX1*). The TF-target regulatory network (Figure 6) was constructed and included 166 nodes and 288 interaction pairs (Supplementary Table 5). The top 20 nodes with the highest degree are listed in Table 3, including the six TFs described above and 14 other DEGs, such as ectodermal-neural cortex 1, fibronectin type III domain-containing 3A, and midline 1, which were coregulated by the six TFs.

4. Discussion

PD is the second most common age-related neurodegenerative disease. However, the pathogenesis and genes involved in PD are not well known [42]. In this study, we performed a comprehensive bioinformatics analysis of the blood gene expression profile using the GSE72267 dataset. The results suggested that four key pathways (metabolic pathways, TNF signaling pathway, rRNA processing, and cytoplasm), the key gene *ICAM1*, three miRNAs (hsa-miR-7-5p, hsa-miR-433-3p, and hsa-miR-133b), and six TFs (*ZBTB7A, OVOL1, GATA3, TFDP1, SMAD1,* and *QSOX*) might play important roles in PD development.

Our results revealed that the upregulated DEGs were enriched in the KEGG pathway "metabolic pathways" and the

GO term "rRNA processing," and the downregulated DEGs were enriched in the KEGG pathway "TNF signaling pathway" and the GO term "cytoplasm." A previous study [43] demonstrated that some metabolic patterns were altered in patients with advanced PD. Multiple metabolic pathways are also involved in PD [44], which supports our study results. Cytoplasmic inclusions are a pathological hallmark of PD [45]. Lewy body pathology is involved [46, 47], and glial cytoplasmic inclusions are associated with Lewy bodies [48]. Thus, the GO term "cytoplasm" may play a role in PD. Furthermore, TNF receptor-associated protein is excluded from the nucleolus and is sequestered to the cytoplasm by TNF receptor-associated factor 6, thereby altering ribosomal RNA (rRNA) biogenesis [49]. The TNF signaling pathway is also involved in PD [50], and rRNA transcription is repressed in patients with PD [51]. Therefore, the GO term "rRNA processing" and the KEGG pathway "TNF signaling pathway" may play important roles in PD. Altogether, the metabolic pathways, TNF signaling pathway, rRNA processing, and cytoplasm are essentially involved in PD pathogenesis.

ICAM1 was among the top 10 DEGs in the PPI network. Moreover, *ICAM1* gene was involved in six KEGG pathways for subnetwork c. *ICAM1* is involved in the adhesion and transmigration of leukocytes across the endothelium, promoting brain inflammation and resulting in brain diseases [52]. T helper 17 cells can exert a neurotoxic effect in the brain parenchyma of patients with PD by interacting with *ICAM1* and leukocyte function-associated antigen 1 [53]. In addition, *ICAM1* is involved in persistent inflammation in PD [54]. Our results from the KEGG pathway analysis for genes in subnetworks revealed that *ICAM1* might play roles in viral myocarditis and CAMs and thus contributed to PD.

The miRNA-target regulatory network analysis identified three miRNAs involved in PD, namely, hsa-miR-7-5p, hsa-miR-433-3p, and hsa-miR-133b. A study described miR-7-2 dysregulation (the stem loop of hsa-miR-7-5p) in Parkinson's patient's leukocytes [55] and revealed that hsa-miR-7-5p expression decreased in PD, possibly upregulating *α-SYN*, a PD-related gene [56]. The variation of the hsa-miR-433- (the stem loop of hsa-miR-433-3p-) binding site of fibroblast growth factor 20 can lead to *α-SYN* overexpression, increasing the risk for PD [57]. hsa-miR-133b expression is increased in the cerebrospinal fluid of patients with PD [58]; however, its expression levels in serum is decreased, which is related to low serum ceruloplasmin levels [59]. hsa-miR-133b is also deficient in the midbrain tissue of patients with PD and is associated with the maturation and function of midbrain dopaminergic neurons [60]. Notably, reduced circulating levels of miR-433 and miR-133b are considered as promising biomarkers for PD [61]. Therefore, we speculate that the three miRNAs, including hsa-miR-7-5p, hsa-miR-433-3p, and hsa-miR-133b may play important roles in PD.

TFs are important regulators of target gene expressions [53, 62]. In this study, we analyzed DEGs in the PPI network to screen TFs involved in PD. Among the 83 TFs identified in the PPI network, six were found to be differentially expressed. *ZBTB7A*, *OVOL1*, and *GATA3* were upregulated in patients with PD compared with those in healthy matched controls, whereas *TFDP1*, *SMAD1*, and *QSOX1* were downregulated. *ZBTB7A* is a tumor suppressor, which is involved in several cancers such as prostate and nonsmall cell lung cancers [63–65]. *OVOL1*, encoding a zinc finger protein, is expressed in embryonic epidermal progenitor cells and is an inducer of mesenchymal-to-epithelial transition in human cancers [66, 67]. *GATA3*, a member of the GATA family, is a regulator of T-cell development and plays roles in endothelial cells [68, 69]. *TFDP1* is involved in the cell cycle and contributes to hepatocellular carcinomas [70, 71], *SMAD1* is involved in multiple pathways [72, 73], and *QSOX1* plays roles in some cancers such as breast cancer and neuroblastoma [74–76]. However, there are few reports regarding the involvement of these TFs in PD. Hence,

further studies regarding the associations between the TFs identified in this study and PD are warranted.

In conclusion, our data demonstrated that the metabolic pathways, TNF signaling pathway, rRNA processing, and cytoplasm play important roles in PD pathogenesis; *ICAM1* might also play a vital role. Besides six TFs, three miRNAs, including hsa-miR-7-5p, hsa-miR-433-3p, and hsa-miR-133b, may be involved in PD. However, because of the study limitations, further investigation remains to be performed in the future.

Acknowledgments

This study was supported by the Construction of Accurate Technology Innovation Centers of Nervous System Disease, Jilin Province (no. 20170623006TC), and Study on the Mechanism of the Parkinson lncrna, Jilin Provincial Department of Finance Project.

References

[1] W. Dauer and S. Przedborski, "Parkinson's disease: mechanisms and models," *Neuron*, vol. 39, no. 6, pp. 889–909, 2003.

[2] A. E. Lang and A. M. Lozano, "Parkinson's disease. Second of two parts," *New England Journal of Medicine*, vol. 339, no. 16, pp. 1130–1143, 1998.

[3] A. E. Lang and A. M. Lozano, "Parkinson's disease," *New England Journal of Medicine*, vol. 37, p. 198, 1998.

[4] L. V. Kalia and A. E. Lang, "Parkinson's disease," *Lancet*, vol. 386, no. 9996, pp. 896–912, 2015.

[5] D. J. Moore, A. B. West, V. L. Dawson, and T. M. Dawson, "Molecular pathophysiology of Parkinson's disease," *Annual Review of Neuroscience*, vol. 28, no. 1, pp. 57–87, 2005.

[6] S. K. Bae, C. H. Heo, D. J. Choi et al., "A ratiometric two-photon fluorescent probe reveals reduction in mitochondrial H2S production in Parkinson's disease gene knockout astrocytes," *Journal of the American Chemical Society*, vol. 135, no. 26, pp. 9915–9923, 2013.

[7] R. Calligaris, M. Banica, P. Roncaglia et al., "Blood transcriptomics of drug-naïve sporadic Parkinson's disease patients," *BMC Genomics*, vol. 16, no. 1, pp. 1–14, 2015.

[8] L. Gong, Q. L. Zhang, N. Zhang et al., "Neuroprotection by urate on 6-OHDA-lesioned rat model of Parkinson's disease: linking to Akt/GSK3β signaling pathway," *Journal of Neurochemistry*, vol. 123, no. 5, pp. 876–885, 2012.

[9] K. U. Tufekci, E. C. Bayin, S. Genc, and K. Genc, "The Nrf2/ARE pathway: a promising target to counteract mitochondrial dysfunction in Parkinson's disease," *Parkinson's Disease*, vol. 2011, Article ID 314082, 14 pages, 2011.

[10] D. Cheng, A. M. Jenner, G. Shui et al., "Lipid pathway alterations in Parkinson's disease primary visual cortex," *PLoS One*, vol. 6, Article ID e17299, 2011.

[11] R. Deumens, A. Blokland, and J. Prickaerts, "Modeling Parkinson's disease in rats: an evaluation of 6-OHDA lesions of the nigrostriatal pathway," *Experimental Neurology*, vol. 175, no. 2, pp. 303–317, 2002.

[12] E. Leroy, R. Boyer, G. Auburger et al., "The ubiquitin pathway in Parkinson's disease," *Nature*, vol. 395, no. 6701, pp. 451-452, 1998.

[13] T. Pan, S. Kondo, W. Le, and J. Jankovic, "The role of autophagy-lysosome pathway in neurodegeneration associated with Parkinson's disease," *Brain*, vol. 131, no. 8, pp. 1969–1978, 2008.

[14] R. M. Perrett, Z. Alexopoulou, and G. K. Tofaris, "The endosomal pathway in Parkinson's disease," *Molecular & Cellular Neurosciences*, vol. 66, pp. 21-28, 2015.

[15] A. L. Whone, R. Y. Moore, P. P. Piccini, and D. J. Brooks, "Plasticity of the nigropallidal pathway in Parkinson's disease," *Annals of Neurology*, vol. 53, no. 2, pp. 206–213, 2003.

[16] B. D. Cholewa, X. Liu, and N. Ahmad, "The role of polo-like kinase 1 in carcinogenesis: cause or consequence?," *Cancer Research*, vol. 73, no. 23, pp. 6848–6855, 2013.

[17] E. Miñonesmoyano, S. Porta, G. Escaramís et al., "MicroRNA profiling of Parkinson's disease brains identifies early downregulation of miR-34b/c which modulate mitochondrial function," *Human Molecular Genetics*, vol. 20, no. 15, p. 3067, 2011.

[18] M. L. De, E. Coto, L. F. Cardo et al., "Analysis of the Micro-RNA-133 and PITX3 genes in Parkinson's disease," *American Journal of Medical Genetics Part B Neuropsychiatric genetics: The Official Publication of the International Society of Psychiatric Genetics*, vol. 153B, no. 6, pp. 1234–1239, 2010.

[19] S. Li, X. Lv, K. Zhai et al., "MicroRNA-7 inhibits neuronal apoptosis in a cellular Parkinson's disease model by targeting Bax and Sirt2," *American Journal of Translational Research*, vol. 8, no. 2, pp. 993–1004, 2016.

[20] Y. Zhou, M. Lu, R. H. Du et al., "MicroRNA-7 targets Nod-like receptor protein 3 inflammasome to modulate neuroinflammation in the pathogenesis of Parkinson's disease," *Molecular Neurodegeneration*, vol. 11, no. 1, p. 28, 2016.

[21] W. Le, D. Nguyen, X. W. Lin et al., "Transcription factor PITX3 gene in Parkinson's disease," *Neurobiology of Aging*, vol. 32, no. 4, pp. 750–753, 2011.

[22] J. Li, J. A. Dani, and W. Le, "The role of transcription factor Pitx3 in dopamine neuron development and Parkinson's disease," *Current Topics in Medicinal Chemistry*, vol. 9, no. 10, pp. 855–859, 2009.

[23] X. Xie, H. Liu, and Y. Gao, "Expression changes of transcription factor EN1 in the midbrain of mice model of Parkinson's disease," *Chinese Journal of Rehabilitation Medicine*, vol. 27, pp. 197–200, 2012.

[24] A. Cuadrado, P. Morenomurciano, and J. Pedrazachaverri, "The transcription factor Nrf2 as a new therapeutic target in Parkinson's disease," *Expert Opinion on Therapeutic Targets*, vol. 13, no. 3, pp. 319–329, 2009.

[25] P. M. Flood, L. Qian, L. J. Peterson et al., "Transcriptional factor NF-κB as a target for therapy in Parkinson's disease," *Parkinson's Disease*, vol. 2011, Article ID 216298, 8 pages, 2011.

[26] M. Kurzawski, M. Białecka, J. Sławek, G. Kłodowskaduda, and M. Droździk, "Association study of GATA-2 transcription factor gene (GATA2) polymorphism and Parkinson's disease," *Parkinsonism & Related Disorders*, vol. 16, no. 4, pp. 284–287, 2009.

[27] N. V. Soshnikova, N. E. Vorob'Eva, A. A. Kolacheva et al., "Ratio of transcription factor PHF10 splice variants in lymphocytes as a molecular marker of Parkinson's disease," *Molecular Biology*, vol. 50, no. 4, pp. 695–702, 2016.

[28] T. Barrett, T. O. Suzek, D. B. Troup et al., "NCBI GEO: mining millions of expression profiles—database and tools," *Nucleic Acids Research*, vol. 33, pp. D562-D566, 2005.

[29] L. Gautier, L. Cope, B. M. Bolstad, and R. A. Irizarry, "affy—analysis of Affymetrix GeneChip data at the probe level," *Bioinformatics*, vol. 20, no. 3, pp. 307–315, 2004.

[30] G. Smyth and G. K. Smyth, "Limma: linear models for microarray data," *Bioinformatics and Computational Biology Solution Using R and Bioconductor*, Springer, Berlin, Germany, 2005.

[31] I. Hulsegge, A. Kommadath, and M. A. Smits, "Globaltest and GOEAST: two different approaches for Gene Ontology analysis," *BMC Proceedings*, vol. 3, no. 4, p. S10, 2009.

[32] T. G. O. Consortium, M. Ashburner, C. A. Ball et al., "Gene ontology: tool for the unification of biology," *Nature Genetics*, vol. 25, no. 1, pp. 25–29, 2000.

[33] M. Kanehisa and S. Goto, "KEGG: Kyoto Encyclopedia of Genes and Genomes," *Nucleic Acids Research*, vol. 27, no. 1, pp. 27–30, 1999.

[34] D. W. Huang, B. T. Sherman, and R. A. Lempicki, "Systematic and integrative analysis of large gene lists using DAVID bioinformatics resources," *Nature Protocol*, vol. 4, no. 1, pp. 44–57, 2009.

[35] D. Szklarczyk, A. Franceschini, S. Wyder et al., "STRING v10: protein-protein interaction networks, integrated over the tree of life," *Nucleic Acids Research*, vol. 43, pp. D1-D447, 2015.

[36] P. Shannon, A. Markiel, O. Ozier et al., "Cytoscape: a software environment for integrated models of biomolecular interaction networks," *Genome Research*, vol. 13, no. 11, pp. 2498–2504, 2003.

[37] Y. Tang, M. Li, J. Wang, Y. Pan, and F. X. Wu, "CytoNCA: a cytoscape plugin for centrality analysis and evaluation of protein interaction networks," *Bio Systems*, vol. 127, pp. 67–72, 2014.

[38] W. P. Bandettini, P. Kellman, C. Mancini et al., "Multi-Contrast Delayed Enhancement (MCODE) improves detection of subendocardial myocardial infarction by late gadolinium enhancement cardiovascular magnetic resonance: a clinical validation study," *Journal of Cardiovascular Magnetic Resonance*, vol. 14, no. 1, p. 83, 2012.

[39] Q. Jiang, Y. Wang, Y. Hao et al., "miR2Disease: a manually curated database for microRNA deregulation in human disease," *Nucleic Acids Research*, vol. 37, pp. D98-104, 2009.

[40] H. Dweep and N. Gretz, "miRWalk2.0: a comprehensive atlas of microRNA-target interactions," *Nature Methods*, vol. 12, no. 8, p. 697, 2015.

[41] R. Janky, A. Verfaillie, H. Imrichová et al., "iRegulon: from a gene list to a gene regulatory network using large motif and track collections," *Plos Computational Biology*, vol. 10, no. 7, p. e1003731, 2014.

[42] Y. Feng, J. Jankovic, and Y. C. Wu, "Epigenetic mechanisms in Parkinson's disease," *Journal of the Neurological Sciences*, vol. 349, no. 1-2, pp. 3–9, 2015.

[43] M. G. Moreno, C. Sánchez, G. Vazquez, J. Altamirano, and M. Avilarodriguez, "Metabolic mismatch patterns in patients with advanced Parkinson's disease on ^{18}F-FDOPA, ^{11}C-Raclopride and ^{11}C-DTBZ PET/CT," *Journal of Nuclear Medicine*, vol. 56, no. 3, p. 1890, 2015.

[44] M. Bonin, S. Poths, H. Osaka, YL. Wang, K. Wada, and O. Riess, "Microarray expression analysis of gad mice

implicates involvement of Parkinson's disease associated UCH-L1 in multiple metabolic pathways," *Molecular Brain Research*, vol. 126, no. 1, pp. 88–97, 2004.

[45] M. Ihara, H. Tomimoto, H. Kitayama et al., "Association of the cytoskeletal GTP-binding protein Sept4/H5 with cytoplasmic inclusions found in Parkinson's disease and other synucleinopathies," *Journal of Biological Chemistry*, vol. 278, no. 26, pp. 24095–24102, 2003.

[46] K. A. Mills, Z. Mari, C. Bakker et al., "Gait function and locus coeruleus Lewy body pathology in 51 Parkinson's disease patients," *Parkinsonism & Related Disorders*, vol. 33, pp. 102–106, 2016.

[47] Y. Saito, A. Shioya, T. Sano, H. Sumikura, M. Murata, and S. Murayama, "Lewy body pathology involves the olfactory cells in Parkinson's disease and related disorders," *Movement Disorders Official Journal of the Movement Disorder Society*, vol. 31, no. 1, pp. 135–138, 2016.

[48] A. Mochizuki, Y. Komatsuzaki, and S. I. Shoji, "Association of Lewy bodies and glial cytoplasmic inclusions in the brain of Parkinson's disease," *Acta Neuropathologica*, vol. 104, pp. 534–537, 2002.

[49] S. Vilotti, M. Codrich, M. D. Ferro et al., "Parkinson's disease DJ-1 L166P alters rRNA biogenesis by exclusion of TTRAP from the nucleolus and sequestration into cytoplasmic aggregates via TRAF6," *PLoS One*, vol. 7, no. 4, Article ID e35051, 2012.

[50] T. N. Martinez, "Neuroinflammation, TNF, and ceramide signaling: putative pathways for neurotoxicity in Parkinson's disease," *Diss.*, 2010.

[51] H. Kang and J. H. Shin, "Repression of rRNA transcription by PARIS contributes to Parkinson's disease," *Neurobiology of Disease*, vol. 73, pp. 220–228, 2015.

[52] J. Y. Choi and S. A. Jo, "KDM7A histone demethylase mediates TNF-α-induced ICAM1 protein upregulation by modulating lysosomal activity," *Biochemical & Biophysical Research Communications*, vol. 478, no. 3, pp. 1355–1362, 2016.

[53] Q. Zhao, H. Liu, C. Yao, J. Shuai, and X. Sun, "Effect of dynamic interaction between microRNA and transcription factor on gene expression," *Biomed Research International*, vol. 2016, Article ID 2676282, 10 pages, 2016.

[54] J. Miklossy, D. D. Doudet, C. Schwab, S. Yu, E. G. Mcgeer, and P. L. Mcgeer, "Role of ICAM-1 in persisting inflammation in Parkinson disease and MPTP monkeys," *Experimental Neurology*, vol. 197, no. 2, pp. 275–283, 2006.

[55] L. Soreq, M. Bronstein, D. S. Greenberg et al., "Small RNA sequencing-microarray analyses in Parkinson leukocytes reveal deep brain stimulation-induced splicing changes that classify brain region transcriptomes," *Frontiers in Molecular Neuroscience*, vol. 6, p. 10, 2013.

[56] E. Junn, K. W. Lee, B. S. Jeong, T. W. Chan, J. Y. Im, and M. M. Mouradian, "Repression of alpha-synuclein expression and toxicity by microRNA-7," *Proceedings of the National Academy of Sciences of the United States of America*, vol. 106, no. 31, pp. 13052–13507, 2009.

[57] G. Wang, J. van der Walt, Y. Li et al., "Variation in the miRNA-433 binding site of FGF20 confers risk for Parkinson disease by overexpression of alpha-synuclein," *American Journal of Human Genetics*, vol. 82, no. 2, pp. 283–289, 2008.

[58] X. Ma, J. Ren, Y. Jiao, J. Yang, F. Xu, and Y. Song, "Expression of miR-133b and its clinical significance in cerebrospinal fluid of patients with Parkinson's disease," *Modern Journal of Integrated Traditional Chinese & Western Medicine*, vol. 23, no. 24, pp. 2656–2658, 2014.

[59] N. Zhao, L. Jin, G. Fei, Z. Zheng, and C. Zhong, "Serum microRNA-133b is associated with low ceruloplasmin levels in Parkinson's disease," *Parkinsonism & Related Disorders*, vol. 20, no. 11, pp. 1177–1180, 2014.

[60] J. Kim, K. Inoue, J. Ishii et al., "A MicroRNA feedback circuit in midbrain dopamine neurons," *Science*, vol. 317, no. 5842, pp. 1220–1224, 2007.

[61] X. Zhang, R. Yang, B. L. Hu et al., "Reduced circulating levels of miR-433 and miR-133b are potential biomarkers for Parkinson's disease," *Frontiers in Cellular Neuroscience*, vol. 11, p. 170, 2017.

[62] N. J. Martinez and A. J. Walhout, "The interplay between transcription factors and microRNAs in genome-scale regulatory networks," *Bioessays*, vol. 31, no. 4, pp. 435–445, 2009.

[63] K. Apostolopoulou, I. S. Pateras, K. Evangelou et al., "Gene amplification is a relatively frequent event leading to ZBTB7A (Pokemon) overexpression in non-small cell lung cancer," *Journal of Pathology*, vol. 213, no. 3, pp. 294–302, 2007.

[64] X. S. Liu, J. E. Haines, E. K. Mehanna et al., "ZBTB7A acts as a tumor suppressor through the transcriptional repression of glycolysis," *Genes & Development*, vol. 28, no. 17, pp. 1917–1928, 2014.

[65] G. Wang, A. Lunardi, J. Zhang et al., "Zbtb7a suppresses prostate cancer through repression of a Sox9-dependent pathway for cellular senescence bypass and tumor invasion," *Nature Genetics*, vol. 45, no. 7, pp. 739–746, 2013.

[66] M. Nair, A. Teng, V. Bilanchone, A. Agrawal, B. Li, and X. Dai, "Ovol1 regulates the growth arrest of embryonic epidermal progenitor cells and represses c-myc transcription," *Journal of Cell Biology*, vol. 173, no. 2, pp. 253–264, 2006.

[67] H. Roca, J. Hernandez, S. Weidner et al., "Transcription factors OVOL1 and OVOL2 induce the mesenchymal to epithelial transition in human cancer," *PLoS One*, vol. 8, no. 10, Article ID e76773, 2013.

[68] I. C. Ho, T. S. Tai, and S. Y. Pai, "GATA3 and the T-cell lineage: essential functions before and after T-helper-2-cell differentiation," *Nature Reviews Immunology*, vol. 9, no. 2, pp. 125–135, 2009.

[69] H. Song, J. Suehiro, Y. Kanki et al., "Critical role for GATA3 in mediating Tie2 expression and function in large vessel endothelial cells," *Journal of Biological Chemistry*, vol. 284, no. 42, pp. 29109–29124, 2009.

[70] X. Lu, X. D. Lv, Y. H. Ren et al., "Dysregulation of TFDP1 and of the cell cycle pathway in high-grade glioblastoma multiforme: a bioinformatic analysis," *Genetics & Molecular Research*, vol. 15, no. 2, 2016.

[71] K. Yasui, H. Okamoto, S. Arii, and J. Inazawa, "Association of over-expressed TFDP1 with progression of hepatocellular carcinomas," *Journal of Human Genetics*, vol. 48, no. 12, pp. 609–613, 2003.

[72] LC. Fuentealba, E. Eivers, A. Ikeda et al., "Integrating patterning signals: Wnt/GSK3 regulates the duration of the BMP/Smad1 signal," *Cell*, vol. 131, no. 5, pp. 980–993, 2007.

[73] M. MacíAssilva, P. A. Hoodless, S. J. Tang, M. Buchwald, and J. L. Wrana, "Specific activation of Smad1 signaling pathways by the BMP7 type I receptor, ALK2," *Journal of Biological Chemistry*, vol. 273, no. 40, pp. 25628–25636, 1998.

[74] D. Araújo and L. Nakao, "Expression level of quiescin sulfhydryl oxidase 1 (QSOX1) in neuroblastomas," *European Journal of Histochemistry*, vol. 58, no. 1, p. 2228, 2014.

[75] D. F. Lake and D. O. Faigel, "The emerging role of QSOX1 in cancer," *Antioxid Redox Signal*, vol. 21, no. 3, pp. 485–496, 2014.

12

The Effect of Parkinson's Disease on Patients Undergoing Lumbar Spine Surgery

Jeremy Steinberger,[1] Jeffrey Gilligan ⓘ,[1] Branko Skovrlj,[2] Christopher A. Sarkiss,[1] Javier Z. Guzman,[3] Samuel K. Cho,[3] and John M. Caridi[1]

[1]Department of Neurosurgery, Icahn School of Medicine at Mount Sinai, New York, NY, USA
[2]Department of Neurosurgery, North Jersey Spine Group, Wayne, NJ, USA
[3]Department of Orthopaedics, Icahn School of Medicine at Mount Sinai, New York, NY, USA

Correspondence should be addressed to Jeffrey Gilligan; Jeffreygilligan18@gmail.com

Academic Editor: Giovanni Mirabella

Study Design. Retrospective Database Analysis. *Objective*. The purpose of this study was to assess characteristics and outcomes of patients with Parkinson's disease (PD) undergoing lumbar spine surgery for degenerative conditions. *Methods*. The Nationwide Inpatient Sample was examined from 2002 to 2011. Patients were included for study based on ICD-9-CM procedural codes for lumbar spine surgery and substratified to degenerative diagnoses. Incidence and baseline patient characteristics were determined. Multivariable analysis was performed to determine independent risk factors increasing incidence of lumbar fusion revision in PD patients. *Results*. PD patients account for 0.9% of all degenerative lumbar procedures. At baseline, PD patients are older (70.7 versus 58.9, $p < 0.0001$) and more likely to be male (58.6% male, $p < 160.0001$). Mean length of stay (LOS) was increased in PD patients undergoing lumbar fusion (5.1 days versus 4.0 days, $p < 0.0001$) and lumbar fusion revision (6.2 days versus 4.8 days, $p < 180.0001$). Costs were 7.9% ($p < 0.0001$) higher for lumbar fusion and 25.2% ($p < 0.0001$) higher for lumbar fusion revision in PD patients. Multivariable analysis indicates that osteoporosis, fluid/electrolyte disorders, blood loss anemia, and insurance status are significant independent predictors of lumbar fusion revision in patients with PD. *Conclusion*. PD patients undergoing lumbar surgery for degenerative conditions have increased LOS and costs when compared to patients without PD.

1. Introduction

Parkinson's disease (PD) is a neurodegenerative disorder characterized by resting tremors, rigidity, bradykinesia, postural instability, and gait disturbances [1]. The prevalence of PD in industrialized countries is estimated at 0.3% of the entire population with approximately 7 million people affected worldwide [2]. PD is an age-related disease which is rare before the age of 50, with a prevalence of about 1% in people over the age of 60 and up to 4% in people over the age of 80 [3, 4].

Apart from the neurodegenerative symptoms, patients with PD suffer from a wide variety of systemic and musculoskeletal dysfunctions. They are predisposed to falls due to a high incidence of visual impairment and autonomic dysfunction separate from neurodegenerative symptoms [5]. Epidemiologic studies suggest that approximately half of PD patients fall at least once as compared with a third of healthy ambulatory subjects greater than 60 years of age [6, 7]. These patients also suffer from osteoporosis, thus increasing their risk of bone fractures [8]. Musculoskeletal dysfunction in patients with PD leads to an increased incidence of muscle weakness and degenerative spondylarthroses resulting in scoliosis, thoracic kyphosis, and cervical deformity [9].

PD is increasingly recognized as an important cause of spinal disorders requiring surgical intervention [9]. However, spinal procedures can be complicated by underlying osteoporosis and severe musculoskeletal dysfunction in this population.

In this study, we investigate the effect of PD on patients undergoing lumbar spine surgery. The aim of this study is to identify the incidence, trend, risk factors, outcomes, and cost of lumbar spinal surgery for degenerative disease in PD patients.

2. Materials and Methods

The Nationwide Inpatient Sample (NIS) database, under the auspices of the Healthcare Cost and Utilization Project (HCUP) and administered by the Agency for Healthcare Research and Quality, was queried from 2002 to 2011 [10]. The NIS, which comprises a 20% stratified samples of all hospital discharges, is the largest all-payer hospital inpatient database in the US. This sample comprises approximately 8 million hospitalizations, and when sample weights are applied, it comprises approximately 40 million hospitalizations or 96% of all US hospital discharges each year. The NIS data contain patient demographics (e.g., race, age, and gender), hospital characteristics (e.g., teaching status, location, and size), and clinical outcomes (e.g., mortality, costs, and length of stay).

2.1. Sample Selection. PD was identified by the International Classification of Diseases, Ninth Revision, Clinical Modification (ICD-9-CM) code 332.0, which applies Parkinsonism characterized in the following forms: primary, idiopathic, or not otherwise specified. Patients were separated into two cohorts: patients with PD and those without PD. Hospitalizations were selected for the study based on ICD-9-CM procedural codes for lumbar spine procedures and further stratified to include only procedures for degenerative conditions of the lumbar spine. Only patients with hospitalizations that contained all of the demographics and clinical outcome measures were included. Since our search was conducted in this fashion, it is not known the amount of patients who had incomplete data that were excluded. The procedural codes used in this study are outlined in Table 1. Procedures were organized into three groups: lumbar fusion, lumbar fusion revision, and lumbar decompression without fusion.

2.2. Outcome Measures. Demographic data was analyzed, which included age, pay schedule, gender, race, modified Elixhauser Comorbidity Index, hospital characteristics, and surgical procedure. We chose the Elixhauser index for its ability to adjust for each single comorbidity's independent association with hospital death and its significant association with short- and long-term mortality as well as burden of diseases [11–13]. We have modified the Elixhauser index to exclude the point value of the neurological comorbidity as this includes the ICD-9-CM code for PD when utilizing the validated and updated comorbidity software provided by HCUP.

Perioperative complications were also chosen based on ICD-9-CM diagnosis codes (Supplementary Appendix A). We further analyzed hospitalization outcomes such as length of stay (LOS), costs, and mortality rates. All hospital charges were adjusted for inflation using the US Bureau of Labor statistics' yearly inflation calculator to represent charges in the year 2011 and converted into costs with the HCUP costs to charge ratio tool [14, 15].

TABLE 1: ICD-9-CM procedural and diagnosis codes used.

ICD-9-CM procedural and diagnosis codes	
Procedural codes	
81.04	Dorsal and dorsolumbar fusion, anterior technique
81.05	Dorsal or dorsolumbar fusion, posterior technique
81.06	Lumbar and lumbosacral fusion, anterior technique
81.07	Lumbar and lumbosacral fusion, lateral transverse process technique
81.08	Lumbar and lumbosacral fusion, posterior technique
81.34	Refusion of dorsal and dorsolumbar spine, anterior technique
81.35	Refusion of dorsal and dorsolumbar spine, posterior technique
81.36	Refusion of lumbar and lumbosacral spine, anterior technique
81.37	Refusion of lumbar and lumbosacral spine, lateral transverse process technique
81.38	Refusion of lumbar and lumbosacral spine, posterior technique
03.09	Posterior lumbar decompression without fusion
Diagnosis codes	
721.3	Lumbosacral spondylosis without myelopathy
721.42	Lumbar region, spondylogenic compression of lumbar spinal cord
722.1	Lumbar intervertebral disc without myelopathy
722.52	Lumbar or lumbosacral intervertebral disc
722.73	Lumbar region, intervertebral disc disorder with myelopathy
722.83	Lumbar region, postlaminectomy syndrome
722.93	Lumbar region, other and unspecified disc disorder
724.02	Lumbar region, spinal stenosis

ICD-9-CM: International Classification of Diseases, Ninth Edition, Clinical Modification.

2.3. Data Analysis. Statistical analysis was performed using SAS version 9.3 (SAS Institute, Cary, NC, USA). Chi-squared test was used for analysis of categorical variables and Student's *t*-test was used for continuous variables. Analysis took into account the complex survey design of the NIS and procedures such as *surveyfreq*, *surveymeans*, and *surveylogistic* being used for data analysis. Discharge weights, NIS stratum, and cluster (hospital identification) variables were included to correctly estimate variance and to produce national estimates from the stratified sample. Regression modeling for acute complications adjusting for PD, gender, race, hospital bed size, hospital region, and hospital location and modified Elixhauser index was performed to examine odds ratios for complications referencing PD patients to those without PD.

Multivariate analysis was performed to assess factors associated with lumbar fusion revision in the PD patient population. Factors included in multivariate analysis for lumbar fusion revision included the following: osteoporosis, age, race, gender, hospital size, region and location, insurance, and modified Elixhauser index. Two separate multivariate analyses not isolating the PD patient population but including all lumbar patients looked at the role PD +/− 6 osteoporosis had on lumbar fusion revision. These analyses included the same variables as the model isolating the PD patient population. Cochran–Armitage trend test was performed to assess PD trend of prevalence over time in patients undergoing

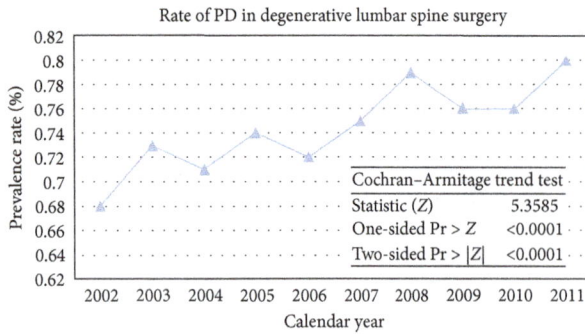

FIGURE 1: Stock plot demonstrating increased prevalence of Parkinson's disease patients undergoing lumbar spine surgery for degenerative conditions between the years 2002 and 2011.

degenerative lumbar spine surgery. Statistical significance was maintained at $p < 0.05$.

No Institutional Board Review approval was required for this study.

3. Results

A total of 19,211 PD patients underwent elective spine surgery from 2002 to 2011, with the prevalence significantly increasing over time ($p < 0.0001$) (Figure 1). Patients with PD were significantly older (70.7 versus 58.9, $p < 0.0001$) and more likely to be male (58.6% versus 47.1%, $p < 0.0001$) (Table 2). A greater proportion of PD patients had Medicare than non-PD patients (77.7% versus 41.1%, $p < 0.0001$) and more PD patients underwent lumbar decompression without fusion and lumbar fusion revision when compared to non-PD patients ($p < 0.0001$) (Table 2).

PD patients undergoing lumbar spine surgery had more comorbidities than those without PD (Table 3). Notably, patients with PD were more likely to have osteoporosis (7.9% versus 4.0%, $p < 0.0001$) and congestive heart failure (3.6% versus 1.9%, $p < 0.0001$). Despite the general pattern of greater comorbidities in patients with PD, this did not hold true for chronic pulmonary disease, rheumatoid arthritis, or obesity (Table 3).

Adjusted regression modeling for postoperative complications showed genitourinary complications' odds ratio (OR) = 1.5, confidence interval (CI) = 1.5–1.9, $p = 0.001$ and postoperative hemorrhage (OR = 1.3, CI = 1.2–1.5, $p \leq 0.0001$) as having significantly increased adjusted odds ratios amongst the complications analyzed (Table 4). As seen in Table 5, PD patients have significantly increased LOS with all procedures analyzed. When compared to non-PD patients, costs were significantly increased in lumbar fusion ($29,427 versus $27,272, $p < 0.0001$) and lumbar fusion revision ($39,885 versus $31,866, $p < 0.0001$). PD was not found to be associated with increased mortality in patients undergoing lumbar spine surgery (0.13% versus 0.11%, $p = 0.810$).

Multivariate analysis performed on the PD patient population identified several independent factors that increase the odds of revision surgery (Table 6). Of note, PD patients with a diagnosis of osteoporosis (OR = 2.0, $p = 0.029$) and Medicare (OR = 1.4, $p < 0.0001$) had increased likelihood of revision. Uninsured patients showed the most dramatic increased

TABLE 2: Patients with and without PD undergoing lumbar spine surgery.

Demographics	No PD	PD	p value
Mean age	58.9	70.7	<0.0001
Age groups			<0.0001
0–44	18.53	0.45	
45–64	42.09	21.57	
>65	39.31	77.94	
Gender			<0.0001
Male	47.07	58.61	<0.0001
Female	52.93	41.39	<0.0001
Race			<0.0001
White	65.08	69.81	
Black	4.87	1.42	
Hispanic	4.17	3.75	
Asian	0.78	1.31	
Native American	0.29	0.15	
Other	1.75	1.62	
Missing	23.06	21.93	
Insurance			<0.0001
Medicare	41.13	77.66	
Medicaid	6.37	3.50	
Private	41.96	17.04	
Uninsured	0.83	0.34	
Other	9.52	1.35	
Missing	0.19	0.11	
Procedures			
Lumbar fusion	53.98	40.56	<0.0001
Lumbar decompression without fusion	42.23	55.42	<0.0001
Lumbar fusion revision	3.79	4.02	0.488
Modified Elixhauser index	0.32	0.70	<0.0001

PD: Parkinson's disease.

likelihood of revision surgery (OR = 9.84, $p < 0.0001$). Similar multivariate analysis on all patients undergoing degenerative lumbar spine surgery including PD patients also identified osteoporosis (OR = 1.3, CI = 1.2–1.4, $p < 0.0001$) as having increased odds of revision surgery (Supplementary Appendix B). However, a diagnosis of PD was not an independent risk factor for revision surgery. The combined diagnoses of PD and osteoporosis showed a significantly increased risk for lumbar fusion revision surgery (OR = 1.8, CI = 1.03–3.2, $p = 0.040$) (Supplementary Appendix C).

4. Discussion

Adults older than 50 years are projected to be the fastest growing segment of the adult population. It is estimated that by 2050, a third of the American population will be over the age of 55 and 20% will be over 65 [16]. As such, a growing number of patients undergoing treatment for degenerative spinal conditions will have PD.

Despite its increasing disease burden, only six studies investigating spine surgery in the PD population exist presently [9, 17–21]. In this combined cohort of only 95 patients, complications were reported in 59% of all cases with 71% of patients achieving successful fusion following index surgery and 45% requiring revision surgery [22].

TABLE 3: Comorbidities of patients with and without PD.

Comorbidities	No PD	PD	p value
Congestive heart failure	1.94	3.61	<0.0001
Valvular heart disease	2.86	4.34	<0.0001
Pulmonary circulation disease	0.51	0.87	0.001
Peripheral vascular disease	2.43	3.12	0.006
Hypertension	49.50	55.53	<0.0001
Paralysis	1.65	2.73	<0.0001
Chronic pulmonary disease	13.99	10.62	<0.0001
Diabetes w/o chronic complications	14.88	14.22	0.276
Diabetes w/chronic complications	1.54	2.26	0.000
Hypothyroidism	9.56	12.99	<0.0001
Renal failure	1.68	2.39	0.001
Liver disease	0.76	0.33	0.002
Peptic ulcer disease	0.02	0.05	0.160
Acquired immune deficiency syndrome	0.03	0.05	0.544
Lymphoma	0.23	0.22	0.869
Metastatic cancer	0.16	0.16	0.916
Solid tumor w/o metastasis	0.35	0.76	<0.0001
Rheumatoid arthritis	2.82	2.61	0.438
Coagulopathy	1.21	2.16	<0.0001
Obesity	10.18	5.79	<0.0001
Weight loss	0.38	0.91	<0.0001
Fluid and electrolyte disorders	6.15	8.46	<0.0001
Chronic blood loss anemia	0.87	1.01	0.374
Deficiency anemia	6.89	8.69	<0.0001
Alcohol abuse	0.92	0.54	0.014
Drug abuse	0.79	0.50	0.041
Psychoses	1.69	2.79	<0.0001
Depression	10.94	12.46	0.002
Osteoporosis	3.95	7.89	<0.0001

PD: Parkinson's disease.

In patients who underwent decompression surgery alone, 100% required revision multilevel-instrumented fusion [22]. Satisfactory surgical outcome was noted in only 63% of patients [22].

Babat et al. [17] were the first to report on 14 patients with PD who underwent lumbar spine surgery and found an overall reoperation rate of 86% with hardware failure reported in 29% of patients. The authors opined that the primary mechanisms of failure were relentless kyphosis or segmental instability at the operated levels.

Kaspar et al. [19] assessed the postoperative complications in 24 PD patients undergoing all types of spinal surgery and reported a 21% revision rate, including 2 cases of pseudoarthrosis and 2 patients with recurrent stenosis. The authors concluded that symptoms and functional deficits of spinal disease were often masked by PD, which posed difficulties in diagnosis. However, in their series, the complication rates in PD patients were comparable to those in the general population, and it was the authors' opinion that spine symptoms improved concomitantly with successful surgery, unless the PD symptoms progressed or significant complications ensued.

Moon et al. [9] reported postoperative outcomes in twenty patients with PD undergoing lumbar fusion surgery for degenerative disease. In their series, only one patient (5%) had a satisfactory outcome. The average postoperative visual analog pain scale (VAS, 0 to 100 mm) was 55.2, whereas the mean preoperative VAS was 53.9. Radiological assessment showed

successful fusion in 15 (75%) patients. The authors concluded that a poor surgical outcome might be inevitable due to the progressive natural history of PD and that surgical indications in patients with PD and spinal stenosis should be exercised with caution. It was the authors' opinion that even though implementing the proper surgical intervention is crucial in treating spinal disease in PD patients, the most important factor in the management of PD patients should be medical and/or surgical treatment of PD itself.

In the present study, a total of 19,211 patients with PD underwent elective lumbar spine surgery for degenerative diagnoses. There was an increasing national trend of PD patients undergoing lumbar spine surgery. The overall prevalence of PD is 1.6% in the population over age of 65 years 6 and 3.5% in those over age of 85 years [23] Additionally, PD patients were more often White males, which is in 7 accordance with the current epidemiologic data on PD [2, 24–26].

A larger proportion of patients with PD who underwent surgery had Medicare as their insurance (77.7 versus 41.1, $p < 0.0001$) compared to other patients, a finding which is not surprising given the older age of PD patients. Compared to non-PD patients, those with PD underwent a greater number of noninstrumented, lumbar decompression-only surgeries (55.4 versus 42.2, $p < 0.0001$). This could be explained by the increased age and greater number of comorbidities in PD patients, forcing surgeons to perform shorter, less complicated, and potentially safer surgeries on these patients.

Of all postoperative complications, only genitourinary (GU) and hemorrhagic complications were found to be significantly increased in the PD population. GU dysfunction predisposes to urinary retention and is one of the most common autonomic disorders in patients with PD, making this patient population increasingly vulnerable to postoperative GU complications [27]. Hypertension is a common perioperative problem in PD patients that has been associated with increased risk of intracerebral hemorrhage in patients undergoing deep brain stimulator implantation [28, 29]. The increased risk for hemorrhagic complications in our study suggest a need for tight perioperative pressure control with an increased role for surgical drains to decrease hemorrhagic complications in PD patients undergoing lumbar spine surgery.

Additionally, we found that PD patients undergoing lumbar spine surgery had greater LOS and hospitalization costs associated with fusion and fusion revision surgery but not lumbar decompression surgery. While a greater percentage of PD patients underwent decompression surgery without fusion, it is important to decipher whether those patients who undergo decompression surgery alone have higher incidence of revision surgery as has been the finding of previously published studies [22].

Multivariate analysis assessing risk factors associated with lumbar revision surgery in PD patients found that insurance status and osteoporosis were associated with revision following the index procedure. In terms of insurance, uninsured patients were found to have a significantly increased odds ratio of revision surgery (OR = 9.84, $p < 0.0001$). Uninsured patients, secondary to decreased access to

TABLE 4: Adjusted complication odds ratio in PD patients undergoing lumbar surgery*.

Complications	Odds ratio	Low 95% CI	High 95% CI	p value
Cerebrovascular accident	0.49	0.07	3.58	0.484
Respiratory complication	0.85	0.56	1.29	0.444
Cardiac complication	1.01	0.72	1.43	0.940
Deep venous thrombosis	1.76	0.98	3.17	0.061
Peripheral vascular disease	1.38	0.45	4.31	0.575
Neurological complication	2.03	0.99	4.16	0.052
Genitourinary complication	1.47	1.16	1.87	0.001
Postoperative shock	1.24	0.40	3.87	0.716
Wound complication	0.88	0.12	6.47	0.904
Pulmonary embolism	<0.001	<0.001	<0.001	<0.0001
Postoperative infection	1.48	0.90	2.43	0.123
Postoperative hemorrhage	1.30	1.16	1.47	<0.0001
Postoperative pneumonia	0.39	0.05	2.85	0.354
Myocardial infarction	1.16	0.42	3.15	0.778
Arrhythmia	0.99	0.62	1.60	0.977
Death	0.53	0.17	1.667	0.277

PD: Parkinson's disease. *Regression modeling adjusting for gender, race, hospital (bed size, region, and location), and modified Elixhauser index—reference for PD patients without PD.

TABLE 5: Length of stay and costs for patients with PD undergoing degenerative lumbar spine surgery.

	Length of stay (LOS)			Costs ($USD)		
	No PD	PD	p value	No PD	PD	p value
Lumbar fusion	4.00	5.13	<0.0001	$27,272	$29,427	<0.0001
Lumbar decompression	3.28	4.15	<0.0001	$12,366	$12,469	0.717
Lumbar fusion revision	4.80	6.24	<0.0001	$31,866	$39,885	<0.0001

PD: Parkinson's disease.

TABLE 6: Multivariate analysis assessing risk factors associated with lumbar revision surgery in patients with PD.

Risk factor	Odds ratio	Low 95% CI	High 95% CI	p value
Osteoporosis	1.98	1.07	3.65	0.029
Black	0.26	0.03	2.52	<0.0001
Hispanic	0.94	0.33	2.67	<0.0001
Asian	<0.001	<0.001	<0.001	<0.0001
Native American	<0.001	<0.001	<0.001	<0.0001
Other	0.57	0.18	1.80	<0.0001
Female	1.07	0.72	1.58	0.750
Age	0.95	0.93	0.97	<0.0001
Small hospital	0.92	0.36	2.40	0.953
Medium hospital	0.81	0.49	1.33	0.591
Teaching hospital	1.40	0.92	2.14	0.118
Midwest	1.22	0.51	2.87	0.653
South	1.59	0.75	3.38	0.350
West	1.72	0.79	3.75	0.209
Urban hospital	1.02	0.43	2.42	0.964
Modified Elixhauser index	1.01	0.95	1.06	0.856
Medicare	1.37	0.80	2.35	<0.0001
Medicaid	0.92	0.38	2.23	<0.0001
Uninsured	9.84	1.31	73.87	<0.0001
Other	0.97	0.21	4.48	0.004
Missing	<0.001	<0.001	<0.001	<0.0001

Race reference: white; hospital reference: large hospital; region reference: northeast; insurance reference: private.

healthcare, likely present with advanced PD, multiple untreated comorbidities, and more severe spinal pathology requiring complex procedures with higher failure rates. As was theorized by other authors on this topic, adequate medical and surgical control of PD is of great importance as

it may significantly affect postoperative outcomes in patients undergoing spine surgery [9].

Multiple studies have confirmed the association between osteoporosis and PD [30, 31]. This is not only associated with increased age but also with disorders of bone metabolism

[32]. This factor is especially aggravated in women, as most women with PD are also postmenopausal [18]. Studies have shown that low bone mineral density values in PD patients are closely correlated with disease severity, increased bone turnover, vitamin D deficiency, and poor nutritional status [33–35]. Low vitamin D levels are associated with increased fracture risk, poor musculoskeletal coordination, and poor muscle tone [9]. When taken together, these factors are important reasons for poor surgical outcomes in PD patients.

This study found that a diagnosis of PD was not found to be an independent risk factor for revision lumbar fusion surgery. However, a combined diagnosis of PD and osteoporosis was found to significantly increase the likelihood of lumbar fusion revision surgery. The poor bone quality in osteoporotic individuals together with the severe musculoskeletal dysfunction associated with PD appears to have significant negative effects on the likelihood of a positive spinal fusion outcome in PD patients, a finding which was also emphasized by Moon et al. [9].

5. Conclusion

This study was able to evaluate the characteristics and outcomes of patients with PD undergoing lumbar spine surgery for degenerative conditions using a large national database. PD patients had increased LOS and overall costs but did not have an increased risk of postoperative mortality. PD in itself was not found to be a risk factor for revision lumbar fusion surgery; however, PD and a diagnosis of osteoporosis significantly increased the likelihood of fusion revision. While the national trend in PD patient's undergoing elective lumbar surgery is rising, surgeons must be aware of the less favorable outcomes of lumbar spine surgery in patients with PD. PD patients should be treated with greater caution than the general population, and adequate medical and surgical control of PD prior to spine surgery may allow for improved diagnosis and better outcomes in this patient population. Though not investigated in this study, future research could inspect if the rate of readmissions and functional outcomes following surgical intervention differs in the PD patient population. As further data are collected to study the various complications associated with PD, more work can be done to establish strategies and protocols to reduce these complications and help optimize the care and outcomes of PD patients.

Disclosure

The manuscript was presented as an abstract in "2015 Annual Meeting of AANS/CNS Section on Disorders of the Spine and Peripheral Nerves, Phoenix, Arizona, March 4–7, 2015."

References

[1] J. Jankovic, "Etiology and pathogenesis of Parkinson disease," in *UpToDate*, H. Hurtig, Ed., UpToDate, Waltham, MA, USA, 2014.

[2] L. M. de Lau and M. M. Breteler, "Epidemiology of Parkinson's disease," *The Lancet Neurology*, vol. 5, no. 6, pp. 525–535, 2006.

[3] M. C. de Rijk, M. M. Breteler, G. A. Graveland et al., "Prevalence of Parkinson's disease in the elderly: the Rotterdam Study," *Neurology*, vol. 45, no. 12, pp. 2143–2146, 1995.

[4] S. K. Van den Eeden, C. M. Tanner, A. L. Bernstein et al., "Incidence of Parkinson's disease: variation by age, gender, and race/ethnicity," *American Journal of Epidemiology*, vol. 157, no. 11, pp. 1015–1022, 2003.

[5] M. Pandya, C. S. Kubu, and M. L. Giroux, "Parkinson disease: not just a movement disorder," *Cleveland Clinic Journal of Medicine*, vol. 75, no. 12, pp. 856–864, 2008.

[6] G. W. Paulson, K. Schafer, and B. Hallum, "Avoiding mental changes and falls in older Parkinson's patients," *Geriatrics*, vol. 41, pp. 59–67, 1986.

[7] W. C. Koller, S. Glatt, B. Vetere-Overfield et al., "Falls in Parkinson's disease," *Clinical Neuropharmacology*, vol. 2, pp. 98–105, 1989.

[8] F. van den Bos, A. D. Speelman, M. Samson et al., "Parkinson's disease and osteoporosis," *Age Ageing*, vol. 42, no. 2, pp. 156–162, 2013.

[9] S. H. Moon, H. M. Lee, H. J. Chun et al., "Surgical outcome of lumbar fusion surgery in patients with Parkinson's disease," *Journal of Spinal Disorders & Techniques*, vol. 25, no. 7, pp. 351–355, 2012.

[10] HCUP Nationwide Inpatient Sample (NIS), *Healthcare Cost and Utilization Project (HCUP), 2002-2011*, Agency for Healthcare Research and Quality, Rockville, MD, USA, 2011, http://www.hcup-us.ahrq.gov/nisoverview.jsp.

[11] C. van Walraven, P. C. Austin, A. Jennings et al., "A modification of the Elixhauser comorbidity measures into a point system for hospital death using administrative data," *Medical Care*, vol. 47, no. 6, pp. 626–633, 2009.

[12] A. Elixhauser, C. Steiner, D. R. Harris et al., "Comorbidity measures for use with administrative data," *Medical Care*, vol. 36, no. 1, pp. 8–27, 1998.

[13] M. T. Sharabiani, P. Aylin, and A. Bottle, "A systematic review of comorbidity indices for administrative data," *Medical Care*, vol. 50, no. 12, pp. 1109–1118, 2012.

[14] HCUP Cost-to-Ratio Files (CCR), *Healthcare Cost and Utilization Project (HCUP), 2002-2011*, Agency for Healthcare Research and Quality, Rockville, MD, USA, 2011.

[15] Bureau of Labor Statistics, *CPI Inflation Calculator*, Washington, DC, USA, 2014, http://data.bls.gov/cgi-bin/cpicalc.pl.

[16] Institute for the Ages, *Demographic Transition Facts*, Sarasota, FL, USA, 2014, http://www.institutefortheages.org/facts-on-aging/.

[17] L. B. Babat, R. F. McLain, W. Bingaman, I. Kalfas, P. Young, and C. Rufo-Smith, "Spinal surgery in patients with Parkinson's disease: construct failure and progressive deformity," *Spine*, vol. 29, no. 18, pp. 2006–2012, 2004.

[18] A. Bourghli, P. Guerin, J. M. Vital et al., "Posterior spinal fusion from T2 to the sacrum for the management of major deformities in patients with Parkinson disease: a retrospective review with analysis of complications," *ournal of Spinal Disorders & Techniques*, vol. 25, no. 3, pp. E53–E60, 2012.

[19] S. Kaspar, L. Riley, D. Cohen, D. Long, J. Kostuik, and H. Hassanzadeh, "Spine surgery in Parkinson's," *Journal of Bone and Joint Surgery*, vol. 87, p. 292, 2005.

[20] H. Koller, F. Acosta, J. Zenner et al., "Spinal surgery in patients with Parkinson's disease: experiences with the challenges posed by sagittal imbalance and the Parkinson's spine," *European Spine Journal*, vol. 19, no. 10, pp. 1785–1794, 2010.

[21] P. M. Wadia, G. Tan, R. P. Munhoz, S. H. Fox, S. J. Lewis, and A. E. Lang, "Surgical correction of kyphosis in patients with camptocormia due to Parkinson's disease: a retrospective evaluation," *Journal of Neurology, Neurosurgery & Psychiatry*, vol. 82, no. 4, pp. 364–368, 2011.

[22] B. Skovrlj, C. A. Sarkiss, J. Z. Guzman, S. K. Cho, and J. M. Caridi, "A literature review of spine surgery outcomes in patients with Parkinson's disease," in *Proceedings of the Cervical Spine Research Society European Section Annual Meeting*, Pamplona, Spain, June 2014.

[23] M. C. deRijk, C. Tzourio, M. M. Breteler et al., "Prevalence of parkinsonism and Parkinson' disease in Europe; the EUROPARKINSON Collaborative Study. European Community concerted action on the epidemiology of Parkinson's disease," *Journal of Neurology, Neurosurgery & Psychiatry*, vol. 62, no. 1, pp. 10–15, 1997.

[24] A. Wright Willis, B. A. Evanoff, M. Lian, S. R. Criswell, and B. A. Racette, "Geographic and ethnic variation in Parkinson disease: a population-based study of US Medicare beneficiaries," *Neuroepidemiology*, vol. 34, no. 3, pp. 143–151, 2010.

[25] J. F. Kurtzke and I. D. Goldberg, "Parkinsonism death rates by race, sex, and geography," *Neurology*, vol. 38, no. 10, pp. 1558–1561, 1988.

[26] D. E. Lilienfeld, D. Sekkor, S. Simpson et al., "Parkinsonism death rates by race, sex and geography: a 1980s update," *Neuroepidemiology*, vol. 9, no. 5, pp. 243–247, 1990.

[27] R. Sakakibara, T. Uchiyama, T. Yamanishi, and M. Kishi, "Genitourinary dysfunction in Parkinson's disease," *Movement Disorders*, vol. 25, no. 1, pp. 2–12, 2010.

[28] R. Khatib, Z. Ebrahim, A. Rezai et al., "Perioperative events during deep brain stimulation: the experience at Cleveland clinic," *Journal of Neurosurgical Anesthesiology*, vol. 20, no. 1, pp. 36–40, 2008.

[29] D. K. Binder, G. M. Rau, and P. A. Starr, "Risk factors for hemorrhage during microelectrode-guided deep brain stimulator implantation for movement disorders," *Neurosurgery*, vol. 56, no. 4, pp. 722–732, 2005.

[30] C. H. Kao, C. C. Chen, S. J. Wang, L. G. Chia, and S. H. Yeh, "Bone mineral density in patients with Parkinson's disease measured by dual photon absorptimetry," *Nuclear Medicine Communications*, vol. 15, no. 3, pp. 172–177, 1994.

[31] F. Ishizaki, T. Harada, S. Katayama, H. Abe, and S. Nakamura, "Relationship between osteopenia and clinical characteristics of Parkinson's disease," *Movement Disorders*, vol. 8, no. 4, pp. 507–511, 1993.

[32] Y. Sato, M. Kikuyama, and K. Oizumi, "High prevalence of vitamin D deficiency and reduced bone mass in Parkinson's disease," *Neurology*, vol. 49, no. 5, pp. 1273–1278, 1997.

[33] N. Vaserman, "Parkinson's disease and osteoporosis," *Joint Bone Spine*, vol. 72, no. 6, pp. 484–488, 2005.

[34] H. Taggart and V. Crawford, "Reduced bone density of the hip in elderly patients with Parkinson's disease," *Age Ageing*, vol. 24, no. 4, pp. 326–328, 1995.

[35] J. M. Sheard, S. Ash, P. A. Silburn, and G. K. Kerr, "Prevalence of malnutrition in Parkinson's disease: a systematic review," *Nutrition Reviews*, vol. 69, no. 9, pp. 520–532, 2011.

13

Serum Homocysteine Level in Parkinson's Disease and its Association with Duration, Cardinal Manifestation, and Severity of Disease

Payam Saadat,[1] Alijan Ahmadi Ahangar ⓘ,[1] Seyed Ehsan Samaei ⓘ,[2] Alireza Firozjaie,[3] Fatemeh Abbaspour,[4] Sorrayya Khafri ⓘ,[5] and Azam Khoddami[4]

[1]Mobility Impairment Research Center, Health Research Institute, Babol University of Medical Sciences, Babol, Iran
[2]Social Determinants of Health Research Center, Health Research Institute, Babol University of Medical Sciences, Babol, Iran
[3]Cellular and Molecular Biology Research Center, Health Research Institute, Babol University of Medical Sciences, Babol, Iran
[4]Clinical Research Development Center, Ayatollah Rohani Hospital, Babol University of Medical Sciences, Babol, Iran
[5]Department of Statistic and Epidmiology, School of Medicine, Babol University of Medical Sciences, Babol, Iran

Correspondence should be addressed to Alijan Ahmadi Ahangar; ahmadiahangaralijan@yahoo.com

Academic Editor: Jan Aasly

Background and Purpose. Due to the high prevalence of Parkinson's disease (PD) in the elderly, a large financial burden is imposed on the families and health systems of countries in addition to the problems related to the mobility impairment caused by the disease for the patients. Studies on controversial issues in this disease are taken into consideration, and one of these cases is the role of serum homocysteine level in Parkinson's patients. In this study, the serum level of homocysteine and its association with various variables in relation to this disease was compared with healthy individuals. *Materials and Methods.* In this study, 100 patients with PD and 100 healthy individuals as control group were investigated. Serum homocysteine level and demographic and clinical data were included in the checklist. Data were analyzed by SPSS version 23. In all tests, the significance level was below 0.05. *Results.* The mean level of serum homocysteine in case and control groups was 14.93 ± 8.30 and 11.52 ± 2.86 μmol/L, respectively (95% CI: 1.68; 5.14, $P < 0.001$). In total patients, 85 had normal serum homocysteine level, while 15 had high serum homocysteine level. In controls, the homocysteine level was 98 and 2, respectively ($P = 0.002$). In multivariate logistic regression analysis, serum homocysteine level higher than 20 μmol/L was accompanied by 8.64-fold in Parkinson's disease involvement (95% CI: 1.92; 38.90, $P = 0.005$). *Conclusion.* Increasing serum homocysteine level elevates the rate to having PD. Serum homocysteine levels did not have any relationship with the duration of the disease, type of cardinal manifestation, and the severity of Parkinson's disease.

1. Introduction

PD is the second progressive neurodegenerative disease and one of the important and common causes of mobility impairment in the elderly that occurs in all races with almost equal gender distribution [1]. Its prevalence is increased with increasing age [2]. This disease often occurs in individuals older than 60 years and is sporadic in most cases, but the incidence of disease in families is also observed in about 15% of cases; genetic and environmental factors are involved in the etiology of the disease [3, 4]. Agricultural pesticides [5] are one of the environmental factors that affect the disease.

On the other hand, cigarette [6] and caffeine [7] seem to have a protective effect. Homocysteine is produced by the metabolism of the methionine amino acid, and there is a possibility of its reuptake by remethylation and converts into methionine. The enzyme that performs the recent reaction requires folate and B12. This enzyme also controls the serum level of homocysteine by coenzymes B12, folate, B6, and choline. Hence, the deficiency of these vitamins leads to the accumulation of homocysteine [8]. The deficiency of folate and B12 leads to atrophy of the neurons of CA1 region of the hippocampus and disruption of cognitive processes with increasing homocysteine [9].

Increasing plasma homocysteine level is associated with elevating the risk of systemic vascular disease through enhancement of the adverse effects of risk factors such as hypertension, smoking, and lipid and lipoprotein metabolism, as well as acceleration of development of inflammation. Increased homocysteine also has been reported during recent decades in neurological diseases without vascular origin such as Alzheimer's disease [10] and idiopathic Parkinson's disease [11, 12].

Furthermore, in the research conducted on PD patients, homocysteine level of cerebrospinal fluid has been reported higher than normal [11]. Homocysteine leads to damage to MPTP-dependent (1-methyl,4-phenyl-1,2,5, and 6 tetrahydropyridine) dopaminergic cells [13].

On the other hand, according to some researchers, high homocysteine level in PD patients may be due to dopamine compound treatment [14]. However, with regard to homocysteine and Parkinson's disease, the available findings are controversial. Due to the high prevalence of PD in the elderly, a large financial burden is imposed on the families and health systems of countries in addition to the problems related to the mobility impairment caused by the disease for these patients. Hence, conducting research projects on different aspects of this disease can be important. Given these issues, there is a controversy about the relationship between homocysteine and PD. Even if there is this relationship, there is vagueness regarding the association between homocysteine with some variables of Parkinson's disease.

Variables such as demographic characteristics of patients and issues such as type of occupation or patients' degree of education may have an impact in the serum level of homocysteine. To answer these questions, this study was designed and carried out. In the case of the existence of relationships between homocysteine and PD and specifically with some of its related variables in this study and its confirmation with other studies, it may be possible to use these results in preventing or treating this disease.

2. Materials and Methods

This cross-sectional and case-control study was conducted at the Neurology Clinic of Ayatollah Rouhani Hospital in Babol during 2015-2016. The proposal of this study was approved by the Research Council of Babol University of Medical Sciences (number 3183) and the Ethics Committee of Research Studies of Babol University of Medical Sciences. One hundred new PD patients who have not received treatment yet were selected as the case group and 100 healthy individuals as the control group. Two groups of case and control were matched according to age and gender.

Inclusion criteria were the definite diagnosis of PD based on the Movement Disorder Society (MDS) Clinical Diagnostic Criteria for Parkinson's Disease [15], with four major cardinal manifestations including tremor, hypokinesia, rigidity, and postural instability [16], under the supervision of a neurologist who is responsible for the study.

Grading of motor impairment was done based on the Movement Disorder Society- (MDS-) sponsored revision of the Unified Parkinson's Disease Rating Scale (MDS-UPDRS) [17]. Scoring severity of disease was done based on modified Hoehn and Yahr staging; thus, the severity of the disease was classified into three classes of 1-2 (mild), 2.5–3 (moderate), and more than 3 (severe) [18].

Demographic information (age, gender, occupation, level of education, and economic status) of PD cases and control groups and clinical status of PD patients (duration, cardinal manifestation, and severity of disease) were determined.

Exclusion criteria were as follows: patients with Parkinson's disease who have already been receiving medical treatment, including levodopa, disease caused by the use of certain neuroleptic drugs or toxins, Parkinsonism associated with other neurologic diseases, and Parkinson's disease patients with renal hepatic failure, pharmaceutical supplement consumption, and patient's dissatisfaction to participate in the study.

Exclusion criteria for control group were individuals having any symptoms or signs of Parkinson's syndrome, renal and hepatic failure, and pharmaceutical supplement consumption. The ages of patients were classified into three classes: under 60, 60–80, and older than 80 years.

In terms of education, patients were divided into two classes: illiterate and literate. Based on type of job, they were classified as an employee, a freelancer (mostly farmers), and an unemployed (including housewives). Duration of the disease was classified into three classes: less than 5 years, between 5 and 10 years, and more than 10 years. For ruling out other diagnoses, brain imaging was performed for the patients. Routine laboratory tests and measurements of serum homocysteine level were done in the laboratory of Ayatollah Rouhani Hospital in Babol. In both the case and control groups, serum homocysteine level was measured by the ELISA method [19]. Heparin plasma samples were centrifuged within 30 minutes in the laboratory to prevent its false increase due to the release of homocysteine from red blood cells. Separation and freezing the samples after collection was done within an hour. Serum homocysteine levels less than 12 μmol/L were desirable, and levels higher than 15 μmol/L were considered at risk of vascular disease [20]. We consider serum homocysteine levels higher than 20 μmol/L associated with an increased risk of PD, and based on this, the serum homocysteine level was classified into two classes: normal (20 μmol/L and less) and high (more than 20 μmol/L).

In addition to the results of serum homocysteine level, demographic information (age, gender, occupation, and level of education) of the case and control groups and clinical status (duration, cardinal manifestation, and severity of disease) of the patient group were entered in the study checklist.

The information and laboratory results obtained from the patients and the control group were entered into SPSS version 23 software and analyzed using the statistical independent t-test and one-way ANOVA. They were also investigated using multivariate logistic regression test by modifying the interfering variables that have a role homocysteine level in Parkinson's disease. In all tests, the significance level was less than 0.05.

TABLE 1: Demographic characteristic of Parkinson's patients and control group.

Variables	Case (%) (n = 100)	Control (%) (n = 100)	P value
Gender			
Male	53 (53%)	50 (50%)	0.777
Female	47 (47%)	50 (50%)	
Age (year)			
<60	16 (16%)	16 (16%)	
60–80	72 (72%)	72 (72%)	1.00
>80	12 (12%)	12 (12%)	
Education			
Literate	39 (39%)	31 (31%)	0.299
Illiterate	69 (69%)	61 (61%)	

TABLE 2: Clinical features of Parkinson's disease.

Features	Patients, n (%)
Duration of the disease	
Less than 5 years	65 (65%)
5–10 years	27 (27%)
More than 10 years	8 (8%)
Cardinal manifestation of the disease	
Tremor	62 (62%)
Rigidity	13 (13%)
Bradykinesia	22 (22%)
Postural instability	3 (3%)
Severity of deterioration of the disease	
(based on modified Hoehn and Yahr staging)	
1-2 (mild)	35 (13%)
2.5-3 (moderate)	44 (44%)
More than 3 (severe)	21 (21%)

3. Results

The mean age of 100 PD cases was 69.72 ± 9.88 years and the control group was 69.37 ± 9.88 years (the age range was 42–97 years in both groups). Male and female in the case group were 53 and 47 years, respectively, and both were 50 years in the control group (Table 1). In terms of age, the patients were as follows: 16 cases were below 60 years, 72 cases were between 60 and 80 years, and 12 individuals were older than 80 years. In relation to the level of literacy, 61 individuals were illiterate and 39 individuals were literate. There was no significant difference between the case and control groups in any of these variables (Table 1).

According to the duration of the disease, 65 individuals involved were less than 5 years ago, 27 were between 5 and 10 years ago, and 8 were more than 10 years ago. In terms of cardinal manifestation of patients, 62 individuals suffer tremor, 13 had rigidity, 22 with bradykinesia, and 3 had postural instability. The severity of the disease of the patients was 1-2 (35 individuals), 2.5-3 (44 individuals), and more than 3 (21 individuals) (Table 2).

Accordingly, 85 patients were with normal serum homocysteine level and 15 patients were with increased serum homocysteine level in the case group. This number was 98 and 2 patients, respectively, in the control group. Accordingly, there was a significant difference between the two groups ($P = 0.002$). The mean of serum homocysteine level was

TABLE 3: (Mean) serum homocysteine level of the case and control groups (μmol/L).

Demographic pattern	(Mean) serum homocysteine level		P value
	Case (n = 100)	Control (n = 100)	
Gender			
Male	14.73 ± 6.46	11.87 ± 2.72	0.005
Female	15.17 ± 10.05	11.18 ± 10.05	0.009
Age (years)			
<60	12.30 ± 3.21	12.01 ± 0.52	0.776
60–80	15.54 ± 8.20	11.78 ± 2.87	0.001
>80	14.79 ± 6.02	11.18 ± 2.15	0.063
Education			
Literate	14.19 ± 8.51	10.96 ± 2.79	0.047
Illiterate	15.41 ± 8.20	11.78 ± 2.87	0.001

$8.30 \pm 14.93 \mu$mol/L in the case group and $2.86 \pm 11.52 \mu$mol/L in the control group (Table 3), and there was a significant difference between the two groups in this regard ($P < 0.001$; 95% CI: 1.68; 514). In the Pearson correlation analysis, the correlation of homocysteine level with the control group and case group was -0.02 and 0.148, respectively, but none of them was statistically significant (P was 0.840 and 0.140, resp.). There was a significant difference in the patient group compared to the control group, male and female, between the age of 60 and 80 years, and in the literate and illiterate individuals in terms of the mean of the serum homocysteine level (P was 0.005, 0.009, 0.001, 0.047, and 0.001, resp.) (Table 3).

The serum homocysteine level has increased with the increasing severity of the disease, but this increase was not statistically significant. At the severity of 2.5–3 of Parkinson's disease compared to other severities, the higher frequency of patients with increased serum homocysteine was observed (8 patients). Nonetheless, this difference was not significant between the three different classes of the severity of Parkinson's disease (Table 4). Homocysteine level in patients with Parkinson's disease increased with increasing duration of the disease, but this difference was not significant between patient groups (Table 4). The serum homocysteine level in patients with Parkinson's disease was not significant in this study according to their cardinal manifestation (Table 4).

The mean level of homocysteine of employed people was $5.39 \pm 13.09 \mu$mol/L, freelancer (farmers) was $7.29 \pm 14.79 \mu$mol/L, and unemployed (housewives) was $9.80 \pm 15.85 \mu$mol/L. Accordingly, the mean level of homocysteine of the farmers and unemployed/housewives was higher than the employed people, but this difference was not statistically significant (Table 5).

The amount of risk of independent factors for Parkinson's disease was investigated using logistic regression analysis by modifying the involved factors such as age and gender. Accordingly, serum homocysteine levels higher than 20μmol/L increased 8.64-fold the chance of having PD ($P = 0.005$, 95% CI: 1.92; 38.90) (Table 6).

4. Discussion

According to this study, the serum homocysteine level in PD patients was significantly higher than the healthy subjects.

TABLE 4: Frequency of different clinical features of Parkinson's disease based on serum levels of homocysteine.

Serum homocysteine level (μmol/L)	Parkinson's disease features				P value
	Duration of the disease (years)				
	≤5	5–10	>10		
≤20	57 (87/7%)	21 (77/8%)	7 (87/5%)		0.572
>20	8 (12.3%)	6 (22.2%)	11 (12.5%)		
	Cardinal manifestation of the disease				
	Postural instability	Tremor	Rigidity	Bradykinesia	
≤20	2 (66.7%)	53 (85.5%)	11 (84/6%)	19 (86.4%)	0.841
>20	1 (33.3%)	9(14.5%)	2 (15.4%)	3 (13.6%)	
	Severity of the disease based on modified Hoehn and Yahr staging				
	1-2 (mild)	2.5-3 (moderate)	>3 (severe)		
≤20	33 (94.3%)	36 (81.8%)	16 (76.2%)		0.154
>20	2 (5.7 %)	8 (18.2%)	5 (23.8%)		

TABLE 5: The mean serum homocysteine level by occupation in the patients group.

Variables	Occupation			P value
	Employed ($n = 22$)	Freelancer (mostly farmers) ($n = 29$)	Unemployed/housewives ($n = 49$)	
Means of homocysteine	13.09 ± 5.39	14.79 ± 7.29	15.85 ± 80	0.433

Although many factors can influence this level difference, all of which may not be considered in our study, it can be said that the risk of getting involved in Parkinson's disease was estimated to be 8.64-fold with increasing the serum homocysteine level more than $20\,\mu$mol/L based on logistic regression multivariate analysis.

One of the most important factors that can affect the serum homocysteine level is the type of diet. Regarding the available data, the type of diet can play an important role in Parkinson's disease; for example, vitamin B12 and folate, whose amount varies in different diets, are involved in controlling serum homocysteine levels [8].

Definitely, how high serum homocysteine level can increase the risk of Parkinson's disease is not clear, and it is even possible that the high serum homocysteine level may be due to the effect of disease on patients rather than that causes PD. In some previous studies, increasing homocysteine level in the general population was associated with the risk of mild cognitive impairment, atherosclerosis, and neurodegenerative diseases such as Alzheimer's disease, vascular dementia, and Parkinson's disease [21–24].

Although the empirical observations confirm this issue, many studies do not confirm this relationship and the role of homocysteine in the pathogenesis of Parkinson's disease is currently unknown. In a study conducted by Rodriguez-Oroz et al. in 2009, the findings showed an increase in serum homocysteine in patients with Parkinson's disease compared to healthy subjects, as in our study [21].

In a study by Song et al. in 2016, the serum homocysteine level in patients with PD was higher than that in healthy subjects [22], which is consistent with our study. They also investigated the effect of levodopa on increasing serum homocysteine in patients, and according to their findings, the patients with levodopa treatment had higher levels of homocysteine than others. In another study conducted by Hu et al. in 2013, findings showed no significant difference in

TABLE 6: Logistic regression multivariate analysis to determine the role of independent risk factors in Parkinson's disease.

Variables		OR	95% CI	P value
Serum homocysteine levels higher than 20		8.64	1.92–38.90	0.005
Severity of illness	1-2	Ref.	Ref.	0.172
	2.5-3	3.67	0.72–18.53	0.116
	>3	5.16	0.9–29.53	0.065

homocysteine level in the untreated patients compared to healthy subjects [14].

According to the findings of our study, there was no significant difference between the male and female PD patients in terms of the mean of serum level of homocysteine, although there was a significant difference between the two groups of patients and healthy subjects in terms of gender. Based on the study of Kocer et al. in 2016, there was a significant difference between the two groups of patients in terms of gender [25]. They report higher serum homocysteine level in men than women, which was not consistent with our study as mentioned; there was no significant difference between serum homocysteine levels in the two genders of the patient group, and our findings were not consistent with these studies. In this regard, we cannot provide an acceptable justification for this inconsistency, but perhaps the small number of patients in our study had led to the lack of significance of the serum homocysteine level in these two groups. Certainly, as mentioned earlier, there was a significant difference between the two groups of patients and controls in terms of men and women and their serum homocysteine level. In other words, the grade of difference of homocysteine serum level in the patient groups in comparison with the control group was higher in women than men.

The mean of serum homocysteine level was not significant based on the degree of education of patients, and also difference between different ages was not significant. In this study, the mean of serum homocysteine level increased in patients with increasing severity of PD. Although this difference was not statistically significant, there was no significant relationship of the increased homocysteine level of patients in terms of duration of the disease in the study of Kocer et al. [9], which was consistent with our study.

Based on the results of this study, there was not a significant difference in terms of the relationship between the duration of involvement of Parkinson's disease patients and their serum homocysteine level; perhaps, the reason is that they did not receive any medical treatment (dopamine compounds). And this hypothesis justifies that the high serum homocysteine level in Parkinson's disease may be due to receiving dopaminergic drugs. In another study conducted by Religa et al. in 2006, serum homocysteine level of patients with Parkinson's disease was higher than healthy subjects; moreover, there was a significant relationship between the duration of the disease and increased serum homocysteine [26]. However, the results of this study were not consistent with the results of our study.

Among other variables studied in this study, serum homocysteine level was based on the type of their employment; accordingly, there was no significant difference between the groups of patients and control and different variables studied in patients with Parkinson's disease. In the previous studies conducted, the effect of different occupations on Parkinson's disease had been due to the effects of occupational factors such as agricultural pesticides [5] or industrial toxins such as metals, solvents, and organophosphate compounds on this disease [27], and the results of this study also show that the effect of the type of occupation on PD is not due to its direct effect on serum homocysteine level.

There was not a significant difference between changes in serum homocysteine levels in patients with Parkinson's disease in terms of the type of their cardinal manifestation. The results of the few studies that were conducted and searched were also similar to the results of our study [23, 25]. One of the interesting aspects in Parkinson's disease is its association with the digestive tract. Intestinal dysfunction occurs in most patients before the onset of motor manifestations of the disease; it can be indicative of a possible contribution of intestinal dysfunction in the pathogenesis of PD.

High α-synuclein protein that is present in the intestines of PD patients increases intestinal permeability, resulting in synucleinopathy in the intestines of these individuals; this happens before the occurrence of cardinal manifestation in PD patients. Regarding these and many other findings, the association between the digestive tract and Parkinson's disease (the gut axis in PD patients) has been very much considered in the recent study [28].

The strengths of this study were selection of patients with Parkinson's disease who were not under any medical treatment so far and investigation of changes in the serum homocysteine level in patients with Parkinson's disease due to the type of their cardinal manifestation and some other variables, although the small number of cases and control groups studied was the limitation of this study.

Our small sample size might have led to loss of the power statistical analysis. To determine more precisely the relationship between homocysteine and PD, the study of measurement of serum homocysteine level in patients with Parkinson's diagnosis with more cases, and more healthy controls, and also the study on the patient group with Parkinson's disease diagnosis with and without dopamine compounds treatment are recommended.

5. Conclusion

According to this study, an increase in serum homocysteine level in PD patients has been observed, which can be one of the factors associated with to the disease. High age was one of the factors associated with increased serum homocysteine level in patients. There was no relationship between the severity of the disease and the serum homocysteine level. The mean of serum homocysteine level increased in patients with increasing severity of Parkinson's disease.

There was not a significant difference in terms of the relationship between the duration of involvement in Parkinson's disease patients with their serum homocysteine level. Moreover, there was no significant relationship between serum homocysteine level of patients in terms of duration of the disease. There is no exact mechanism for increasing serum homocysteine level in Parkinson's disease patients, and more studies must be conducted to clarify this issue. By clearing up these issues, measuring serum homocysteine level can be suggested in the laboratory screening test to identify the patients at risk for Parkinson's disease. In the future, modification of serum homocysteine level may play a role in preventive methods or treatment of Parkinson's disease.

Acknowledgments

The authors wish to express their sincere gratitude to the Deputy for Research and Technology of Babol University of Medical Sciences and Mobility Impairment Research Center for approving the proposal of this study and its implementation. The authors also thank Dr. Vanji for the English revision of the manuscript.

References

[1] L. Hirsch, N. Jette, A. Frolkis, T. Steeves, and T. Pringsheim, "The incidence of Parkinson's disease: a systematic review and meta-analysis," *Neuroepidemiology*, vol. 46, no. 4, pp. 292–300, 2016.

[2] G. W. Ross and R. D. Abbott, "Living and dying with Parkinson's disease," *Movement Disorders*, vol. 29, no. 13, pp. 1571–1573, 2014.

[3] A. B. Singleton, M. J. Farrer, and V. Bonifati, "The genetics of Parkinson's disease: progress and therapeutic implications," *Movement Disorders*, vol. 28, no. 1, pp. 14–23, 2013.

[4] M. Białecka, P. Robowski, K. Honczarenko, A. Roszmann, and J. Sławek, "Genetic and environmental factors for

hyperhomocysteinaemia and its clinical implications in Parkinson's disease," *Neurologia i Neurochirurgia Polska*, vol. 43, pp. 272–285, 2009.

[5] F. Moisan, J. Spinosi, L. Delabre et al., "Association of Parkinson's disease and its subtypes with agricultural pesticide exposures in men: a case–control study in France," *Environmental Health Perspectives*, vol. 123, no. 11, 2015.

[6] E. L. Thacker, E. J. O'Reilly, M. G. Weisskopf et al., "Temporal relationship between cigarette smoking and risk of Parkinson disease," *Neurology*, vol. 68, no. 10, pp. 764–768, 2007.

[7] M. H. Madeira, R. Boia, A. F. Ambrósio, and A. R. Santiago, "Having a coffee break: the impact of caffeine consumption on microglia-mediated inflammation in neurodegenerative diseases," *Mediators of Inflammation*, vol. 2017, Article ID 4761081, 12 pages, 2017.

[8] K. T. Williams and K. L. Schalinske, "Homocysteine metabolism and its relation to health and disease," *Biofactors*, vol. 36, no. 1, pp. 19–24, 2010.

[9] B. Kocer, H. Guven, I. Conkbayir, S. S. Comoglu, and S. Delibas, "The effect of hyperhomocysteinemia on motor symptoms, cognitive status, and vascular risk in patients with Parkinson's disease," *Parkinson's Disease*, vol. 2016, pp. 1–7, 2016.

[10] S. Seshadri, A. Beiser, J. Selhub et al., "Plasma homocysteine as a risk factor for dementia and Alzheimer's disease," *New England Journal of Medicine*, vol. 346, no. 7, pp. 476–483, 2002.

[11] C. Isobe, T. Murata, C. Sato, and Y. Terayama, "Increase of total homocysteine concentration in cerebrospinal fluid in patients with Alzheimer's disease and Parkinson's disease," *Life Sciences*, vol. 77, no. 15, pp. 1836–1843, 2005.

[12] R. Ansari, A. Mahta, E. Mallack, and J. J. Luo, "Hyperhomocysteinemia and neurologic disorders: a review," *Journal of Clinical Neurology*, vol. 10, no. 4, pp. 281–288, 2014.

[13] P. E. O'Suilleabhain, R. Oberle, C. Bartis, R. B. Dewey, T. Bottiglieri, and R. Diaz-Arrastia, "Clinical course in Parkinson's disease with elevated homocysteine," *Parkinsonism and Related Disorders*, vol. 12, no. 2, pp. 103–107, 2006.

[14] X. W. Hu, S. M. Qin, D. Li, L. F. Hu, and C. F. Liu, "Elevated homocysteine levels in levodopa-treated idiopathic Parkinson's disease: a meta-analysis," *Acta Neurologica Scandinavica*, vol. 128, no. 2, pp. 73–82, 2013.

[15] R. B. Postuma, D. Berg, M. Stern et al., "MDS clinical diagnostic criteria for Parkinson's disease," *Movement Disorders*, vol. 30, no. 12, pp. 1591–1601, 2015.

[16] J. Jankovic, "Parkinson's disease: clinical features and diagnosis," *Journal of Neurology, Neurosurgery and Psychiatry*, vol. 79, no. 4, pp. 368–376, 2008.

[17] C. G. Goetz, B. C. Tilley, S. R. Shaftman et al., "Movement Disorder Society-sponsored revision of the Unified Parkinson's Disease Rating Scale (MDS-UPDRS): scale presentation and clinimetric testing results," *Movement Disorders*, vol. 23, no. 15, pp. 2129–2170, 2008.

[18] C. G. Goetz, W. Poewe, O. Rascol et al., "Movement Disorder Society Task Force report on the Hoehn and Yahr staging scale: status and recommendations. The Movement Disorder Society Task Force on rating scales for Parkinson's disease," *Movement Disorders*, vol. 19, no. 9, pp. 1020–1028, 2004.

[19] S. Ramakrishnan and K. N. Sulohana, *Manual of Medical Laboratory Techniques*, Jaypee Brothers Medical Publishers Pvt. Ltd., New Delhi, India, 2012.

[20] P. S. Sachdev, "Homocysteine and brain atrophy," *Progress in Neuro-Psychopharmacology and Biological Psychiatry*, vol. 29, no. 7, pp. 1152–1161, 2005.

[21] M. C. Rodriguez-Oroz, P. M. Lage, J. Sanchez-Mut et al., "Homocysteine and cognitive impairment in Parkinson's disease: a biochemical, neuroimaging, and genetic study," *Movement Disorders*, vol. 24, no. 10, pp. 1437–1444, 2009.

[22] I. U. Song, T. W. Kim, I. Yoo, Y. A. Chung, and K. S. Lee, "Can COMT-inhibitor delay the clinical progression of Parkinson's disease? 2 years follow up pilot study," *International Journal of Imaging Systems and Technology*, vol. 26, no. 1, pp. 38–42, 2016.

[23] I.-U. Song, J.-S. Kim, I.-S. Park et al., "Clinical significance of homocysteine (Hcy) on dementia in Parkinson's disease (PD)," *Archives of Gerontology and Geriatrics*, vol. 57, no. 3, pp. 288–291, 2013.

[24] K. R. Chaudhuri, D. G. Healy, and A. H. Schapira, "Non-motor symptoms of Parkinson's disease: diagnosis and management," *The Lancet Neurology*, vol. 5, no. 3, pp. 235–236, 2006.

[25] B. Kocer, H. Guven, and S. S. Comoglu, "Homocysteine levels in Parkinson's disease: is entacapone effective?," *BioMed Research International*, vol. 2016, Article ID 7563705, 6 pages, 2016.

[26] D. Religa, K. Czyzewski, M. Styczynska et al., "Hyperhomocysteinemia and methylenetetrahydrofolatereductase polymorphism in patients with Parkinson's disease," *Neuroscience Letters*, vol. 404, no. 1, pp. 56–60, 2006.

[27] W. M. Caudle, T. S. Guillot, C. R. Lazo, and G. W. Miller, "Miller industrial toxicants and Parkinson's disease," *Neurotoxicology*, vol. 33, no. 2, pp. 178–188, 2012.

[28] C. Madelyn and M. G. Tansey, "The gut-brain axis: is intestinal inflammation a silent driver of Parkinson's disease pathogenesis?," *NPJ Parkinson's Disease*, vol. 11, no. 1, p. 3, 2017.

14

Festination Correlates with SNCA Polymorphism in Chinese Patients with Parkinson's Disease

Jinhua Zheng, Xinglong Yang, Quanzhen Zhao, Sijia Tian, Hongyan Huang, Yalan Chen, and Yanming Xu

Department of Neurology, West China Hospital, Sichuan University, 37 Guo Xue Xiang, Chengdu, Sichuan Province 610041, China

Correspondence should be addressed to Yanming Xu; neuroxym999@163.com

Academic Editor: Jan Aasly

The genetic basis of festination, a common motor symptom in Parkinson's disease (PD), remains unclear. Since polymorphism in the alpha-synuclein (SNCA) gene is associated with PD phenotype, we examined whether such polymorphism is also associated with festination. SNCA polymorphisms rs11931074 and rs894278 were genotyped in a consecutive series of 258 patients with PD, of whom 122 (47.3%) suffered festination. Univariate analysis revealed significant differences in genotype and minor allele frequencies at rs11931074 or rs894278 between patients with festination and those without it (all $p < 0.05$). Based on logistic regression, a GG or GT genotype at rs11931074 was associated with higher risk of festination among patients with PD (OR 2.077, 95% CI 1.111–3.883, $p = 0.022$), as was the TT genotype at rs894278 (OR 2.271, 95% CI 1.246–4.139, $p = 0.007$). Therefore, we conclude that festination is associated with polymorphism at rs11931074 or rs894278 among patients with PD.

1. Introduction

Parkinson's disease (PD) is the most common neurodegenerative movement disorder, affecting approximately 1% of people aged 65 or older worldwide [1]. Clinical manifestations of PD include motor deficits such as rigidity, slowness in movement (bradykinesia), postural instability, and a characteristic tremor at rest [1]. Motor symptoms of PD result from the selective loss of dopaminergic neurons in the pars compacta of the substantia nigra (SN) in the midbrain, as well as their axon terminals, which project to the dorsal striatum [2].

A neuropathological hallmark of PD is the presence of intraneuronal proteinaceous inclusions, termed Lewy bodies (LBs) or Lewy neurites. These structures are enriched in filamentous forms of the synaptic protein α-synuclein [3]. The gene that encodes the protein α-synuclein is alpha-synuclein (*SNCA*). Missense mutations within the *SNCA* gene or genetic duplication or triplication of the *SNCA* locus can lead to autosomal dominant forms of PD [4–6]. In addition to these rare *SNCA* gene mutations, some common genetic variations at the *SNCA* locus, including single-nucleotide polymorphisms (SNPs), are associated with higher risk of PD in the general population [7–9]. In Chinese populations,

SNCA polymorphism has been associated with PD onset or progression. The T allele at rs11931074 and the G allele at rs894278 have been associated with significantly higher risk of PD [10], while the minor allele G at rs11931074 has been reported to reduce the risk of PD progression [10]. The TT genotype at rs11931074 may increase the risk of hyposmia [11].

Advanced PD commonly manifests with festination [12–14], which refers to the shortening of each step in a long gait sequence together with an increase in gait speed and involuntary forward-leaning of the trunk [15]. Festination in patients with PD may be associated with gait freezing and with PD duration or severity [13, 14, 16]. The genetic basis of festination is unclear, leading us in the present study to examine whether two loci linked to PD risk (rs11931074 and rs894278) are also linked to festination in Chinese patients with PD.

2. Methods

2.1. Study Population. The study protocol was approved by West China Hospital, Sichuan University. Written informed consent was obtained from all study participants. A consecutive sample of 258 Han Chinese patients was recruited from the PD clinic at our hospital between September

2009 and June 2014. All patients were diagnosed with sporadic PD based on Queen Square Brain Bank Criteria [17]. Patients were excluded from the study if they had other neurodegenerative disorders, severe medical illness, a history of schizophrenia, or bipolar disorder. Patients were also excluded if they had at least one relative with PD.

Patients were divided into those with festination (defined as described [15]) and those without it. Patients were classified as showing festination if it was observed by experienced neurologists during a visit to our PD clinic or if the patient, family member, or caregiver reported that it had occurred more than once during the previous week anywhere outside the hospital.

2.2. Clinical Assessment. We collected patient data on age, sex, and symptoms at PD onset, PD duration, and Hoehn and Yahr stage of PD severity [18]. Primary onset symptoms were classified as tremor or as akinetic-rigid (bradykinesia or rigidity), based on patient self-report. If the patient experienced tremor as well as akinetic-rigid symptoms at PD onset, he or she was asked to indicate which predominated.

2.3. SNCA Genotyping. Genomic DNA was obtained from peripheral leukocytes using classical phenol-chloroform extraction. The single-nucleotide polymorphisms (SNPs) rs11931074 and rs894278 in the *SNCA* gene were genotyped by the Shanghai Biowing Applied Biotechnology Company using the ligase detection reaction [19]. To ensure genotyping accuracy and reliability, genotyping technicians were blinded to sample identity, and 20% of samples were regenotyped by a different technician selected at random. The replication rate was 100%.

2.4. Statistical Analysis. Statistical analyses were performed using SPSS 16.0 (IBM, Chicago, IL, USA). Intergroup differences were assessed for significance using Student's t-test in the case of continuous variables or the chi-squared or Fisher's exact tests in the case of categorical variables. Logistic regression was used to test the association between SNPs and festination in PD. Results of multivariate analyses were presented as odds ratios (ORs) with 95% confidence intervals (CIs) and p values. All tests were 2-sided, and the threshold of significance was $p < 0.05$.

3. Results

The study involved 258 patients with PD, of whom 122 (47.3%) suffered festination, which was reported by the patient, family member, or caregiver in 113 cases (93%) or observed directly by neurologists in the remaining 9 cases (7%). Genotype frequencies at rs11931074 and rs894278 were consistent with Hardy-Weinberg equilibrium across all patients. Patients with festination were significantly older, they had suffered PD longer, and their PD was at a more advanced Hoehn and Yahr stage (Table 1). Univariate analysis suggested that polymorphism at rs11931074 affected risk of festination according to a dominant genetic model, while polymorphism at rs894278 affected risk according to a recessive model.

Next we performed logistic regression with the following covariates: sex, age, age and symptoms at PD onset, PD duration, Hoehn and Yahr stage (≤2 versus >2), genotype at rs11931074 (GG+GT versus TT), and genotype at rs894278 (TT versus GG+GT). Variables were selected using a forward logistic regression procedure. The analysis identified the following associated factors (Table 2): PD duration, onset symptom, Hoehn and Yahr stage, GG/GT genotype at rs11931074, and TT genotype at rs894278.

4. Discussion

This study provides the first evidence that, at least among Han Chinese patients with PD, *SCNA* polymorphism significantly increases risk of festination, specifically the GG/GT genotype at rs11931074 and TT genotype at rs894278. Our data also indicate that occurrence of festination is related to PD duration, Hoehn and Yahr stage, and onset symptoms. Further study is needed to clarify the molecular mechanisms behind these apparent associations.

Our data associate the T allele at rs11931074 and the G allele at rs894278 with lower risk of festination, while the same alleles have previously been linked to greater risk of PD in Han Chinese [10]. These results are not contradictory, since one study examined risk of PD and the other examined risk of festination in patients with the disease.

Our finding that longer disease duration is associated with higher risk of festination is consistent with results of studies in Israeli patients [14] and Han Chinese patients [13]. Our finding that more severe PD is associated with higher risk of festination is also consistent with both of those studies [13, 14]. A greater proportion of patients in our study had festination than in those two previous studies, perhaps reflecting differences in how patients were classified as experiencing festination or not.

Our data suggest that patients who experience bradykinesia or rigidity as the primary symptoms at PD onset are more likely to experience festination than patients with other onset symptoms. This is, to our knowledge, the first report of such an association, so this result should be verified in studies with larger samples and other ethnic groups.

Since nearly all cases of festination in our study were based on patient or caregiver report, our study may be affected by recall bias given the infrequent, episodic nature of festination. In addition, we did not systematically analyze possible nongenetic confounders, such as medication history or gait freezing. Nevertheless, we were able to show that the association between festination and *SNCA* polymorphism remained after adjusting for possible confounders of sex, age, and onset age. While we were able to observe an association between festination and disease duration, consistent with previous studies, we did not collect data allowing us to explore whether festination correlated with disease duration prior to onset of festination, which may help determine whether festination is linked to genetic variation per se or simply to longer disease progression and development of motor symptoms. Future studies should examine this question. Lastly, our patients came from a single medical center, albeit the largest one in western China that draws patients from Sichuan and neighboring provinces.

TABLE 1: Characteristics of Han Chinese patients with Parkinson's disease in the presence or absence of festination.

Variable	Festination ($n = 122$)	No festination ($n = 136$)	p
Males	78 (63.9)	75 (55.1)	0.151
Mean age, yr	64.8 ± 9.2	59.3 ± 11.9	0.000
<60	36 (29.5)	59 (43.4)	0.021
≥60	86 (7.05)	77 (56.6)	
Mean age at onset, yr	58.9 ± 10.2	55.9 ± 11.9	0.033
<55	44 (36.1)	54 (39.7)	0.548
≥55	78 (63.9)	82 (60.3)	
Disease duration ≥ 5 yr	63 (51.6)	28 (20.6)	0.000
Onset symptoms			0.129
Tremor	63 (51.6)	83 (61.0)	
Akinetic-rigid	59 (48.4)	53 (39.0)	
Hoehn and Yahr stage ≤ 2	38 (31.1)	82 (60.3)	0.000
rs11931074			
Genotype frequencies			0.015
GG	24 (19.7)	16 (11.8)	
GT	65 (53.3)	61 (44.9)	
TT	33 (27.0)	59 (43.4)	
MAF (G)	113 (46.3)	93 (34.2)	0.005
Dominant model (GG + GT)	89 (73.0)	77 (56.6)	0.006
Recessive model (GG)	24 (19.7)	16 (11.8)	0.080
rs894278			
Genotype frequencies			0.003
TT	61 (50.0)	40 (29.4)	
GT	51 (41.8)	78 (57.4)	
GG	10 (8.2)	18 (13.2)	
MAF (G)	71 (29.1)	114 (41.9)	0.002
Dominant model (TT+GT)	112 (91.8)	118 (86.8)	0.194
Recessive model (TT)	61 (50.0)	40 (29.4)	0.001

Results are shown as mean ± SD or n (%).
MAF: minor allele frequency.

TABLE 2: Logistic regression to identify factors associated with risk of festination in Han Chinese patients with PD.

Factor	p	OR	95% CI
Disease duration < 5 yr	0.000	0.224	0.116–0.435
Tremor as onset symptom	0.019	0.505	0.285–0.895
Hoehn and Yahr stage ≤ 2	0.007	0.439	0.242–0.798
rs11931074 (GG/GT)	0.022	2.077	1.111–3.883
rs894278 (TT)	0.007	2.271	1.246–4.139

5. Conclusions

Despite these limitations, our study is the first to provide evidence that festination is associated with *SNCA* polymorphism at rs11931074 or rs894278. Our results should be verified and extended in larger studies, preferably involving multiple sites and ethnic groups.

Acknowledgments

This research was supported by the Sichuan Key Project of Science and Technology (no. 2010SZ0086). The authors also thank the patients involved in this study. The authors wish to thank Shanghai Biowing Applied Biotechnology Company for their excellent technical support.

References

[1] L. V. Kalia and A. E. Lang, "Parkinson's disease," *The Lancet*, vol. 386, no. 9996, article no. 70, pp. 896–912, 2015.

[2] O. Hornykiewicz, "Dopamine (3-hydroxytyramine) in the central nervous system and its relation to the Parkinson syndrome in man," *Deutsche Medizinische Wochenschrift*, vol. 87, pp. 1807–

1810, 1962.

[3] M. G. Spillantini, M. L. Schmidt, V. M.-Y. Lee, J. Q. Trojanowski, R. Jakes, and M. Goedert, "α-synuclein in Lewy bodies," *Nature*, vol. 388, no. 6645, pp. 839–840, 1997.

[4] M. H. Polymeropoulos, J. J. Higgins, L. I. Golbe et al., "Mapping of a gene for Parkinson's disease to chromosome 4q21-q23," *Science*, vol. 274, no. 5290, pp. 1197–1199, 1996.

[5] A. B. Singleton, M. Farrer, J. Johnson et al., "α-synuclein locus triplication causes Parkinson's disease," *Science*, vol. 302, no. 5646, p. 841, 2003.

[6] M.-C. Chartier-Harlin, J. Kachergus, C. Roumier et al., "α-synuclein locus duplication as a cause of familial Parkinson's disease," *The Lancet*, vol. 364, no. 9440, pp. 1167–1169, 2004.

[7] M. A. Nalls, N. Pankratz, C. M. Lill et al., "Large-scale meta-analysis of genome-wide association data identifies six new risk loci for Parkinson's disease," *Nature Genetics*, vol. 46, no. 9, pp. 989–993, 2014.

[8] International Parkinson Disease Genomics Consortium, M. A. Nalls, V. Plagnol et al., "Imputation of sequence variants for identification of genetic risks for Parkinson's disease: a meta-analysis of genome-wide association studies," *The Lancet*, vol. 377, no. 9766, pp. 641–649, 2011.

[9] M. Farrer, D. M. Maraganore, P. Lockhart et al., "α-synuclein gene haplotypes are associated with Parkinson's disease," *Human Molecular Genetics*, vol. 10, no. 17, pp. 1847–1851, 2001.

[10] J. Liu, Q. Xiao, Y. Wang et al., "Analysis of genome-wide association study-linked loci in Parkinson's disease of mainland China," *Movement Disorders*, vol. 28, no. 13, pp. 1892–1895, 2013.

[11] W. Chen, W.-Y. Kang, S. Chen et al., "Hyposmia correlates with SNCA variant and non-motor symptoms in Chinese patients with Parkinson's disease," *Parkinsonism and Related Disorders*, vol. 21, no. 6, pp. 610–614, 2015.

[12] M. E. Morris, "Locomotor training in people with Parkinson disease," *Physical Therapy*, vol. 86, no. 10, pp. 1426–1435, 2006.

[13] R. Ou, X. Guo, Q. Wei et al., "Festination in Chinese patients with Parkinson's disease," *Clinical Neurology and Neurosurgery*, vol. 139, pp. 172–176, 2015.

[14] N. Giladi, H. Shabtai, E. Rozenberg, and E. Shabtai, "Gait festination in Parkinson's disease," *Parkinsonism and Related Disorders*, vol. 7, no. 2, pp. 135–138, 2001.

[15] M. E. Morris, R. Iansek, and B. Galna, "Gait festination and freezing in Parkinson's disease: pathogenesis and rehabilitation," *Movement Disorders*, vol. 23, no. 2, pp. S451–S460, 2008.

[16] R. Iansek, F. Huxham, and J. McGinley, "The sequence effect and gait festination in Parkinson disease: contributors to freezing of gait?" *Movement Disorders*, vol. 21, no. 9, pp. 1419–1424, 2006.

[17] D. B. Calne, B. J. Snow, and C. Lee, "Criteria for diagnosing Parkinson's disease," *Annals of Neurology*, vol. 32, no. 1, pp. S125–S127, 1992.

[18] M. M. Hoehn and M. D. Yahr, "Parkinsonism: onset, progression and mortality," *Neurology*, vol. 17, no. 5, pp. 427–442, 1967.

[19] G. Thomas, R. Sinville, S. Sutton et al., "Capillary and microelectrophoretic separations of ligase detection reaction products produced from low-abundant point mutations in genomic DNA," *Electrophoresis*, vol. 25, no. 10-11, pp. 1668–1677, 2004.

15

Subthalamic Nucleus Deep Brain Stimulation in Early Stage Parkinson's Disease is not Associated with Increased Body Mass Index

Sarah H. Millan, Mallory L. Hacker, Maxim Turchan, Anna L. Molinari, Amanda D. Currie, and David Charles

Department of Neurology, Vanderbilt University Medical Center, 1611 21st Ave S., A-0118 Medical Center North, Nashville, TN 37223-2551, USA

Correspondence should be addressed to David Charles; david.charles@vanderbilt.edu

Academic Editor: Raja Mehanna

Previous studies suggest that deep brain stimulation of the subthalamic nucleus (STN-DBS) for Parkinson's disease (PD) leads to weight gain. This study analyzes changes in body mass index (BMI) in 29 subjects from a prospective, single-blind trial of DBS in early stage PD (age 50–75, Hoehn & Yahr stage II off medication, treated with antiparkinsonian medications for ≥ 6 months but <4 years, and without a history of motor fluctuations, dyskinesias, or dementia). Subjects were randomized to DBS plus optimal drug therapy (DBS+ODT; $n = 15$) or ODT ($n = 14$) and followed for 24 months. Weight and height were recorded at baseline and each follow-up visit and used to calculate BMI. BMIs were compared within and between groups using nonparametric t-tests. Mean BMI at baseline was 29.7 in the ODT group and 32.3 in the DBS+ODT group ($p > 0.05$). BMI change over two years was not different between the groups ($p = 0.62$, ODT = −0.89; DBS+ODT = −0.17). This study suggests that STN-DBS is not associated with weight gain in subjects with early stage PD. This finding will be tested in an upcoming FDA-approved phase III multicenter, randomized, double-blind, placebo-controlled, pivotal clinical trial evaluating DBS in early stage PD (ClinicalTrials.gov identifier NCT00282152).

1. Introduction

Deep brain stimulation of the subthalamic nucleus (STN-DBS) is an FDA-approved adjunctive treatment for Parkinson's disease (PD) when symptoms are no longer adequately controlled by medications. DBS therapy is demonstrated to significantly improve motor symptoms and quality of life for PD patients. Despite its clinical success, isolated studies suggest that STN-DBS is associated with postoperative weight gain and increased body mass index (BMI) [1]. While average weight gain after STN-DBS is reported as a 12.8% increase from preoperative body weight [2], the most significant weight gain typically occurs within the first few months after surgery (8.4% BMI increase [3]), with gradual increases thereafter [1]. These reports of weight gain following STN-DBS are concerning because of the implications for this effective PD therapy leading to additional health complications such as obesity and/or diabetes [4].

STN-DBS is a potent therapy that treats many features of PD that cause weight loss as PD progresses (e.g., dyskinesias and other motor fluctuations and side effects of medical therapy, such as nausea and loss of appetite [5]). For nearly 20 years, DBS has been indicated for advanced stage PD (average disease duration of 10.8 years [6]); this PD patient population has prolonged exposure to the negative effects of the disease progression as well as medication-associated complications leading to considerable weight loss [7]. Therefore, it is not currently clear whether the postoperative weight gain previously reported is due to active STN stimulation or is a consequence of the typical postoperative reduction in medication need and/or the general benefits for PD secondary to DBS therapy.

Vanderbilt University completed a pilot safety and tolerability clinical trial testing STN-DBS in early stage PD (NCT#00282152) [8]. This study offers a unique cohort to evaluate potential postsurgical changes in BMI in early stage

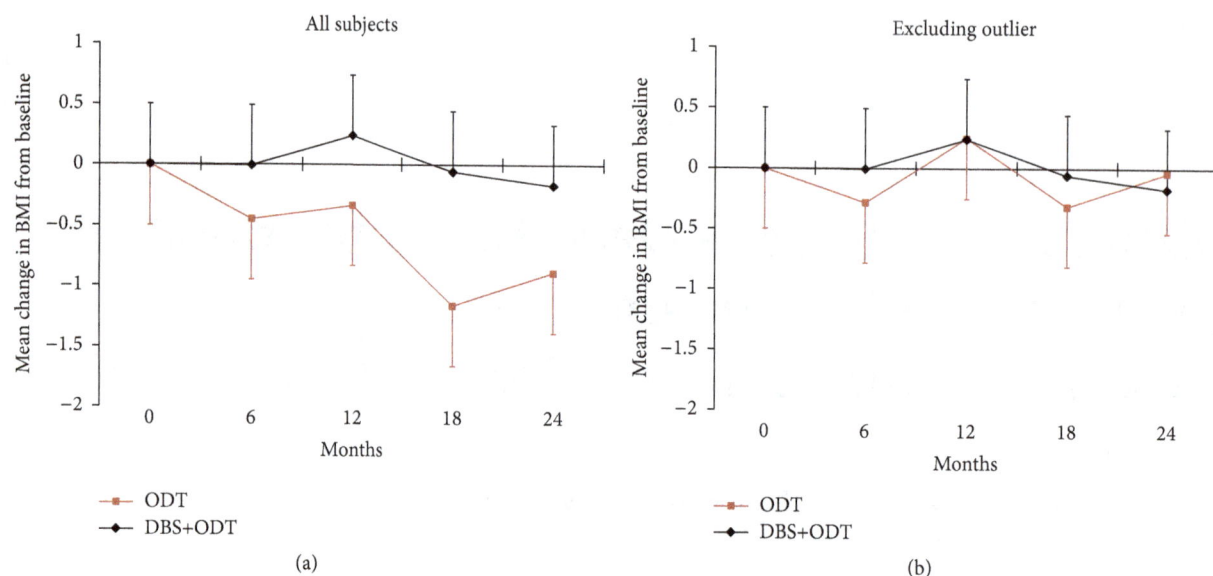

FIGURE 1: Body mass index change from baseline. (a) Average change in BMI from baseline at 6, 12, 18, and 24 months (± SEM). ODT $n = 14$, DBS+ODT $n = 15$. (b) One subject experienced significant weight loss (BMI decreased by 12 points from baseline to 24 months) and was excluded from this secondary analysis. ODT, $n = 13$; DBS+ODT, $n = 15$.

PD patients not yet experiencing many of the negative effects related to PD progression. Here, we investigated changes in BMI in the only prospective, randomized clinical trial of STN-DBS in very early stage PD.

2. Materials and Methods

Thirty subjects with early stage PD enrolled in the pilot clinical trial. The study was approved by the Vanderbilt University Institutional Review Board (IRB#040797) and the FDA (IDE#G050016). Subjects age 50 to 75 were eligible for enrollment into the study if they were diagnosed with idiopathic PD, treated with medications for more than six months and less than four years, Hoehn & Yahr stage II off medication, and without any history of motor fluctuations or dyskinesias [8–10]. Subjects were excluded if they had any major psychiatric illness, previous brain injury or operative intervention, or contraindications to surgery. A multiphased informed consent process ensured subjects' understanding of the study [11].

Subjects were randomized to receive DBS plus optimal drug therapy (DBS+ODT ($n = 15$) or ODT alone ($n = 14$; one subject dropped out after baseline due to family and career-related circumstances)). Subjects' heights and weights were recorded every six months at each week-long Clinical Research Center (CRC) study visit.

BMI was calculated at each visit using the height and weight collected on day one of the week-long antiparkinsonian medication and stimulation washout. Mean BMI for each group at baseline, 6, 12, 18, and 24 months was calculated (Figure 1). All within- and between-group comparisons were carried out with nonparametric t-tests, Wilcoxon Signed Rank test, and Mann-Whitney U test, respectively. Data are reported as mean ± standard deviation (SD) unless otherwise indicated.

3. Results

There was no significant difference in average BMI at baseline between the ODT (29.6 ± 4.2) and DBS+ODT groups (32.3 ± 5.7; Table 1; $p = 0.25$). All but one of the subjects in the pilot trial were overweight or obese at baseline (97%, 28/29 with BMI ≥ 25; Table 1).

Over the two-year study period, BMI change for the DBS+ODT group was not significant ($p = 0.63$; Figure 1). Although there was a reduction in average BMI in the ODT group over the two-year period, it was not a significant change from baseline to 24 months ($p = 0.75$). Additionally, the between-group difference in change in BMI score at 24 months was not significant ($p = 0.62$).

There was no BMI change in patients treated with STN-DBS from baseline to the first follow-up visit at 6 months ($p = 0.65$; Figure 1(a)) (prior studies reported the most rapid weight change after the first few months following surgery [4]). One subject in the ODT group experienced a gastrointestinal disorder unrelated to the study, which led to dramatic weight loss over the course of the trial (BMI was reduced by 32.6% from baseline to 24 months). A secondary analysis, conducted with this subject excluded, demonstrated that the slightly lower change in BMI for the ODT group compared to the DBS+ODT group was driven by this subject's extreme weight loss (Figure 1(b)).

4. Discussion

These results suggest that STN-DBS is not associated with weight gain in early stage Parkinson's disease. There was minimal change in BMI for the DBS+ODT group over two years (average BMI reduction = -0.17 ± 2.3). Although the BMI for the ODT group decreased slightly over two years (average BMI reduction = -0.89 ± 3.6), this change did not reach

TABLE 1: Characteristics at baseline[a].

Characteristic	ODT ($n = 14$)	DBS + ODT ($n = 15$)
Gender		
Male	12	14
Female	2	1
Age (years)		
Mean	60 ± 7.0	60 ± 6.8
Range	51–69	52–74
Baseline medicine use		
Mean duration (years)	2.1 ± 1.1	2.2 ± 1.4
Mean L-dopa equivalents (mg/day)	569 ± 389	451 ± 304
BMI category		
Healthy ($18.5 < \text{BMI} \leq 24.9$)	1	0
Overweight ($24.9 < \text{BMI} < 30$)	7	7
Obese ($\text{BMI} \geq 30$)	6	8
BMI (kg/m^2)	29.7 ± 4.3	32.3 ± 5.7

[a]Modified Table 1 from [10]. Mean ± SD.

significance ($p = 0.75$) and was largely driven by one patient who experienced dramatic weight loss from a gastrointestinal disorder unrelated to the study (Figure 1(b)). These findings suggest that weight gain previously observed in advanced PD patients [1] may not be due to STN stimulation but instead may result from the magnitude of symptom improvement that DBS provides in patients with a more advanced stage of PD.

It is well known that many PD patients experience weight loss with disease progression, and reduced BMI is correlated with increased disease severity [12]. There are many features of advanced PD that likely contribute to weight loss, including increased muscle rigidity, levodopa-induced dyskinesia with increased energy expenditure, and/or depression [5, 7]. Therefore, the great degree of improvement that advanced PD patients experience after STN-DBS therapy more likely explains the weight gain observed in previous isolated studies.

Here, we analyzed an early stage cohort not yet suffering from disabling features of PD that can lead to weight loss, and there was no significant change in BMI after STN-DBS for early stage PD patients. Because this study was open-label, it is possible that BMI changes were influenced by the subjects' awareness of their treatment allocation. Limitations for this study also include the study's small sample size and gender imbalance. It is also important to note that a majority of subjects were overweight or obese at baseline (28/29, Table 1).

Despite its superior clinical benefit over medications alone, one of the *perceived drawbacks* of STN-DBS therapy in advanced PD is its stimulation-associated weight gain [1]. This weight gain is likely due to a variety of factors including postoperative decreased energy expenditure [1] and dosage reduction in PD medications [2]. Since symptoms are typically mild in early stage PD, difference in pre- and postoperative energy expenditure is not expected to change as much as with advanced stage PD.

5. Conclusion

These results suggest that STN-DBS does not cause increased BMI in early stage PD. More study is needed to confirm these findings and the FDA has approved a phase III multicenter, randomized, double-blind, placebo-controlled, pivotal clinical trial evaluating DBS in early stage PD.

Disclosure

Medtronic representatives did not take part in data collection, management, analysis, or interpretation of the data or in preparation, review, or approval of the manuscript.

Acknowledgments

The authors thank their study coordinator, Odessa Lankford, for her dedication and commitment to the trial. Research reported in this publication was supported by Medtronic, Inc., by Vanderbilt CTSA Grant UL1TR000445 from the National Center for Advancing Translational Sciences (NCATS), by NCATS/NIH award UL1TR000011, by NIH R01 EB006136, by private donations, and by The Michael J. Fox Foundation for Parkinson's Research.

References

[1] M. Barichella, A. M. Marczewska, C. Mariani, A. Landi, A. Vairo, and G. Pezzoli, "Body weight gain rate in patients with Parkinson's disease and deep brain stimulation," *Movement Disorders*, vol. 18, no. 11, pp. 1337–1340, 2003.

[2] E. Moro, M. Scerrati, L. M. A. Romito, R. Roselli, P. Tonali, and A. Albanese, "Chronic subthalamic nucleus stimulation reduces medication requirements in Parkinson's disease," *Neurology*, vol. 53, no. 1, pp. 85–90, 1999.

[3] P. Sauleau, E. Leray, T. Rouaud et al., "Comparison of weight gain and energy intake after subthalamic versus pallidal stimulation in Parkinson's disease," *Movement Disorders*, vol. 24, no. 14, pp. 2149–2155, 2009.

[4] I. Rieu, P. Derost, M. Ulla et al., "Body weight gain and deep brain stimulation," *Journal of the Neurological Sciences*, vol. 310, no. 1-2, pp. 267–270, 2011.

[5] C. G. Bachmann and C. Trenkwalde, "Body weight in patients with Parkinson's disease," *Movement Disorders*, vol. 21, no. 11, pp. 1824–1830, 2006.

[6] F. M. Weaver and K. Follett, "Bilateral deep brain stimulation vs best medical therapy for patients with advanced parkinson disease: a randomized controlled trial," *Journal of the American Medical Association*, vol. 301, no. 1, pp. 63–73, 2009.

[7] K. Kashihara, "Weight loss in Parkinson's disease," *Journal of Neurology*, vol. 253, no. 7, pp. VII/38–VII/41, 2006.

[8] D. Charles, P. E. Konrad, J. S. Neimat et al., "Subthalamic nucleus deep brain stimulation in early stage Parkinson's disease," *Parkinsonism and Related Disorders*, vol. 20, no. 7, pp. 731–737, 2014.

[9] D. Charles, C. Tolleson, T. L. Davis et al., "Pilot study assessing the feasibility of applying bilateral subthalamic nucleus deep brain stimulation in very early stage Parkinson's disease: study design and rationale," *Journal of Parkinson's Disease*, vol. 2, no. 3, pp. 215–223, 2012.

[10] P. D. Charles, R. M. Dolhun, C. E. Gill et al., "Deep brain stimulation in early Parkinson's disease: enrollment experience from a pilot trial," *Parkinsonism and Related Disorders*, vol. 18, no. 3, pp. 268–273, 2012.

[11] S. G. Finder, M. J. Bliton, C. E. Gill, T. L. Davis, P. E. Konrad, and P. D. Charles, "Potential subjects' responses to an ethics questionnaire in a Phase I study of deep brain stimulation in early Parkinson's disease," *Journal of Clinical Ethics*, vol. 23, no. 3, pp. 207–216, 2012.

[12] M. A. Van der Marck, H. C. Dicke, E. Y. Uc et al., "Body mass index in Parkinson's disease: a meta-analysis," *Parkinsonism and Related Disorders*, vol. 18, no. 3, pp. 263–267, 2012.

16

Analysis of *LRRK2*, *SNCA*, and *ITGA8* Gene Variants with Sporadic Parkinson's Disease Susceptibility in Chinese Han Population

Jie Fang,[1] Kehui Yi,[2] Mingwei Guo,[3] Xingkai An,[1] Hongli Qu,[1] Qing Lin,[1] Min Bi,[1] and Qilin Ma[1,2]

[1]*Department of Neurology, The First Affiliated Hospital of Xiamen University, Xiamen, China*
[2]*The First Clinical Medical College of Fujian Medical University, Fuzhou, China*
[3]*Department of Neurology, The First Affiliated Hospital of Gannan Medical University, Ganzhou, China*

Correspondence should be addressed to Qilin Ma; qilinma@yeah.net

Academic Editor: Eng King Tan

Background. Parkinson's disease (PD) is an age-related neurodegenerative disease affected by multiple genetic and environmental factors. We performed a case-control study on candidate gene to scrutinize whether genetic variants in *LRRK2*, *SNCA*, and *ITGA8* genes could be associated with sporadic PD in Chinese Han population. *Methods.* Five single-nucleotide polymorphisms (SNPs) of *LRRK2* (rs1491942), *SNCA* (rs2301134, rs2301135, and rs356221), and *ITGA8* (rs7077361) were selected and genotyped among 583 unrelated PD patients and 558 healthy controls. *Results.* Rs1491942 of *LRRK2* gene had a significantly higher genotype frequency ($P = 3.543E - 09$) and allelic G/C frequencies ($P = 2.601E - 10$) in PD patients than controls. Rs2301135 of *SNCA* gene also showed an obvious difference in genotype frequency ($P = 4.394E - 07$) and allelic G/C frequencies ($P = 9.116E - 13$) between PD patients and controls. SNPs rs2301134 and rs356221 of *SNCA* gene and rs7077361 of *ITGA8* gene lacked the significant association with the susceptibility of PD in Chinese Han population. *Conclusions.* Our study firstly expresses that rs1491942 of *LRRK2* and rs2301135 of *SNCA* gene are substantially associated with sporadic Parkinson's disease in Chinese Han population.

1. Introduction

Parkinson's disease (PD), the second most common neurodegenerative disease after Alzheimer's disease, consists of two major pathological hallmarks: loss of dopaminergic neurons and the presence of Lewy bodies (LB). The classic manifestations of PD are characterized by resting tremor, rigidity, bradykinesia, and impairment of postural reflexes. In addition, some untypical nonmotor features, such as sleep disturbances, mood disorders, autonomic dysfunction, sensory problems, and cognitive impairment, are highly concerned recently. Even when treated with effective therapies, PD is progressive and somehow leads to disability or even mortality.

Increasing evidence supports that complex factors contribute a lot to the susceptibility of PD, which includes genetic and environmental factors [1–3]. In the past decades, a large number of Genome-Wide Association Studies (GWAS),

Candidate Gene Replication Study (CGRS), and subsequent meta-analysis studies have found that a number of potential genes and single-nucleotide polymorphisms (SNPs) associated with PD, including both risk variants and protective variants [4]. In addition, the previous candidate genetic studies provided conclusive evidence showing SNPs in *LRRK2*, *SNCA*, and *ITGA8* genes significantly impact PD susceptibility and disease characteristics.

Several variations of *LRRK2* gene were identified as risk factors for PD. For example, rs34778348 (G2385R, c.7153G>A) and rs33949390 (R1628P, c.4883G>C) were seen to associate with PD in Asian population [5, 6]. Another novel SNP within *LRRK2*, rs1491942, was found to be responsible for PD in Caucasian populations [7, 8]. However, it was never reported in Chinese Han population before.

SNCA, as the first pathogenic gene identified in PD, encodes α-synuclein, the primary component of LB, the pathological hallmark of PD. From then on, several SNPs of

TABLE 1: Demographic characteristics of Parkinson's disease (PD) cases and controls.

Characteristics	Cases = 583		Controls = 553	
Gender (n, %)*				
Female	320	54.9	286	51.7
Male	263	45.1	267	48.3
Age at collection (mean, SD)†	65.10	8.90	65.37	9.03
Age at onset (n, %)				
<50	131	22.5	n.a.	n.a.
≥50	452	77.5	n.a.	n.a.

All the subjects were ethnic Hans; * PD compared with controls by gender: $P > 0.05$; † PD compared with controls by age: $P > 0.05$; n.a.: not applicable.

SNCA were highly considered as the genetic risk factors for sporadic PD. Located in the promoter region of SNCA, two SNPs (rs2301134 and rs2301135) with high allele frequency were reported in some studies as PD-related SNPs in European and Taiwanese cohorts [9, 10]. One SNP (rs356221) in the 3'UTR region of SNCA gene showed association with susceptibility to sporadic PD in Japanese and Taiwanese cohorts [10, 11]. All these three SNPs of SNCA (rs2301134, rs2301135, and rs356221) have not been investigated in Han population on the Mainland of China.

While ITGA8 (encoding integrin alpha 8, a type-I transmembrane protein) gene was firstly proved to connect with idiopathic PD in Caucasian population in Simón-Sánchez's study [4], it was not featured as a PD relevant gene until Lill's study revealed its potential association with PD [8]. Additional studies are needed to screen the potential pathogenic variants within this gene and assess the potential role of these variants in PD pathogenesis.

There are no study that explores the association of the three genes and their SNPs with Parkinson's disease in Chinese Han population. Here, we perform the first SNP replication study on previously published SNPs within SNCA (rs356221, rs2301134, and rs2301135), LRRK2 (rs1491942), and ITGA8 (rs7077361) gene in Chinese Han population to explore the ethnic differences and recognize predictive factors for the diagnosis of PD.

2. Methods

2.1. Subjects. This study recruits 1136 cases in the Neurology Department of the First Affiliated Hospital of Xiamen University, which includes 583 Chinese Han sporadic PD patients and 553 matched healthy controls. PD diagnosis coincided well with the diagnostic criteria of UK Parkinson's Disease Society Brain Bank [12]. Among all the PD patients, the mean age is 65.10 ± 8.90 and the ratio of male to female patients is 320 : 263. The group of controls consists of healthy volunteers from the Medical Center of the First Affiliated Hospital of Xiamen University, the mean age of which is 65.37 ± 9.03, and the ratio of male to female patients is 286 : 267 (Table 1). All subjects are Han population, and the two groups are matched for age, gender, ethnicity, and area of residence. Moreover,

TABLE 2: PCR and Snapshot probe primer sequences.

Polymorphisms	Primers	Sequence 5' → 3'
LRRK2		
rs1491942	Forward	CAGGCTTGGGCAATTTCTAA
	Reverse	GCCTATTGTGCTTCCTGCTC
	Probe	40Ts+CAGGCTCCCCTGGGTT
SNCA		
rs2301134	Forward	ATCACGCTGGATTTGTCTCC
	Reverse	CACGGTCACAGGTTACAACG
	Probe	41Ts+GACTCTTCCTTAGTAG-TCTCCC
rs356221	Forward	TGCCATAGAAACAACGAGGA
	Reverse	TTGAAGAACCCAAAATGCAA
	Probe	24Ts+AAGAGAAGCCATCCTAGT
rs2301135	Forward	ACTTAACGTGAGGCGCAAAA
	Reverse	CGTCCTCCTCCTCCTAGTCC
	Probe	54Ts+CCGGGAGAGGGGCGGG
IGTA8		
rs7077361	Forward	TGCGAAAACTATTTGGTGAAA
	Reverse	CCCACCCACCAAATCTCTAA
	Probe	31Ts+GAAATCATCTAGGGGATA

this study has gained approval of the local ethics committees, and all patients and controls signed informed consents.

2.2. Genetic Analysis. Venous blood specimens are collected directly from all PD patients and the healthy controls with ethylene diamine tetraacetic acid (EDTA) anticoagulant. Genomic DNA is extracted from the blood samples with the QIAamp DNA Mini Kit (Qiagen, Hilden, Germany) under the manufacturer's instructions and stored at −20°C. The five SNPs are genotyped by Multiplex Snapshot technique (Applied Biosystems by Life Technologies, Foster City, CA, USA). The primers are designed for each SNP locus using Primer 5 and listed in Table 2. Multiplex PCR reactions are performed to amplify target regions containing the selected SNPs. All products are analyzed by the ABI PRISM 3730 DNA Sequence, of which the sequence analyses are conducted by DNA Sequencing Analysis software, GeneMapper4.0. To confirm the results, 10% patients and 10% controls are randomly selected for Sanger sequencing approaches. The concordance rate for replicate approaches was 100%.

2.3. Statistical Analysis. The statistical analyses are processed with SPSS, version 20.0 (IBM, Armonk, NY, USA). The clinical data are expressed as the means ± standard deviation (SD) for the continuous variables and as numbers (percentage) for the quantitative variables. Student's t-test is used to compare the age variables between the patients and controls. The gender variables are assessed by the chi-square test. Differences in frequencies of the alleles and genotypes between cases and controls are tested for each SNP through Pearson's chi-square test and Fisher's exact test. The criterion for significance is set at $P < 0.05$ based on two sides for all of the tests. The statistical power is calculated by Power and Sample Size Calculations version 3.1.2. The Hardy-Weinberg equilibrium (HWE) is tested by adopting the public statistics web tool (http://ihg.gsf.de/cgi-bin/hw/hwa1.pl). The Haploview program [13] is used for the calculation of linkage disequilibrium (LD) among the three SNPs in *SNCA*.

3. Results

Genotype and allele frequencies of each SNP of all 1136 subjects (583 patients and 553 healthy controls) are shown in Table 3. Among PD patients, 131 (22%) had an early age of onset (<50 years) and around 77% of the patients were LOPD (≥50 years). The age ($P = 0.860$) and gender ($P = 0.284$) show no statistical difference between the PD patients and the controls in our study. All the subjects were ethnic Hans.

Linkage disequilibrium between the *SNCA* SNPs rs2301134 and rs356221 is $r^2 = 0.235$, while for rs356221 and rs2301135 it is $r^2 = 0.066$ and for rs2301134 and rs2301135 it is $r^2 = 0.127$. This shows weakly correlation with in rs2301134, rs2301135, and rs356221.

Single marker analysis showed a number of significantly statistical associations in our study. Two SNPs from *SNCA* and *LRRK2* genes displayed P values < 0.05 prior to correction, both of which were estimated ORs > 1.4. The best P value SNPs from both *LRRK2* and *SNCA* genes were further analyzed for age stratification.

Between all PD patients and controls, *LRRK2* gene showed a significant difference in the genotype frequency of variant rs1491942 ($P = 3.543E − 09$) and allelic G/C frequencies ($P = 2.601E − 10$, OR = 1.884, and 95% CI: 1.55–2.30). In the three SNPs of *SNCA* gene, only variant rs2301135 met the statistics standard in genotype frequencies ($P = 4.39E − 07$) and the allelic G/C frequencies ($P = 9.116E − 13$, OR = 7.857, and 95% CI: 4.05–15.26). The *ITGA8* variant rs7077361 failed to show significant difference in this group ($P > 0.05$).

In the subgroup of EOPD patients and the controls (age < 50 years), the differences were still obvious in the genotype frequencies of variant rs1491942 of *LRRK2* gene ($P = 1.200E − 02$) and allelic G/C frequencies ($P = 3.028E − 03$, OR = 1.924, and 95% CI: 1.24–2.98). Three SNPs of *SNCA* gene ($P > 0.05$) and one SNP of *ITGA8* gene ($P > 0.05$) failed to show significant difference in this group. Our statistic data of the LOPD patients and controls aged ≥ 50 years also surpassed the significance thresholds. The variant rs1491942 of *LRRK2* gene showed a P value of 2.538E-07 in genotype frequencies. And the allelic G/C frequencies have a P value of 2.459E-08 while the OR is 1.874, and the 95% CI ranged from 1.50 to 2.34. The difference is obvious in the variant rs2301135 of *SNCA* gene in the genotype frequencies ($P = 5.561E − 07$) and allelic G/C frequencies ($P = 1.45E − 12$, OR = 7.846, and 95% CI: 4.03–15.29) in the subgroup. All SNPs in our study met Hardy-Weinberg equilibrium except for the rs2301135 of *SNCA* gene, shown in Table 3.

4. Discussion

Since the first Genome-Wide Association Study on sporadic Parkinson's disease was performed in 2005, a new era starts to gain attention in the genetic basis of Parkinson's disease [14]. Advances in genotyping technology and meta-analysis have allowed researchers to rapidly identify common variants related to PD in different populations [4]. Though some of the previously nominated PD risk genes were firstly reported in familiar Parkinson's disease (such as *SNCA* and *LRRK2*), both of them were successfully replicated in unrelated sporadic PD patients [15]. Additional associated studies and subsequent meta-analysis contributed a lot to identifying the unnoticed variants that can also drive PD risk, *ITGA8* as an example [8].

LRRK2 gene was firstly featured as a PD-related gene in Zimprich's study of families with autosomal-dominant, late-onset Parkinsonism in 2004 [16]. Variants in different domains of *LRRK2* have been identified in both familial and sporadic PD in different populations [17–19]. Rs1494942 in *LRRK2* was previously found associated with PD in US and European series [8, 20]. Our result, being consistent with previous studies, suggests that polymorphism rs1491942 of *LRRK2* is a risk loci of sporadic PD, and the variant carriers may share a similar pathomechanism in different populations. As it is reported, *LRRK2* variant carriers share similar clinical and pathological features, including a wild range of onset ages, typical Parkinsonism presentation, and sensitivity to L-dopa therapy [21]. In our PD patients, the rs1491942 shows significantly higher frequencies in both EOPD and LOPD subgroups compared with matched controls. These suggest that rs1491942 does not influence the onset age but contributes to the pathogenesis of EOPD and LOPD in a similar way.

SNCA is the first identified causal gene in familial PD [22]. Our findings are partly consistent with previous reports of the association of polymorphisms in *SNCA* with the susceptibility of PD in US, Norway, and Italian studies [23–25]. The linkage disequilibrium of three SNPs of *SNCA* gene showed that those SNPs are independent. Only one SNP near the promoter region (rs2301135) shows significant differences between PD patients and the controls in Chinese Han population. Concerning the age of onset, rs2301135 is more likely to associate with late-onset PD in our study, while another study in UK suggested that *SNCA* risk alleles for PD may associate with earlier onset of PD [26]. Given that genotype frequencies and allelic frequencies of rs2301135 of *SNCA* gene do not follow the Hardy-Weinberg equilibrium in our study, this suggests the possibility of inappropriate population stratification and selection or other confounding factors in our study. Therefore, these results should be interpreted carefully.

ITGA8 expressing in brain mediates cell-cell interactions and regulates neurite outgrowth of sensory and motor neurons [8]. *ITGA8* gene was firstly shown associated with PD in Caucasian population in Simón-Sánchez's study but failed to replicate in other studies of Greece, Irish, and Polish series [4, 19, 20]. *ITGA8* variant rs7077361 showed no evidence of relation to PD in our population. In patients and controls, the observed MAFs of the SNP rs7077361 were similar to those reported in the 1000 genomes Southern Han Chinese (CHS) population. However, there is insufficient power to detect the association of rs7077361 with PD in the current sample size. The lack of association of the rs7077361 in Chinese

TABLE 3: Comparison of the genotype frequencies and the allele frequencies of *LRRK2*, *SNCA*, and *ITGA8* polymorphisms.

Gene SNP	Group	Genotype n% CC	Genotype n% GC	Genotype n% GG	P_{HWE}	Allele Min/Maj	MAF[a]	MAF[b]	OR (95% CI)	P	Power[c]
LRRK2											
rs1491942		*CC*	*GC*	*GG*		*G/C*					
	Patients total	291 49.9	240 41.2	52 8.9	0.84	344/822	0.30	0.36	1.884 (1.546–2.297)	2.60E − 10*	1.00
	Controls total	372 67.3	161 29.1	20 3.6	0.67	201/905	0.18				
	EOPD	65 49.6	54 41.2	12 9.2	0.84	78/184			1.924 (1.244–2.976)	3.03E − 03*	
	Controls < 50 y	74 68.5	29 26.9	5 4.6	0.33	39/177					
	LOPD	226 50.0	186 41.2	40 8.8	0.82	266/638			1.874 (1.500–2.340)	2.46E − 08*	
	Controls ≧ 50 y	298 67.0	132 29.7	15 3.4	0.87	162/728					
SNCA											
rs2301134		*GG*	*AG*	*AA*		*A/G*					
	Patients total	437 75.0	132 22.6	14 2.4	0.29	160/1006	0.14	0.20	1.237 (0.964–1.588)	9.43E − 02	0.42
	Controls total	436 78.8	108 19.5	9 1.6	0.40	126/980	0.11				
	EOPD	97 74.0	32 24.4	2 1.5	1.00	36/226			1.561 (0.875–2.786)	1.29E − 01	
	Controls < 50 y	88 81.5	20 18.5	0 0.0	0.59	20/196					
	LOPD	340 75.2	100 22.1	12 2.7	0.16	124/780			1.176 (0.891–1.552)	2.52E − 01	
	Controls ≧ 50 y	348 78.2	88 19.8	9 2.0	0.25	106/784					
rs356221		*AA*	*TA*	*TT*		*T/A*					
	Patients total	210 36.0	282 48.4	91 15.6	0.86	464/702	0.40	0.40	1.167 (0.985–1.382)	7.50E − 02	0.45
	Controls total	231 41.8	244 44.1	78 14.1	0.31	400/706	0.36				
	EOPD	43 32.8	67 51.1	21 16.0	0.59	109/153			1.286 (0.887–1.864)	1.84E − 01	
	Controls < 50 y	46 42.6	47 43.5	15 13.9	0.67	77/139					
	LOPD	167 36.9	215 47.6	70 15.5	1.00	355/549			1.135 (0.938–1.374)	1.93E − 01	
	Controls ≧ 50 y	185 41.6	197 44.3	63 14.2	0.36	323/567					
rs2301135		*CC*	*GC*	*GG*		*G/C*					
	Patients total	544 93.3	39 6.7		<0.05	78/1088	0.07	0.19	7.857 (4.046–15.258)	9.12E − 13*	1.00
	Controls total	548 99.1	5 0.9		<0.05	10/1096	0.01				
	EOPD	129 98.5	2 1.5		<0.05	4/258			1.016 (1.000–1.031)	1.30E − 01	
	Controls < 50 y	108 100.0	0 0.0		<0.05	0/216					
	LOPD	415 91.8	37 8.2		<0.05	74/830			7.846 (4.026–15.288)	1.45E − 12*	
	Controls ≧ 50 y	440 98.9	5 1.1		<0.05	10/880					
ITGA8											
rs7077361		*TT*	*CT*	*CC*		*C/T*					
	Patients total	580 99.5	3 0.5		1.00	3/1163	0.00	0.00	2.85 (0.296–27.443)	6.25E − 01	0.34
	Controls total	552 99.8	1 0.2		1.00	1/1105	0.00				
	EOPD	131 100.0	0 0.0		<0.05	0/262			0.995 (0.986–1.004)	4.52E − 01	
	Controls < 50 y	107 99.1	1 0.9		1.00	0/0					
	LOPD	449 99.3	3 0.7		1.00	3/449			1.003 (1.000–1.007)	2.50E − 01	
	Controls ≧ 50 y	445 100.0	0 0.0		<0.05	0/445					

EOPD: early onset Parkinson's disease; LOPD: late-onset Parkinson's disease; P_{HWE}: *P* value obtained in the Hardy-Weinberg equilibrium (HWE) test; *: significant *P* value obtained in the case-control analysis; Min: minor; Maj: major; MAF: minor allele frequency; a: this study; b: 1000 genomes (Southern Han Chinese); c: power was calculated by Power and Sample Size Calculations version 3.1.2.

Han population could be ascribed to the limited sample size and the rare existence of this SNP in Chinese population. Large-sample trials from multicenter are required to better understand the contribution of rs7077361 in *ITGA8* to PD susceptibility.

In conclusion, the present study provides considerable evidence to support the significant influence of genetic variants on PD risk. It does not replicate the susceptibility of rs2301134 and rs356221 in *SNCA* and rs7077361 in *ITGA8* for PD but confirms that single-nucleotide polymorphisms rs1491942 of *LRRK2* and rs2301135 of *SNCA* gene are susceptible to sporadic PD in Chinese Han population. Certain variants are responsible for the incidence of this disease, while other variants may modify the onset age, which suggests that distinct aspects of PD have a specific genetic architecture. Further studies are required to enrich genetic architecture of PD.

Authors' Contributions

Jie Fang and Kehui Yi contributed equally to this work as first authors.

Acknowledgments

The authors would like to thank all the patients and control subjects who participated in this study. The authors would like to show many thanks to Jingjing Yin, a teacher from New Oriental English training school (E-mail: yinjingjing@xdf.cn), for the substantial English editing. This work was supported by the Fujian Medical Technology Innovation Programs (no. 2014-CXB-33), Xiamen Important Joint Research Project of Major Diseases (no. 3502Z20149028), Science and Technology Program of Xiamen (no. 3502Z20154014), National Natural Science Foundation of China (no. 81400912), and Natural Science Foundation of Fujian Province (no. 2015J01544).

References

[1] M. A. Nalls, N. Pankratz, C. M. Lill et al., "Large-scale meta-analysis of genome-wide association data identifies six new risk loci for Parkinson's disease," *Nature Genetics*, vol. 46, no. 9, pp. 989–993, 2014.

[2] A. L. McCormack, M. Thiruchelvam, A. B. Manning-Bog et al., "Environmental risk factors and Parkinson's disease: selective degeneration of nigral dopaminergic neurons caused by the herbicide paraquat," *Neurobiology of Disease*, vol. 10, no. 2, pp. 119–127, 2002.

[3] K. Kalinderi, S. Bostantjopoulou, and L. Fidani, "The genetic background of Parkinson's disease: current progress and future prospects," *Acta Neurologica Scandinavica*, 2016.

[4] J. Simón-Sánchez, C. Schulte, J. M. Bras et al., "Genome-wide association study reveals genetic risk underlying Parkinson's disease," *Nature Genetics*, vol. 41, pp. 1308–1312, 2009.

[5] M. J. Farrer, J. T. Stone, C.-H. Lin et al., "Lrrk2 G2385R is an ancestral risk factor for Parkinson's disease in Asia," *Parkinsonism & Related Disorders*, vol. 13, no. 2, pp. 89–92, 2007.

[6] O. A. Ross, Y.-R. Wu, M.-C. Lee et al., "Analysis of Lrrk2 R1628P as a risk factor for Parkinson's disease," *Annals of Neurology*, vol. 64, no. 1, pp. 88–92, 2008.

[7] M. A. Nalls, V. Plagnol, D. G. Hernandez et al., "Imputation of sequence variants for identification of genetic risks for Parkinson's disease: a meta-analysis of genome-wide association studies," *The Lancet*, vol. 377, no. 9766, pp. 641–649, 2011.

[8] C. M. Lill, J. T. Roehr, M. B. McQueen et al., "Comprehensive research synopsis and systematic meta-analyses in Parkinson's disease genetics: the PDgene database," *PLoS Genetics*, vol. 8, no. 3, Article ID e1002548, 2012.

[9] S. Winkler, J. Hagenah, S. Lincoln et al., "α-Synuclein and Parkinson disease susceptibility," *Neurology*, vol. 69, no. 18, pp. 1745–1750, 2007.

[10] Y.-H. Wu-Chou, Y.-T. Chen, T.-H. Yeh et al., "Genetic variants of SNCA and LRRK2 genes are associated with sporadic PD susceptibility: a replication study in a Taiwanese cohort," *Parkinsonism and Related Disorders*, vol. 19, no. 2, pp. 251–255, 2013.

[11] I. Mizuta, W. Satake, Y. Nakabayashi et al., "Multiple candidate gene analysis identifies α-synuclein as a susceptibility gene for sporadic Parkinson's disease," *Human Molecular Genetics*, vol. 15, no. 7, pp. 1151–1158, 2006.

[12] D. B. Calne, B. J. Snow, and C. Lee, "Criteria for diagnosing Parkinson's disease," *Annals of Neurology*, vol. 32, pp. S125–S127, 1992.

[13] J. C. Barrett, B. Fry, J. Maller, and M. J. Daly, "Haploview: analysis and visualization of LD and haplotype maps," *Bioinformatics*, vol. 21, no. 2, pp. 263–265, 2005.

[14] D. M. Maraganore, M. De Andrade, T. C. Lesnick et al., "High-resolution whole-genome association study of Parkinson disease," *The American Journal of Human Genetics*, vol. 77, no. 5, pp. 685–693, 2005.

[15] O. A. Ross, D. Gosal, J. T. Stone et al., "Familial genes in sporadic disease: common variants of α-synuclein gene associate with Parkinson's disease," *Mechanisms of Ageing and Development*, vol. 128, no. 5-6, pp. 378–382, 2007.

[16] A. Zimprich, S. Biskup, P. Leitner et al., "Mutations in LRRK2 cause autosomal-dominant parkinsonism with pleomorphic pathology," *Neuron*, vol. 44, no. 4, pp. 601–607, 2004.

[17] L. J. Ozelius, G. Senthil, R. Saunders-Pullman et al., "LRRK2 G2019S as a cause of Parkinson's disease in Ashkenazi Jews," *The New England Journal of Medicine*, vol. 354, no. 4, pp. 424–425, 2006.

[18] S. Lesage, A. Dürr, M. Tazir et al., "LRRK2 G2019S as a cause of Parkinson's disease in North African Arabs," *The New England Journal of Medicine*, vol. 354, no. 4, pp. 422–423, 2006.

[19] E. Kara, G. Xiromerisiou, C. Spanaki et al., "Assessment of Parkinson's disease risk loci in Greece," *Neurobiology of Aging*, vol. 35, no. 2, pp. 442.e9–442.e16, 2014.

[20] A. I. Soto-Ortolaza, M. G. Heckman, C. Labbé et al., "GWAS risk factors in Parkinson's disease: LRRK2 coding variation and genetic interaction with PARK16," *American Journal of Neurodegenerative Disease*, vol. 2, pp. 287–299, 2013.

[21] J. C. Dächsel and M. J. Farrer, "LRRK2 and Parkinson disease," *Archives of Neurology*, vol. 67, no. 5, pp. 542–547, 2010.

[22] S. Lesage and A. Brice, "Parkinson's disease: from monogenic forms to genetic susceptibility factors," *Human Molecular Genetics*, vol. 18, no. 1, pp. R48–R59, 2009.

[23] A. A. Davis, K. M. Andruska, B. A. Benitez, B. A. Racette, J. S. Perlmutter, and C. Cruchaga, "Variants in GBA, SNCA, and MAPT influence Parkinson disease risk, age at onset, and progression," *Neurobiology of Aging*, vol. 37, pp. 209.e1–209.e7, 2016.

[24] R. Myhre, M. Toft, J. Kachergus et al., "Multiple alpha-synuclein gene polymorphisms are associated with Parkinson's disease in a Norwegian population," *Acta Neurologica Scandinavica*, vol. 118, no. 5, pp. 320–327, 2008.

[25] L. Trotta, I. Guella, G. Soldà et al., "SNCA and MAPT genes: independent and joint effects in Parkinson disease in the Italian population," *Parkinsonism and Related Disorders*, vol. 18, no. 3, pp. 257–262, 2012.

[26] C. C. Spencer, V. Plagnol, A. Strange et al., "Dissection of the genetics of Parkinson's disease identifies an additional association 5′ of SNCA and multiple associated haplotypes at 17q21," *Human Molecular Genetics*, vol. 20, no. 2, pp. 345–353, 2011.

17

DBS Programming: An Evolving Approach for Patients with Parkinson's Disease

Aparna Wagle Shukla,[1] Pam Zeilman,[1] Hubert Fernandez,[2]
Jawad A. Bajwa,[3] and Raja Mehanna[4]

[1]Center for Movement Disorders and Neurorestoration, Department of Neurology, University of Florida, Gainesville, FL, USA
[2]Center for Neurological Restoration, Cleveland Clinic, Cleveland, OH, USA
[3]Parkinson's Disease, Movement Disorders and Neurorestoration Program, National Neuroscience Institute, King Fahad Medical City, Riyadh, Saudi Arabia
[4]University of Texas Health Science Center, McGovern Medical School, Houston, TX, USA

Correspondence should be addressed to Aparna Wagle Shukla; aparna.shukla@neurology.ufl.edu

Academic Editor: Jan Aasly

Deep brain stimulation (DBS) surgery is a well-established therapy for control of motor symptoms in Parkinson's disease. Despite an appropriate targeting and an accurate placement of DBS lead, a thorough and efficient programming is critical for a successful clinical outcome. DBS programming is a time consuming and laborious manual process. The current approach involves use of general guidelines involving determination of the lead type, electrode configuration, impedance check, and battery check. However there are no validated and well-established programming protocols. In this review, we will discuss the current practice and the recent advances in DBS programming including the use of interleaving, fractionated current, directional steering of current, and the use of novel DBS pulses. These technological improvements are focused on achieving a more efficient control of clinical symptoms with the least possible side effects. Other promising advances include the introduction of computer guided programming which will likely impact the efficiency of programming for the clinicians and the possibility of remote Internet based programming which will improve access to DBS care for the patients.

1. Introduction

Deep brain stimulation (DBS) therapy was approved by the US Federal Drug Administration (FDA) in the year 2002 for treatment of motor symptoms in Parkinson's disease [1]. The efficacy of DBS has been well established through randomized controlled studies involving several hundreds of Parkinson's disease patients [2]. DBS is effective for control of tremors that are refractory to dopaminergic medications, motor fluctuations, and levodopa induced dyskinesia that are bothersome to patients. The success of DBS is dependent on many factors including selection of appropriate patients, accurate placement of DBS lead, and a thorough programming process to identify the optimal stimulation parameters [3]. Selection of appropriate patients is based on many factors including the age of the patient, disease

stage, disease duration, comorbidities, and responsiveness to levodopa medication. These factors are discussed by an interdisciplinary team consisting of neurologist, neurosurgeon, psychiatrist, neuropsychologist, rehab specialist, and sometimes a social worker. Once the DBS lead is placed in an appropriate target using standard surgical technique, DBS programming is initiated which in most cases is a time and labor intensive manual process involving multiple patient visits [4]. DBS programming is generally performed by movement disorder neurologists (including fellows in training), neurosurgeons, nurses, nurse practitioners, or physician assistants who have acquired training and experience for this procedure. Although there are general guidelines available for programming, there are no clear, validated, and established programming protocols. An inefficient programming can result in suboptimal clinical outcomes and lead to side effects which becomes a source of frustration for Parkinson's disease patients and caregivers as well as healthcare providers [3]. These patients are then referred to as "DBS failures" and referrals are placed to advanced DBS centers for consideration of a lead revision surgery. In a retrospective analysis of 41 patients who presented to two academic DBS centers for management of "DBS failures," over a period of two years, 15 patients (37%) were identified as inadequately programmed and they improved significantly after reprogramming. There were 6 additional patients (15%) who benefitted partially from expert reprogramming, and 21 patients (51%) failed to improve despite a detailed reprogramming. There were also seven (17%) patients who did not demonstrate clinical improvement due to poor access to programming [5]. Thus lead revision is potentially avoidable when a careful and systematic algorithm based programming is employed.

2. Current Approach to DBS Programming

2.1. Initiation of Programming. In Parkinson's disease, a successful DBS programming is usually accomplished over a period of three to six months. Programming is usually not initiated immediately after the placement of a lead; instead a time frame of 2–4 weeks is allowed for the microlesion effects to fade away. These microlesion effects are believed to arise from the trauma of the DBS lead implantation rather than from the stimulation of the targeted brain structure. As a result, there is temporary improvement in clinical symptoms. Thus, for an accurate assessment of stimulation benefits, it is recommended that DBS programming gets initiated only when the initial benefits fade away [6]. In a large randomized controlled DBS study, the mean medication "on" time in patients randomized to receive delayed stimulation therapy was observed to improve at three months after surgery attributed to the microlesion effects. Nearly 40% of this group responded with an improvement of more than 2 hours of "on" time compared to the case before surgery [7]. There are some DBS centers that advocate initiation of programming at an earlier stage while the patients are still hospitalized as this method is more patient convenient and avoids an extra programming visit [8]. In addition to the microlesion effect confounding the initial results, impedance fluctuations in the tissue surrounding the DBS lead can also contribute to inaccurate assessment. Impedances are observed to be increased immediately after placement of a lead, as a consequence of edema, and they tend to decrease and stabilize over the first few weeks [9]. In these situations, DBS therapy delivered through constant-voltage stimulation is avoidable as the current delivered depends on the impedance. Instead, a constant-current stimulation that allows the current to adapt to changes in the impedance is recommended.

2.2. Lead Type, Impedance Check, Programming Thresholds, and Battery Check. In order to utilize effective stimulation parameters at the bedside, it is important for the DBS programmer to be aware of the lead type which refers to the size of the contacts and the distance between them. With the Medtronic system, the commonly used lead models are

the 3387 and the 3389. The 3387 model is a 40 cm long and 1.27 mm wide cylindrical lead with 4 cylindrical electrodes that are 1.5 mm in length each and placed 1.5 mm apart. The 3389 model carries the same specifications except for electrode spacing of 0.5 mm. The Boston Scientific DBS lead has 8 cylindrical contacts that are 1.3 mm in diameter and 1.5 mm in length, placed 2 mm apart and covering a span of 15.5 mm. The Boston Scientific DBS system also offers a directional lead in which the middle two levels are split into three segments spanning approximately 120 degrees and the highest and the lowest level contain ring shaped electrodes. The Boston Scientific system is currently not FDA approved; however trials are underway. The St Jude Infinity DBS system (now called Abbott's Infinity DBS system) that has segmented electrodes and a wireless mobile platform for programming recently received FDA approval.

It is also necessary to confirm the location of the DBS lead prior to initiation of programming. At our center, we routinely obtain a postoperative CT brain that is coregistered with the preoperative MRI scan. Another important step is to gather intraoperative records for review of stimulation parameters used for testing immediately after the implantation. Once these steps are completed, the programming healthcare professional records the impedance at each of the contacts to establish a baseline for future reference. Compared to intraoperative parameters (influenced by edema), the impedance recorded is often different. If an impedance recording suggests a short circuit or an open circuit then the impedance is rechecked at higher voltages to ensure accuracy of the reading. The older Soletra® and Kinetra® Medtronic models require the provider to manually select the higher voltage for the repeat impedance check, whereas the Activa® SC/RC/PC will automatically check at 1.5 V and 3.0 V if open circuit is noted at 0.7 V stimulation. If there is a short circuit (which is extremely low impedance < 250 ohms) then the provider is not required to check at higher voltages. When a short circuit is identified, it is recommended to avoid the involved contacts as these are not dependable. There is generally faster battery depletion or there is sometimes a sudden loss of benefit. A common reason identified for short circuit has been anchoring of DBS lead with a miniplate [10]. High impedance, for example, 2000 ohms for the Soletra and 4000 ohms for the Kinetra, should be in general seen concurrently with unipolar and bipolar review. If the impedances are high in the bipolar contacts but normal in the unipolar contacts then there may not be an open circuit. Decisions regarding open circuit findings need to be evaluated on a case-by-case basis. The high impedance (open circuit) will be generated in the Activa SC/PC/RC when >10000 ohms in unipolar and bipolar configuration is noted [11]. The St Jude DBS system will show a message of "high" (read as 31 with older version and with newer one as >3000) when there is an open circuit. Lead fractures are common reasons for open circuits with an overall incidence of 5.1%, clinically presenting as electrical shocks reported by patients or lack of a therapeutic benefit. In the context of Parkinson's disease, it is also important to consider head jerking from cervical dystonia or a twiddler's syndrome, in which the patients who have developed dopaminergic medication induced impulse control disorder subconsciously spin the neurostimulator in the chest wall which results in lead fractures [12]. In a series of 226 DBS patients, three patients identified to have a twiddler's syndrome presented with reemergence of Parkinson's disease symptoms and pain along the path of the hardware. In these patients, twisting/fracture of DBS extension was identified radiographically and was treated surgically by securing the neurostimulator in the chest wall [13, 14].

Once the electrical intactness of the system is established, thresholds of stimulation parameters that elicit benefits and induce side effects are determined. Initially, each electrode contact on the lead is tested in a monopolar configuration with the electrode as negative (cathode) and the neurostimulator case as positive (anode), a process referred to as monopolar review. The main stimulation parameters include the voltage, the frequency, and the pulse width. Amplitude controls the intensity of the stimulation, pulse width refers to the duration of each electrical pulse delivered, and frequency is the rate of stimulation employed in programming. The Medtronic system for the Soletra and Kinetra is only available in amplitudes of voltage (V). The Medtronic system for the Activa SC/RC/PC is available in either amplitudes of V or milliamps (mA). The St Jude and Boston Scientific systems are available only in amplitudes of mA. With a fixed frequency and pulse width, each of the electrode contacts is separately examined with amplitude delivered at increasing increments of 0.5 V or mA until there is elicitation of adverse effect (objective or subjective) that stays persistent with continued stimulation. This establishes a stimulation threshold for the adverse effects. Then the efficacy of stimulation at this contact is examined using an amplitude reduction by 0.1–1.0 V or mA below the stimulation threshold for side effects [15]. As the amplitude is reduced, the lowest threshold for inducing the best clinical benefits is determined. On the other hand, some centers first identify the threshold for clinical benefit and then increase the amplitude to identify the threshold for side effects. The electrode contact with the widest therapeutic window (wider difference between the threshold for inducing side effects and the threshold for clinical benefits) is selected for chronic stimulation. Both clinical effects and side effects depend on the direction of spread of current stimulating the anatomical structures as described in detail in the Table 1. If there is inadequate control of motor symptoms with single monopolar configuration, the next choice is to employ double monopolar stimulation with the two stimulation contacts as negative and the neurostimulator case as positive. There is no fixed time interval on taking this decision but most programmers wait few weeks or couple of programming sessions before switching to a bipolar configuration. Alternate method is to stay in monopolar stimulation but adjust the frequency or the pulse width. Bipolar configuration (most effective contact is negative and the adjacent contact is positive) is sought if side effects with monopolar configuration are induced at low amplitudes. With bipolar configuration, higher stimulation intensities are sometimes required to achieve the same clinical benefit.

In theory, DBS programming for a Medtronic device involves thousands of possible parameter combinations considering the range of programmable amplitudes (>90 possible), pulse widths (>10 possible), frequencies (>25 possible), interleaving settings, and configuration of anodes and cathodes. However since the recommended limit for charge density is $30\,mC/cm^2$ which is calculated by dividing the product of the voltage and the pulse width by the product of the impedance and the geometric surface area of the DBS electrode ($0.06\,cm^2$) it limits the number of possible combinations [16]. There is a wide variation in the final stimulation parameters selected for DBS programming which is driven by multiple factors such as patient characteristics, the specific Parkinson's disease phenotype, and the lead position. In Parkinson's disease, the stimulation parameters used with a Medtronic system consist of a range of pulse widths (60 to $450\,\mu s$), frequencies (60 to 160 Hz), and voltages or currents (1 V to highest tolerated value). In most clinical DBS studies for Parkinson's disease, voltage in the range 2.4 to 4.4 V, frequency in the range 143 to 173 Hz, and pulse width in the range 67 to $138\,\mu s$ have been found to effectively control the motor symptoms [17]. For efficient management of motor symptoms few published algorithms are available. In one study from Grenoble, France, with several combinations of stimulation settings that were systematically evaluated in patients with Parkinson's disease, the most important factors for alleviation of motor symptoms were identified as the voltage followed by the frequency [18]. In a recent study, an algorithm was proposed to specifically address the speech issue, gait impairment, and stimulation induced dyskinesia. The authors suggested lowering of stimulation frequency once other considerations including reduction of voltage, stimulation with bipolar configuration, and interleaving pattern had been tried with no clinical improvements. Caution should be exercised while using low frequency DBS as there is a possibility of worsening of appendicular rigidity, bradykinesia, and tremor [3].

2.3. Programming Visits. The initial programming visit can be often long lasting nearly 60–90 minutes. During this visit, it is important to provide patient education on several matters that are pertinent for a successful DBS programming. These include the knowledge on potential stimulation induced side effects, the use of the patient programmer (how to turn on and turn off the stimulator or go between patient group settings or programs if provided or adjusting parameters provided to the patient), and the safety precautions that need to be followed such as avoidance of strong magnetic fields and the use of diathermy during surgical procedures. Thus, family and friends are encouraged to accompany the patients during this initial programming visit. The programming is usually performed in the morning in an off-dopaminergic medication state. The rationale for holding medications is that dopaminergic medications can potentially obscure the stimulation induced benefits. Patients are instructed to hold the medications overnight or to miss at least a couple of doses so that they present to clinic in the "off-" medication state. If off-medication symptoms are intolerably severe or there is a lack of family support for outpatient management, inpatient programming is recommended. Alternately, patients are allowed to present in an on-medication state and they are

TABLE 1: Clinical effects of stimulating individual targets employed in Parkinson's disease depend on spread of current.

	Optimal location stimulation	Medial spread of current	Lateral spread of current	Anterior spread of current	Posterior spread of current	Dorsal or superior spread of current	Ventral or inferior spread of current
Subthalamic nucleus							
Anatomical structure stimulated	Dorsolateral aspect of subthalamic nucleus (motor territory)	Cranial nerve III Red nucleus Limbic aspect	Corticospinal tract/internal capsule Frontal eye field fibers of internal capsule	Corticospinal tract/internal capsule Hypothalamus	Medial lemniscus	Internal capsule Thalamus Zona incerta	Substantia nigra reticulata Internal capsule fibers
Clinical effects	Control of tremors, bradykinesia, and rigidity	Diplopia, eye deviation, dizziness Sweating, nausea, paresthesia, warm sensation Personality change Depression, impulsivity	Facial pulling Limb contraction contralateral side Contralateral deviation of gaze	Facial pulling Limb contraction contralateral side Autonomic symptoms Sweating, nausea	Paresthesia (tingling, electrical sensation, numbness)	Contralateral muscle contraction Improvement of dyskinesia/tremor Improvement of dyskinesia/tremor	Mood changes Depression Muscle contractions
Globus pallidum							
Anatomical structure stimulated	Posteroventral aspect of globus pallidum	Internal capsule posterior limb	Globus pallidum externus Putamen	Globus pallidum externus Putamen	Internal capsule posterior limb	Globus pallidum externus	Optic tract
Clinical effects	Reduction of bradykinesia, rigidity, and dystonia	Contralateral muscle contractions	No effect	No effect	Contralateral muscle contractions	Putamen No effect	Phosphenes
Thalamus							
Anatomical structure stimulated	Ventral intermedius nucleus located in the middle of thalamus	Medial aspect of nucleus, centromedian nucleus/parafascicular nucleus	Internal capsule posterior limb	Ventral oralis anterior Ventral oralis posterior	Ventral caudalis nucleus	Dorsal aspect of thalamic nucleus Internal capsule fibers	Zona incerta Medial lemniscus Brachium conjunctivum
Clinical effects	Tremor control	Dysarthria	Dysarthria Contralateral muscle contractions	No effect Reduction of tremor	Paresthesia	No effect Dysarthria	Improvement of tremor/dyskinesia Paresthesia ataxia

examined once the medications effects show signs of wearing off (suboptimal on-medication) [17]. Standardized motor tasks of the Unified Parkinson's Disease Rating Scale are used for clinical assessment. Amongst all the cardinal motor symptoms of Parkinson's disease, tremors and rigidity are found to respond very quickly, usually within seconds to minutes of stimulation, whereas there is a variable time delay for improvement in bradykinesia. The clinical response to DBS depends on several factors such as disease characteristics, DBS lead position, stimulation parameters, and individual patient profile. Since patient participation is critical, factors such as patient fatigue, patient comfort, patient anxiety, and training contribute significantly to the outcome.

Once the off-medication state programming is completed, patients are given their usual dopaminergic dose to further determine stimulation parameters for control of levodopa induced dyskinesia. It is noteworthy that levodopa induced dyskinesia does not necessarily emerge immediately after the first dose of medication, sometimes requiring the cumulative effects of two or three doses to develop, and is most often seen in the afternoon. The best electrode configuration is the one that adequately improves off-medication parkinsonism and reasonably suppresses on-medication dyskinesia. A challenge that arises in relation to subthalamic nucleus DBS is stimulation induced dyskinesia when the DBS lead is well-positioned in the motor territory. In these circumstances, a gradual reduction of stimulation voltage is recommended to achieve balance between control of parkinsonism and control of dyskinesia. On the other hand, stimulation of the dorsal globus pallidum may show differential effects on control of dyskinesia based on the specific anatomical region stimulated. There are reports that stimulation of dorsal globus pallidus internus induces dyskinesia which may be confused with medication related dyskinesia. When stimulation contact is shifted ventrally, dyskinesia becomes suppressed and bradykinesia tends to worsen [19].

DBS programming requires multiple patient visits. During the initial six months after surgery, patients are followed every month. Once the optimal programing settings are determined, patients are then followed on an annual basis for clinical performance, troubleshooting, and battery checks. An earlier follow-up is scheduled if the disease status worsens at a faster pace.

2.4. Battery and Programming. During the follow-up of DBS patients, estimation of battery life is critical. Battery drain is dependent on many factors including manufacturing tolerances, battery usage, battery chemistry, and variations in tissue impedance. The electrode surface area (small surface areas result in larger impedances) and the number of contacts used for stimulation affect the tissue impedance [20, 21]. With the Medtronic Soletra system, the battery life starts at a voltage of 3.69–3.74 V with an end of life (EOL) reached when the battery drains to about 2.5 V. In general with Soletra battery the voltage stays the same over a period of time; however as the battery nears the end of longevity, a slow drop in voltage may occur followed eventually by a more rapid depletion. Some patients notice worsening of symptoms when the battery is depleting and thus waiting to reach 2.5 V

is not necessary to plan replacement of the DBS battery. With the Medtronic Kinetra system, the starting battery voltage is 3.2 V and the EOL is reached around 1.97 V. The Kinetra battery voltage reading slowly decreases over time; sometimes the Kinetra battery will stop showing a decline in the battery voltage for several visits; however if the patient complains of return in symptoms then it is important to make plans to replace the DBS battery. The current consumption with Kinetra is linear, unlike Soletra where the voltage doubler or tripler circuit is activated once the voltage parameter delivered for clinical stimulation increases to 3.6 V leading to a faster drain of battery [22]. In addition to the battery status indicator available in each device, battery life can be estimated through helplines/website made available locally or through Medtronic Inc [20]. Newer generation DBS systems offer rechargeable neurostimulators such as the Activa RC through the Medtronic (expected lifespan of about 9 years) or Vercise® system through the Boston Scientific (expected lifespan of about 25 years). The Abbott Infinity® system has a battery life of 3–5 years (Saint Paul, MN, USA) [23]. Medtronic Activa RC, Boston Scientific Vercise (not approved by FDA yet), and Abbott Brio all offer rechargeable DBS batteries. The Abbott Infinity 5 and Infinity 7 batteries show a status of either "battery okay," "battery low," or "battery depleted." Further details on battery life and impedance details are provided in Table 2. Future advances in DBS technology such as closed loop DBS will increase battery life and advances in DBS programming like remote and Internet based programming will increase patient comfort and convenience [24].

3. Recent Advances in DBS Programming

The electrical field delivered through the DBS contact in monopolar configuration is spherical with intensity of field decreasing in proportion to distance from the electrode. Large diameter myelinated axons have the lowest threshold for activation compared to dendrites and soma and also respond to shorter pulse widths. With bipolar configuration, the intensity of field decreases to one-quarter when the distance from electrode doubles. The intensity of electrical field increases as the distance between cathode and anode increases with wider bipolar configuration giving higher intensity field compared to narrow configuration. The conventional DBS however has limited capabilities with regard to modulating the shape of electrical field and tailoring the intensity of stimulation to maximally stimulate the neuronal pathways of interest and minimize the unintended spread to anatomical structures leading to side effects. Over the last few years, several novel technologies have developed in the field of DBS therapy. Current-based programming, interleaved programming, fractionated current, and directional current steering are important examples. The following sections will discuss these recent developments which are important advances in the field of DBS programming.

3.1. Interleaved Programming. Interleaving strategy is applied when conventional programming techniques, such as bipolar, double monopolar, or tripolar settings, and use of alternative pulse widths and frequencies fail to achieve desired clinical

TABLE 2: DBS system battery life and impedance limit.

DBS system company model	Battery type	Battery life (average)	Impedance limit for open circuit in ohms.	Impedance limit for short circuit in ohms
Medtronic Soletra™ (no longer manufactured)	Single chamber Nonrechargeable battery	3 to 5 years	If it is >2,000 ohms for bipolar and corresponding monopolar configurations and current is less than 10 uamps then it is likely open circuit.	<250 ohms
Medtronic Kinetra™ (no longer manufactured)	Dual chamber Nonrechargeable battery	3 to 5 years	If it is >4,000 ohms for bipolar and corresponding monopolar configurations and current is less than 10 uamps then it is likely open circuit.	<250 ohms
Medtronic Activa SC	Single chamber Nonrechargeable battery	3 to 5 years	If it is 5000–9000 ohms for bipolar and corresponding monopolar configurations suspect possible threatened open circuit. If it is >10000 ohms for bipolar and corresponding monopolar configurations then there is high suspicion of open circuit. If it is >40000 likely there is fracture in system.	<250 ohms
Medtronic Activa PC	Dual chamber Nonrechargeable battery	3 to 5 years	Same as Activa SC.	<250 ohms
Medtronic Activa RC	Dual chamber Rechargeable battery	8 years	Same as Activa SC.	<250 ohms
St Jude Libra™ (no longer manufactured)	Single chamber Nonrechargeable battery	3 to 5 years	High (31) is an open circuit.	
Abbott Infinity 5™	Dual chamber Nonrechargeable battery	3 to 4 years	>3000 Ohms.	
Abbott Infinity 7™	Dual chamber Nonrechargeable battery	4 to 5 years	>3000 Ohms.	

results. Interleaving is also useful when stimulation induced side effects are elicited at lower voltages. Interleaving consists of a rapid and alternate activation of two electrode contacts with two distinct voltages and pulse widths but with an identical frequency, up to maximum of 125 Hz in the Medtronic Activa system (interleaving not available with St Jude and Boston Scientific). Thus a limitation in modulation of frequency potentially interferes with simultaneous control of tremors and other motor symptoms as tremors tend to respond to a higher frequency [25]. Interleaving is not the same as simultaneous double monopolar stimulation as the pulses at each of the two contacts could be potentially offset by 4 ms (125 Hz equals 8 ms interpulse interval). With interleaving, an area of overlap that receives stimulation from both the electrical fields at double the frequency is seen and this area is speculated to contribute to stimulation induced chronic side effects. Interleaving is also useful when two contacts require different voltages for control of two different symptoms. For example, interleaving allowed treatment of tremors and bradykinesia through stimulation of the subregions of subthalamic nucleus and the adjacent zona incerta [26]. In another case, interleaving was used to deliver pulses to the ventral intermedius nucleus of the thalamus as well as the subthalamic nucleus region in a patient who presented with coexisting diagnosis of essential tremor and Parkinson's disease [27]. The main drawback of interleaving to keep in mind is the possibility of an increased battery drain which is a concern if Parkinson's disease patient symptoms of dystonia require high stimulation voltages and pulse widths [25].

3.2. Directional Stimulation.

With the advent of directional lead technology, it is now possible to steer different shapes of current at the stimulation contact instead of providing the conventional spherical shape of current. A major advantage of this technology is steering current to the desired structures and avoidance of unintended stimulation of the neighboring anatomical structures. This new technology facilitates achievement of greater efficacy and fewer side effects [28]. This is especially desirable when small and complex brain regions are targeted [29], such as the pedunculopontine nucleus [30], or other fiber bundle targets, such as the medial forebrain bundle. Direct STN Acute (Aleva Neurotherapeutics SA) that incorporates six directional contacts with three directional contacts on each of the two levels was investigated in a recent pilot study of Parkinson's disease patients who underwent subthalamic nucleus lead implantation. This lead also had two omnidirectional electrodes proximal to the directional contacts. The directional contacts were each $1 \, mm \times 1 \, mm$ in dimension, with a longitudinal spacing of 0.5 mm. The investigators compared the effects of directional stimulation to omnidirectional stimulation in an intraoperative setting, focusing specifically on the volume of tissue activated. They found that the volume of tissue activated with directional stimulation ($4.2 \, mm^3$) was substantially lower compared to the omnidirectional stimulation ($10.5 \, mm^3$). As a consequence, the therapeutic window was significantly wider (43% wider) and the side effects were much lower with directional stimulation [28]. Another parallel study tested a

novel 32 contact lead (formerly Sapiens Steering Brain Stimulation BV, Eindhoven, the Netherlands, now called Medtronic Eindhoven Design Center). These contacts could be activated independently in clusters, allowing for directional steering of the stimulation field and directional recording of local field potentials. In this study, thresholds for therapeutic benefit and side effects determined intraoperatively in 8 patients with Parkinson's disease were noted to be increased and the therapeutic window widened [31]. Recently Vercise directional lead (Boston Scientific, Valencia, CA), which has eight-contact leads and a pulse generator capable of multiple independent current source, was tested in seven Parkinson's disease patients. This novel lead with four electrode levels had two middle level electrodes split into three segments spanning approximately 120 degrees each and ring shaped electrodes in the highest and the lowest level. An extended monopolar review session was performed during the first week after the placement of leads. The current thresholds for control of rigidity and stimulation induced adverse effects were determined using either directional or ring-mode settings. Similar to the previous two studies, the investigators reported an expansion of the therapeutic window with this novel system [32]. The benefits of directional stimulation were best appreciated when the lead was suboptimally placed and the therapeutic window was narrow, for example, when the subthalamic nucleus lead was laterally placed close to the internal capsule. While these results are promising, larger studies are warranted for further confirmation.

3.3. Current-Based Programming and Fractionalization of Current.

For several years, DBS therapy involved the use of voltage based programming. However the fluctuations in the impedance at the level of electrode-tissue interface were noted to contribute to an instability of voltages delivered to the target neural tissue [33]. As a result, stimulation parameters required frequent adjustments especially during the initial programming period after the DBS lead has been placed. These undesirable fluctuations also led to the understimulation or overstimulation of the intended target. These factors prompted the development of current-controlled DBS that regulated the current delivered to the targeted neural tissue regardless of the impedance. With a constant-current device, the need for programming adjustments was expected to reduce and the outcomes of DBS programming were expected to be more reliable. In a randomized multicenter controlled study, a constant-current device was examined in Parkinson's disease patients who underwent bilateral subthalamic nucleus implantation [7]. Subjects participating received either immediate stimulation or a delayed stimulation which was initiated three months after surgery (control group). The primary outcome of the study was the mean increase in the amount of medication ON time, and it was significantly increased in the immediate stimulation group (4.27 h versus 1.77 h, $p = 0.003$). The immediate stimulation group also performed better than the control group in the off-medication/on-stimulation assessment of Unified Parkinson's Disease Rating Scale motor score (40% improvement in the immediate stimulation group). The study was not primarily designed to determine the frequency of programming adjustments or compare constant-current with constant-voltage neurostimulation. In another crossover study of 8 Parkinson's disease cases, patients were randomized to constant-current and constant-voltage setting at about two years after subthalamic nucleus DBS surgery [33]. In both groups, the improvements in the motor scores, the reduction in levodopa dose, and the quality of life improvement were equivalent. The study concluded that constant-current stimulation programming was not necessarily superior to constant-voltage stimulation.

An accurate DBS targeting is critical for successful control of motor symptoms, and a slight error in lead location can sometime significantly impact clinical outcomes. In these circumstances, the delivery of small amounts of stimulation to multiple contacts is desirable. Until now, the DBS system consisted of a single source stimulation device. In the recent VANTAGE study, a multiple source delivery of fractionalized currents (Vercise DBS system, Boston Scientific) was examined in 40 Parkinson's disease patients who underwent bilateral subthalamic nucleus DBS surgery [23]. The Vercise DBS lead consisted of 8 contact rings one above the other on each side; each contact was 1.5 mm in length with 0.5 mm spacing between the contacts. A fractionated current with a well-defined shape of the electrical field allowed an enhanced and reliable motor response with minimized stimulation induced side effects. Once the healthcare programmer identified the contact that provided the best clinical benefits, the current was fractionalized between the best and the next best contact. Patients were then sent home with an ability to make adjustments at a preset stimulation range. In this open label study, Parkinson's disease patients were noted to improve by nearly 60% when comparing the baseline UPDRS motor scores (37.4 ± 8.9) with the six months postoperative scores (13.5 ± 6.8). There were also improvements in the quality of life, increase in the time spent in the medication on state, and reduction of the overall dose of dopaminergic medications. These outcomes were regarded better in comparison to other DBS trials and the incidence of adverse effects was in the acceptable range. Thus fractionalization of current is an important contribution to advanced DBS programming that will be soon applied in many more clinical studies.

3.4. Closed Loop DBS.
There is an increasing enthusiasm for the use of closed loop DBS or adaptive DBS which represents a real-time change of DBS parameters in response to underlying physiological signals. The real-time change enables a more efficient control of clinical symptoms and at the same time there is a lesser use of battery [34]. However several questions have been raised over the best possible underlying physiological signal. In Parkinson's disease, these signals could be potentially recorded from the cortex, basal ganglia, and the skin surface over the affected body part (e.g., surface EMG) [35]. Local field potentials (LFPs) recorded from the basal ganglia are promising markers. LFPs indicate the oscillatory activity of a neuronal population surrounding the recording electrode and are usually clustered into specific frequency bands. The beta band frequency (11–30 Hz) is regarded as antikinetic, contributing to the bradykinesia and freezing of gait [36], whereas gamma band frequencies

(>60 Hz) have a prokinetic role [37]. Beta band oscillations recorded from the subthalamic nucleus are found to be modulated by dopaminergic medication [38] and electrical stimulation [39]. They have been found to correlate with movement preparation and execution [40], akinesia [41], and the freezing of gait [42]. In a proof-of-principle study, LFP-based adaptive DBS was investigated in 8 patients with advanced PD who underwent subthalamic nucleus DBS [43]. The investigators applied an arbitrary threshold to the LFP power recorded from the subthalamic nucleus with DBS programmed to switch off if the beta power fell below threshold. Adaptive DBS was found to lead to a 30% greater motor improvement compared to continuous DBS therapy. Another source of physiological signals for adaptive programming is the cortex. Cortical signals recorded with electrocorticography have been frequently used for detection of seizures. In a primate model of Parkinson's disease, there was alleviation of akinesia when short stimulation trains (130 Hz) were delivered to the globus pallidus internus at fixed latency following an action potential recorded from the primary motor cortex area [44]. In another example of Parkinson's disease patient, there was improvement in rigidity when the phase amplitude coupling between beta and gamma oscillations of the cortical signals was observed to be decreased [45]. Closed loop stimulation will be increasingly utilized as the clinical advantages become established in patients with Parkinson's disease.

3.5. Applying Novel DBS Pulse for Programming.
The conventional DBS therapy is a continuous delivery of charge-balanced, square waveform, cathodic pulse at specific voltages, and pulse widths that are within the limits of FDA recommended safety guidelines (30 mC/cm^2). The square waveform DBS pulse has an active high-amplitude, short-duration stimulation phase, and an exponential passive low-amplitude, long-duration recharge phase that prevents tissue damage. However Hofmann et al. found that when the initial cathodic phase was followed by a short gap of time prior to introduction of an anodic phase, the neural activation and entrainment became more effective [46]. Foutz and McIntyre examined the effects of novel pulse shapes such as Gaussian, exponential, triangular, and sinusoidal pulses in both intracellular and extracellular environment to find that neural effects were elicited at lower energy consumption [47]. However, using biphasic pulse DBS therapy in which charge-balanced square-wave pulse with active recharge was used for patients with Parkinson's disease led to greater clinical benefits but at the cost of an increased battery drain [48]. Nevertheless, these applications of novel pulse shapes are promising and warrant further testing in a clinical population.

4. Guided Programming

4.1. Computer Guidance.
Until now, DBS programming is mostly a time consuming and labor intensive manual process. DBS programming is also inconvenient to many patients as the DBS centers are few for meeting the needs of an increasing number of patients (more than 140,000 DBS surgeries performed worldwide) and often far away from a patient's

home [5]. The complexities involved in clinical programming are perceived as burdensome by many healthcare providers [49]. Therefore, there are growing efforts to develop computer guided programming in conjunction with a sensor-based technology for feedback. Motion sensor-based feedback has been found to result in a better clinical outcome compared to subjective assessment [50]. The feasibility of computer guided DBS programming and automated motion sensor-based assessment, requiring minimal physician involvement, has been examined in a pilot study [5]. In this study, once the software performed the initial monopolar review, multiple iterations were conducted based on the automated feedback. The software then applied an algorithm to determine the final stimulation settings required to achieve control of symptoms and at the same time minimize the side effects and the battery usage [49]. The investigators concluded that significant improvement in tremors and bradykinesia could be achieved with minimal clinician involvement. Even though these findings are promising, they will require further confirmation in the clinical settings.

4.2. Visual Guidance. DBS programming is regarded as an "empirical" and "blind" technique. The clinician empirically inputs the electrical parameters and awaits the patient response as the output. Over the last few years, computational models have been developed that incorporate individual patient neuroanatomy to facilitate visual programming. Recently, these models were tested with an iPad application interface (ImageVis3D Mobile) that provided a mobile environment for a visual feedback on the interaction of the stimulation parameters with the surrounding anatomy [51]. Aside from clear advantage in visual feedback, programming time reduced from over 4 hours to less than 2 minutes (>99% saving in time) with computational model [51]. Diffusion tensor imaging and other advanced MRI sequences can potentially contribute to improved visually guided programming. Commercial programming platforms available through the Boston Scientific (Boston Scientific Guide DBS) and Medtronic (Medtronic Optivise) should be soon available for visually guided programming [24].

In summary, the success of DBS is dependent on numerous factors including appropriate selection of patients, appropriate patient expectations, accurate placement of DBS lead, and a thorough programming to identify the optimal stimulation parameters. Although there are general guidelines available for programming, there are no protocols that are validated and clearly established. Identifying the lead type, electrode configuration, impedance in the electrical system, and battery check are key elements for programming visits. There are growing efforts to advance the current approach to DBS programming. With the advent of fractionated current technology, it is now possible to distribute current to electrodes in fractions for a broader capture of motor symptoms. Directional lead steers different shapes of current to stimulate the desired structures and avoid unintended stimulation of the neighboring anatomical structures. Since DBS programming is a time consuming and labor intensive manual process, there is increasing interest to develop computer and visually guided protocol. Programming is also not a

comfortable experience for the patient as it requires frequent clinic visits and programming facilities may not necessarily be close to the patient home. However remote and Internet based programming are likely to resolve these issues in the near future.

Acknowledgments

This work was supported by NIH K23 NS092957-01A1 (Aparna Wagle Shukla).

References

[1] A. Wagle Shukla and M. S. Okun, "Surgical treatment of Parkinson's disease: patients, targets, devices, and approaches," *Neurotherapeutics*, vol. 11, no. 1, pp. 47–59, 2014.

[2] A. Wagle Shukla and M. S. Okun, "State of the art for deep brain stimulation therapy in movement disorders: A clinical and technological perspective," *IEEE Reviews in Biomedical Engineering*, vol. 9, pp. 219–233, 2016.

[3] M. Picillo, A. M. Lozano, N. Kou, R. Puppi Munhoz, and A. Fasano, "Programming Deep Brain Stimulation for Parkinson's Disease: The Toronto Western Hospital Algorithms," *Brain Stimulation*, vol. 9, no. 3, pp. 425–437, 2016.

[4] A. M. Kuncel and W. M. Grill, "Selection of stimulus parameters for deep brain stimulation," *Clinical Neurophysiology*, vol. 115, no. 11, pp. 2431–2441, 2004.

[5] M. S. Okun, M. Tagliati, M. Pourfar et al., "Management of referred deep brain stimulation failures: A retrospective analysis from 2 Movement Disorders Centers," *Archives of Neurology*, vol. 62, no. 8, pp. 1250–1255, 2005.

[6] G. Kleiner-Fisman, D. N. Fisman, E. Sime, J. A. Saint-Cyr, A. M. Lozano, and A. E. Lang, "Long-term follow up of bilateral deep brain stimulation of the subthalamic nucleus in patients with advanced Parkinson disease," *Journal of Neurosurgery*, vol. 99, no. 3, pp. 489–495, 2003.

[7] M. S. Okun, B. V. Gallo, G. Mandybur et al., "Subthalamic deep brain stimulation with a constant-current device in Parkinson's disease: an open-label randomised controlled trial," *The Lancet Neurology*, vol. 11, no. 2, pp. 140–149, 2012.

[8] D. B. Cohen, M. Y. Oh, S. M. Baser et al., "Fast-Track Programming and Rehabilitation Model: A Novel Approach to Postoperative Deep Brain Stimulation Patient Care," *Archives of Physical Medicine and Rehabilitation*, vol. 88, no. 10, pp. 1320–1324, 2007.

[9] S. F. Lempka, S. Miocinovic, M. D. Johnson, J. L. Vitek, and C. C. McIntyre, "In vivo impedance spectroscopy of deep brain stimulation electrodes," *Journal of Neural Engineering*, vol. 6, no. 4, Article ID 046001, 2009.

[10] K. Samura, Y. Miyagi, T. Okamoto et al., "Short circuit in deep brain stimulation," *Journal of Neurosurgery*, vol. 117, no. 5, pp. 955–961, 2012.

[11] I. Medtronic, "N'Vision clinician programmer with software. Activa® PC, Activa®RC and Activa®SC neurostimulation systems for deep brain stimulation, 2008".

[12] P. Blomstedt and M. I. Hariz, "Hardware-related complications of deep brain stimulation: A ten year experience," *Acta Neurochirurgica*, vol. 147, no. 10, pp. 1061–1064, 2005.

[13] G. Geissinger and J. H. Neal, "Spontaneous twiddler's syndrome

in a patient with a deep brain stimulator," *Surgical Neurology*, vol. 68, no. 4, pp. 454–456, 2007.

[14] A. P. Burdick, M. S. Okun, I. U. Haq et al., "Prevalence of twiddler's syndrome as a cause of deep brain stimulation hardware failure," *Stereotactic and Functional Neurosurgery*, vol. 88, no. 6, pp. 353–359, 2010.

[15] J. Volkmann, J. Herzog, F. Kopper, and G. Geuschl, "Introduction to the programming of deep brain stimulators," *Movement Disorders*, vol. 17, no. 3, pp. S181–S187, 2002.

[16] A. M. Kuncel, S. E. Cooper, B. R. Wolgamuth, and W. M. Grill, "Amplitude- and frequency-dependent changes in neuronal regularity parallel changes in tremor with thalamic deep brain stimulation," *IEEE Transactions on Neural Systems and Rehabilitation Engineering*, vol. 15, no. 2, pp. 190–197, 2007.

[17] A. Wagle Shukla, A. Bona, and R. Walz, *Troubleshooting*, Nova Science Publishers, 2015.

[18] E. Moro, R. J. A. Esselink, J. Xie, M. Hommel, A. L. Benabid, and P. Pollak, "The impact on Parkinson's disease of electrical parameter settings in STN stimulation," *Neurology*, vol. 59, no. 5, pp. 706–713, 2002.

[19] R. Kumar, "Methods for programming and patient management with deep brain stimulation of the globus pallidus for the treatment of advanced parkinson's disease and dystonia," *Movement Disorders*, vol. 17, no. 3, pp. S198–S207, 2002.

[20] K. Fakhar, E. Hastings, C. R. Butson, K. D. Foote, P. Zeilman, and M. S. Okun, "Management of Deep Brain Stimulator Battery Failure: Battery Estimators, Charge Density, and Importance of Clinical Symptoms," *PLoS ONE*, vol. 8, no. 3, Article ID e58665, 2013.

[21] M. A. Montuno, A. B. Kohner, K. D. Foote, and M. S. Okun, "An algorithm for management of deep brain stimulation battery replacements: Devising a web-based battery estimator and clinical symptom approach," *Neuromodulation*, vol. 16, no. 2, pp. 147–153, 2013.

[22] J. Volkmann, N. Allert, J. Voges, V. Sturm, A. Schnitzler, and H.-J. Freund, "Long-term results of bilateral pallidal stimulation in Parkinson's disease," *Annals of Neurology*, vol. 55, no. 6, pp. 871–875, 2004.

[23] L. Timmermann, R. Jain, L. Chen et al., "Multiple-source current steering in subthalamic nucleus deep brain stimulation for Parkinson's disease (the VANTAGE study): A non-randomised, prospective, multicentre, open-label study," *The Lancet Neurology*, vol. 14, no. 7, pp. 693–701, 2015.

[24] A. Fasano and A. M. Lozano, "Deep brain stimulation for movement disorders: 2015 and beyond," *Current Opinion in Neurology*, vol. 28, no. 4, pp. 423–436, 2015.

[25] S. Miocinovic, P. Khemani, R. Whiddon et al., "Outcomes, management, and potential mechanisms of interleaving deep brain stimulation settings," *Parkinsonism and Related Disorders*, vol. 20, no. 12, pp. 1434–1437, 2014.

[26] L. Wojtecki, J. Vesper, and A. Schnitzler, "Interleaving programming of subthalamic deep brain stimulation to reduce side effects with good motor outcome in a patient with Parkinson's disease," *Parkinsonism and Related Disorders*, vol. 17, no. 4, pp. 293-294, 2011.

[27] C. R. Baumann, L. L. Imbach, M. Baumann-Vogel, M. Uhl, J. Sarnthein, and O. Sürücü, "Interleaving deep brain stimulation for a patient with both Parkinson's disease and essential tremor," *Movement Disorders*, vol. 27, no. 13, pp. 1700-1701, 2012.

[28] C. Pollo, A. Kaelin-Lang, M. F. Oertel et al., "Directional deep brain stimulation: An intraoperative double-blind pilot study," *Brain*, vol. 137, no. 7, pp. 2015–2026, 2014.

[29] A. Peppe, A. Gasbarra, A. Stefani et al., "Deep brain stimulation of CM/PF of thalamus could be the new elective target for tremor in advanced Parkinson's Disease?" *Parkinsonism and Related Disorders*, vol. 14, no. 6, pp. 501–504, 2008.

[30] W. Thevathasan, T. J. Coyne, J. A. Hyam et al., "Pedunculopontine nucleus stimulation improves gait freezing in parkinson disease," *Neurosurgery*, vol. 69, no. 6, pp. 1248–1253, 2011.

[31] M. F. Contarino, L. J. Bour, R. Verhagen et al., "Directional steering: A novel approach to deep brain stimulation," *Neurology*, vol. 83, no. 13, pp. 1163–1169, 2014.

[32] F. Steigerwald, L. Müller, S. Johannes, C. Matthies, and J. Volkmann, "Directional deep brain stimulation of the subthalamic nucleus: A pilot study using a novel neurostimulation device," *Movement Disorders*, vol. 31, no. 8, pp. 1240–1243, 2016.

[33] C. B. Maks, C. R. Butson, B. L. Walter, J. L. Vitek, and C. C. McIntyre, "Deep brain stimulation activation volumes and their association with neurophysiological mapping and therapeutic outcomes," *Journal of Neurology, Neurosurgery and Psychiatry*, vol. 80, no. 6, pp. 659–666, 2009.

[34] M. Arlotti, M. Rosa, S. Marceglia, S. Barbieri, and A. Priori, "The adaptive deep brain stimulation challenge," *Parkinsonism and Related Disorders*, vol. 28, pp. 12–17, 2016.

[35] I. Basu, D. Graupe, D. Tuninetti et al., "Pathological tremor prediction using surface electromyogram and acceleration: Potential use in 'ON-OFF' demand driven deep brain stimulator design," *Journal of Neural Engineering*, vol. 10, no. 3, Article ID 036019, 2013.

[36] P. Brown, "Oscillatory nature of human basal ganglia activity: Relationship to the pathophysiology of parkinson's disease," *Movement Disorders*, vol. 18, no. 4, pp. 357–363, 2003.

[37] E. Florin, R. Erasmi, C. Reck et al., "Does increased gamma activity in patients suffering from Parkinson's disease counteract the movement inhibiting beta activity?" *Neuroscience*, vol. 237, pp. 42–50, 2013.

[38] A. Priori, G. Foffani, A. Pesenti et al., "Rhythm-specific pharmacological modulation of subthalamic activity in Parkinson's disease," *Experimental Neurology*, vol. 189, no. 2, pp. 369–379, 2004.

[39] A. Eusebio, W. Thevathasan, L. Doyle Gaynor et al., "Deep brain stimulation can suppress pathological synchronisation in parkinsonian patients," *Journal of Neurology, Neurosurgery and Psychiatry*, vol. 82, no. 5, pp. 569–573, 2011.

[40] G. Foffani, G. Ardolino, B. Meda et al., "Altered subthalamo-pallidal synchronisation in parkinsonian dyskinesias," *Journal of Neurology, Neurosurgery and Psychiatry*, vol. 76, no. 3, pp. 426–428, 2005.

[41] A. A. Kühn, A. Tsui, T. Aziz et al., "Pathological synchronisation in the subthalamic nucleus of patients with Parkinson's disease relates to both bradykinesia and rigidity," *Experimental Neurology*, vol. 215, no. 2, pp. 380–387, 2009.

[42] J. B. Toledo, J. López-Azcárate, D. Garcia-Garcia et al., "High beta activity in the subthalamic nucleus and freezing of gait in Parkinson's disease," *Neurobiology of Disease*, vol. 64, pp. 60–65, 2014.

[43] S. Little, A. Pogosyan, S. Neal et al., "Adaptive deep brain stimulation in advanced Parkinson disease," *Annals of Neurology*, vol. 74, no. 3, pp. 449–457, 2013.

[44] B. Rosin, M. Slovik, R. Mitelman et al., "Closed-loop deep brain stimulation is superior in ameliorating parkinsonism," *Neuron*, vol. 72, no. 2, pp. 370–384, 2011.

[45] C. De Hemptinne, N. C. Swann, J. L. Ostrem et al., "Therapeutic deep brain stimulation reduces cortical phase-amplitude coupling in Parkinson's disease," *Nature Neuroscience*, vol. 18, no. 5, pp. 779–786, 2015.

[46] L. Hofmann, M. Ebert, P. A. Tass, and C. Hauptmann, "Modified pulse shapes for effective neural stimulation," *Frontiers in Neuroengineering*, no. SEPTEMBER, pp. 1–10, 2011.

[47] T. J. Foutz and C. C. McIntyre, "Evaluation of novel stimulus waveforms for deep brain stimulation," *Journal of Neural Engineering*, vol. 7, no. 6, Article ID 066008, 2010.

[48] U. Akbar, R. S. Raike, N. Hack et al., "Randomized, Blinded Pilot Testing of Nonconventional Stimulation Patterns and Shapes in Parkinson's Disease and Essential Tremor: Evidence for Further Evaluating Narrow and Biphasic Pulses," *Neuromodulation*, vol. 19, no. 4, pp. 343–356, 2016.

[49] D. A. Heldman, C. L. Pulliam, E. Urrea Mendoza et al., "Computer-Guided Deep Brain Stimulation Programming for Parkinson's Disease," *Neuromodulation*, vol. 19, no. 2, pp. 127–131, 2016.

[50] C. L. Pulliam, D. A. Heldman, T. H. Orcutt, T. O. Mera, J. P. Giuffrida, and J. L. Vitek, "Motion sensor strategies for automated optimization of deep brain stimulation in Parkinson's disease," *Parkinsonism and Related Disorders*, vol. 21, no. 4, pp. 378–382, 2015.

[51] C. R. Butson, G. Tamm, S. Jain, T. Fogal, and J. Krüger, "Evaluation of interactive visualization on mobile computing platforms for selection of deep brain stimulation parameters," *IEEE Transactions on Visualization and Computer Graphics*, vol. 19, no. 1, pp. 108–117, 2013.

18

Bridging the Gaps in Patient Education for DBS Surgery in Parkinson's Disease

Colleen D. Knoop,[1] Robert Kadish,[2] Kathy Hager,[3] Michael C. Park,[4] Paul D. Loprinzi,[5] and Kathrin LaFaver[2]

[1]*Ochsner Health System, Division of Movement Disorders, 1514 Jefferson Highway, New Orleans, LA 70121, USA*
[2]*Department of Neurology, University of Louisville, 220 Abraham Flexner Way, Suite 606, Louisville, KY 40202, USA*
[3]*Bellarmine University, 2001 Newburg Road, Miles Hall 301, Louisville, KY 40205, USA*
[4]*Department of Neurosurgery and Neurology, University of Minnesota, 420 Delaware Street SE, MMC 96, Minneapolis, MN 55455, USA*
[5]*University of Mississippi, 229 Turner Center, Oxford, MS 38677, USA*

Correspondence should be addressed to Kathrin LaFaver; kathrin.lafaver@louisville.edu

Academic Editor: Jawad A. Bajwa

Introduction. Improvements in quality of life, tremor, and other motor features have been recognized as superior in patients with advanced Parkinson's disease (PD) treated with deep brain stimulation (DBS) surgery versus best medical therapy. We studied a group of patients with PD after undergoing DBS surgery in regard to expectations and satisfaction with DBS outcomes to determine gaps in patient education. *Methods.* This study was a retrospective, single academic center chart review and outcome questionnaire sent to patients with PD who had undergone DBS surgery between 2007 and 2014. *Results.* All patients surveyed indicated that benefit from DBS surgery met their overall expectations at least partially, but only 46.4% (*SE: 9.6%*) were in complete agreement. 3.6% (*SE: 3.6%*) of participants strongly disagreed that preoperative education prepared them adequately for the procedure and 17.9% (*SE: 7.4%*) only somewhat agreed. *Conclusions.* Our findings demonstrate that patients' expectations of DBS surgery in PD were at least partially met. However, there was a considerable percentage of patients who did not feel adequately prepared for the procedure. A structured, multidisciplinary team approach in educating PD patients throughout the different stages of DBS surgery may be helpful in optimizing patients' experience and satisfaction with surgery outcomes.

1. Introduction

Parkinson's disease (PD) is a progressive neurological disorder in which the cardinal signs are resting tremor, bradykinesia, rigidity, and loss of postural reflexes [1]. In 2002, the FDA approved deep brain stimulation (DBS) in the subthalamic nucleus (STN) for patients with levodopa-responsive PD [2]. The proposed mechanisms that explain the therapeutic benefit of DBS include local and network-wide electrical and neurochemical effects of stimulation, modulation of oscillatory activity, synaptic plasticity, neuroprotection, and neurogenesis [3–8]. Motor benefits have been documented as long as 10 years after implantation [9].

A good DBS surgical candidate is considered to be a patient with idiopathic PD and good response to levodopa, who is experiencing motor fluctuations, dyskinesias, or refractory tremor despite the best medical therapy and does not suffer from significant cognitive impairment. Prospective DBS candidates need to have an adequate understanding of expected benefits and possible adverse effects from DBS. This is best accomplished through a thorough educational process that spans the pre- to postoperative period. Few studies have been specifically conducted to explore the patient expectations and satisfaction from DBS surgery in relation to the education received by the multidisciplinary treatment team (neurosurgeon, movement disorder specialist, nurses, and neuropsychologists).

Multiple studies have addressed both motor and nonmotor quality-of-life issues after DBS surgery (see Appendix 1 in the Supplementary Material available online at https://doi.org/10.1155/2017/9360354) [10–15]. While motor aspects of PD consistently show improvement with DBS, changes in quality of life (QoL) and mental health are less frequently documented in the literature. Montel and Bungener [12] conducted a study comparing patients undergoing DBS surgery with the best medical therapy alone. The authors found that depression and anxiety were not significantly impacted by the type of therapy received. Those with DBS therapy scored higher in coping techniques, with no particular strategy showing significant differences. The DBS treatment group also experienced decreased QoL measures related to dysarthria.

Ferrara et al. [11] looked at health-related quality of life (HRQoL) and health satisfaction (HS) following DBS surgery. The findings revealed improvements in various HRQoL issues, especially motor function and independence measures. Life satisfaction following DBS did not improve perceived function at work, personal relationships, leisure activities, or living conditions. Social, emotional, and cognitive factors tended to be better predictors of quality of life. Following DBS, energy level and life enjoyment improved significantly. The authors suggested studying HRQoL and HS in subsequent studies, focusing on the enhancement of the patient selection process and consideration of predictive clinical variables.

In a study by Lezcano et al. [13], patients were followed up for five years following DBS surgery. The overall QoL was found to be significantly improved one year after surgery but regressed back to baseline at five years in most measures. Floden et al. [10] retrospectively studied the predictability of QoL measures in 85 patients after STN DBS. They found that QoL improved on 39-item PD questionnaire (PDQ-39) measures for motor function, mood, and self-consciousness but not for speech, cognitive function, and hallucinations. Patients who reported reduced QoL before surgery did not experience a significant increase in QoL after surgery. The authors concluded that DBS increases or preserves QoL in most patients. Hasegawa et al. [16] studied the correlation between patient expectations with satisfaction and outcomes in STN DBS for PD and concluded that pre- and postoperative expectations may play an important role in patient satisfaction and overall success of STN DBS.

The goal of our study was to determine the degree to which patients' expectations from DBS surgery were met postoperatively. Additionally, we sought to gain information that could aid in improving patient education for DBS and creating a patient-centered experience.

2. Methods

A retrospective, single academic center study was conducted to evaluate patients' postoperative expectations of DBS. The study was IRB-approved and followed ethical guidelines. A twenty-seven-item questionnaire was developed (Appendix 2 in the Supplementary Material) and administered to patients and a retrospective chart review was performed. Study subjects were identified by using billing codes for PD and DBS from 2007 to 2014. Fifty-two patients were contacted. Patients who had devices removed for any reason were

TABLE 1: Patient demographics and clinical characteristics.

Gender	21 M/8 F
Race	100% Caucasian
Disease duration (mean ± SD)	15.1 ± 8.59 years
Age at surgery (mean ± SD)	66.8 ± 10.8 years
Education	43% high school/GED 43% associates degree or higher
DBS targets	STN bilateral 62.1% STN unilateral 17.4% GPi bilateral 13.8% VIM unilateral 6.9%

included, regardless of whether they had been reimplanted or not. Initially, patients were recruited via mail. The questionnaire was designed to evaluate patients' expectations, preoperative education, and overall satisfaction with DBS surgery. Most items were evaluated using a Likert scale, but several free response questions were included. Patients' charts were reviewed to identify documentation about DBS education. Additional information gathered included gender, date of birth, education level, ethnicity, age at symptom onset, age at PD diagnosis, age at implant(s), most troublesome symptom(s) prompting DBS, and implanted target area of the brain. Analysis of data was done with STATA, version 12.

3. Results

Among the 52 questionnaires mailed, 32 were returned and 29 were included in the analysis, yielding a response rate of 55.8%. One survey was returned unanswered. One subject was excluded from analysis as chart review revealed a diagnosis of essential tremor, rather than PD. The age at DBS surgery ranged from 36 to 86 years with a mean of 66.8 (SD: 10.8) years (Table 1). The majority of patients were males (71%) and the range of disease duration was 2–32 years with a mean of 15.1 (SD: 8.6) years.

The most commonly cited symptoms from the patients' perspective prompting consideration for DBS were tremor (79.3%), dyskinesias (24.1%), and rigidity (13.8%). Another 6.9% of patients reported inadequate on-time and complex medication schedules. Other reasons cited for seeking DBS surgery included walking problems (10.3%), reduced quality of life (10.3%), balance problems (3.4%), freezing of gait (3.4%), and impaired handwriting (3.4%). When participants were asked to identify their sources of DBS education, 96.4% indicated having received information from the provider managing their PD, 60.7% from the neurosurgeon, 46.4% from industry device representatives, 14.3% from nurses or other ancillary staff members, 46.4% from the Internet, and 14.3% from other sources (i.e., support groups, seminars).

71.4% of the participants reported having been asked about their expectations from DBS prior to surgery; however, a discussion of patient expectations was only documented in medical charts in 48.3%. Postoperatively, 100% of subjects were in at least some agreement that their expectations

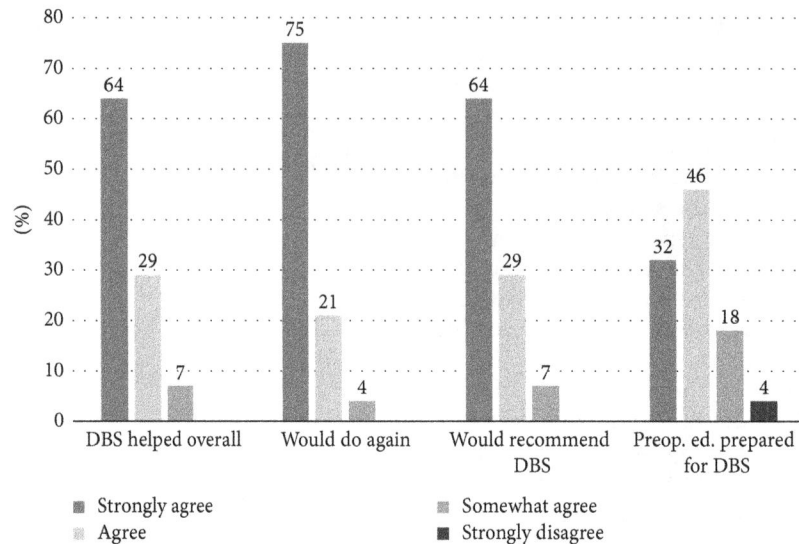

FIGURE 1: Patient satisfaction with DBS outcomes and preoperative education.

TABLE 2: Percentage of patients having their motor expectations met after DBS surgery.

Symptom (% of any agreement)	Strongly agree % (SE)	Agree % (SE)	Somewhat agree % (SE)	Neither agree nor disagree % (SE)	Somewhat disagree % (SE)	Disagree % (SE)	Strongly disagree % (SE)	N/A % (SE)
Tremor N = 29 (82)	61 (9.0)	14 (7.0)	7.0 (5.0)	0	0	0	0	18 (7.0)
Rigidity N = 29 (82)	32 (9.0)	29 (9.0)	21 (8.0)	4.0 (4.0)	4.0 (4.0)	0	0	10 (6.0)
Slowness N = 29 (75)	29 (9.0)	21 (8.0)	25 (8.0)	7.0 (5.0)	4.0 (4.0)	7.0 (5.0)	0	7.0 (5.0)
On-time N = 28 (85)	39 (9.0)	25 (8.0)	21 (8.0)	11 (1.1)	0	0	0	4.0 (4.0)
Dyskinesia N = 29 (82)	36 (9.0)	25 (8.0)	21 (8.0)	7.0 (5.0)	0	0	0	10 (6.0)
Dystonia N = 29 (62)	21 (8.0)	29 (9.0)	18 (7.0)	7.0 (5.0)	0	0	0	25 (8.0)

from DBS surgery were met. More specifically, 46.4% (SE: 9.6%) strongly agreed, 39.3% agreed (SE: 9.4%), and 14.3% (SE: 6.7%) somewhat agreed. Furthermore, 100% of patients surveyed agreed that DBS was overall helpful with 64.3% (SE: 9.2%) in strong agreement, 28.6% (SE: 8.7%) in agreement, and 7.1% (SE: 5%) somewhat in agreement. 100% of participants would elect to undergo DBS surgery again, with 75% (SE: 8.3%) in strong agreement, 21.4% (SE: 7.9%) in agreement, and 3.6% (SE: 3.6%) in some agreement. Similarly, 100% of participants would recommend DBS to someone else with PD, with 64.3% (SE: 9.2%) in strong agreement, 28.6% (SE: 8.7%) in agreement, and 7.1% (SE: 5%) in some agreement. When asked whether preoperative education prepared them adequately about the limitations of DBS, 32.1% (SE: 8.9%) strongly agreed, 46.4% (SE: 9.6%) agreed, 17.9% (SE: 7.4%) somewhat agreed, and 3.6% (SE: 3.6%) strongly disagreed (Figure 1).

We also investigated the level to which DBS outcomes met patients' expectations for improvement of various PD symptoms. Expectations were defined as met if the participants strongly agreed, agreed, or somewhat agreed. Overall, patients felt their expectations of symptom improvement were met by DBS (Table 2). Specifically, 82% of patients agreed that their expectations were met for improvement of tremor, rigidity, and dyskinesias, 75% for improvement of bradykinesia, 85% for improvement of "on-time," and 68% for dystonia.

Table 3 shows data on pre- and postoperative patient expectations across all symptoms and the degree to which expectations were met. Reduction of tremor was identified as the expected outcome by 75% of participants, yet this was only documented in 34.5% of reviewed charts. 79.3% of the participants reported that their expectation for tremor improvement was met. Medication reduction was documented as an expected outcome in 31% of chart reviews,

TABLE 3: A comparison of pre- and postoperative patient expectations from DBS surgery. Expectations listed under "A" are deemed realistic expectations with good chances for improvement following DBS surgery. Reducing PD medications ("B") following DBS surgery is a realistic expectation depending on the target for electrode placement. Symptoms listed under "C" may or may not improve following DBS surgery.

	Feature	Preop. expectation documented N = 14 % (SE)	Desired expectation for having DBS N = 29 % (SE)	Expectation met N = 28 % (SE)	Expectation somewhat met N = 28 % (SE)	Expectation not met N = 28 % (SE)
A	Tremor	35 (9.0)	75 (8.3)	79 (7.7)	3.4 (3.4)	—
	Rigidity	10 (5.8)	8.8 (7.4)	10 (5.8)	—	3.4 (3.4)
	Slowness	—	7.1 (5.0)	3.4 (3.4)	3.4 (3.4)	—
	On-time	21 (7.7)	21 (7.9)	17 (7.1)	3.4 (3.4)	—
	Dyskinesias	17 (7.1)	18 (7.4)	21 (7.7)	3.4 (3.4)	—
	Dystonia	3.4 (3.4)	7.1 (5.0)	3.4 (3.4)	3.4 (3.4)	—
B	Reduce medications	31 (8.7)	21 (7.9)	14 (6.5)	3.4 (3.4)	3.4 (3.4)
C	Sleep	10 (5.8)	3.6 (3.6)	3.4 (3.4)	—	—
	Freezing of gait	6.9 (4.8)	3.6 (3.6)	—	—	—
	Speech	—	3.6 (3.6)	—	—	3.4 (3.4)
	Balance	3.4 (3.4)	3.6 (3.6)	—	—	3.4 (3.4)
	Walking	6.9 (4.8)	14 (6.7)	6.9 (4.8)	—	10 (5.8)
	Writing	—	11 (6.0)	14 (6.5)	—	—
	QoL	—	21 (7.9)	17 (7.1)	—	3.4 (3.4)
	Reduce pain	—	7.1 (5.0)	—	3.4 (3.4)	3.4 (3.4)
	Eat w/utensils	—	3.6 (3.6)	6.9 (4.8)	—	—
	Use tools	—	—	—	3.4 (3.4)	—
	Improve PD	—	11 (6.0)	6.9 (4.8)	3.4 (3.4)	—
	Ride bike	—	3.6 (3.6)	3.4 (3.4)	—	—
	Use of arm	—	3.6 (3.6)	3.4 (3.4)	—	—
	Normal life	—	3.6 (3.6)	3.4 (3.4)	—	—
	Other	24 (8.1)	3.6 (3.6)	3.4 (3.4)	—	—

while 21.4% identified this as a desired expectation of DBS on the questionnaire. This expectation was met in 13.8%, whereas 3.4% reported that the expectation was somewhat met, and 3.4% did not have their expectation met. Other patient expectations were felt to be more problematic (C in Table 3), such as improvements in sleep which was cited by 10.3% of participants. In summary, we identified considerable discrepancies in documentations of expected symptom improvements per chart review with patient self-reported expectations on retrospective questionnaire as well as the absence of consistent documentation of patient expectations in medical charts.

4. Discussion

The aim of this study was to determine whether patient expectations from DBS surgery in PD were met and to identify gaps in patient education. Data from patient outcome questionnaires showed that a majority of patients (79%) listed tremor as the main reason for pursuing DBS, a symptom that is highly associated with improvement after surgery [17]. Over 96% of the study participants noted that they received DBS education by a PD specialist, but far fewer (61%) recalled

having received education from a neurosurgeon. Frequently, patients sought education on their own, with 46% reporting education from Internet sources. While the lower reported rate of education by neurosurgeons may be related to less time spent with the patient throughout the process, it highlights an area for improvement, especially considering the possibility of surgical complications [18]. The large portion of patients receiving information from the Internet highlights the need for providers to guide patients towards reliable sources for information online. A considerable discrepancy between documentation of preoperative patient expectations in charts compared to patient reports of having discussed expectation with providers indicates a need for improvements in documentation of DBS education and following a standard format for this purpose.

Overall, patients had high satisfaction with DBS outcomes and 100% of the participants in our study were in at least partial agreement that their postoperative expectations for DBS surgery were met. Although 96% of the participants were in at least partial agreement when asked whether preoperative education prepared them for DBS surgery, 3.6% strongly disagreed, suggesting a need to optimize the educational process for DBS surgery.

Breit et al. [19] described unmet patient expectations as adverse DBS effects, negatively affecting the stimulation therapy. This is of special concern if the primary patient goals from surgery are not deemed realistic. Family members may also have unrealistic expectations that should be addressed whenever possible. Some patients or families may have unrealistic goals sparked as a result of media depictions of DBS or making generalizations from outcomes observed on other patients [20, 21].

Clinical practice guidelines state that patient education should begin early in the preoperative evaluation process. What can realistically be expected from surgery should be described [17]. Thorough preoperative education should be mandatory, including potential surgical complications [18]. Patients and medical providers should clearly document patient expectations, so that this can be reviewed postoperatively for a more meaningful assessment of goal attainment [22].

As well documented in the literature, most motor symptoms show improvement after DBS surgery. In our sample, 62 to 82% of patients had their expectations of motor-symptom improvements met. Of note, "slowness," for which 11% of patients disagreed about any improvements postoperatively, is a broad encompassing symptom that may have different meanings. It may be interpreted both in a psychosocial context and in relation to axial signs, which have been documented to relate to dissatisfaction with DBS, especially if present preoperatively [23]. Medication reduction, which often can be accomplished especially after STN-DBS [9, 13, 18, 24], was an expectation that was met for the majority of patients. Expectations for improvement in nonmotor symptoms such as sleep, gait freezing, and handwriting were relatively infrequently mentioned in our survey which likely reflects adequate patient education about the uncertainty of expected benefits from DBS for these symptoms.

Our study has several limitations. This is a retrospective study with a relatively small sample size collected over a seven-year period. Our survey instrument was not evaluated for reliability or validity and was developed as there are currently no established scales to measure patient expectation and satisfaction from DBS surgery. Different practitioners provided the patient with education and documentation in charts was lacking in many instances. There was no protocol in place for a standardized approach to patient education on DBS surgery. The study was performed at a single institution and may not reflect experience with DBS patient education at other centers.

5. Conclusions

Despite overall satisfaction in our patient sample with outcomes from DBS, patient expectations should be further explored in a systematic manner. We found considerable discrepancies of documented patient education versus patient reported education on expected symptom improvement. Patient education on DBS should be improved and follow a standardized protocol, ideally involving a multidisciplinary team. Involvement of a nurse educator, a DBS support group, and tailored information over several visits may assist patients in reaching realistic expectations about surgery outcomes and improving their overall satisfaction with DBS surgery. Additional longitudinal studies are needed to further understand the patient-centered experience.

Disclosure

This study has previously been presented as a poster presentation at Ochsner Medical Center and was the capstone project for the doctoral degree in nursing for Colleen D. Knoop, DNP, APRN.

Acknowledgments

The authors would like to thank all the patients and involved family members for participating in this study.

References

[1] J. Jankovic, "Parkinson's disease: Clinical features and diagnosis," *Journal of Neurology, Neurosurgery and Psychiatry*, vol. 79, no. 4, pp. 368–376, 2008.

[2] R. J. Coffey, "Deep brain stimulation devices: A brief technical history and review," *Artificial Organs*, vol. 33, no. 3, pp. 208–220, 2009.

[3] M. Filali, W. D. Hutchison, V. N. Palter, A. M. Lozano, and J. O. Dostrovsky, "Stimulation-induced inhibition of neuronal firing in human subthalamic nucleus," *Experimental Brain Research*, vol. 156, no. 3, pp. 274–281, 2004.

[4] S. Maesawa, Y. Kaneoke, Y. Kajita et al., "Long-term stimulation of the subthalamic nucleus in hemiparkinsonian rats: Neuroprotection of dopaminergic neurons," *Journal of Neurosurgery*, vol. 100, no. 4, pp. 679–687, 2004.

[5] B. Piallat, A. Benazzouz, and A. L. Benabid, "Subthalamic nucleus lesion in rats prevents dopaminergic nigral neuron degeneration after striatal 6-OHDA injection: Behavioural and immunohistochemical studies," *European Journal of Neuroscience*, vol. 8, no. 7, pp. 1408–1414, 1996.

[6] K.-Z. Shen, Z.-T. Zhu, A. Munhall, and S. W. Johnson, "Synaptic Plasticity in Rat Subthalamic Nucleus Induced by High-Frequency Stimulation," *Synapse*, vol. 50, no. 4, pp. 314–319, 2003.

[7] M.-L. Welter, J.-L. Houeto, A.-M. Bonnet et al., "Effects of High-Frequency Stimulation on Subthalamic Neuronal Activity in Parkinsonian Patients," *Archives of Neurology*, vol. 61, no. 1, pp. 89–96, 2004.

[8] A. Zaidel, A. Spivak, B. Grieb, H. Bergman, and Z. Israel, "Subthalamic span of β oscillations predicts deep brain stimulation efficacy for patients with Parkinson's disease," *Brain*, vol. 133, no. 7, pp. 2007–2021, 2010.

[9] A. Castrioto, A. M. Lozano, Y.-Y. Poon, A. E. Lang, M. Fallis, and E. Moro, "Ten-year outcome of subthalamic stimulation in Parkinson disease: A blinded evaluation," *Archives of Neurology*, vol. 68, no. 12, pp. 1550–1556, 2011.

[10] D. Floden, S. E. Cooper, S. D. Griffith, and A. G. Machado, "Predicting quality of life outcomes after subthalamic nucleus deep brain stimulation," *Neurology*, vol. 83, no. 18, pp. 1627–1633, 2014.

[11] J. Ferrara et al., "Impact of STN-DBS on life and health satisfaction in patients with Parkinson's disease," *Journal of Neurology, Neurosurgery & Psychiatry*, vol. 81, no. 3, pp. 315–319, 2009.

[12] S. R. Montel and C. Bungener, "Coping and quality of life of patients with Parkinson disease who have undergone deep brain stimulation of the subthalamic nucleus," *Surgical Neurology*, vol. 72, no. 2, pp. 105–110, 2009.

[13] E. Lezcano, J. C. Gómez-Esteban, B. Tijero et al., "Long-term impact on quality of life of subthalamic nucleus stimulation in Parkinson's disease," *Journal of Neurology*, vol. 263, no. 5, pp. 895–905, 2016.

[14] C. S. Kubu et al., "Insights gleaned by measuring patients' stated goals for DBS: More than tremor," *Neurology*, vol. 88, no. 2, pp. 124–130, 2017.

[15] G.-M. Hariz, P. Limousin, and K. Hamberg, ""dBS means everything - For some time". Patients' perspectives on daily life with deep brain stimulation for Parkinson's disease," *Journal of Parkinson's Disease*, vol. 6, no. 2, pp. 335–347, 2016.

[16] H. Hasegawa, M. Samuel, A. Douiri, and K. Ashkan, "Patients' expectations in subthalamic nucleus deep brain stimulation surgery for Parkinson disease," *World Neurosurgery*, vol. 82, no. 6, pp. 1295–1299.E2, 2014.

[17] C. Ward, S. Heath, V. Janovsky, E. Lanier, R. Franks, and S. O'Connor, *Care of the movement disorder patient with deep brain stimulation: AANN clinical practice guideline series*, 2009.

[18] J. M. Bronstein, M. Tagliati, R. L. Alterman et al., "Deep brain stimulation for Parkinson disease an expert consensus and review of key issues," *Archives of Neurology*, vol. 68, no. 2, pp. 165–171, 2011.

[19] S. Breit, J. B. Schulz, and A.-L. Benabid, "Deep brain stimulation," *Cell and Tissue Research*, vol. 318, no. 1, pp. 275–288, 2004.

[20] M. K. Sanghera, M. J. Desaloms, and M. R. Stewart, "High-Frequency stimulation of the subthalamic nucleus for the treatment of Parkinson's disease-a team perspective," *Journal of Neuroscience Nursing*, vol. 36, no. 6, pp. 301–311, 2004.

[21] R. J. Uitti, "Surgical treatments for Parkinson's disease," *Can Fam Physician*, vol. 46, pp. 368–373, 2000.

[22] W. J. Marks, *Deep Brain Stimulation Management*, Cambridge University Press, Cambridge, NY, USA, 2011.

[23] F. Maier, C. J. Lewis, N. Horstkoetter et al., "Subjective perceived outcome of subthalamic deep brain stimulation in Parkinson's disease one year after surgery," *Parkinsonism and Related Disorders*, vol. 24, pp. 41–47, 2016.

[24] M. Piper, G. M. Abrams, and W. J. Marks Jr., "Deep brain stimulation for the treatment of Parkinson's disease: overview and impact on gait and mobility," *NeuroRehabilitation*, vol. 20, no. 3, pp. 223–232, 2005.

19

Physiotherapy in Parkinson's Disease: Building ParkinsonNet in Czechia

Ota Gal,[1] Martin Srp,[1] Romana Konvalinkova,[1] Martina Hoskovcova,[1] Vaclav Capek,[2] Jan Roth,[1] and Evzen Ruzicka[1]

[1]Department of Neurology and Centre of Clinical Neuroscience, First Faculty of Medicine and General University Hospital, Charles University in Prague, Katerinska 30, 128 21 Prague, Czech Republic
[2]Applied Neurosciences and Brain Imaging, National Institute of Mental Health, Topolova 748, 250 67 Klecany, Czech Republic

Correspondence should be addressed to Ota Gal; ota.gal@vfn.cz

Academic Editor: Jan Aasly

Objective. We conducted a questionnaire survey to investigate the availability and quality of physiotherapy (PT) for Parkinson's disease (PD). *Background.* Despite evidence about the benefits of PT, there is no data regarding its use in Czechia. *Methods.* Questionnaires were sent to 368 PD patients seen in a single movement disorders centre within two years (inclusion criteria: idiopathic PD, Hoehn and Yahr stage <5, and residence in Prague) and to 211 physical therapists (PTs) registered in Prague. The patient questionnaire evaluated limitations in 6 core areas and in activities of daily living and inquired about experience with PT. The PTs questionnaire evaluated knowledge about PD, number of PD patients treated yearly, and details of therapy. *Results.* Questionnaires were returned by 248 patients and 157 PTs. PT was prescribed to 70/248 patients. The effects were satisfactory in 79% and lasted >3 months in 60/64. About half of the PTs have no experience with PD patients, 26% reported <3, and 5% see >10 yearly. The most widely used techniques were neurodevelopmental treatments. *Conclusion.* Present PD healthcare model in Czechia is suboptimal (low PT prescription, non-evidence-based PT). Implementation of European PT Guidelines for PD and the introduction of an efficient model of care are needed.

1. Introduction

The prevalence of Parkinson's disease (PD) is increasing [1, 2], paralleled by growing healthcare expenses [3]. PD is a complex disorder, for which interprofessional care is appropriate [3–6]. Despite increasing evidence about the benefits of physiotherapy [7–15], detailed insight into the current provision of physiotherapy, as well as barriers and facilitators for optimal care, is lacking in Czechia. However, the Dutch model for Community Healthcare is available and has proven both being cost effective and providing greater patient satisfaction [16, 17]. The authors of this model have developed stepwise recommendations for the application of such model in other countries [3]. As the first step they recommend gaining insight into current healthcare, that is, patient utilization, and satisfaction with provided allied healthcare as well as allied healthcare provider's expertise and volume of PD patients treated. Moreover, this healthcare model is recommended

by the European Physiotherapy Guideline for PD (EPGPD) [9], which is binding for Czechia, and the Czech Union of Physical therapist (UNIFY) took part in their development. Consequently, we conducted a questionnaire survey to investigate the quality and availability of physiotherapy for PD patients in Czechia based on previously published studies [18, 19].

2. Methods

Questionnaires approved by the Ethics Committee of General University Hospital in Prague were sent to 368 PD patients seen in April 2013–April 2015 in our department. Inclusion criteria were idiopathic PD, Hoehn and Yahr stage <5, and residence in Prague. The questionnaire evaluated the patients' limitations in activities of daily living (PADLS) [20], frequency of falls, limitations in 6 core areas (gait, transfers, manual dexterity, stability and falls, posture, and physical condition), their relative importance to the patient, and the patient's motivation to improve in them. Patients, who were referred to a physiotherapist (PT) because of PD, were also asked about the specifics of the therapy. Finally they were asked to estimate the time willing to travel to a PT specialized in PD.

A second questionnaire was delivered to 211 PTs working in a central district of Prague (Prague 2). PTs were first asked to provide details on their involvement in the healthcare system, years of experience, knowledge, interest, and education in PD treatment. Questions related to the PTs' knowledge about PD treatment addressed physiotherapy, occupational therapy, speech therapy, nursing, and neurological care. Consequently the questionnaire evaluated number of PD patients treated yearly, most frequent reasons for referral and medical specialization of the referring physician. Also, PTs were asked to provide opinion on the rightfulness of referral, on the importance of individual core areas, on the quality of communication in their team, and on most important barriers in the improvement of PD specific healthcare in Czechia. Details on the provided physiotherapy were required.

Responses from both questionnaires were, due to their nature, analysed using nonparametric statistical methods. Ordinal variables were compared among groups using a Mann-Whitney U test in case of comparisons of two groups and using a Kruskal-Wallis ANOVA in case of more than two groups. Categorical variables were subject to contingency tables and a Fisher exact test of independence in contingency tables. For expressing a relation of two ordinal variables, a Spearman correlation coefficient was evaluated. Moreover, a factor and cluster analyses were performed; details of these two methods are given in a text further. p values less than 0.05 were considered as statistically significant. Analyses were conducted using R statistical package, version 3.2.3.

3. Results

Questionnaires were returned by 248 patients and 157 PTs. Not all questionnaires were completely filled, so the sample size differs in some questions. Patients reported no or mild difficulties in ADL in 59% (147/248) and a high level of difficulties or extreme difficulties in 19% (47/248). Nearly 20% (48/247) were repeat fallers and 30% (73/247) very frequent fallers [21], while 38% (94/247) reported no falls in the last year. Impairment in all core areas, as well as the motivation to improve, referral to physiotherapy because of the respective core areas, and the marked average order of importance of the core areas are given in Table 1. Only 28% of the patients had experience with physiotherapy prescribed because of PD (Figure 1(a)). These patients reported at least partial satisfaction with the quality of explanation of the possibilities of physiotherapy by the referring physician in nearly 96% and sufficient satisfaction with the explanation by a PT in nearly 60%. The quality of explanation by physicians and by PTs was the same ($p = 0.078$, Spearman's correlation coefficient $\rho = 0.413$, $p = 0.000$). On a subjective scale from 0 (no benefit) to 10 (maximal benefit) the median of the effect of the therapy was 5 (IQR 3–7) with the effect that lasted less than one month in 25%, 3 months in 38%,

6 months in 12%, and one year in 16%. In 9% the patients felt no effect (Figure 1(b)). The overall expected duration of the effect was 4.9 months. The patients' expectations were rather or completely met in 79%. Mean of the time patients are willing to spend travelling to a PT specialist was estimated to be 36 minutes (for details see Figure 1(c)).

A factor analysis was used to analyse all answers related to impairment in core areas, answers related to patients' will to improve and the number of falls in the last year. The main goal of a factor analysis is to reveal and calculate hidden or not directly measured factor/factors that influence behaviour of the subjects. The analysis was performed with an Ordinary Least Squares factoring method and a Varimax rotation. It showed that the patients' answers were determined by two factors, actual impairment and will to improve. These factors explain 57% of the variability of the data. The will to travel far to a PD specialized PT diminishes with severity of impairment ($p = 0.000$) but increases with will to improve ($p = 0.000$). We also showed correlation of time willing to spend travelling to a PT specialist with PADLS ($\rho = -0.372$, $p = 0.000$). Patients who had high level of difficulties or extreme difficulties in ADL were willing to travel 13 minutes, while those with no or moderate difficulties were willing to travel 41 minutes.

A cluster analysis was performed to find and describe groups of patients that are somehow similar in their actual impairment and will to improve. We used a K-Means Clustering method and showed that our patients could be divided into three not particularly distinct groups: (1) patients with both above average impairment and will to improve, (2) patients with below average impairment but above average will to improve, and (3) patients with both below average impairment and will to improve (Figure 2).

PTs that filled the second questionnaire were in 58% involved in hospital care, were relatively equally distributed in groups according to years of experience, and claimed to have interest in PD in 70%. This interest depends on number of PD patients treated yearly ($p = 0.003$) but does not depend on the length of PTs' practice ($p = 0.310$) or their knowledge about PD ($p = 0.262$). In 93% they did not attend any PD specialized course. PTs marked their knowledge about physiotherapy in PD as substandard in 25%, standard in 63%, and above standard in 13%. The situation in case of PD specific occupational therapy, speech therapy, nursing, and neurological care was similar, but slightly more shifted towards substandard knowledge. Generally, knowledge about these forms of PD care strongly correlated with knowledge about physiotherapy in PD ($p = 0.000$ in all cases). The attendance of a PD specific physiotherapy course did not correlate with increased knowledge about PD ($p = 0.362$). PTs reported in 52% that they see no PD patients per year and in 26% less than 3 and only 5% of them take care of more than 10. The mean estimate of PD patients treated yearly was for this group 2.63. The number of PD patients treated yearly correlated with knowledge about PD ($p = 0.000$). Those PTs in our group who treat at least 3 PD patients yearly had significantly greater interest in PD ($p = 0.003$). PTs reported similar referral rates from neurologists, rehabilitation physicians, and geriatrists ($p = 0.073$). Most frequent reasons for referral and

TABLE 1: Selected data from the PD patients and PT's questionnaires.

	Gait	Transfers	Manual dexterity	Stability and falls	Posture	Physical condition
Importance (patient opinion): average order ($n = 248$)	1.91	3.35	3.71	3.56	4.43	3.99
Importance (PT opinion): average order ($n = 91$)	2.22	2.95	4.13	2.25	4.85	4.60
Most frequent reasons for referral ($n = 92$)	25% ($n = 58$)	3.45% ($n = 8$)	6.03% ($n = 14$)	27.59% ($n = 64$)	16.38% ($n = 38$)	10.78% ($n = 25$)
Limitations	$n = 248$	$n = 248$	$n = 248$	$n = 248$	$n = 248$	$n = 248$
(i) No difficulties	(i) 4.8% ($n = 12$)	(i) 14.1% ($n = 35$)	(i) 8.5% ($n = 21$)	(i) 17.7% ($n = 44$)	(i) 10.1% ($n = 25$)	(i) 10.1% ($n = 25$)
(ii) Mild difficulties	(ii) 24.6% ($n = 61$)	(ii) 22.6% ($n = 56$)	(ii) 31.0% ($n = 77$)	(ii) 35.1% ($n = 87$)	(ii) 31.0% ($n = 77$)	(ii) 23.4% ($n = 58$)
(iii) Moderate difficulties	(iii) 37.5% ($n = 93$)	(iii) 36.3% ($n = 90$)	(iii) 36.7% ($n = 91$)	(iii) 19.0% ($n = 47$)	(iii) 35.5% ($n = 88$)	(iii) 35.9% ($n = 89$)
(iv) Severe difficulties	(iv) 21.4% ($n = 53$)	(iv) 19.3% ($n = 48$)	(iv) 17.3% ($n = 43$)	(iv) 16.9% ($n = 42$)	(iv) 18.6% ($n = 46$)	(iv) 18.5% ($n = 46$)
(v) Extreme difficulties	(v) 11.7% ($n = 29$)	(v) 7.7% ($n = 19$)	(v) 6.5% ($n = 16$)	(v) 11.3% ($n = 28$)	(v) 4.8 ($n = 12$)	(v) 12.1% ($n = 30$)
Motivation to improve	$n = 248$	$n = 248$	$n = 247$	$n = 248$	$n = 248$	$n = 248$
(i) No interest	(i) 2.8% ($n = 7$)	(i) 5.6% ($n = 14$)	(i) 2.0% ($n = 5$)	(i) 7.3% ($n = 18$)	(i) 6.4% ($n = 16$)	(i) 3.6% ($n = 9$)
(ii) Slight interest	(ii) 0.4% ($n = 1$)	(ii) 1.2% ($n = 3$)	(ii) 0.8% ($n = 2$)	(ii) 0.8% ($n = 2$)	(ii) 1.6% ($n = 4$)	(ii) 0.4% ($n = 1$)
(iii) Neutral	(iii) 12.1% ($n = 30$)	(iii) 11.7% ($n = 29$)	(iii) 13.8% ($n = 34$)	(iii) 10.9% ($n = 27$)	(iii) 9.7% ($n = 24$)	(iii) 9.3% ($n = 23$)
(iv) Rather interested	(iv) 19.8% ($n = 49$)	(iv) 21.8% ($n = 54$)	(iv) 19.0% ($n = 47$)	(iv) 19.7% ($n = 49$)	(iv) 18.2% ($n = 45$)	(iv) 22.6% ($n = 56$)
(v) Interested	(v) 64.9% ($n = 161$)	(v) 59.7% ($n = 148$)	(v) 64.4% ($n = 159$)	(v) 61.3% ($n = 152$)	(v) 64.1% ($n = 159$)	(v) 64.1% ($n = 159$)
Referral to PT	$n = 248$	$n = 248$	$n = 248$	$n = 248$	$n = 248$	$n = 248$
(i) Yes	(i) 20.6% ($n = 51$)	(i) 17.7% ($n = 44$)	(i) 13.7% ($n = 34$)	(i) 15.7% ($n = 39$)	(i) 16.9% ($n = 42$)	(i) 14.1% ($n = 35$)
(ii) No	(ii) 79.4% ($n = 197$)	(ii) 82.3% ($n = 204$)	(ii) 86.3% ($n = 214$)	(ii) 84.3% ($n = 209$)	(ii) 83.1% ($n = 206$)	(ii) 85.9% ($n = 213$)

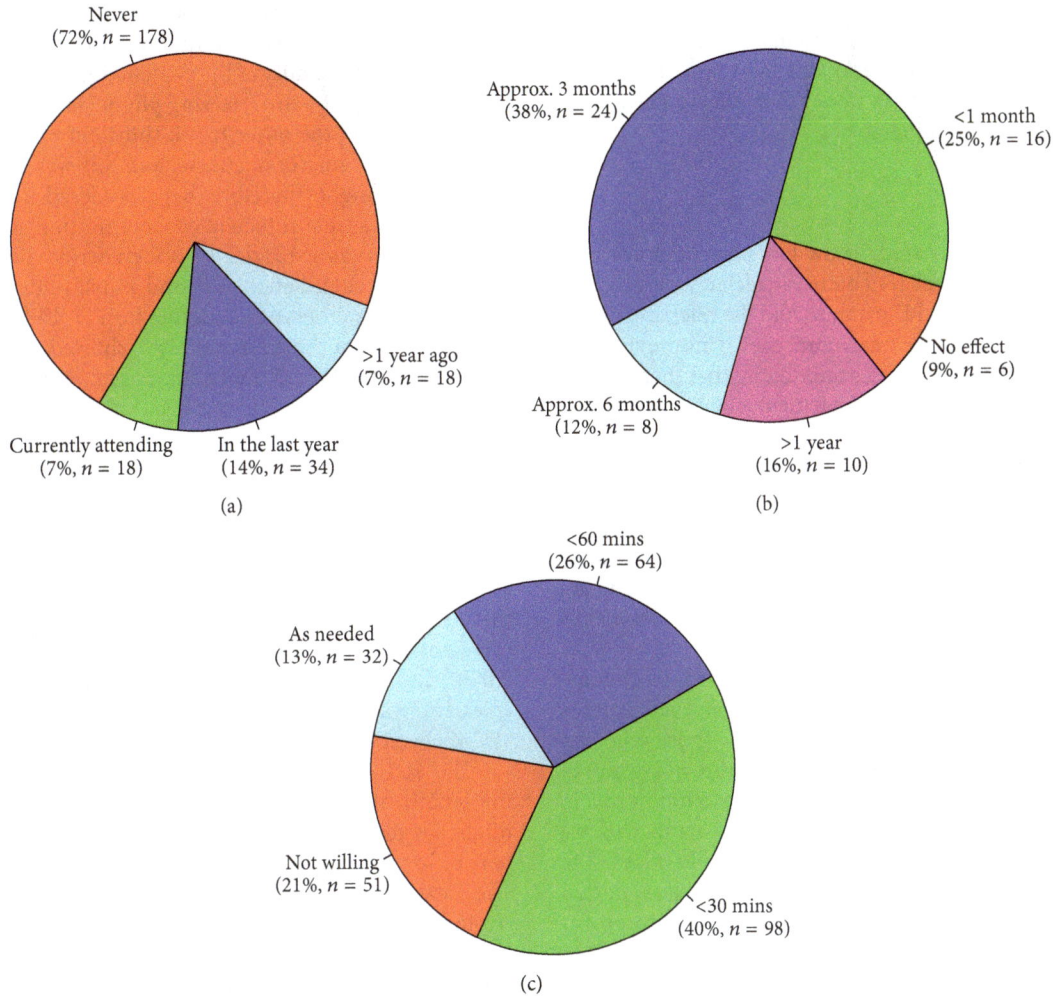

FIGURE 1: (a) Experience with PD specific physiotherapy ($n = 248$). (b) Duration of the effect of physiotherapy ($n = 64$). (c) Time patients are willing to travel to PT ($n = 245$).

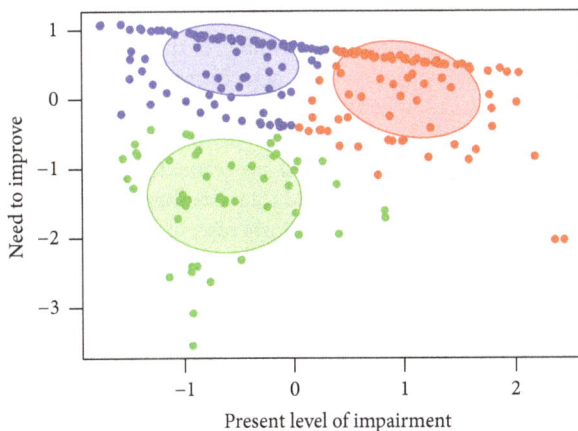

FIGURE 2

the average order of importance of the core areas for patients are given in Table 1. PTs do not value all core areas the same ($p = 0.000$). The comparison of the order of importance of the core areas as reported by PTs, PD patients, and the referring physicians (based on the reported reason of referral; see Table 1) showed significant differences in priorities of all three groups ($p = 0.000$).

PTs found the communication in their team rather adequate or adequate in 53% and 31% of them marked the small amount of PD patients treated yearly as the most important barrier in the improvement of PD specific healthcare in the Czech Republic, followed by insufficient communication between healthcare professionals in 24%. The median of the length of therapy provided was 30 minutes (IQR 30–45) and the median of the total number of therapy sessions was eight (IQR 6.25–10). The length and total number of therapy did not correlate with PD specific physiotherapy course attendance ($p = 0.438$ and $p = 0.882$, resp.). Neither did they correlate with the PTs' knowledge about physiotherapy in PD ($p = 0.544$ and $p = 0.723$, resp.). PTs work with PD patients individually in 82% which correlated neither with knowledge about physiotherapy in PD ($p = 1.000$), nor with PD specific physiotherapy course attendance ($p = 0.400$). The most widely used physiotherapy techniques were neurodevelopmental treatments (NDTs) like the Bobath concept or Proprioceptive neuromuscular facilitation in 20%, followed by gait training (in 11%) and soft tissue therapy (in 10%). Techniques used by PTs were not related to knowledge about PD specific physiotherapy ($p = 0.063$).

4. Discussion

The main results of our study show low physiotherapy prescription rate, small number of patients treated yearly by PTs, discrepancy among PTs, PD patients, and the referring physicians in prioritizing core areas, and use of non-evidence-based physiotherapy techniques and finally that there are no patients with above average impairment but below average motivation. Other results show interesting findings about correlations among different PTs' characteristics (interest, length of practice, knowledge, and PD specific physiotherapy course attendance) and therapy parameters (length and number of therapy sessions, effect duration, and used techniques) and finally about most important barriers for optimal care and about communication among healthcare professionals and PD patients.

Results showing low prescription rate of physiotherapy need interpretation. One could object that not all patients in our group needed physiotherapy, that is, those who did not perceive any problem or those who did not want to improve. In order to gain insight into the prescription rate in case of patients who were both impaired and motivated, we adopted the concept of a patient-relevant problem [19]. The prescription rate in this subgroup (i.e., in those who reported impairment in a core area and declared interest in improvement) ranged between 15 and 22% which is comparable to the rate in the whole group of patients (14–21%). We did not find any dependence of prescription on current impairment in case of gait ($p = 0.358$), manual dexterity ($p = 0.068$), posture ($p = 0.116$), and physical condition ($p = 0.128$) and on the patient's motivation in all core areas (p values ranging from 0.088 to 0.638). Such prescription rate is lower than those reported in previous studies [19, 22, 23]. The chance for receiving physiotherapy for the three most important core areas for PD patients (gait, transfers, balance, and falls) is nearly three times lower than it was in Netherlands in 2009 [19]. The prescription rate for instability and falls was only approximately 18% in our study group although 62% of the patients reported at least one fall in the last year and PD patients are four times more endangered by hip fractures than healthy controls [24].

Those of our patients who received physiotherapy (median 30 minutes, 8x) reported high effect with expectations met or rather met in 79% and with a surprisingly long duration estimate (4.9 months). This seems to be overestimated when compared to available data from systematic reviews and meta-analyses of various physiotherapy modalities (resistance and aerobic training), which report lower or similar effect duration but with much longer and frequent therapy sessions [11, 25–27]. On the other hand the follow-up examination in these studies was performed exactly after 3 or 6 months, respectively, so the effect could have lasted longer here as well. A careful interpretation of our data is thus

necessary as the reported duration was not tested objectively and patients may overstate duration of the effect.

The reported quality of the explanation of the possibilities of physiotherapy by the referring physician might be viewed as sufficient. On the other hand, sufficient explanation by a PT should be a matter of course, and this was reported only in 60%. It might therefore be considered relatively low especially because insufficient communication about therapy was described as a barrier in adherence to physiotherapy and patients' compliance [28] and is paid attention in the European Physiotherapy Guideline for PD (EPGPD) [9].

The results of the cluster analysis showed that there were almost no patients with above average impairment but below average motivation. This means that even though some patients with below average impairment are not motivated for physiotherapy, they will be when their condition worsens. However, the later the training starts, the less efficient it is [9]. This result of our study may therefore be used as a motivational tool for poorly motivated patients with below average impairment. This might be also illustrated by our further finding that the importance of stability and falls increases in patients with above average impairment ($p = 0.000$), and they should be therefore motivated to partake in an early physiotherapy balance programme. Such training has already been shown to be effective [29].

The fact that PTs' interest in PD does not depend on the length of their practice or their knowledge about PD might suggest that the necessary education in PD which is a part of implementation of ParkinsonNet can aim at all PTs. The established correlation of the number of PD patients treated yearly with knowledge about PD supports the need to increase the volume of yearly treated patients to gain expertise [3]. Lack of group therapy sessions in our study cohort is probably based on local habitual practice and their implementation might be a way to increase the volume of patients treated yearly as well as to make the therapy more entertaining, thus promoting long-term adherence [9].

The surprising lack of correlation between attendance of a PD specific physiotherapy course with increased knowledge about PD or length and total number of therapy, is given by the fact that there is in fact no such course in Czechia. Those PTs who claimed to have attended such a course actually referred to either the Bobath concept course (which focuses on stroke rehabilitation) or their pregraduate studies.

No correlation of length and total number of therapy with the PTs' knowledge about physiotherapy in PD suggests that the median of 30 minutes of a therapy session repeated eight times was mainly given by custom and not by the PTs' lack of knowledge about the continuum of care recommended by the EPGPD [9]. In theory, the Czech healthcare system has no limits regarding the number and length of physiotherapy sessions, if therapy is reasonably prescribed by a physician (regardless of specialization) and such therapy is generally fully covered by the health insurance, which is obligatory in Czechia. On the other hand, physicians risk in the worst case obligation to pay for the prescribed therapy from their own budget, if they overly exceed the prescription rate from previous years. From this perspective, the Czech healthcare system is at least demotivating. A further explanation might be insufficient knowledge of the physicians about the necessary amount and length of physiotherapy sessions. The EPGPD may provide a useful educational tool as it also entails information for clinicians with detailed description of physiotherapy referral [9].

The most commonly used physiotherapy techniques (NDTs) are not explicitly mentioned anywhere in EPGPD [9]. Based on the definition of conventional therapy [9], NDTs might be implicitly considered a part of it. Nevertheless, strong GRADE-based recommendations for using conventional physiotherapy are based on studies that did not use NDTs but other types of intervention [9]. Moreover, some impairments such as freezing of gait, balance performance, and quality of life have weak recommendation against using conventional physiotherapy to improve them. This suggests that NDTs should not be the most widely used physiotherapy techniques in PD. Similarly, the 3rd most widely used technique, that is, soft tissue or neuromuscular therapy, has only weak recommendation to improve patient-based treatment effect [9]. Other techniques used, that is, gait and balance training, aerobic and resistant training, cueing, and respiratory physiotherapy, were used appropriately [9], but too rarely. Other types of intervention recommended by EPGPD [9] were not mentioned by any of the PTs. The fact that techniques used by PTs did not correlate with knowledge about PD specific physiotherapy ($p = 0.063$) is surprising and probably shows their arbitrary or customary choice. It is therefore again necessary to start evidence-based education in Czechia, which is an integral part of the ParkinsonNet project [3].

Differences in priorities of core areas as reported by patients, PTs, and referring physicians points to the need of better communication between both healthcare professionals and their patients. Even though PTs reported satisfaction with the communication in their team, the quality of this communication can be doubted. Other studies [18, 19] also reported that referring physicians lack information about the benefits of physiotherapy in PD.

The most important barriers for optimal care in Czechia as reported by PTs were few patients treated yearly, insufficient communication, absence of specialized physiotherapy course, and absence of guidelines. These reasons are in accord with previously published Dutch studies [18, 19]. This suggests that implementation of ParkinsonNet should be effective also in Czechia as it was originally designed to overcome these barriers [3] and also proven to be effective in it [16].

5. Conclusions

Our data suggest that the present Czech healthcare model for PD patients is suboptimal (low PT prescription rate, small number of patients treated yearly, non-evidence-based physiotherapy, and insufficient communication between healthcare professionals and PD patients). Implementation of EPGPD and the introduction of an efficient model of care such as ParkinsonNet are needed to improve the awareness of the referring neurologists of the benefits of physiotherapy in PD, the prescription rate, and number of PD patients treated yearly by PTs.

Acknowledgments

The authors acknowledge support from the Ministry of Health of the Czech Republic [MZ ČR 16-28119A] used for statistic processing of the data.

References

[1] T. Pringsheim, N. Jette, A. Frolkis, and T. D. L. Steeves, "The prevalence of Parkinson's disease: a systematic review and meta-analysis," *Movement Disorders*, vol. 29, no. 13, pp. 1583–1590, 2014.

[2] C.-L. Ma, L. Su, J.-J. Xie, J.-X. Long, P. Wu, and L. Gu, "The prevalence and incidence of Parkinson's disease in China: a systematic review and meta-analysis," *Journal of Neural Transmission*, vol. 121, no. 2, pp. 123–134, 2014.

[3] S. H. J. Keus, L. B. Oude Nijhuis, M. J. Nijkrake, B. R. Bloem, and M. Munneke, "Improving community healthcare for patients with Parkinson's disease: the Dutch model," *Parkinson's Disease*, vol. 2012, Article ID 543426, 7 pages, 2012.

[4] M. Monticone, E. Ambrosini, A. Laurini, B. Rocca, and C. Foti, "In-patient multidisciplinary rehabilitation for Parkinson's disease: a randomized controlled trial," *Movement Disorders*, vol. 30, no. 8, pp. 1050–1058, 2015.

[5] M. J. Nijkrake, "Allied health care interventions and complementary therapies in Parkinson's disease," *Parkinsonism & Amp; Related Disorders*, vol. 13, pp. S488-S494, 2007.

[6] M. A. van der Marck, "Multidisciplinary care for patients with Parkinson's disease," *Parkinsonism & Amp; Related Disorders*, no. 15, pp. S219-S223.

[7] C. G. Canning, C. Sherrington, S. R. Lord et al., "Exercise for falls prevention in Parkinson disease: A randomized controlled trial," *Neurology*, vol. 84, no. 3, pp. 304–312, 2015.

[8] A. Carvalho, D. Barbirato, N. Araujo et al., "Comparison of strength training, aerobic training, and additional physical therapy as supplementary treatments for Parkinson's disease: pilot study," *Clinical Interventions in Aging*, vol. 10, pp. 183–191, 2015.

[9] S. H. J. Keus and et al, *European Physiotherapy Guideline for Parkinson's Disease*, KNGF/ParkinsonNet, Nijmegen, The Netherlands, 2014.

[10] J. Mehrholz, J. Kugler, A. Storch, M. Pohl, K. Hirsch, and B. Elsner, "Treadmill training for patients with Parkinson's disease," *Cochrane Database of Systematic Reviews*, no. 9, 2015.

[11] L. Roeder, J. T. Costello, S. S. Smith, I. B. Stewart, and G. K. Kerr, "Effects of resistance training on measures of muscular strength in people with Parkinson's disease: a systematic review and meta-analysis," *PLoS ONE*, vol. 10, no. 7, Article ID e0132135, 2015.

[12] C. L. Tomlinson et al., "Physiotherapy for Parkinson's disease: a comparison of techniques," *Cochrane Database of Systematic Reviews*, 2014.

[13] C. L. Tomlinson, S. Patel, C. Meek et al., "Physiotherapy intervention in Parkinson's disease: systematic review and meta-analysis," *The BMJ*, vol. 345, article ID e5004, 2012.

[14] C. L. Tomlinson, S. Patel, C. Meek et al., "Physiotherapy versus placebo or no intervention in Parkinson's disease," *Cochrane Database of Systematic Reviews*, no. 9, 2013.

[15] A. Uhrbrand, E. Stenager, M. S. Pedersen, and U. Dalgas, "Parkinson's disease and intensive exercise therapy—a systematic review and meta-analysis of randomized controlled trials," *Journal of the Neurological Sciences*, vol. 353, no. 1-2, pp. 9–19, 2015.

[16] B. R. Bloem and M. Munneke, "Revolutionising management of chronic disease: the ParkinsonNet approach," *The BMJ*, vol. 348, Article ID g1838, 2014.

[17] M. Munneke, M. J. Nijkrake, S. H. Keus et al., "Efficacy of community-based physiotherapy networks for patients with Parkinson's disease: a cluster-randomised trial," *The Lancet Neurology*, vol. 9, no. 1, pp. 46–54, 2010.

[18] S. H. J. Keus, B. R. Bloem, D. Verbaan et al., "Physiotherapy in Parkinson's disease: utilisation and patient satisfaction," *Journal of Neurology*, vol. 251, no. 6, pp. 680–687, 2004.

[19] M. J. Nijkrake, S. H. J. Keus, R. A. B. Oostendorp et al., "Allied health care in Parkinson's disease: referral, consultation, and professional expertise," *Movement Disorders*, vol. 24, no. 2, pp. 282–286, 2009.

[20] J. P. Hobson, N. I. Edwards, and R. J. Meara, "The Parkinson's Disease Activities of Daily Living Scale: a new simple and brief subjective measure of disability in Parkinson's disease," *Clinical Rehabilitation*, vol. 15, no. 3, pp. 241–246, 2001.

[21] E. L. Stack and H. C. Roberts, "Slow down and concentrate: time for a paradigm shift in fall prevention among people with Parkinson's disease?" *Parkinson's Disease*, Article ID 704237, 2013.

[22] A. G. E. M. De Boer, M. A. G. Sprangers, H. D. Speelman, and H. C. J. M. De Haes, "Predictors of health care use in patients with Parkinson's disease: a longitudinal study," *Movement Disorders*, vol. 14, no. 5, pp. 772–779, 1999.

[23] T. C. S. O. Physiotherapy, "Neurology: Parkinson's disease, multiple sclerosis and severe traumatic brain injury," *Physiotherapy Effectiveness Bulletin*, vol. 2, no. 3, 2001.

[24] R. W. Walker, A. Chaplin, R. L. Hancock, R. Rutherford, and W. K. Gray, "Hip fractures in people with idiopathic Parkinson's disease: incidence and outcomes," *Movement Disorders*, vol. 28, no. 3, pp. 334–340, 2013.

[25] F. Li, P. Harmer, K. Fitzgerald et al., "Tai chi and postural stability in patients with Parkinson's disease," *The New England Journal of Medicine*, vol. 366, no. 6, pp. 511–519, 2012.

[26] H.-F. Shu, T. Yang, S.-X. Yu et al., "Aerobic exercise for Parkinson's disease: a systematic review and meta-analysis of randomized controlled trials," *PLoS ONE*, vol. 9, no. 7, Article ID e100503, 2014.

[27] I. Miyai, Y. Fujimoto, H. Yamamoto et al., "Long-term effect of body weight-supported treadmill training in Parkinson's disease: a randomized controlled trial," *Archives of Physical Medicine and Rehabilitation*, vol. 83, no. 10, pp. 1370–1373, 2002.

[28] K. Jack, S. M. McLean, J. K. Moffett, and E. Gardiner, "Barriers to treatment adherence in physiotherapy outpatient clinics: a systematic review," *Manual Therapy*, vol. 15, no. 3, pp. 220–228, 2010.

[29] I. S. Wong-Yu and M. K. Y. Mak, "Multi-dimensional balance training programme improves balance and gait performance in people with Parkinson's disease: a pragmatic randomized controlled trial with 12-month follow-up," *Parkinsonism & Related Disorders*, vol. 21, no. 6, pp. 615–621, 2015.

20

Technology-Assisted Rehabilitation of Writing Skills in Parkinson's Disease: Visual Cueing versus Intelligent Feedback

Evelien Nackaerts,[1] Alice Nieuwboer,[1] and Elisabetta Farella[2]

[1]*Neuromotor Rehabilitation Research Group, Department of Rehabilitation Sciences, KU Leuven, Leuven, Belgium*
[2]*E3DA Research Unit, ICT Center, Fondazione Bruno Kessler, Trento, Italy*

Correspondence should be addressed to Evelien Nackaerts; evelien.nackaerts@kuleuven.be

Academic Editor: Hélio Teive

Recent research showed that visual cueing can have both beneficial and detrimental effects on handwriting of patients with Parkinson's disease (PD) and healthy controls depending on the circumstances. Hence, using other sensory modalities to deliver cueing or feedback may be a valuable alternative. Therefore, the current study compared the effects of short-term training with either continuous visual cues or intermittent intelligent verbal feedback. Ten PD patients and nine healthy controls were randomly assigned to one of these training modes. To assess transfer of learning, writing performance was assessed in the absence of cueing and feedback on both trained and untrained writing sequences. The feedback pen and a touch-sensitive writing tablet were used for testing. Both training types resulted in improved writing amplitudes for the trained and untrained sequences. In conclusion, these results suggest that the feedback pen is a valuable tool to implement writing training in a tailor-made fashion for people with PD. Future studies should include larger sample sizes and different subgroups of PD for long-term training with the feedback pen.

1. Introduction

Parkinson's disease (PD) is a neurodegenerative disorder characterized by the loss of dopaminergic neurons in the basal ganglia leading to a combination of motor and non-motor symptoms [1]. In addition to the primary symptoms, that is, tremor, rigidity, bradykinesia, and postural instability, micrographia is a frequently occurring problem [1]. Micrographia is defined as "an impairment of a fine motor skill manifesting mainly as a progressive reduction in amplitude during a writing task" [2]. For treatment of PD, dopaminergic medication is the gold standard, though not all symptoms respond equally well [3]. Therefore, motor rehabilitation is often a necessary therapeutic supplement [4]. Several studies have shown that motor learning is possible in PD, although learning occurs more slowly and with less automaticity (for reviews see [5, 6]). Motor performance and the learning potential in PD can be further improved by means of cueing and feedback strategies [7, 8]. Cues are defined as a reference or trigger for movement generation [9]. Feedback refers to the provision of external information which supplements the internal sensory pathways to guide learning online or after performance [10]. The beneficial effects of both types of input are often attributed to the fact that they induce a shift in motor control from a habitual to a goal-directed modus or, in other words, induce redirection from more to less affected neural circuits [11].

The benefits of cueing and feedback have mainly been shown for gait in PD [12, 13]. Unlike gait, handwriting incorporates both automated and controlled processes [14]. As such, cueing and feedback strategies may have an alternate effect. Several studies have shown benefits of short-term training with visual cues [15, 16]. However, recently, it was shown that visual cues sometimes hamper handwriting, especially when cueing smaller writing sizes, as such introducing an additional accuracy constraint [17]. As a result, the visual system may have become overloaded, increasing difficulty [18]. Hence, using other sensory modalities to deliver cueing or feedback should be considered. Providing supplementary sensory information may aid motor learning as well as motor performance [19]. In contrast, when cueing or feedback was removed, motor performance worsened in PD [20, 21].

Similarly, when feedback was provided too frequently during motor learning, that is, in 100% of the trials, it caused dependency and lack of transfer [22, 23]. To counteract this drawback, providing external input intermittently may be a valuable alternative. With recent technological advances, it is possible to realize individualized and intelligent feedback adjusted to performance outcomes [24–28]. To the best of our knowledge, this has not been studied for upper limb tasks such as writing in PD.

Therefore, an intelligent pen that can provide real-time feedback in an intermittent manner was developed to address micrographia. The current proof-of-concept study was designed to compare the effects of short-term training (one session) with continuous visual cues with intermittent intelligent feedback. We expected that training with the continuous visual cue would lead to more dependency and less improvement of writing amplitude compared to training with intelligent feedback.

2. Methods

2.1. Participants and Experimental Protocol. In this cross-sectional study, 10 patients with PD and 10 healthy controls (CT) were assessed for eligibility. Inclusion criteria for patients were (i) diagnosis of PD according to the UK Brain Bank Criteria [29]; (ii) Hoehn and Yahr (H&Y) stages I–III in the on-phase of the medication cycle [30]; and (iii) being on stable medication. Exclusion criteria for both groups were (i) cognitive impairment (Mini-Mental State Examination, MMSE < 24) [31] and (ii) interfering upper limb problems. As such, one healthy control was excluded from the analyses due to MMSE < 24.

Participants were randomly assigned to one of two training programs, that is, either continuous cueing with visual target zones (Cue), or (ii) intermittent intelligent feedback, that is, providing verbal corrections during writing when it deteriorated (Feedback). The session started with assessment of baseline writing performance. This was followed by a short training period using one of the two training methods. After the training session, writing performance was assessed again. In addition to the writing tests, disease-specific features were determined using the Movement Disorder Society Unified Parkinson's Disease Rating Scale (MDS-UPDRS) part III [32], New Freezing of Gait (NFOG) questionnaire [33], and Levodopa Equivalent Dose (LED) [34]. In addition, the Manual Ability Measure (MAM-16) [35] and Edinburgh Handedness Inventory [36] were completed by both patients and controls. For patients, testing of writing performance and disease-specific characteristics occurred during the on-phase of the medication cycle, that is, approximately 1 h after medication intake.

The study design and protocol were approved by the local Ethics Committee of the University Hospitals Leuven and were in accordance with the code of Ethics of the World Medical Association (Declaration of Helsinki, 1967). After explanation of the study protocol, written informed consent was obtained from all participants prior to participation in the study.

2.2. Writing Assessment. Writing performance was assessed before and after a short training period, both on a touch-sensitive writing tablet (Figure 1(a)) [37] and with a custom-made feedback pen (Figure 1(e)) in a counterbalanced order. Three exercises were performed: (i) writing of continuous loops, resembling the letter "e" (0.6 cm) (Figures 1(b) and 1(f)); (ii) writing of continuous loops, resembling the letter "l" (1.0 cm) (Figures 1(c) and 1(g)); and writing of a figure of 8-like movement (1.0 cm) (Figures 1(d) and 1(h)). Both continuous loops were practiced during the training period (i.e., trained tasks), while the figure of 8-like movement was not (i.e., untrained task) to study short-term transfer effects. All tests were previously used in studies using a touch-sensitive writing tablet [38, 39] and were performed in the absence of visual cueing and intelligent feedback to assess transfer.

2.3. Intervention. The training session lasted approximately 30 min including short breaks. All participants performed a minimum of eight and maximum of 12 writing exercises, depending on the subjective reporting of fatigue. Each exercise consisted of writing different types of preletters for a duration of 90 s. A training session included two exercises with the letter "e," two exercises with the letter "l," and four to eight exercises with alternative preletters (e.g., resembling the letter "v" or "n"). Training with continuous visual cueing was performed on the tablet. Visual cues consisted of colored visual target zones indicating the requested writing size, similar to the ones used in the study by Nackaerts et al. [17]. While in the latter study visual cues were merely offered, participants in the present study were encouraged to increase their amplitude using the cues. The intelligent feedback was provided using a newly developed feedback pen and exercises were performed on regular paper. Feedback was provided intermittently, that is, every 6 s, and consisted of one of five types of feedback messages depending on the writers' performance: (i) good; (ii) try to write larger; (iii) try to write smaller; (iv) try to write slower; and (v) try to write faster. As micrographia was the focus of this study, priority was given to feedback messages with respect to writing amplitude over writing speed. Subjects were instructed to attend to the feedback and alter their performance accordingly.

It is important to note that cued training was only performed on the tablet and not on paper, while feedback training was only performed on paper and not on the tablet.

2.4. System Design. The requirements of the feedback pen were as follows: (i) to accurately capture and process spatial and temporal coordinates of the written trace of a ball-point pen on a regular sheet of paper and (ii) to provide verbal information in real time on a specific writing feature (e.g., amplitude or speed). Therefore, a prototype was developed based on a commercially available digital pen, augmented with appropriate hardware and firmware. The final system consisted of a digital pen with a microcontroller-based add-on board, designed to enable feature extraction and audio feedback. We selected the Staedtler Digital Pen 990 (Staedtler Mars GmbH & Co., Nuremberg, Germany) for its characteristics in terms of working area ($166 \times 125 \text{ mm}^2$),

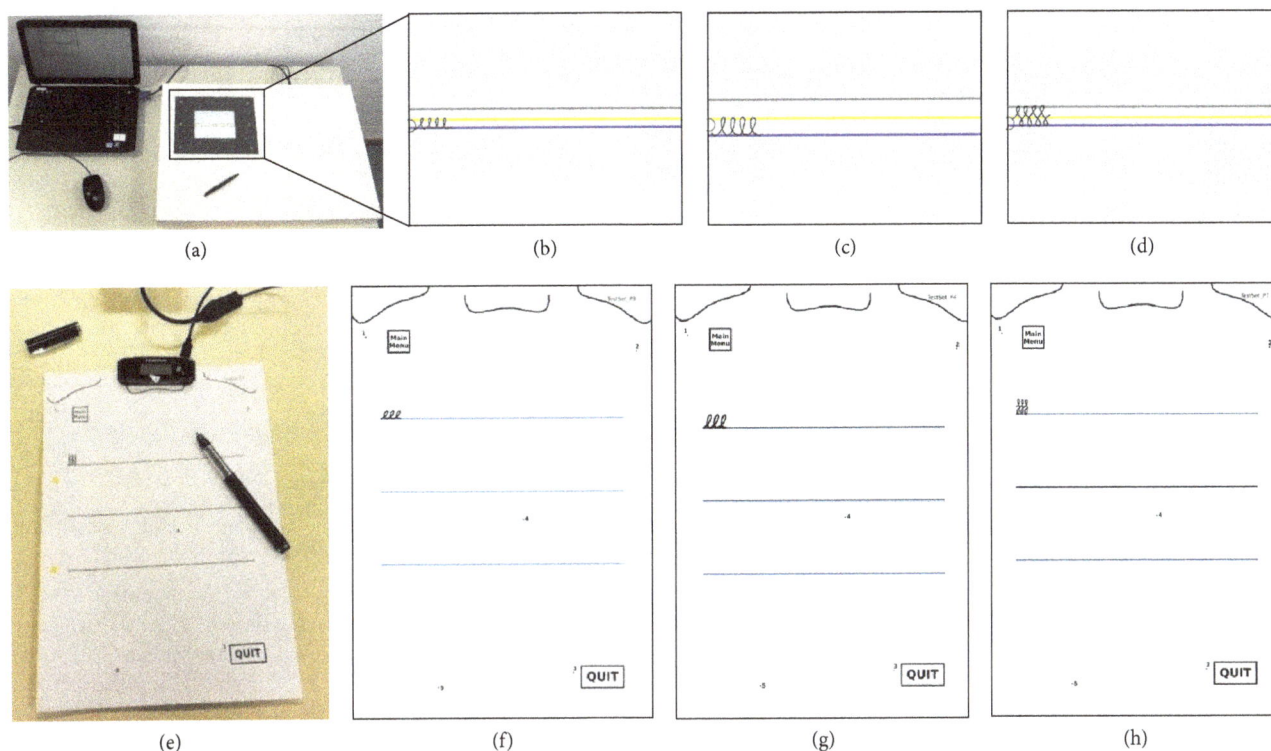

FIGURE 1: *Touch-sensitive tablet and feedback pen system.* (a) Setup of the tablet; (b–d) examples of the small trained (b), large trained (c), and untrained (d) task with visual cues. It has to be noted that testing was performed in the absence of the yellow (middle) and upper (grey) line. (e) Setup of the pen, receiver, and paper; (f–h) examples of the test sheets for the small trained (f), large trained, (g) and untrained task (h).

sample frequency (66 Hz), and accuracy ($0,126 \times 0,126 \, mm^2$ /point) when used in pen mode. More detailed technical information is presented in Guardati et al., 2015 [40].

The final system consisted of three main parts. A first part is the preprinted paper, consisting of a specific exercise (examples in Figure 1). On each paper, possible locations for the receiver of the pen were included for convenience of the user. In addition, the paper also served as an interface, allowing interactive calibration. The second part consisted of the Staedtler Digital Pen and receiver. This receiver collected the coordinates and sent them via USB to the third part, that is, the add-on board. The add-on board was the novelty of the system, as it allows correct interpretation of data based on a calibration process and real-time processing of the writing features. The board was based on a Cortex M4 microcontroller, working at 168 Mhz, with 1024 Kb of flash memory and 192 Kb of RAM. It included an audio Codec, an SD card reader, and a loudspeaker. A real-time operative system, Nuttx RTOS (http://nuttx.org/), ran on the microcontroller providing a flexible and modular environment for easy development and debugging. Libraries for interfacing with the various parts of the system were implemented, in particular to communicate with the pen. On top of that, it ran the firmware based on FiMoSDK (Fine Movement Software Development Kit), a custom library in C++ that implements the handwriting exercises.

The first purpose of the board was to calibrate the system in order to avoid problems with the interpretation of data

as a result of misalignment between the expected and actual position of the receiver on the paper. Therefore, the user was requested to put the pen at five calibration points by means of an audio-guided start-up. These points, watermarked on the paper (Figure 1), were compared with the "default" reference system that was determined in controlled conditions. This allowed a rototranslation to align the reference system. Although three points would be sufficient, we chose a redundancy approach to be able to discard up to two points in case of noise or errors during the acquisition. As such, requests for repeating the calibration to the user were minimized.

The second main functionality of the add-on board was to generate audio feedback. The system could be configured in three different modalities: (i) no feedback; (ii) continuous reminder (not included in the current study); and (iii) intelligent feedback. The first modality was used to assess handwriting without the provision of additional information. The continuous reminder was a periodic signal that did not depend on user performance and just reminded the subject to write in a certain manner (e.g., remember to write big). The intelligent feedback depended on the user performance, measured in real time. In this third modality, a certain feature, such as writing amplitude or speed, was detected while the user was writing and compared to a preset target performance value. The allowed deviation from this target needed to be defined in advance. Comparison between the target value and the actual performance determined the kind of feedback (e.g.,

TABLE 1: General characteristics: median and interquartile ranges are displayed.

	Cue ($N = 10$)	Feedback ($N = 9$)	p-value
PD/CT	6/4	4/5	0.498
Age (years)	66.5 (55.0, 69.0)	52.0 (50.5, 68.5)	0.356
Gender (M/F)	6/4	4/5	0.498
Handedness (R/L)	9/1	7/2	0.842
MMSE (0–30)	28.5 (26.5, 30.0)	29.0 (28.5, 30.0)	0.447
MAM-16 (0–64)	60.0 (52.5, 63.3)	64.0 (61.0, 64.0)	0.065
PD specific			
Disease duration (years)	12.0 (7.3, 21.3)	5.5 (2.0, 9.0)	0.114
LED (mg/24 h)	740.0 (180.2, 1081.7)	482.5 (345.0, 515.0)	0.476
MDS-UPDRS-III (0–132)	35.5 (31.5, 44.0)	22.0 (13.3, 33.0)	0.067
NFOG-Q (0–24)	0.0 (0.0, 12.3)	0.0 (0.0, 9.0)	0.914

CT = healthy control; F = female; L = left; LED = Levodopa Equivalent Dose; M = male; MAM-16 = Manual Ability Measure; MMSE = Mini-Mental State Examination; R = right; MDS-UPDRS-III = Movement Disorder Society Unified Parkinson's Disease Rating Scale part III; PD = Parkinson's disease; NFOG-Q = New Freezing of Gait Questionnaire.

"good" and "try to write larger"). Detailed specifications were explained in Guardati et al., 2015 [40].

2.5. Data Processing and Statistical Analysis. All data from the pen and tablet were filtered at 7 Hz with a 4th-order Butterworth filter and further processed using Matlab R2011b. Writing amplitude (cm) was determined by calculating the differences between the local minima and maxima of each individual stroke [37].

Statistical analysis was performed using SPSS (IBM SPSS statistics version 24). Normality of the data was assessed by means of the Shapiro-Wilk test. The Mann–Whitney U and the Pearson Chi Square test were used to compare differences in demographic characteristics between both training types. Paired t-tests were used to look for systematic differences between writing performance on the tablet and with the pen. To investigate the effect of training, a repeated measures analysis of variance (ANOVA) was performed, with training type (Cue versus Feedback) and group (PD versus CT) as between-subject factors and time (pre versus post) as a within-subject factor. This analysis was performed for the three tasks separately with both measurement tools. Effect sizes were measured by means of the partial eta-squared.

2.6. Feasibility and User Satisfaction. At the end of the session, all patients filled out a questionnaire on how much they wrote in daily life and whether they were familiar with the use of a laptop, tablet, or smartphone. In addition, they were asked whether they were interested in training with the system at home, if so how frequently and whether they had suggestions for improvement.

3. Results

3.1. General Characteristics and Tool Comparison. General group characteristics did not differ significantly between training types (Table 1). Additionally, there was no significant difference in the amount of exercises performed during training ($t = 0.980$, $p = 0.341$).

For writing at the smaller size (letter "e"), no differences were found between writing with the pen and on the tablet ($t = 0.450$, $p = 0.659$). For the larger writing sizes, a systematic difference was found for the letter "l" ($t = 4.148$, $p = 0.001$) and to a lesser extent for the figure of 8-like movement ($t = 1.849$, $p = 0.082$), showing that writing amplitude with the pen was smaller than when assessed with the tablet.

3.2. The Effect of Training on Writing Amplitude. For the test with the trained letter "e," main effects of time were found during both writing tests on the tablet ($F = 3.461$, $p = 0.083$; $\eta^2 = 0.187$) and writing tests with the pen ($F = 6.692$, $p = 0.023$; $\eta^2 = 0.340$). Although the former only revealed a tendency, both test methods exposed an increased writing amplitude after training regardless of the training type (Figures 2(a) and 2(b)). For the trained letter "l," a main effect of time was found for writing assessed on the tablet only ($F = 5.423$, $p = 0.034$; $\eta^2 = 0.266$), showing a larger amplitude after training. However, there was also a strong trend towards an interaction between training type and time in this condition ($F = 3.975$, $p = 0.065$; $\eta^2 = 0.209$). Exploratory post hoc analysis revealed that only the group that received feedback training improved significantly from baseline to posttraining ($p = 0.036$, Bonferroni-corrected) (Figure 2(c)). Finally, main effects of time were found for the untrained task and this for both writing on the tablet ($F = 7.129$, $p = 0.017$; $\eta^2 = 0.322$) and writing with the pen ($F = 6.470$, $p = 0.026$; $\eta^2 = 0.350$). Both displayed an increase in amplitude from baseline to posttraining (Figures 2(e) and 2(f)).

3.3. Feasibility and User Satisfaction. All patients were computer-literate and five were also employing a tablet or smartphone. Across training types, patients were interested in a long-term training program at home, if the exercises would not only include preletters but would become gradually more difficult. Two patients reported problems with the grip of the pen, one in the cue and one in the feedback group. Furthermore, the calibration of the exercise sheets for use of the feedback pen should be addressed to ensure that a new calibration

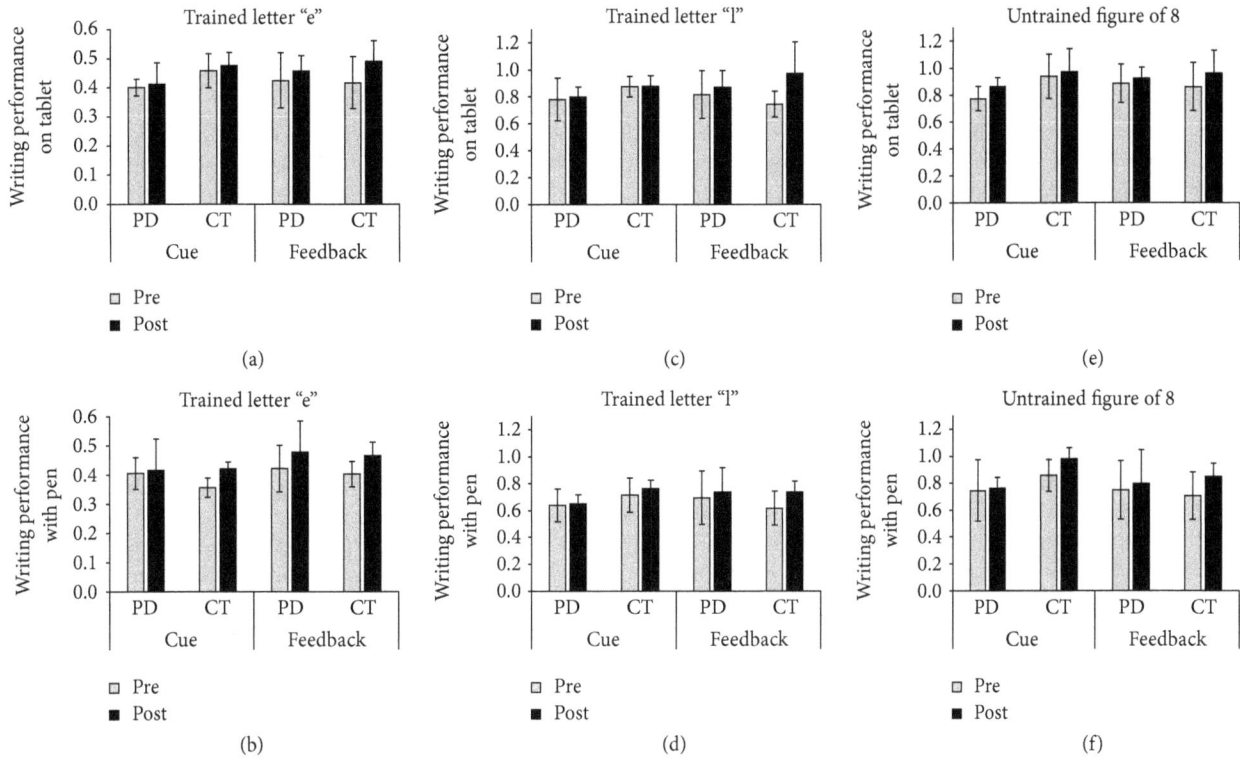

FIGURE 2: *The effects of short-term training with visual cues or intelligent feedback.* Results are displayed for the different tasks and groups, performed both on the touch-sensitive writing tablet and with the feedback pen.

is not necessary at the beginning of each exercise. Participants had no suggestions to improve the delivery of the cues or feedback.

4. Discussion

In the present study, the effects of continuous visual cueing and intermittent intelligent feedback on handwriting were compared for the first time. Results revealed that short-term training with both cueing and feedback can improve writing amplitude in both patients with PD and healthy controls for different writing amplitudes. Contrary to the immediate detrimental effects of visual cueing on writing at small amplitudes (0.6 cm) [17], the current study therefore suggests that the accuracy constraints of visual cueing can be overcome with proper training and that participants can learn how to use the cues to their advantage. As improvements were found for both the trained and untrained tasks and for both measurement tools, these results also suggest transfer of learning, in line with previous work [39]. Furthermore, amplitude improvements were found in the absence of cues or feedback. This is contrary to the guidance hypothesis of motor learning, stating that augmented sensory information during the acquisition phase of motor learning can cause dependency, leading to worse performance when cueing or feedback is withdrawn [19].

However, a strong tendency towards an interaction between training type and time for the large trained task depicts a more refined view. Patients and healthy controls did not deteriorate their writing amplitude during uncued tests after continuous visual cueing, but they did not improve either. On the other hand, after training with the feedback pen, amplitude increased, reflecting the absence of dependency and a possible advantage of training with an intermittent type of feedback [22]. Although the sample size was too small to draw definitive conclusions, the intelligent feedback likely forced participants to pay attention to specific aspects of the task, stimulating cognitive engagement and less habitual control [11, 41]. Future study in a larger sample needs to confirm whether this will lead to more robust learning. Also, training with the intelligent feedback pen could therefore be used to facilitate transfer of practice to daily life in more advanced stages of PD, which was shown to be more difficult in a previous study [42]. Another advantage of using the feedback pen is that is resembles writing in daily life better as it relies on pen and paper, rather than a tablet environment.

PD patients partaking in this study were all technology-literate and expressed an interest in undertaking a long-term training program using either the touch-sensitive tablet or the feedback pen. Both applications were well-tolerated and perceived as user-friendly tools by all participants, albeit that calibration procedures and pen grip will need further refinement. This points to the potential of both methods to serve as training tools for home use, offering the advantage that patients can practice fine motor skills without requiring transport to a rehabilitation clinic.

5. Limitations and Suggestions for Future Research

The current study has several limitations that may have influenced the outcomes. The most important drawback is the small sample size, which likely limited statistical power. As such, future studies should include larger sample sizes to investigate the specific benefit of intermittent intelligent feedback for patients with differences in disease severity. In this regard, the feedback pen has the additional advantage that it also allows gradual withdrawal of feedback, as the time between feedback messages can be easily altered. Though this was not applied in the current study, future research should investigate whether this approach can be used to further reduce cue- and feedback-dependency in PD [23]. Secondly, a systematic difference between performance with the pen and on the tablet was detected, indicating a tendency to write smaller with the pen. One possible explanation is that writing with the pen resembled more natural handwriting, as the typical friction between pen and paper is increased compared to the smoother surface of the touch-sensitive tablet [43, 44]. This may have led to better transfer at the expense of performance. In this regard, it would be interesting if future research could combine and compare different types of cueing and feedback delivery, that is, cued training on both a touch-sensitive tablet and on paper and feedback training on both paper and a touch-sensitive tablet.

6. Conclusion

In summary, the current study presented a novel feedback pen and compared it to visually cued writing training. The pen made it possible to receive personalized verbal feedback intermittently during writing practice. Online verbal corrections during writing practice proved to have a more robust beneficial learning effect than training supported by continuous visual cueing. This suggests that the feedback pen is a valuable tool to implement writing training in a tailor-made fashion for people with PD. As such, the findings are encouraging and future research should focus on including larger sample sizes and different subgroups of PD for long-term training.

Acknowledgments

The authors are grateful to all participants in this study. They would like to thank Ir. Leonardo Guardati and Ir. Filippo Casamassima for the development of the feedback system and Ir. Marc Beirinckx for development of the touch-sensitive tablet. This work was supported by the Research Foundation-Flanders (FWO), where E. Nackaerts is a Ph.D. fellow.

References

[1] J. Jankovic, "Parkinson's disease: Clinical features and diagnosis," *Journal of Neurology, Neurosurgery and Psychiatry*, vol. 79, no. 4, pp. 368–376, 2008.

[2] A. W. Shukla, S. Ounpraseuth, M. S. Okun, V. Gray, J. Schwankhaus, and W. S. Metzer, "Micrographia and related deficits in Parkinson's disease: a cross-sectional study," *BMJ Open*, vol. 2, no. 3, Article ID e000628, 2012.

[3] A. A. Moustafa, S. Chakravarthy, J. R. Phillips et al., "Motor symptoms in Parkinson's disease: a unified framework," *Neuroscience and Biobehavioral Reviews*, vol. 68, pp. 727–740, 2016.

[4] C. L. Tomlinson, S. Patel, C. Meek et al., "Physiotherapy versus placebo or no intervention in Parkinson's disease," *The Cochrane Database of Systematic Reviews*, vol. 9, Article ID CD002817, 2013.

[5] G. Abbruzzese, R. Marchese, L. Avanzino, and E. Pelosin, "Rehabilitation for Parkinson's disease: current outlook and future challenges," *Parkinsonism and Related Disorders*, vol. 22, supplement 1, pp. S60–S64, 2016.

[6] T. Wu, M. Hallett, and P. Chan, "Motor automaticity in Parkinson's disease," *Neurobiology of Disease*, vol. 82, pp. 226–234, 2015.

[7] C. Cassimatis, K. P. Y. Liu, P. Fahey, and M. Bissett, "The effectiveness of external sensory cues in improving functional performance in individuals with Parkinson's disease: A systematic review with meta-analysis," *International Journal of Rehabilitation Research*, vol. 39, no. 3, pp. 211–218, 2016.

[8] A. Nieuwboer, L. Rochester, L. Müncks, and S. P. Swinnen, "Motor learning in Parkinson's disease: limitations and potential for rehabilitation," *Parkinsonism and Related Disorders*, vol. 15, supplement 3, pp. S53–S58, 2009.

[9] A. Nieuwboer, G. Kwakkel, L. Rochester et al., "Cueing training in the home improves gait-related mobility in Parkinson's disease: the RESCUE trial," *Journal of Neurology, Neurosurgery and Psychiatry*, vol. 78, no. 2, pp. 134–140, 2007.

[10] R. A. Schmidt and T. D. Lee, *Motor control and learning: a behavioral emphasis*, *Champaign: Human kinetics*, Champaign, Human kinetics, 5th edition, 2011.

[11] P. Redgrave, M. Rodriguez, Y. Smith et al., "Goal-directed and habitual control in the basal ganglia: implications for Parkinson's disease," *Nature Reviews Neuroscience*, vol. 11, no. 11, pp. 760–772, 2010.

[12] P. A. Rocha, G. M. Porfírio, H. B. Ferraz, and V. F. M. Trevisani, "Effects of external cues on gait parameters of Parkinson's disease patients: a systematic review," *Clinical Neurology and Neurosurgery*, vol. 124, pp. 127–134, 2014.

[13] S. J. Spaulding, B. Barber, M. Colby, B. Cormack, T. Mick, and M. E. Jenkins, "Cueing and gait improvement among people with Parkinson's disease: a meta-analysis," *Archives of Physical Medicine and Rehabilitation*, vol. 94, no. 3, pp. 562–570, 2013.

[14] O. Tucha, L. Mecklinger, S. Walitza, and K. W. Lange, "Attention and movement execution during handwriting," *Human Movement Science*, vol. 25, no. 4-5, pp. 536–552, 2006, Advances in Graphonomics: Studies on Fine Motor Control, Its Development and Disorders.

[15] M. S. Bryant, D. H. Rintala, E. C. Lai, and E. J. Protas, "An investigation of two interventions for micrographia in individuals with Parkinson's disease," *Clinical Rehabilitation*, vol. 24, no. 11, pp. 1021–1026, 2010.

[16] R. M. Oliveira, J. M. Gurd, P. Nixon, J. C. Marshall, and R. E. Passingham, "Micrographia in Parkinson's disease: the effect of providing external cues," *Journal of Neurology Neurosurgery and Psychiatry*, vol. 63, no. 4, pp. 429–433, 1997.

[17] E. Nackaerts, A. Nieuwboer, S. Broeder et al., "Opposite Effects of Visual Cueing during Writing-Like Movements of Different

Amplitudes in Parkinson's Disease," *Neurorehabilitation and Neural Repair*, vol. 30, no. 5, pp. 431–439, 2015.

[18] J. Danna and J.-L. Velay, "Basic and supplementary sensory feedback in handwriting," *Frontiers in Psychology*, vol. 6, article no. 169, 2015.

[19] A. W. Salmoni, R. A. Schmidt, and C. B. Walter, "Knowledge of results and motor learning: a review and critical reappraisal," *Psychological Bulletin*, vol. 95, no. 3, pp. 355–386, 1984.

[20] S. Vercruysse, J. Spildooren, E. Heremans et al., "Abnormalities and cue dependence of rhythmical upper-limb movements in Parkinson patients with freezing of gait," *Neurorehabilitation and Neural Repair*, vol. 26, no. 6, pp. 636–645, 2012.

[21] S. M. P. Verschueren, S. P. Swinnen, R. Dom, and W. De Weerdt, "Interlimb coordination in patients with parkinson's disease: motor learning deficits and the importance of augmented information feedback," *Experimental Brain Research*, vol. 113, no. 3, pp. 497–508, 1997.

[22] S. Chiviacowsky, T. Campos, and M. R. Domingues, "Reduced frequency of knowledge of results enhances learning in persons with Parkinson's disease," *Frontiers in Psychology*, vol. 1, Article ID Article 226, 2010.

[23] S. Onla-Or and C. J. Winstein, "Determining the optimal challenge point for motor skill learning in adults with moderately severe Parkinson's disease," *Neurorehabilitation and Neural Repair*, vol. 22, no. 4, pp. 385–395, 2008.

[24] Y. Baram, J. Aharon-Peretz, S. Badarny, Z. Susel, and I. Schlesinger, "Closed-loop auditory feedback for the improvement of gait in patients with Parkinson's disease," *Journal of the Neurological Sciences*, vol. 363, pp. 104–106, 2016.

[25] F. Casamassima, A. Ferrari, B. Milosevic, P. Ginis, E. Farella, and L. Rocchi, "A wearable system for gait training in subjects with Parkinson's disease," *Sensors*, vol. 14, no. 4, pp. 6229–6246, 2014.

[26] M. S. Ekker, S. Janssen, J. Nonnekes, B. R. Bloem, and M. de Vries, "Neurorehabilitation for Parkinson's disease: future perspectives for behavioural adaptation," *Parkinsonism Relat Disord*, vol. 22, Supplement 1, pp. S73–S77, 2016.

[27] P. Ginis, A. Nieuwboer, M. Dorfman et al., "Feasibility and effects of home-based smartphone-delivered automated feedback training for gait in people with Parkinson's disease: a pilot randomized controlled trial," *Parkinsonism and Related Disorders*, vol. 22, pp. 28–34, 2016.

[28] V. S. Huang, A. Haith, P. Mazzoni, and J. W. Krakauer, "Rethinking motor learning and savings in adaptation paradigms: model-free memory for successful actions combines with internal models," *Neuron*, vol. 70, no. 4, pp. 787–801, 2011.

[29] A. J. Hughes, S. E. Daniel, L. Kilford, and A. J. Lees, "Accuracy of clinical diagnosis of idiopathic parkinson's disease: a clinico-pathological study of 100 cases," *Journal of Neurology Neurosurgery and Psychiatry*, vol. 55, no. 3, pp. 181–184, 1992.

[30] M. M. Hoehn and M. D. Yahr, "Parkinsonism: onset, progression and mortality," *Neurology*, vol. 17, no. 5, pp. 427–442, 1967.

[31] M. F. Folstein, S. E. Folstein, and P. R. McHugh, "'Mini mental state'. A practical method for grading the cognitive state of patients for the clinician," *Journal of Psychiatric Research*, vol. 12, no. 3, pp. 189–198, 1975.

[32] C. G. Goetz, B. C. Tilley, S. R. Shaftman et al., "Movement disorder society-sponsored revision of the unified parkinson's disease rating scale (mds-updrs): scale presentation and clinimetric testing results," *Movement Disorders*, vol. 23, no. 15, pp. 2129–2170, 2008.

[33] A. Nieuwboer, L. Rochester, T. Herman et al., "Reliability of the new freezing of gait questionnaire: agreement between patients with Parkinson's disease and their carers," *Gait and Posture*, vol. 30, no. 4, pp. 459–463, 2009.

[34] C. L. Tomlinson, R. Stowe, S. Patel, C. Rick, R. Gray, and C. E. Clarke, "Systematic review of levodopa dose equivalency reporting in Parkinson's disease," *Movement Disorders*, vol. 25, no. 15, pp. 2649–2653, 2010.

[35] C. C. Chen, C. V. Granger, C. A. Peimer, O. J. Moy, and S. Wald, "Manual ability measure (MAM-16): A preliminary report on a new patient-centred and task-oriented outcome measure of hand function," *Journal of Hand Surgery*, vol. 30, no. 2, pp. 207–216, 2005.

[36] R. C. Oldfield, "The assessment and analysis of handedness: the Edinburgh inventory," *Neuropsychologia*, vol. 9, no. 1, pp. 97–113, 1971.

[37] S. Broeder, E. Nackaerts, A. Nieuwboer, B. C. M. Smits-Engelsman, S. P. Swinnen, and E. Heremans, "The effects of dual tasking on handwriting in patients with Parkinson's disease," *Neuroscience*, vol. 263, pp. 193–202, 2014.

[38] E. Heremans, E. Nackaerts, S. Broeder, G. Vervoort, S. P. Swinnen, and A. Nieuwboer, "Handwriting Impairments in People with Parkinson's Disease and Freezing of Gait," *Neurorehabilitation and Neural Repair*, vol. 30, no. 10, pp. 911–919, 2016.

[39] E. Nackaerts, E. Heremans, G. Vervoort et al., "Relearning of writing skills in Parkinson's disease after intensive amplitude training," *Movement Disorders*, 2016.

[40] L. Guardati, F. Casamassima, E. Farella, and L. Benini, "Paper, pen and ink: An innovative system and software framework to assist writing rehabilitation," in *Proceedings of the 2015 Design, Automation and Test in Europe Conference and Exhibition, DATE 2015*, pp. 1473–1478, fra, March 2015.

[41] G. M. Petzinger, B. E. Fisher, S. McEwen, J. A. Beeler, J. P. Walsh, and M. W. Jakowec, "Exercise-enhanced neuroplasticity targeting motor and cognitive circuitry in Parkinson's disease," *The Lancet Neurology*, vol. 12, no. 7, pp. 716–726, 2013.

[42] E. Heremans, E. Nackaerts, G. Vervoort, S. Broeder, S. P. Swinnen, and A. Nieuwboer, "Impaired retention of motor learning of writing skills in patients with Parkinson's disease with freezing of gait," *PLoS ONE*, vol. 11, no. 2, Article ID e0148933, 2016.

[43] S. Gerth, T. Dolk, A. Klassert et al., "Adapting to the surface: a comparison of handwriting measures when writing on a tablet computer and on paper," *Human Movement Science*, vol. 48, pp. 62–73, 2016.

[44] J. J. van der Gon Denier and J. P. Thuring, "The guiding of human writing movements," *Kybernetik*, vol. 2, no. 4, pp. 145–148, 1965.

21

Dynamic Changes in the Nigrostriatal Pathway in the MPTP Mouse Model of Parkinson's Disease

Dongping Huang,[1] Jing Xu,[2] Jinghui Wang,[1] Jiabin Tong,[1] Xiaochen Bai,[1] Heng Li,[1] Zishan Wang,[1] Yulu Huang,[3] Yufei Wu,[3] Mei Yu,[1] and Fang Huang[1]

[1]*The State Key Laboratory of Medical Neurobiology, The Institutes of Brain Science and the Collaborative Innovation Center for Brain Science, Shanghai Medical College, Fudan University, 138 Yixueyuan Road, Shanghai 200032, China*
[2]*School of Life Science and Technology, Tongji University, 1239 Siping Road, Shanghai 200092, China*
[3]*School of Basic Medical Sciences, Fudan University, 138 Yixueyuan Road, Shanghai 200032, China*

Correspondence should be addressed to Mei Yu; yumei@fudan.edu.cn and Fang Huang; huangf@shmu.edu.cn

Academic Editor: Ivan Bodis-Wollner

The characteristic brain pathology and motor and nonmotor symptoms of Parkinson's disease (PD) are well established. However, the details regarding the causes of the disease and its course are much less clear. Animal models have significantly enriched our current understanding of the progression of this disease. Among various neurotoxin-based models of PD, 1-methyl-4-phenyl-1,2,3,6-tetrahydropyridine (MPTP) mouse model is the most commonly studied model. Here, we provide an overview of the dynamic changes in the nigrostriatal pathway in the MPTP mouse model of PD. Pathophysiological events, such as reductions in the striatal dopamine (DA) concentrations and levels of the tyrosine hydroxylase (TH) protein, depletion of TH-positive nerve fibers, a decrease in the number of TH-positive neurons in the substantia nigra pars compacta (SNpc), and glial activation, are addressed. This article will assist with the development of interventions or therapeutic strategies for PD.

1. Introduction

Parkinson's disease (PD) is the second most common neurodegenerative disorder, which is prevalent among the elderly [1, 2]. An anatomical circuit, the nigrostriatal pathway, is required for the fine tuning of basal ganglion function. This pathway is preferentially damaged in patients with PD and subsequently contributes to the clinical motor abnormalities, including tremor, muscle stiffness, a paucity of voluntary movements, and postural instability [3]. The main neuropathological features of PD are the loss of dopaminergic neurons in the substantia nigra pars compacta (SNpc) and their projections into the caudate nucleus, as well as the cytoplasmic accumulation of proteinaceous aggregates, Lewy bodies (LBs), which were named after the neurologist Frederic Lewy [4]. During a 200-year period, the characteristic brain pathology and motor and nonmotor symptoms of PD have been well described. However, the etiology and pathogenesis of PD remain unclear [5, 6]. Based on abundant

studies of postmortem tissue and various genetic or neurotoxic animal models, the death of dopaminergic neurons has been linked to mitochondrial dysfunction, oxidative stress, neuroinflammation, and insufficient protein degradation [7]. Since the first synthesis of MPTP in the 1970s, MPTP-based animal models have greatly improved our understanding of the cause and course of the disease [8, 9]. Here, we provide a brief review of the dynamic changes observed in the nigrostriatal pathway in the MPTP mouse model of PD.

2. Microglia, Astrocytes, and Neurons in the Nigrostriatal Pathway

Microglia and astrocytes are categorized as glial cell populations. In contrast to other glial cells and neurons, which are of neuroectodermal origin, microglia are derived from primitive hematopoiesis in the fetal yolk sac and migrate into the brain during early fetal development [10, 11]. Using ablation approaches in the adult brains, microglia have been shown to possess a repopulation capacity; approximately 1 week after depletion, microglia are restored to their normal density [12–14]. Microglia constitute 5–20% of the total glial cell population in the rodent brains. The basal ganglia and substantia nigra (SN) are among the most densely populated areas [15]. Acting as primary cells that respond to pathogen infection and injury, microglial cells play the roles of resident macrophages in the central nervous system (CNS) [10, 16, 17]. By adopting an "amoeboid" phenotype, activated microglia produce many proinflammatory mediators, including cytokines, chemokines, reactive oxygen species (ROS), and nitric oxide (NO) [10]. The presence of reactive microglia in the SNpc of postmortem human brain tissue was first revealed as early as in 1988, suggesting the involvement of neuroinflammation in the pathogenesis of PD [18, 19].

Astrocytes represent the most abundant glial cell type in the adult brain [20]. The most important functions of astrocytes include the maintenance of water and ion homeostasis, participation in the tripartite synapse, and the formation of the blood brain barrier (BBB) [21]. Proteins that are generally used as astrocyte markers are the intermediate filament protein, glial fibrillary acidic protein (GFAP), the glutamate transporter, GLAST, and the aldehyde dehydrogenase 1 family member L1 (Aldh1L1) [22, 23]. Like microglia, astrocytes respond to inflammatory stimuli such as LPS, IL-1β, and TNF-α by producing an array of pro- and anti-inflammatory mediators, antioxidants, and neurotrophic factors. Reactive astrogliosis, which is characterized by increased expression levels of GFAP and hypertrophy of the cell body and its extensions, has been observed in affected brain regions of patients with PD [24, 25], indicating the involvement of astrocytes in the immune processes in PD [19].

Under physiological conditions, the crosstalk among neurons, astrocytes, and microglial cells are essential for the homeostasis of the nigrostriatal axis. Astrocytes promote the survival and maintenance of dopaminergic neurons by secreting various neurotrophic factors in the SN. Microglial cells survey the cerebral microenvironment and engulf cell debris. Therefore, both astrocytes and microglia are required for neuronal protection. However, astrocytes and microglial cells are not sufficient for the protection of dopaminergic neurons. Microglia and astrocytes are the main components of the innate immune system in the CNS [26, 27]. When the homeostasis of neurons, astrocytes, and microglial cells is disrupted with the administration of dopaminergic neurotoxins, such as MPTP and 6-hydroxydopamine (6-OHDA), neuroinflammatory activities mediated by activated microglia and reactive astrocytes promote neurodegeneration. Glial activation is indexed as an increase in the number and size of glial cells, as well as the induction of morphological changes.

The effects of exaggerated inflammatory responses on microglia are mainly considered deleterious [28]. Inhibition or attenuation of microglial activation is related to dopaminergic neuroprotection [29–32], with the exception of the report on IL-6 knockout mice [33]. However, the effects of reactive astrocytes are still controversial. Reactive astrocytes have been implicated in inducing oxidative stress and inflammation, therefore triggering the degeneration of dopaminergic neurons [27]. In contrast, astrocyte activation

may suppress neuroinflammation and improve the resistance of dopaminergic neurons in animal models of PD. Many of the results have been revealed using gene targeting strategies in animals in combination with the neurotoxin-based PD models. Genes and their products per se are not necessarily beneficial or detrimental. In glial cells, the expressed proteome coordinately implements glial functions. The ablation of certain genes alters responses to glial activation. For example, a glial deficiency of dopamine D1 receptor or an astrocytic deficiency of dopamine D2 receptor exacerbates dopaminergic neuronal loss in MPTP-challenged mice [34, 35], whereas the activation of glial cells lacking major histocompatibility complex II (MHC II) or Lipocalin-2 (LCN2) is inhibited in mice, and the dopaminergic system is subsequently protected following the MPTP treatment [31, 32].

Astrocytes are activated by damaged dopaminergic neurons [32, 36] or activated microglial cells [28, 31, 37]. Moreover, reactive astrocytes also secrete soluble factors that stimulate microglial activation [10, 27]. Interestingly, the status of astrocyte activation is correlated with dopaminergic neurodegeneration in MPTP mouse models: stronger astrocyte activation is associated with more severe damage to the nigrostriatal pathway [35, 36]; attenuated astrocyte activation is correlated with less dopaminergic neuronal loss [32]; and a lack of astrocyte activation is accompanied by nondopaminergic neurodegeneration [31].

3. The MPTP Mouse Model of Parkinson's Disease

Neurotoxins, such as MPTP, 6-OHDA, rotenone, paraquat, paraquat combined with manganese ethylenebisdithiocarbamate (Maneb), reserpine, and lipopolysaccharide (LPS), induce dopaminergic neurodegeneration in animals [7, 38]. Neurotoxic effects of MPTP on humans, monkeys, rodents, zebrafish, and C. elegans have been observed. For decades, the MPTP mouse model has been the most commonly used model for elucidating damage to the nigrostriatal pathway in PD.

MPTP is systemically administered to mice. Due to its lipophilic property, it easily crosses the BBB. Inside the brain, MPTP is converted to the intermediate 1-methyl-4-phenyl-2,3-dihydropyridinium species (MPDP$^+$) by glial monoamine oxidase-B (MAO-B) [39, 40]. MPDP$^+$ is subsequently oxidized to the toxic metabolite 1-methyl-4-phenylpyridinium (MPP$^+$) [41]. MPP$^+$ is released from the astrocytes through the organic cation transporter 3 into the extracellular space, where it is taken up by the dopaminergic neurons and terminals via the plasma membrane dopamine transporter [7, 38, 42, 43]. Once MPP$^+$ accumulates in dopaminergic neurons, it induces neurotoxicity primarily by inhibiting complex I of the mitochondrial electron transport chain [44], resulting in ATP depletion and oxidative stress mediated by superoxide and NO, followed by neuronal death [3].

The inbred strain C57BL/6 with high MAO-B activity is sensitive to MPTP toxicity. Following exposure to MPTP, the striatal MPP$^+$ content reaches the highest value within 2 h and the metabolite is cleared from the brain within 12 h

[29, 45–48]. In 1995, Jackson-Lewis and Przedborski developed the acute regimen [49], which is widely adopted in the study of PD. In this case, dynamic changes in the nigrostriatal pathway are examined in the acute MPTP mouse model (four injections of MPTP-HCl at a dose of 18–20 mg/kg with 2 h intervals between injections, 1 mg of MPTP-HCl equal to 0.826 mg of free base MPTP). C57BL/6 mice are euthanized at 90 min to 12 h, 1 day to 9 days, and 42 days to 90 days after the last MPTP administration to analyze immediate, early, and late effects, respectively.

4. Immediate Effects of MPTP on the Nigrostriatal Pathway

Following an acute MPTP treatment, the striatal concentrations of DA and its metabolite DOPAC are dramatically reduced to approximately 10% of the control level at 90 min after injection. No changes in the striatal HVA, 5-HT, or 5-HIAA levels are observed. At this time point, 67% of the TH-positive (TH^+) nerve fibers remained intact in the striatum. Thus, the inhibition of the enzymatic activity of TH by MPP^+ is more dramatic than the degeneration of TH^+ terminals. Using a stereological counting method, MPTP was shown to cause a slight decrease in the number of TH^+ neurons in the SNpc (87% of the control). Levels of the TH protein in the SN were comparable between the control and MPTP-injured mice [50]. These findings are consistent with the well-known concept that the striatal TH^+ fibers have a different sensitivity to the toxin MPTP compared to TH^+ soma in the SNpc [51–54]. Microglial activation, which is characterized by an increase in the number of microglia and changes in morphology, was detected in the striatum at 90 min after the last MPTP injection [50] (Figure 1). Microglial activation in the striatum and the SN was confirmed 12 h after the acute MPTP treatment in many other studies [55, 56]. Collectively, in the acute MPTP model, systemic injections of MPTP result in a rapid onset of neuroinflammatory responses in the striatum and the SN, and microglial activation and proliferation precede the death of dopaminergic neurons [50, 57].

5. Early Effects of MPTP on the Nigrostriatal Pathway

Reductions in striatal levels of the TH protein and the depletion of TH^+ nerve fibers are observed 1 day after MPTP intoxication. According to studies performing immuno-histochemical staining of the midbrain and stereological counting, the numbers of TH^+ neurons and Nissl-positive neurons are significantly decreased in the MPTP-lesioned SNpc. Notably, TH protein expression is not detected in the Fluoro-Jade B-positive degenerating neurons [50, 58]. At this time point, MPTP induces widespread microglial activation in the nigrostriatal pathway, as indicated by an increase in the number and size of $Iba1^+$ microglial cells and morphological changes, such as hypertrophy [50, 59]. At 7 days after injection, a remarkable number of microglial cells were still activated in the SN of young [35, 57] and

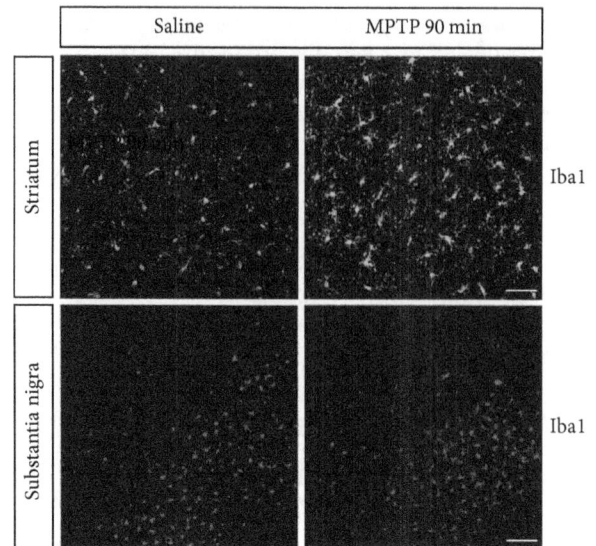

FIGURE 1: *Microglial cells in the nigrostriatal pathway at 90 min after acute MPTP treatment.* Immunofluorescence staining for Iba1 (green) in the striatum (scale bar: 0.05 mm) and immunofluorescence staining for Iba1 (red) in the SN (scale bar: 0.1 mm) were shown. This figure is adapted from Liu et al., *scientific reports* 5:15720 [50].

old mice [60]. One day after MPTP treatment, the striatal levels of the GFAP protein did not change, suggesting the astrocytes might still be at the resting state [58]. In another study, Muramatsu et al. observed a marked increase in the number of GFAP-positive astrocytes (exhibiting a ramified form with many fine processes) in both the striatum and the SN at 3 and 7 days after MPTP treatment [61]. Eight days after MPTP administration, the striatal levels of the GFAP protein were significantly increased [58]. Compared to the responses of microglia and neurons in the acute MPTP model, astrocytes manifest a delayed reaction, which is also involved in mediating the neuroinflammation [57].

At 9 days after the MPTP challenge, the striatal DA concentration reached 17% of the control, which was elevated compared with the value observed at 90 min [50]. The reductions in striatal levels of the TH protein, the depletion of TH^+ nerve fibers, and the decrease in the number of TH^+ neurons in the SNpc were maintained. At this time point, the activation of microglia in the nigrostriatal pathway autonomously decreased to a level similar to the resting state [50] (Figure 2).

6. Late Effects of MPTP on the Nigrostriatal Pathway

The entire nigrostriatal pathway undergoes a process of recovery 2-3 weeks after the acute MPTP treatment. At 42 days after the last MPTP injection, progressive striatal dopaminergic reinnervation was confirmed by DAT immunoreactivity and [^{3}H] dopamine uptake [55]. The striatal levels of the TH protein, the intensity of TH^+ nerve fibers, and the number of TH^+ neurons in the SNpc were still significantly reduced

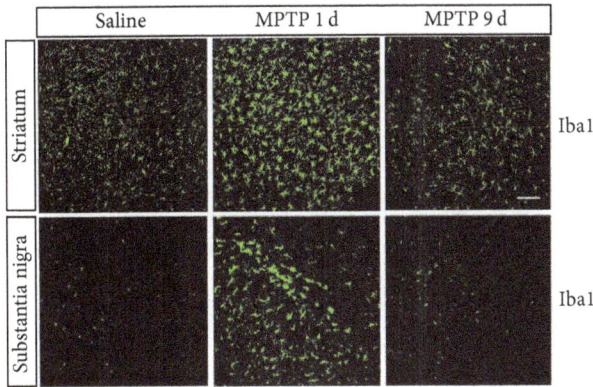

FIGURE 2: *Microglial cells in the nigrostriatal pathway at 1 and 9 days after acute MPTP treatment*. Immunofluorescence staining for Iba1 (green) in the striatum and in the SN was shown. Scale bar: 0.1 mm. This figure is adapted from Liu et al., scientific reports 5:15720 [50].

(unpublished data). These phenomena are maintained for 90 days after MPTP intoxication. Activated astrocytes are detected in the nigrostriatal pathway at 42 days (unpublished data), 65 days [62], and 90 days after injection (unpublished data).

7. Dynamic Changes in the Nigrostriatal Pathway in Subacute, Subchronic, and Chronic MPTP Mouse Models

In mice, acute MPTP treatment primarily damages the nigrostriatal dopaminergic pathway [3]. However, dopaminergic neurons die quickly and little progression in the loss of nigrostriatal DA is observed [46]. According to the study question, different MPTP regimens are applied in different studies [63]. The time course of the deleterious events and the magnitude of the lesion depend on the regimen of administration [52, 64]. Other commonly used MPTP regimens include the following:

(1) Presymptomatic PD model: an acute single MPTP application at low dose (1×10–20 mg/kg)

(2) Subacute PD model: repetitive subacute MPTP applications at intermediate doses (4×15–25 mg/kg at 6 or 12 h intervals within two days)

(3) Subchronic PD model: daily MPTP injections at doses of approximately 20–30 mg/kg for up to 4-5 consecutive days

(4) Progressive chronic PD model: daily injections of low doses (4 mg/kg) of MPTP over 20 days.

In the subacute PD regimen, adult male C57BL/6 mice were challenged with MPTP (24 mg/kg, every 12 h for 2 d). Mice were euthanized at different time points after the last dose. TH protein expression in both the striatum and the SN is noticeably decreased. According to the statistical analysis, the levels of TH protein in the striatum at 18, 36, and 72 h after injection were 38%, 45%, and 31% of the saline group, respectively, and the levels in the SN were 60%, 38%, and

67% of the control, respectively [65]. The dose of MPTP administered to 12-month-old mice was reduced to 15 mg/kg. Four weeks after the MPTP treatment, the level of striatal TH protein decreased by 59% compared with saline-treated mice, whereas the striatal DA concentration after the MPTP treatment decreased by 79%. Approximately 63% of dopaminergic neurons in the SN were lost following the MPTP treatment. The striatal GFAP level increased by 3.7-fold at 3 days after MPTP administration, and this level was maintained for 4 weeks in old mice [36].

The different responses observed in young and old mice have been repeatedly measured, but with some variation. The dosages of MPTP and the age are likely the main determining factors. Young (9–12 weeks old) and old (11–13 months old) mice were intraperitoneally injected with MPTP twice a day at 12 h intervals for 2 days. The dosage of MPTP was 20 mg/kg for young mice and 15 mg/kg for old animals. One or 3 days after the last MPTP injection, MPTP elicited an approximately 90% (1 day) to 55% (3 days) decrease in the striatal levels of the TH protein in young mice. In old mice, MPTP induced a nearly 70% (1 day or 3 days) decrease. On the 8th day, MPTP elicited a 57% decrease in the striatal levels of the TH protein. Approximately 80% and 70% losses of TH$^+$ fibers were observed in young mice 1 day or 3 days after MPTP intoxication. Meanwhile, MPTP caused an approximately 66% (1 day) to 58% (3 days) decrease in the density of TH$^+$ fibers in old mice. In the SN, MPTP elicited approximately 41% (1 day) to 38% (3 days) and 50% (1 day) to 53% (3 days) loss of TH$^+$ neurons in young and old mice, respectively. Based on electron microscopic analyses, MPTP induced a significant increase in the number of structurally altered mitochondria in the SNpc neurons of young mice at 3 days after injection; these alterations comprised numerous vacuoles and fragmented cristae. According to the quantitative analysis, the SNpc neurons exhibited a significantly higher percentage of damaged mitochondria (51.3%) [54]. In a study with cHS4I-hIL-1βP-Luc transgenic mice, in which the expression of luciferase reporter gene is controlled by the human *IL-1β* gene promoter [66], both old male and female mice were monitored following subacute MPTP intoxication. MPTP induced elevated expression of the IL-1β transcript in the cortex, striatum, and ventral midbrain at 2 h after treatment. Luciferase expression was significantly elevated at 2, 8, 32, and 49 h in MPTP-treated male mice, the inducible signals peaked at 8 h. The old female mice showed a marked increase in luciferase expression at 4 and 26 h after MPTP administration. At 96 h after the last MPTP injection, striatal levels of the GFAP protein were robustly increased. As expected, MPTP elicited less dopaminergic toxicity in old female than in male mice [67].

In the subchronic PD regimen (30 mg/kg/day for 5 consecutive days), MPTP induced the depletion of more than 90% of the TH protein in the striatum and reduced the number of TH$^+$ neurons in the SNpc by 30% at 24 h after injection. Notably, MPTP administration significantly increased the expression of α-synuclein in the striatum ([68] and unpublished data). The observation of reactive gliosis is also compelling in this model. A significantly higher number of Iba 1-positive cells were observed in the SNpc at 1 day [31]

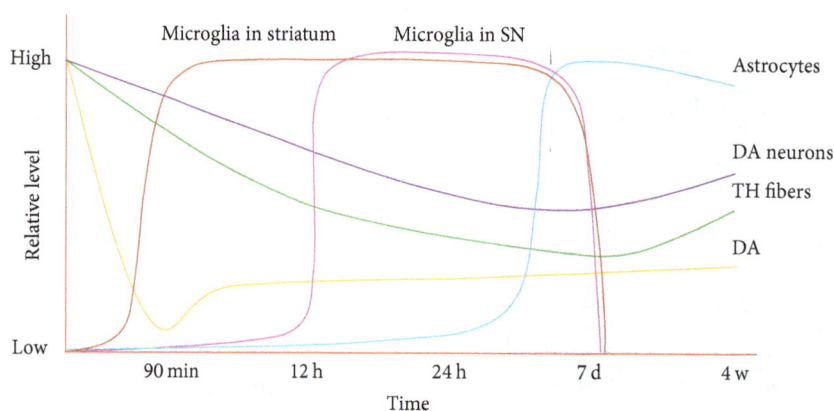

FIGURE 3: Dynamic changes in the nigrostriatal pathway in the acute MPTP mouse model of Parkinson's disease.

or 2 days [30], after MPTP treatment. However, at 2 days after injection, astrogliosis is not consistently detected [30, 31]. Three weeks after the injection, the striatal DA level was reduced to 17% of the control level by the MPTP treatment [31], whereas 42% of the TH^+ neurons in the SNpc and 14% of TH^+ fibers (by density assay) in the striatum were preserved and the astroglial cell count increased [30].

In summary, the specific and reproducible neurotoxic effect on the nigrostriatal system are a strength of MPTP induced PD models. However, MPTP mouse models exhibit an apparent lack of Lewy body-like inclusions bodies in the midbrain [46, 69]. Here, the communication between the CNS and immune system, which also contributes to the progression of PD, should be mentioned. Peripheral immune cells play an important role during the course of neuroinflammation in the mouse MPTP models, with reports of $CD4^+$ and $CD8^+$ T-lymphocytes infiltrating the SN [70].

8. Conclusions

The nigrostriatal pathway plays an important role in regulating the functions of the basal ganglion. Under physiological conditions, neurons, astrocytes, and microglia support each other and maintain a triple "win-win" relationship. When exposed to environmental or endogenous toxins, which may be combined with genetic susceptibility, this circuit is damaged, causing motor symptoms in patients with PD. The strengths and limitations of MPTP mouse models of PD are both remarkable. Microglial activation precedes the degeneration of dopaminergic neurons and astrocyte activation in the nigrostriatal pathway of the acute MPTP mouse model. The dynamic changes observed in the nigrostriatal pathway are summarized in Figure 3. A better understanding of the time course of pathophysiological events will benefit studies developing interventions or therapeutic strategies for PD.

Authors' Contributions

Dongping Huang and Jing Xu contributed equally to this paper.

Acknowledgments

This work was supported by grants from the National Natural Science Foundation of China (31671043, 81371412, and 81400992) and the Open Project of State Key Laboratory of Medical Neurobiology (SKLMN2015005).

References

[1] R. L. Mosley, J. A. Hutter-Saunders, D. K. Stone, and H. E. Gendelman, "Inflammation and adaptive immunity in Parkinson's disease," *Cold Spring Harbor Perspectives in Medicine*, vol. 2, no. 1, 2012.

[2] T. M. Dawson, H. S. Ko, and V. L. Dawson, "Genetic animal models of Parkinson's disease," *Neuron*, vol. 66, no. 5, pp. 646–661, 2010.

[3] W. Dauer and S. Przedborski, "Parkinson's disease: mechanisms and models," *Neuron*, vol. 39, no. 6, pp. 889–909, 2003.

[4] L. S. Forno, "Neuropathology of Parkinson's disease," *Journal of Neuropathology and Experimental Neurology*, vol. 55, no. 3, pp. 259–272, 1996.

[5] L. Drew, "Two hundred steps," *Nature*, vol. 538, no. 7626, pp. S2–S3, 2016.

[6] S. Deweerdt, "Parkinson's disease: 4 big questions," *Nature*, vol. 538, no. 7626, p. S17, 2016.

[7] K. Tieu, "A guide to neurotoxic animal models of Parkinson's disease," *Cold Spring Harbor perspectives in medicine*, vol. 1, no. 1, p. a009316, 2011.

[8] G. C. Davis, A. C. Williams, S. P. Markey et al., "Chronic parkinsonism secondary to intravenous injection of meperidine analogues," *Psychiatry Research*, vol. 1, no. 3, pp. 249–254, 1979.

[9] J. W. Langston, P. Ballard, J. W. Tetrud, and I. Irwin, "Chronic parkinsonism in humans due to a product of meperidine-analog synthesis," *Science*, vol. 219, no. 4587, pp. 979-980, 1983.

[10] K. Saijo and C. K. Glass, "Microglial cell origin and phenotypes in health and disease," *Nature Reviews Immunology*, vol. 11, no. 11, pp. 775–787, 2011.

[11] F. Alliot, I. Godin, and B. Pessac, "Microglia derive from progenitors, originating from the yolk sac, and which proliferate in the brain," *Developmental Brain Research*, vol. 117, no. 2, pp. 145–152, 1999.

[12] M. R. P. Elmore, A. R. Najafi, M. A. Koike et al., "Colony-stimulating factor 1 receptor signaling is necessary for microglia viability, unmasking a microglia progenitor cell in the adult brain," *Neuron*, vol. 82, pp. 380–397, 2014.

[13] J. Bruttger, K. Karram, S. Wörtge et al., "Genetic cell ablation reveals clusters of local self-renewing microglia in the mammalian central nervous system," *Immunity*, vol. 43, no. 1, pp. 92–107, 2015.

[14] S. Jäkel and L. Dimou, "Glial cells and their function in the adult brain: a journey through the history of their ablation," *Frontiers in Cellular Neuroscience*, vol. 11, 24 pages, 2017.

[15] L. J. Lawson, V. H. Perry, P. Dri, and S. Gordon, "Heterogeneity in the distribution and morphology of microglia in the normal adult mouse brain," *Neuroscience*, vol. 39, no. 1, pp. 151–170, 1990.

[16] H. Kettenmann, U. K. Hanisch, M. Noda, and A. Verkhratsky, "Physiology of microglia," *Physiological Reviews*, vol. 91, no. 2, pp. 461–553, 2011.

[17] A. Suzumura, "Neuron-microglia interaction in neuroinflammation," *Current Protein and Peptide Science*, vol. 14, no. 1, pp. 16–20, 2013.

[18] P. L. McGeer, S. Itagaki, B. E. Boyes, and E. G. McGeer, "Reactive microglia are positive for HLA-DR in the substantia nigra of Parkinson's and Alzheimer's disease brains," *Neurology*, vol. 38, no. 8, pp. 1285–1291, 1988.

[19] Q. Wang, Y. Liu, and J. Zhou, "Neuroinflammation in Parkinson's disease and its potential as therapeutic target," *Neurodegeneration*, vol. 4, article 19, 2015.

[20] S. Lee, J.-Y. Park, W.-H. Lee et al., "Lipocalin-2 is an autocrine mediator of reactive astrocytosis," *Journal of Neuroscience*, vol. 29, no. 1, pp. 234–249, 2009.

[21] H. K. Kimelberg and M. Nedergaard, "Functions of astrocytes and their potential as therapeutic targets," *Neurotherapeutics*, vol. 7, no. 4, pp. 338–353, 2010.

[22] R. Srinivasan, T.-Y. Lu, H. Chai et al., "New Transgenic Mouse Lines for Selectively Targeting Astrocytes and Studying Calcium Signals in Astrocyte Processes In Situ and In Vivo," *Neuron*, vol. 92, no. 6, pp. 1181–1195, 2016.

[23] H. M. Jahn, A. Scheller, and F. Kirchhoff, "Genetic control of astrocyte function in neural circuits," *Frontiers in Cellular Neuroscience*, vol. 9, no. AUGUST, article no. 310, 2015.

[24] J. W. Langston, L. S. Forno, J. Tetrud, A. G. Reeves, J. A. Kaplan, and D. Karluk, "Evidence of active nerve cell degeneration in the substantia nigra of humans years after 1-methyl-4-phenyl-1,2,3,6-tetrahydropyridine exposure," *Annals of Neurology*, vol. 46, no. 4, pp. 598–605, 1999.

[25] T. Yamada, T. Kawamata, D. G. Walker, and P. L. McGeer, "Vimentin immunoreactivity in normal and pathological human brain tissue," *Acta Neuropathologica*, vol. 84, no. 2, pp. 157–162, 1992.

[26] M. C. O. Rodrigues, P. R. Sanberg, L. E. Cruz, and S. Garbuzova-Davis, "The innate and adaptive immunological aspects in neurodegenerative diseases," *Journal of Neuroimmunology*, vol. 269, no. 1-2, pp. 1–8, 2014.

[27] C. K. Glass, K. Saijo, B. Winner, M. C. Marchetto, and F. H. Gage, "Mechanisms underlying inflammation in neurodegeneration," *Cell*, vol. 140, no. 6, pp. 918–934, 2010.

[28] K. Saijo, B. Winner, C. T. Carson et al., "A Nurr1/CoREST pathway in microglia and astrocytes protects dopaminergic neurons from inflammation-induced death," *Cell*, vol. 137, no. 1, pp. 47–59, 2009.

[29] M. Moon, H. G. Kim, L. Hwang et al., "Blockade of microglial activation is neuroprotective in the 1-methyl-4-phenyl-1,2,3,6-tetrahydropyridine mouse model of Parkinson disease," *Journal of Neuroscience*, vol. 22, no. 5, pp. 1763–1771, 2002.

[30] K. Sathe, W. Maetzler, J. D. Lang et al., "S100B is increased in Parkinson's disease and ablation protects against MPTP-induced toxicity through the RAGE and TNF-α pathway," *Brain*, vol. 135, no. 11, pp. 3336–3347, 2012.

[31] H. L. Martin, M. Santoro, S. Mustafa, G. Riedel, J. V. Forrester, and P. Teismann, "Evidence for a role of adaptive immune response in the disease pathogenesis of the MPTP mouse model of Parkinson's disease," *Glia*, vol. 64, no. 3, pp. 386–395, 2016.

[32] B.-W. Kim, K. H. Jeong, J.-H. Kim et al., "Pathogenic upregulation of glial lipocalin-2 in the parkinsonian dopaminergic system," *Journal of Neuroscience*, vol. 36, no. 20, pp. 5608–5622, 2016.

[33] H. Cardenas and L. M. Bolin, "Compromised reactive microgliosis in MPTP-lesioned IL-6 KO mice," *Brain Research*, vol. 985, no. 1, pp. 89–97, 2003.

[34] Y. Yan, W. Jiang, L. Liu et al., "Dopamine controls systemic inflammation through inhibition of NLRP3 inflammasome," *Cell*, vol. 160, no. 1-2, pp. 62–73, 2015.

[35] W. Shao, S.-Z. Zhang, M. Tang et al., "Suppression of neuroinflammation by astrocytic dopamine D2 receptors via αb-crystallin," *Nature*, vol. 494, no. 7435, pp. 90–94, 2013.

[36] M. Yu, H. Suo, M. Liu et al., "NRSF/REST neuronal deficient mice are more vulnerable to the neurotoxin MPTP," *Neurobiology of Aging*, vol. 34, no. 3, pp. 916–927, 2013.

[37] S. A. Liddelow, K. A. Guttenplan, L. E. Clarke et al., "Neurotoxic reactive astrocytes are induced by activated microglia," *Nature*, vol. 541, no. 7638, pp. 481–487, 2017.

[38] J. Bové and C. Perier, "Neurotoxin-based models of Parkinson's disease," *Neuroscience*, vol. 211, pp. 51–76, 2012.

[39] R. E. Heikkila, L. Manzino, F. S. Cabbat, and R. C. Duvoisin, "Protection against the dopaminergic neurotoxicity of 1-methyl-4-phenyl-1,2, 5,6-tetrahydropyridine by monoamine oxidase inhibitors," *Nature*, vol. 311, no. 5985, pp. 467–469, 1984.

[40] K. Chiba, A. Trevor, and N. Castagnoli Jr., "Metabolism of the neurotoxic tertiary amine, MPTP, by brain monoamine oxidase," *Biochemical and Biophysical Research Communications*, vol. 120, no. 2, pp. 574–578, 1984.

[41] R. Heikkila, A. Hess, and R. Duvoisin, "Dopaminergic neurotoxicity of 1-methyl-4-phenyl-1,2,5,6-tetrahydropyridine in mice," *Science*, vol. 224, no. 4656, pp. 1451–1453, 1984.

[42] S. J. Choi, A. Panhelainen, Y. Schmitz et al., "Changes in neuronal dopamine homeostasis following 1-methyl-4-phenylpyridinium (MPP+) exposure," *Journal of Biological Chemistry*, vol. 290, no. 11, pp. 6799–6809, 2015.

[43] J. A. Javitch, R. J. D'Amato, S. M. Strittmatter, and S. H. Snyder, "Parkinsonism-inducing neurotoxin, N-methyl-4-phenyl-1,2,3,6 -tetrahydropyridine: uptake of the metabolite N-methyl-4-phenylpyridine by dopamine neurons explains selective toxicity," *Proceedings of the National Academy of Sciences of the United States of America*, vol. 82, no. 7, pp. 2173–2177, 1985.

[44] W. J. Nicklas, I. Vyas, and R. E. Heikkila, "Inhibition of NADH-linked oxidation in brain mitochondria by 1-methyl-4-phenyl-pyridine, a metabolite of the neurotoxin, 1-methyl-4-phenyl-1,2,5,6-tetrahydropyridine," *Life Sciences*, vol. 36, no. 26, pp. 2503–2508, 1985.

[45] V. Jackson-Lewis and S. Przedborski, "Protocol for the MPTP mouse model of Parkinson's disease," *Nature Protocols*, vol. 2, no. 1, pp. 141–151, 2007.

[46] G. E. Meredith and D. J. Rademacher, "MPTP mouse models of Parkinson's disease: an update," *Journal of Parkinson's Disease*, vol. 1, no. 1, pp. 19–33, 2011.

[47] T. Kawasaki, Y. Ago, T. Kitao et al., "A neuroprotective agent, T-817MA (1-3-[2-(1-benzothiophen-5-yl)ethoxy]propyl azetidin-3-ol maleate), prevents 1-methyl-4-phenyl-1,2,3,6-tetrahydro-pyridine-induced neurotoxicity in mice," *Neuropharmacology*, vol. 55, no. 5, pp. 654–660, 2008.

[48] Y. C. Chung, S. R. Kim, J. Park et al., "Fluoxetine prevents MPTP-induced loss of dopaminergic neurons by inhibiting microglial activation," *Neuropharmacology*, vol. 60, no. 6, pp. 963–974, 2011.

[49] V. Jackson-Lewis, M. Jakowec, R. E. Burke, and S. Przedborski, "Time course and morphology of dopaminergic neuronal death caused by the neurotoxin 1-methyl-4-phenyl-1,2,3,6-tet-rahydropyridine," *Neurodegeneration*, vol. 4, no. 3, pp. 257–269, 1995.

[50] J. Liu, D. Huang, J. Xu et al., "Tiagabine Protects Dopaminergic Neurons against Neurotoxins by Inhibiting Microglial Activation," *Scientific Reports*, vol. 5, Article ID 15720, 2015.

[51] P. Teismann, K. Tieu, D. K. Choi et al., "Cyclooxygenase-2 is instrumental in Parkinson's disease neurodegeneration," *Proceedings of the National Academy of Sciences of the United States of America*, vol. 100, no. 9, pp. 5473–5478, 2003.

[52] C. Gibrat, M. Saint-Pierre, M. Bousquet, D. Lévesque, C. Rouillard, and F. Cicchetti, "Differences between subacute and chronic MPTP mice models: investigation of dopaminergic neuronal degeneration and α-synuclein inclusions," *Journal of Neurochemistry*, vol. 109, no. 5, pp. 1469–1482, 2009.

[53] G. Costa, L. Frau, J. Wardas, A. Pinna, A. Plumitallo, and M. Morelli, "MPTP-induced dopamine neuron degeneration and glia activation is potentiated in MDMA-pretreated mice," *Movement Disorders*, vol. 28, no. 14, pp. 1957–1965, 2013.

[54] M. Bian, J. Liu, X. Hong et al., "Overexpression of parkin ameliorates dopaminergic neurodegeneration induced by 1-methyl-4-phenyl-1,2,3,6-tetrahydropyridine in mice," *PLoS ONE*, vol. 7, no. 6, Article ID e39953, 2012.

[55] F. L'Episcopo, C. Tirolo, N. Testa et al., "Plasticity of subventricular zone neuroprogenitors in MPTP (1-Methyl-4-Phenyl-1,2,3,6-tetrahydropyridine) mouse model of Parkinson's disease involves cross talk between inflammatory and Wnt/β-catenin signaling pathways: functional consequences for neuroprotection and repair," *Journal of Neuroscience*, vol. 32, no. 6, pp. 2062–2085, 2012.

[56] T. Furuya, H. Hayakawa, M. Yamada et al., "Caspase-11 mediates inflammatory dopaminergic cell death in the 1-methyl-4-phenyl-1,2,3,6-tetrahydropyridine mouse model of Parkinson's disease," *Journal of Neuroscience*, vol. 24, no. 8, pp. 1865–1872, 2004.

[57] M. Kohutnicka, E. Lewandowska, I. Kurkowska-Jastrzebska, A. Członkowski, and A. Członkowska, "Microglial and astrocytic involvement in a murine model of Parkinson's disease induced by 1-methyl-4-phenyl-1,2,3,6-tetrahydropyridine (MPTP)," *Immunopharmacology*, vol. 39, no. 3, pp. 167–180, 1998.

[58] H. Suo, P. Wang, J. Tong et al., "NRSF is an essential mediator for the neuroprotection of trichostatin A in the MPTP mouse model of Parkinson's disease," *Neuropharmacology*, vol. 99, pp. 67–78, 2015.

[59] M. Jin, B. W. Kim, S. Koppula et al., "Molecular effects of activated BV-2 microglia by mitochondrial toxin 1-methyl-4-phenylpyridinium," *NeuroToxicology*, vol. 33, no. 2, pp. 147–155, 2012.

[60] J. Xu, L. Bu, L. Huang et al., "Heart failure having little effect on the progression of Parkinson's disease: Direct evidence from mouse model," *International Journal of Cardiology*, vol. 177, no. 2, pp. 683–689, 2014.

[61] Y. Muramatsu, R. Kurosaki, H. Watanabe et al., "Expression of S-100 protein is related to neuronal damage in MPTP-treated mice," *GLIA*, vol. 42, no. 3, pp. 307–313, 2003.

[62] F. L'Episcopo, C. Tirolo, N. Testa et al., "Wnt/β-catenin signaling is required to rescue midbrain dopaminergic progenitors and promote neurorepair in ageing mouse model of Parkinson's disease," *Stem Cells*, vol. 32, no. 8, pp. 2147–2163, 2014.

[63] V. Machado, T. Zöller, A. Attaai, and B. Spittau, "Microglia-mediated neuroinflammation and neurotrophic factor-induced protection in the MPTP mouse model of parkinson's disease-lessons from transgenic mice," *International Journal of Molecular Sciences*, vol. 17, no. 2, article no. 151, 2016.

[64] S. Przedborski and M. Vila, "The 1-methyl-4-phenyl-1,2,3,6-tetrahydropyridine mouse model: a tool to explore the pathogenesis of Parkinson's disease," *Annals of the New York Academy of Sciences*, vol. 991, pp. 189–198, 2003.

[65] M. Bian, M. Yu, S. Yang et al., "Expression of Cbl-interacting protein of 85 kDa in MPTP mouse model of Parkinson's disease and 1-methyl-4-phenyl-pyridinium ion-treated dopaminergic SH-SY5Y cells," *Acta Biochimica et Biophysica Sinica*, vol. 40, no. 6, pp. 505–512, 2008.

[66] L. Li, Z. Fei, J. Ren et al., "Functional imaging of interleukin 1 beta expression in inflammatory process using bioluminescence imaging in transgenic mice," *BMC Immunology*, vol. 9, article no. 49, 2008.

[67] M.-J. Bian, L.-M. Li, M. Yu, J. Fei, and F. Huang, "Elevated interleukin-1β induced by 1-methyl-4-phenyl-1,2,3,6-tetrahydropyridine aggravating dopaminergic neurodegeneration in old male mice," *Brain Research*, vol. 1302, pp. 256–264, 2009.

[68] M. Xia, M. Bian, Q. Yu et al., "Cold water stress attenuates dopaminergic neurotoxicity induced by 1-methyl-4-phenyl-1,2,3,6-tetrahydropyridine in mice," *Acta Biochimica et Biophysica Sinica*, vol. 43, no. 6, pp. 448–454, 2011.

[69] D. Alvarez-Fischer, S. Guerreiro, S. Hunot et al., "Modelling Parkinson-like neurodegeneration via osmotic minipump delivery of MPTP and probenecid," *Journal of Neurochemistry*, vol. 107, no. 3, pp. 701–711, 2008.

[70] I. Kurkowska-Jastrzebska, A. Wrońska, M. Kohutnicka, A. Czlonkowski, and A. Czlonkowska, "The inflammatory reaction following 1-methyl-4-phenyl-1,2,3,6- tetrahydropyridine intoxication in mouse," *Experimental Neurology*, vol. 156, no. 1, pp. 50–61, 1999.

22

Dual-Task Performance in GBA Parkinson's Disease

Karin Srulijes,[1,2,3] Kathrin Brockmann,[1,2] Senait Ogbamicael,[1,2]
Markus A. Hobert,[1,2,4] Ann-Kathrin Hauser,[1,2] Claudia Schulte,[1,2] Jasmin Fritzen,[1,2]
Michael Schwenk,[3,5] Thomas Gasser,[1,2] Daniela Berg,[1,2,4] and Walter Maetzler[1,2,4]

[1]Department of Neurodegeneration, Hertie Institute for Clinical Brain Research, University of Tübingen, Tübingen, Germany
[2]German Research Center for Neurodegenerative Diseases (DZNE), University of Tübingen, Tübingen, Germany
[3]Department of Geriatrics and Clinic of Geriatric Rehabilitation, Robert-Bosch-Hospital, Stuttgart, Germany
[4]Department of Neurology, Kiel University, Kiel, Germany
[5]Network Aging Research, Heidelberg University, Heidelberg, Germany

Correspondence should be addressed to Walter Maetzler; w.maetzler@neurologie.uni-kiel.de

Academic Editor: Antonio Pisani

Introduction. Parkinson's disease patients carrying a heterozygous mutation in the gene *glucocerebrosidase* (GBA-PD) show faster motor and cognitive decline than idiopathic Parkinson's disease (iPD) patients, but the mechanisms behind this observation are not well understood. Successful dual tasking (DT) requires a smooth integration of motor and nonmotor operations. This study compared the DT performances between GBA-PD and iPD patients. *Methods.* Eleven GBA-PD patients (p.N370S, p.L444P) and eleven matched iPD patients were included. Clinical characterization included a motor score (Unified PD Rating Scale-III, UPDRS-III) and nonmotor scores (Montreal Cognitive Assessment, MoCA, and Beck's Depression Inventory). Quantitative gait analysis during the single-task (ST) and DT assessments was performed using a wearable sensor unit. These parameters corrected for UPDRS and MoCA were then compared between the groups. *Results.* Under the DT condition "walking while checking boxes," GBA-PD patients showed slower gait and box-checking speeds than iPD patients. GBA-PD and iPD patients did not show significant differences regarding dual-task costs. *Conclusion.* This pilot study suggests that DT performance with a secondary motor task is worse in GBA-PD than in iPD patients. This finding may be associated with the known enhanced motor and cognitive deficits in GBA-PD compared to iPD and should motivate further studies.

1. Introduction

Heterozygous mutations in the *glucocerebrosidase (GBA)* gene represent the most common genetic risk factor for PD so far [1]. Moreover, it has been repeatedly shown that patients with such mutations (GBA-PD patients) present with a different phenotype than idiopathic Parkinson's disease (iPD) patients. For example, they suffer from an earlier age of onset and more rapid disease progression, including motor and nonmotor symptoms, such as cognitive, autonomic, and neuropsychiatric impairment [2–6].

However, it is not yet clear whether GBA-PD patients also differ from iPD patients regarding dual-task (DT) performance. Dual tasking—the performance of two tasks simultaneously—is accomplished multitudinously in one's daily routine. It is required, for example, when crossing a street while observing the surrounding traffic or when talking while walking. Malfunction of this performance can impair safe ambulation in complex natural environments and even have fatal consequences, such as falls. Almost half of the falls of PD patients are the result of trying to carry out two or more tasks simultaneously [7]. Associations between impaired DT and increased risk of a future fall in PD have been described recently [8]. The simultaneous performance of two motor tasks seems to be a valuable fall predictor, fitting well with patients' balance complaints when, for example, taking a cup out of the cupboard.

DT performance has also been used to analyze deficits of motor-cognitive interaction in PD [9]. As gait is not a fully automatic motor task but requires attentional performance and executive functioning [10], an analysis of gait under DT conditions can help detect motor-cognitive deficits.

The present work aimed to evaluate whether the known differences in motor and nonmotor impairments between GBA-PD and iPD are also reflected in differences in DT performance.

2. Materials and Methods

2.1. Ethics. The study protocol was approved by the ethical committee of the Medical Faculty of the University of Tuebingen (number 49720091). All participants gave written informed consent.

2.2. Mutational Screening. Of the PD patients from across Germany who donated DNA to our biobank (https://www.hih-tuebingen.de/ueber-uns/core-facilities/biobank/) between 2006 and 2009 and agreed to genetic testing, the two most common mutations of the *GBA* gene (p.N370S, p.L444P) were screened. For detailed information, refer to Brockmann et al. [2].

2.3. Patients. Thirty-three GBA patients with one of the above-mentioned mutations were identified. All were contacted via mail and/or telephone. Eventually, eleven patients were included in this study. Twenty-two patients could not be investigated due to a degree of clinical impairment that prevented participation. To evaluate GBA-PD-specific features, eleven idiopathic PD patients (controlled to have none of the two *GBA* mutations) were matched for age, gender, and disease duration and were included in this analysis.

2.4. Clinical Assessment. PD was diagnosed according to the UK Brain Bank Society Criteria [11]. All assessments were performed in the dopaminergic ON state. Actual medication was assessed and Levodopa dose equivalency calculated [12] (see Table 1). The severity of motor symptoms was assessed using the motor part of the Unified PD Rating Scale (UPDRS-III) [13]. The Montreal Cognitive Assessment (MoCA) was used to screen for cognitive deficits, and a score of <26 out of 30 points was interpreted as indicating the presence of cognitive impairment [14]. By use of the Trail Making Test, cognitive flexibility and working memory were assessed [15]. Mood disturbance was assessed with Beck's Depression Inventory (BDI-II) [16].

2.5. Gait Analysis. All assessments were performed in a straight corridor at least 1.5 meters wide to allow free 20-meter walks. Gait analysis was performed using a wearable sensor unit (DynaPort Hybrid®, McRoberts, The Netherlands) attached via belt to the lower back. The sensor unit contained a triaxial accelerometer and a triaxial gyroscope. Data were transferred to McRoberts for automated gait analysis. Of the 20 m walked, the first and last 15% of the steps were excluded from the analysis to analyze only steady-state gait.

2.6. Single- and Dual-Task Procedure. All participants performed *three ST trials*: walking at a fast speed, checking boxes, and subtracting serial 7s. During the box-checking task, participants were instructed to mark as fast as possible

TABLE 1: Demographics and clinical characteristics.

	GBA-PD	iPD	*p* value
Demographics			
Male (female) [*n*]	9 (2)	9 (2)	1.00
Age [years]	58 (41–70)	62 (41–70)	0.51
Age of onset [years]	50 (28–65)	54 (36–62)	0.22
Disease duration [years]	6 (4–13)	6 (3–10)	0.46
Levodopa dose equivalent	700 (100–1500)	400 (80–800)	0.27
Motor function			
UPDRS-III (0–108)	35 (24–55)	27 (6–51)	**0.01**
Nonmotor function			
MoCA (0–30)	25 (11–29)	28 (23–30)	0.06
TMT A [s]	45 (30–263)	37 (25–66)	0.31
TMT B [s]	95 (47–300)	86 (50–300)	0.37
ΔTMT [s]	44 (16–98)	39 (24–234)	0.89
BDI-II (0–63)	9 (5–27)	9 (1–31)	0.49

Mann-Whitney *U* test. Values are given in median (range). Significance level was set at *p* < 0.05. UPDRS-III = Unified Parkinson's disease rating scale, part III motor score; MoCA = Montreal Cognitive Assessment; TMT = Trail Making Test; ΔTMT = TMT B − TMT A; BDI-II = revised version of the Becks Depression Inventory; GBA-PD = Parkinson's disease patients carrying a heterozygous glucocerebrosidase mutation; iPD = idiopathic Parkinson's disease.

each of the 32 boxes with a pencil on a paper sheet fixed on a clipboard held in their hand. During the subtracting task, subjects were asked to subtract serial 7s from a randomly chosen three-digit number until 10 subtractions were completed as fast as possible.

All participants then performed *two DT trials*: walking while checking boxes and walking while subtracting serial 7s. The following parameters were collected during the tasks: the duration of the tasks, the number of checked boxes, and the number of subtractions during DT. No instruction on prioritization (either walking or secondary task) was given.

2.7. Statistics. Statistical analysis was performed using JMP 11 software (SAS Institute Inc.). Clinical and demographic variables were compared nonparametrically using the Mann-Whitney *U* test (Table 1). Due to slight clinical differences between the GBA-PD and iPD groups (see Table 1), all outcome variables were corrected for UPDRS-III and MoCA by use of a multivariate regression model. Differences were considered significant at *p* < 0.05 (two-sided). Dual-task costs (DTC) were calculated using the formula according to [17, 18].

$$DTC = \frac{(ST - DT)}{ST} * 100. \quad (1)$$

DTC were defined as the percentage change between single- and dual-task performance: ([single-task − dual-task]/single-task) × 100. Therefore, DTC represent the relative difference in performance between ST and DT.

TABLE 2: Single- and dual-task performance.

	GBA-PD ($n = 11$)	iPD ($n = 11$)	p value
Single-task condition			
Walking speed [m/s]	0.85 (0.54–1.13)	1.07 (0.71–1.35)	**0.038**
Checking boxes [1/s]	1.03 (0.53–1.84)	1.56 (0.91–2.29)	0.059
Subtracting [1/s]	0.31 (0.05–0.49)	0.31 (0.16–0.71)	0.134
Dual-task condition			
Walking speed while checking boxes [m/s]	0.75 (0.39–0.95)	0.97 (0.61–1.25)	**0.024**
Checking boxes while walking [1/s]	0.76 (0.00–0.95)	1.33 (0.95–2.17)	**<0.0001**
Walking speed while subtracting [m/s]	0.75 (0.51–0.95)	0.88 (0.63–1.35)	0.115
Subtracting while walking [1/s]	0.40 (0.07–0.71)	0.42 (0.23–0.78)	0.979

Values are given in median (range). A logistic regression analysis, with the motor part of the Unified Parkinson's Disease Rating Scale and the Montreal Cognitive Assessment as covariables, including likelihood ratio was used to calculate p values. Significance level was set at $p < 0.05$. GBA-PD = Parkinson's disease patients carrying a heterozygous glucocerebrosidase mutation; iPD = idiopathic Parkinson's disease.

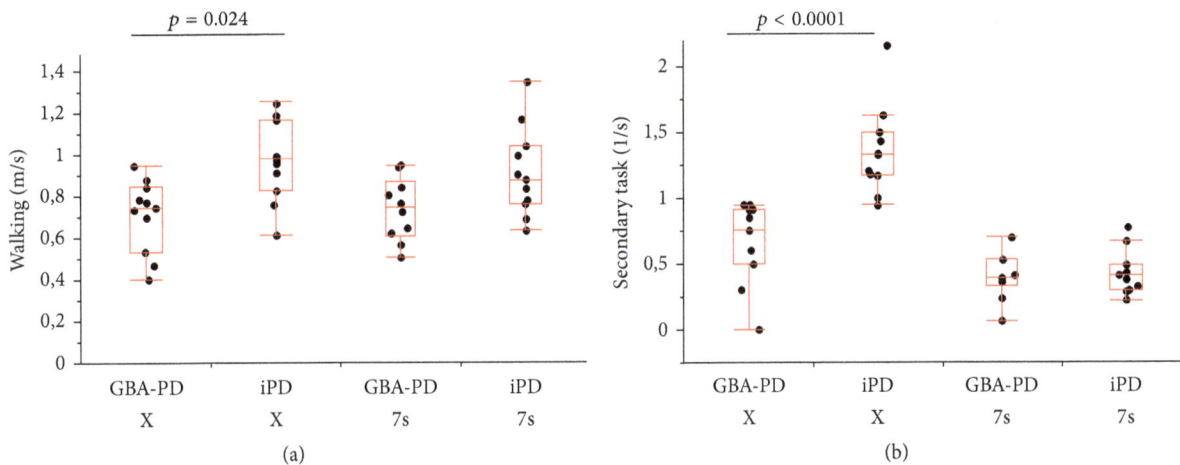

FIGURE 1: (a) Dual-task performance "walking while checking boxes (X) or while subtracting serial 7s (7s)." (b) Dual-task performance "checking boxes (X) or subtracting serial 7s (7s) while walking." A logistic regression analysis, with the motor part of the Unified Parkinson's Disease Rating Scale and the Montreal Cognitive Assessment as covariables, including likelihood ratio was used to calculate p values. Significance level was set at $p < 0.05$. GBA-PD = Parkinson's disease patients carrying a heterozygous glucocerebrosidase mutation; iPD = idiopathic Parkinson's disease.

3. Results

GBA-PD and iPD patients differed significantly regarding UPDRS-III scores (higher in GBA-PD; $p = 0.01$) and showed a trend towards a significant difference in the MoCA values (lower in GBA-PD, $p = 0.06$). Clinical characteristics are shown in Table 1. During the ST conditions, GBA-PD patients walked significantly slower than iPD patients (0.85 m/s versus 1.07 m/s, $p = 0.04$). The groups did not differ significantly regarding the speed of checking boxes and subtracting serial 7s. During the DT condition "walking while checking boxes," GBA-PD patients showed a significantly slower box-checking speed (see below) and walking speed (0.75 m/s versus 0.97 m/s, $p = 0.02$) compared to iPD patients. Remarkably, the box-checking task under the DT condition showed a 100% separation of the groups (checking boxes while walking GBA-PD: 0.76 boxes/sec. (0.00–0.95); iPD: 1.33 boxes/sec. (0.95–2.17, $p < 0.0001$)). In the DT condition "walking and subtracting serial 7s," walking speed and subtraction speed were not significantly different between the

groups. Details are given in Table 2 and Figure 1. Although DT and ST differed between the groups, the DTC of all the speeds were not significantly different between GBA-PD and iPD. Detailed data are provided in Table 3. Sensor-based data of gait (steps, step time, cadence, double support time, and stride time variability) did not add relevantly to these findings.

4. Discussion

GBA-PD patients are known to have more severe motor and nonmotor impairments compared to iPD patients [5]. This phenomenon was also observed in this small study. However, mechanistic aspects with respect to the specific deficits sheading some light on this phenomenon are not well investigated to date. This motivated us to investigate a specific and highly daily-relevant function on the interface of motor and cognitive performance, that is, multitasking. Results from this pilot study suggest that GBA-PD patients have

TABLE 3: Dual-task costs.

	GBA-PD ($n = 11$)	iPD ($n = 11$)	p value
Walking while checking boxes [%]	11 (−11–48)	9 (−0.6–27)	0.88
Checking boxes when walking [%]	25 (−15–100)	12 (−10–44)	0.09
Walking while subtracting [%]	35 (27–59)	40 (33–52)	0.57
Subtracting when walking [%]	−39 (−121–13)	−16 (−78–39)	0.09

Values are given in median (range). A logistic regression analysis, with the motor part of the Unified Parkinson's Disease Rating Scale and the Montreal Cognitive Assessment as covariables, including likelihood ratio was used to calculate p values. Significance level was set at $p < 0.05$. GBA-PD = Parkinson's disease patients carrying a heterozygous glucocerebrosidase mutation; iPD = idiopathic Parkinson's disease.

indeed deficits with respect to this. This group had slower gait speed and box-checking speed under DT conditions (i.e., when performing two motor tasks), even after correction for "general" motor and cognitive deficits.

Previous studies of iPD patients [19–23] have shown that gait speed decreases when gait is simultaneously performed with a secondary task. Secondary tasks involving motor aspects may be more challenging than purely cognitive tasks in particular in patients with parkinsonism [8, 24, 25]. The results of the present study are in line with these findings: walking speed was reduced in both groups under the DT condition. Most notably, also the speed of checking boxes under DT was lower in GBA-PD than in iPD, and it differentiated the groups without any overlap (Figure 1). The findings and our conclusion should be interpreted with caution due to sample size but can motivate the investigation of the observed phenomenon in larger studies.

Importantly, DTC were similar in GBA-PD and iPD patients. The nature of DTC during gait is yet not fully understood. The results of fMRI studies suggest that cortical activity increases under DT conditions. Areas such as the cerebellum, the premotor area, the precuneus, and the prefrontal and parietal cortexes seem to be more active in iPD patients than in healthy individuals under DT [26]. The present results suggest that GBA mutational status does not have a relevant influence on DTC because it is possible that similar networks are activated under the DT condition in both PD groups. It seems that clinically more severely impaired GBA-PD patients show the capability to perform as well as iPD patients under DT conditions, though on a lower level. Whether this is due to pathophysiological differences or motor learning abilities has to be examined in future studies.

There is some evidence that there is a structural and even functional basis of our clinical finding. Cortical areas including the inferior frontal sulcus, middle frontal gyrus, and intraparietal sulcus have been reported to be involved in dual-task performance with increased activation of these areas under increased task complexity [27]. An MRI study [28] found more white matter changes (associated with more and more pronounced clinical deficits) in frontal and interhemispheric corticocortical connections of GBA-PD patients compared to nonmutation carriers and healthy control subjects. Other functional studies using PET showed hypometabolism in frontal and parietooccipital areas of GBA-PD patients [29, 30]. It is thus intriguing to hypothesize that the phenomenological deficit in dual-tasking

performance presented by the GBA-PD patients is associated with the above-mentioned areas.

The effect observed while performing two motor dual tasks was not observed while performing a motor and a cognitive task (i.e., walking while subtracting serial 7s). This lack of difference may be best explained by an insufficient challenge of motor processing capacity. It has previously been hypothesized that (only) the use of the same neural capacities, for example, when performing two motor tasks, can exert group-specific differences [31]. Oscillatory dysfunction in basal ganglia due to dopamine depletion as well as reduced action selection due to dopamine deficiency could to some extent explain this phenomenon [32].

Strengths and Limitations. The small sample size is a limitation of this pilot study, and the reproduction of results in an independent and larger sample is required. Nevertheless, this study is, to the best of our knowledge, the first to present DT measures of GBA patients. All patients were carefully screened, recruited, and examined by specialists in the field of neurodegeneration. Furthermore, iPD patients, screened not to have a *GBA* mutation, were matched for age, gender, and disease duration to allow an adequate comparison between the groups. GBA-PD patients are known for having a more severe PD phenotype than nonmutation carriers do; therefore comparison of disease groups is challenging even when entirely new and daily-relevant parameters are assessed. Thus, we corrected all experimental results for UPDRS and MoCA scores. Further cognitive testing with, for example, the frontal assessment battery, could have added information about cognitive differences between the groups. We chose to examine dual-task performance instead, as it goes beyond the usual clinical investigation adding direct and daily-life-relevant information to our understanding of GBA-PD. We did not check for all pathologic GBA mutations due to logistic reasons. However, any pathologic mutation in our iPD cohort should weaken our results and thus does not argue against the correctness of our results. The DT procedures in this study have been successfully applied in previous work [33] and include different types of secondary (motor and cognitive) tasks.

5. Conclusions

GBA-PD show worse DT performance compared to iPD patients when executing two motor tasks simultaneously. If confirmed in larger studies, this pilot observation could be of relevance for clinical counselling.

Authors' Contributions

Karin Srulijes and Walter Maetzler contributed to design and conceptualization of the study, acquisition of the data, analysis and interpretation of the data, and drafting of the manuscript. Senait Ogbamicael, Ann-Kathrin Hauser, Claudia Schulte, and Jasmin Fritzen contributed to acquisition of the data, analysis and interpretation of the data, and revision of the manuscript. Kathrin Brockmann contributed to design and conceptualization of the study, acquisition of the data, and revision of the manuscript. Markus A. Hobert and Michael Schwenk contributed to analysis and interpretation of the data and revision of the manuscript. Thomas Gasser and Daniela Berg contributed to conceptualization of the study and revision of the manuscript. All authors gave their final approval of the version to be published and agreed to be accountable for all aspects of the work.

Acknowledgments

The authors thank all participants in the study. Dr. Srulijes receives funding from the Robert Bosch Foundation (Grant no. 32.5.1141.0049.0). Mrs. Ogbamicael, Mrs. Hauser, Dr. Schulte, and Dr. Schwenk report no disclosures. Mr. Hobert has received travel grants by Abvie (2015) and Merz (2016). Dr. Brockmann has received a research grant from the University of Tuebingen (TUEFF) and the German Society of Parkinson's Disease (dpv), funding from the Michael J. Fox Foundation (MJFF), travel grants from the Movement Disorders Society, and speaker honoraria from Lundbeck. Professor Gasser has received speaker honoraria from UCB and MedUpdate. He has received grant support from the German Research Foundation (DFG), the German Federal Ministry of Education and Research (BMBF), the European Commission, the Helmholtz Association, the Michael J. Fox Foundation, the Charitable Hertie-Foundation, and Novartis Pharma. Professor Berg has received speaker honoraria from UCB Pharma GmbH and Lundbeck. She is in consultancies and on advisory boards for UCB Pharma GmbH and Lundbeck. She has received grants from the Michael J. Fox Foundation, Janssen Pharmaceutica NV, German Parkinson's Disease Association (Deutsche Parkinson Vereinigung e.V.), BMWi, BMBF, Parkinson Fonds Deutschland GmbH, UCB Pharma GmbH, TEVA Pharma GmbH, EU, Novartis Pharma GmbH, Boehringer Ingelheim Pharma GmbH, and Lundbeck. Professor Maetzler receives funding from the European Union, the Michael J. Fox Foundation, the NeuroAlliance, and Janssen. He has received funding from the Robert Bosch Foundation and speaker honoraria from GlaxoSmithKline, Rölke Pharma, Licher, and UCB.

References

[1] E. Sidransky, M. A. Nalls, J. O. Aasly et al., "Multicenter analysis of glucocerebrosidase mutations in Parkinson's disease," *The New England Journal of Medicine*, vol. 361, no. 17, pp. 1651–1661, 2009.

[2] K. Brockmann, K. Srulijes, A.-K. Hauser et al., "GBA-associated PD presents with nonmotor characteristics," *Neurology*, vol. 77, no. 3, pp. 276–280, 2011.

[3] K. Brockmann, K. Srulijes, S. Pflederer et al., "GBA-associated Parkinson's disease: Reduced survival and more rapid progression in a prospective longitudinal study," *Movement Disorders*, vol. 30, no. 3, pp. 407–411, 2015.

[4] A. McNeill, R. Duran, D. A. Hughes, A. Mehta, and A. H. V. Schapira, "A clinical and family history study of Parkinson's disease in heterozygous glucocerebrosidase mutation carriers," *Journal of Neurology, Neurosurgery and Psychiatry*, vol. 83, no. 8, pp. 853-854, 2012.

[5] J. Neumann, J. Bras, E. Deas et al., "Glucocerebrosidase mutations in clinical and pathologically proven Parkinson's disease," *Brain*, vol. 132, no. 7, pp. 1783–1794, 2009.

[6] E. Sidransky and G. Lopez, "The link between the GBA gene and parkinsonism," *The Lancet Neurology*, vol. 11, no. 11, pp. 986–998, 2012.

[7] M. D. Willemsen, Y. A. M. Grimbergen, M. Slabbekoorn, and B. R. Bloem, "Vallen bij de ziekte van Parkinson: vaker door houdingsinstabiliteit dan door omgevingsfactoren," *Nederlands Tijdschrift voor Geneeskunde*, vol. 144, pp. 2309-2314, 2000.

[8] S. Heinzel, M. Maechtel, S. E. Hasmann et al., "Motor dual-tasking deficits predict falls in Parkinson's disease: A prospective study," *Parkinsonism and Related Disorders*, vol. 26, pp. 73–77, 2016.

[9] R. Morris, S. Lord, J. Bunce, D. Burn, and L. Rochester, "Gait and cognition: Mapping the global and discrete relationships in ageing and neurodegenerative disease," *Neuroscience and Biobehavioral Reviews*, vol. 64, pp. 326–345, 2016.

[10] G. Yogev-Seligmann, J. M. Hausdorff, and N. Giladi, "The role of executive function and attention in gait," *Movement Disorders*, vol. 23, no. 3, pp. 329–342, 2008.

[11] I. Litvan, K. P. Bhatia, D. J. Burn et al., "SIC task force appraisal of clinical diagnostic criteria for parkinsonian disorders," *Movement Disorders*, vol. 18, no. 5, pp. 467–486, 2003.

[12] C. L. Tomlinson, R. Stowe, S. Patel, C. Rick, R. Gray, and C. E. Clarke, "Systematic review of levodopa dose equivalency reporting in Parkinson's disease," *Movement Disorders*, vol. 25, no. 15, pp. 2649–2653, 2010.

[13] C. C. Goetz, "The Unified Parkinson's Disease Rating Scale (UPDRS): status and recommendations," *Movement Disorders*, vol. 18, no. 7, pp. 738–750, 2003.

[14] S. Hoops, S. Nazem, A. D. Siderowf et al., "Validity of the MoCA and MMSE in the detection of MCI and dementia in Parkinson disease," *Neurology*, vol. 73, no. 21, pp. 1738-1745, 2009.

[15] A. Ble, S. Volpato, G. Zuliani et al., "Executive function correlates with walking speed in older persons: the InCHIANTI study," *Journal of the American Geriatrics Society*, vol. 53, no. 3, pp. 410–415, 2005.

[16] C. Kühner, C. Bürger, F. Keller, and M. Hautzinger, "Reliability and validity of the revised Beck Depression Inventory (BDI-II). Results from German samples," *Nervenarzt*, vol. 78, no. 6, pp. 651–656, 2007.

[17] O. Bock, "Dual-task costs while walking increase in old age for some, but not for other tasks: an experimental study of healthy young and elderly persons," *Journal of NeuroEngineering and Rehabilitation*, vol. 5, article 27, 2008.

[18] U. Lindemann, S. Nicolai, D. Beische et al., "Clinical and dual-tasking aspects in frequent and infrequent fallers with progressive supranuclear palsy," *Movement Disorders*, vol. 25, no. 8, pp. 1040–1046, 2010.

[19] B. R. Bloem, Y. A. M. Grimbergen, J. G. van Dijk, and M. Munneke, "The "posture second" strategy: a review of wrong priorities in Parkinson's disease," *Journal of the Neurological Sciences*, vol. 248, no. 1-2, pp. 196–204, 2006.

[20] J. M. Bond and M. Morn's, "Goal-directed secondary motor tasks: their effects on gait in subjects with Parkinson disease," *Archives of Physical Medicine and Rehabilitation*, vol. 81, no. 1, pp. 110–116, 2000.

[21] J. M. Hausdorff, J. Balash, and N. Giladi, "Effects of Cognitive Challenge on Gait Variability in Patients with Parkinson's Disease," *Journal of Geriatric Psychiatry and Neurology*, vol. 16, no. 1, pp. 53–58, 2003.

[22] S. O'Shea, M. E. Morris, and R. Iansek, "Dual task interference during gait in people with Parkinson disease: effects of motor versus cognitive secondary tasks," *Physical Therapy*, vol. 82, no. 9, pp. 888–897, 2002.

[23] L. Rochester, B. Galna, S. Lord, and D. Burn, "The nature of dual-task interference during gait in incident Parkinson's disease," *Neuroscience*, vol. 265, pp. 83–94, 2014.

[24] R. Benecke, J. C. Rothwell, J. P. R. Dick, B. L. Day, and C. D. Marsden, "Performance of simultaneous movements in patients with Parkinson's disease," *Brain*, vol. 109, no. 4, pp. 739–757, 1986.

[25] S. Lord, L. Rochester, V. Hetherington, L. M. Allcock, and D. Burn, "Executive dysfunction and attention contribute to gait interference in 'off' state Parkinson's Disease," *Gait and Posture*, vol. 31, no. 2, pp. 169–174, 2010.

[26] T. Wu and M. Hallett, "Neural correlates of dual task performance in patients with Parkinson's disease," *Journal of Neurology, Neurosurgery and Psychiatry*, vol. 79, no. 7, pp. 760–766, 2008.

[27] A. J. Szameitat, T. Schubert, K. Müller, and D. Y. Von Cramon, "Localization of executive functions in dual-task performance with fMRI," *Journal of Cognitive Neuroscience*, vol. 14, no. 8, pp. 1184–1199, 2002.

[28] F. Agosta, V. S. Kostic, K. Davidovic et al., "White matter abnormalities in Parkinson's disease patients with glucocerebrosidase gene mutations," *Movement Disorders*, vol. 28, no. 6, pp. 772–778, 2013.

[29] S. Kono, Y. Ouchi, T. Terada, H. Ida, M. Suzuki, and H. Miyajima, "Functional brain imaging in glucocerebrosidase mutation carriers with and without parkinsonism," *Movement Disorders*, vol. 25, no. 12, pp. 1823–1829, 2010.

[30] R. Saunders-Pullman, J. Hagenah, V. Dhawan et al., "Gaucher disease ascertained through a Parkinson's center: Imaging and clinical characterization," *Movement Disorders*, vol. 25, no. 10, pp. 1364–1372, 2010.

[31] V. E. Kelly, A. J. Eusterbrock, and A. Shumway-Cook, "A review of dual-task walking deficits in people with Parkinson's disease: Motor and cognitive contributions, mechanisms, and clinical implications," *Parkinson's Disease*, vol. 2012, Article ID 918719, 14 pages, 2012.

[32] M. Weinberger and J. O. Dostrovsky, "A basis for the pathological oscillations in basal ganglia: The crucial role of dopamine," *NeuroReport*, vol. 22, no. 4, pp. 151–156, 2011.

[33] M. A. Hobert, R. Niebler, S. I. Meyer et al., "Poor trail making test performance is directly associated with altered dual task prioritization in the elderly - baseline results from the trend study," *PLoS ONE*, vol. 6, no. 11, Article ID e27831, 2011.

23

Mediating Effect of Mutuality on Health-Related Quality of Life in Patients with Parkinson's Disease

Michaela Karlstedt ⓘ,[1] **Seyed-Mohammad Fereshtehnejad** ⓘ,[1,2] **Dag Aarsland,**[3,4] **and Johan Lökk** ⓘ[1]

[1]*Karolinska Institutet, Department of Neurobiology Care Sciences and Society, Division of Clinical Geriatrics, Floor 7 141 83 Huddinge, Stockholm, Sweden*
[2]*Department of Neurology and Neurosurgery, McGill University, Montreal, QC, Canada*
[3]*Karolinska Institutet, Alzheimer Disease Research Center (KI-ADRC) Novum, Floor 5 SE-141 86, Stockholm, Sweden*
[4]*Department Old Age Psychiatry, Kings College, London, UK*

Correspondence should be addressed to Michaela Karlstedt; michaela.karlstedt@ki.se

Academic Editor: Karsten Witt

The relationship quality, mutuality, has been identified as a protective factor in family care situations, but its role in mediating health-related quality of life (HRQoL) in patients having Parkinson's disease (PD) is not known. Data on patients' and partners' mutuality (MS), motor signs (UPDRS III), non-motor symptoms (NMSQuest), impaired cognition (IQCODE), dependency in activities of daily life (ADL), and HRQoL (PDQ8) were collected from 51 dyads. Structural equation model with manifest variables was applied to explore if the MS score mediated the effect of UPDRS III, NMSQuest, IQCODE, and dependency in ADL on PDQ8. The results suggest that increasing severity of motor and non-motor symptoms decreases patients' mutuality which leads to worse HRQoL. Partners' mutuality mediated the effect of impaired cognition which in turn decreased patients' mutuality. The findings enhance our understanding of how various symptoms may influence PD patients' HRQoL. This may help clinicians to personalize interventions to provide more effective interventions to improve the lives of patients with PD.

1. Introduction

Parkinson's disease (PD) is a complex disorder which often influences several aspects of daily life. It is well known that the combination of motor impairment and a wide variety of non-motor symptoms (NMS) interferes with daily activities and can contribute to impaired health-related quality of life (HRQoL) [1–6]. Living with a chronic condition can invoke many changes in a couple and disrupt social interactions and connectedness [7, 8]. PD patients commonly rely on their partners who often assist them with managing their health. This can lead to an imbalance of the support one receives or gives, resulting in a change of roles and relational dynamics within the dyads [9, 10]. The positive quality of the relationship, defined as mutuality, has been described as having four dimensions: love and affection, shared pleasurable activities, shared values, and reciprocity [11, 12]. In other words, mutuality refers to the quality of the interaction between persons, here a PD patient and a spouse, and involves feelings of closeness, reciprocity of sentiment, understanding of one another, and shared goals and activities. Growing evidence from caregiving research suggests that high mutuality of caregivers is associated with high emotional well-being and acts as a protective factor of negative caregiving outcomes. A review has also shown that mutuality may decrease over the course of a chronic condition [13]. However, research on perceived mutuality of PD patients is scarce and mainly based on small sample sizes. Ricciardi et al. found PD patients to be more depressed and less satisfied with their marriage than their partners [14]. Insecurity and concern if the partner will stay in the relationship or start to resent them as PD advances are feelings that also have been expressed by PD patients in a qualitative interview study [9]. Despite these negative effects,

Mavandadi et al. in a small cross-sectional study found an association between greater marriage quality and perceived benefits or personal growth from having PD [15]. Understanding the interaction between stressors, mediators, and health outcomes often accompanying PD may pave the way for care models and interventions that improve well-being and HRQoL. Guided by the proposed conceptual stress model for individuals with dementia, the aim of the present study was to explore if mutuality acts as a mediator on PD patients' HRQoL [16]. Mediation analysis is often used to test theories regarding a process [17]. In statistics, a mediation model is designed to explain the mechanism that underlies an observed relationship between an independent variable (here PD related symptoms) and a dependent variable (here HRQoL) via the inclusion of a third hypothetical variable, known as a mediator (here mutuality). Rather than a direct causal association, mediation proposes that the independent variable affects the mediator variable, which in turn influences the dependent variable [18].

According to most of the stress process theories, health outcomes are influenced by primary stressors which often refer to disease-related factors or the individuals' appraisal of the situation. These primary stressors can have a direct or indirect effect on health outcomes through different strains (e.g., self-esteem and role strain) or protective factors such as mutuality [16, 19, 20]. In mediation analysis, primary stressors are seen as antecedents of mediators and health outcome variables [17]. We recently showed that primary stressors such as motor and NMS were adversely associated with PD patients' mutuality and PD patients' HRQoL [21] and that patients' mutuality was positively associated with HRQoL, indicating that mutuality may act as a mediator. Also, partners' mutuality was positively associated with patients' mutuality, indicating that partners' mutuality may act as a mediator between significant stressors and patients' mutuality or patients' HRQoL [21]. To our knowledge, there is no published study exploring if mutuality acts as a mediator on PD patients' HRQoL. By testing the mediating effect of mutuality, we will expand our previous research and disentangle different pathways that could explain the effect of PD specific symptoms on patients' HRQoL. Furthermore, the results may also provide new knowledge if mutuality is an effective mechanism to improve PD patients' HRQoL. Guided by the aforementioned theoretical frameworks, we hypothesized that motor symptoms, NMS, impaired cognition, and dependency in ADL act as primary stressors with direct or indirect effects mediated through patients' mutuality and partners' mutuality on patients' HRQoL.

2. Materials and Methods

2.1. Participants. For this cross-sectional study, 51 patients with mild to moderate PD and their partners were recruited through movement disorders clinics at Karolinska University Hospital and through advertisement in the journal of the Swedish Parkinson's Disease Association. The dyads had a well-established relationship and had been living together, on average, for 38.4 years (SD = 14.59). Neither of the

partners were employed as caregivers nor did the dyads rear small children. More details are published elsewhere [21]. The study was approved by the local research ethics committee in Stockholm, Sweden (registration number: 2013/1812-31/3), and was conducted in accordance with the Declaration of Helsinki.

2.2. Measurement. To evaluate severity of PD specific motor signs, the 14-item Unified Parkinson's Disease Rating Scale-Part III (UPDRS III) was used. The scale is answered using a 5-point Likert scale. Higher scores indicate more severe motor signs [22].

To detect PD specific non-motor manifestations in domains such as urinary, cardiovascular, depression/anxiety, memory, sexual function, sleep disorder, digestive, hallucination/delusion, and miscellany, the Non-motor Symptoms Questionnaire (NMSQuest) was used. The scale comprises 30 items scored "yes" or "no." Higher scores indicate higher frequency of non-motor manifestations [23, 24].

The Informant Questionnaire on Cognitive Decline in the Elderly (IQCODE) was used to assess functional changes associated with cognitive status in the patients. The scale is answered using a 5-point Likert scale and comprises 26 items. The individual scores are ranging between 1 and 5 and are calculated by the mean across all item scores. Higher scores (>3) indicate a decline in cognitive functioning. The questionnaire was filled out by the partner. For this scale, Cronbach's alpha has been reported ranging from 0.93 to 0.97 in several studies [25].

The patient's level of dependency in activities of daily life was assessed using a modified form of the extended Katz index [26]. The scale contains items assessing grooming/dressing, bathing, food intake, toileting, walking/transferring, housekeeping, and shopping (0 = need no help to 3 = need all help). The scale was filled out by the partner. A dichotomous variable (0 = independent; 1 = dependent) was created aiming to assess dependency.

The 8-item Parkinson's Disease Questionnaire-short form (PDQ8) was used to measure PD specific HRQoL. The scale covers domains such as mobility, activities of daily life, emotional well-being, stigma, social support, cognitions, communication, and bodily discomfort. The scale is answered using a 5-point Likert scale. A summary index was calculated ranging from 0 to 100. Higher scores indicate worse HRQoL [27].

The 15-item mutuality scale (MS) was used to measure the positive quality of the caregiver-care receiver relationship [11, 12]. The scale is answered using a 5-point Likert scale (0 = not at all to 4 = a great deal). It covers domains such as love and affection (3 items), shared pleasurable activates (4 items), shared values (2 items), and reciprocity (6 items). The individual scores are ranging between 0 and 4 and are calculated by the mean across all item scores. Higher scores indicate higher quality of the mutual relationship between the care-dyads. For the Swedish version of MS, Cronbach's alpha was calculated as 0.936 for PD patients in MS and as 0.933 for PD partners in MS [28].

2.3. Statistical Analysis. Characteristics of the included PD dyads were described using frequency, percentage, means (*m*), and standard deviation (SD).

Two of the participants had one single missing item each within the NMSQuest scale. The individual scores were larger than the sample median. To avoid case-wise deletion and loss of power, these items were imputed with a zero score. To calculate ranking of each NMSQuest domain, the sum of positive responses in each domain was divided by the maximum possible positive responses in the corresponding domain.

To test our mediation hypotheses, structural equation modeling (SEM) with manifest variables was performed. Figure 1 illustrates a schematic model of a simple mediation [17]. At the top in Figure 1, the total effect (path c) can be described as the sum of direct and indirect effects of the primary stressor on the outcome variable or simplified as the effect without the mediator in the equation. Path a (at the bottom in Figure 1) represents the primary stressor's effect on the mediator controlling for the effect of the mediator on the outcome variable (path b). The same applies for path b, which represents the mediator's effect on the outcome variable. The indirect effect is usually calculated as the product of $a \times b$. The direct effect (path c^1) can be described as the effect between the primary stressor and the outcome controlling for the indirect effect [17].

Prior to the analyses, assumptions of multicollinearity were examined through tolerance and variance inflation factor (VIF (1/tolerance)). Tolerance (>0.4) and VIF index (<2.5) were considered acceptable. No influential multivariate outliers were detected using the Mahalanobis and Cooks distance [29]. Based on our prior study and the hypothesis we generated, UPDRS III, NMSQuest, IQCODE, and ADL served as primary stressors (exogenous variables), while patients' HRQoL (PDQ8) served as the outcome variable (endogenous variable) and patients' mutuality and partners' mutuality served as mediators (endogenous variables).

The fit of the models was tested using the Chi-square test, Comparative fit index (CFI), Normed fit index (NFI), Tucker–Lewis index (TLI), Goodness-of-fit statistic (GFI), and the Root-mean-square error of approximation (RMSEA). A model was considered well fitted when the chi-square value was non-significant, TLI, CFI, NFI, and GFI > 0.95, and RMSEA < 0.05 [30]. The square multiple correlation was used to assess how much of the variance in mutuality and HRQoL was explained by the included exogenous variables.

Total, direct, and indirect effects between exogenous and endogenous variables were calculated using maximum likelihood estimation and are presented as standardized path coefficients. An advantage of SEM is that direct and indirect effects (mediation) can be tested simultaneously within the model. To test the indirect effects, the bias-corrected bootstrap method was used [31]. The 95% confidence interval (CI) was determined following 2000 iterations from the sample of 51 participants.

To classify and understand different types of mediation, the proposed typology and interpretation of mediation by

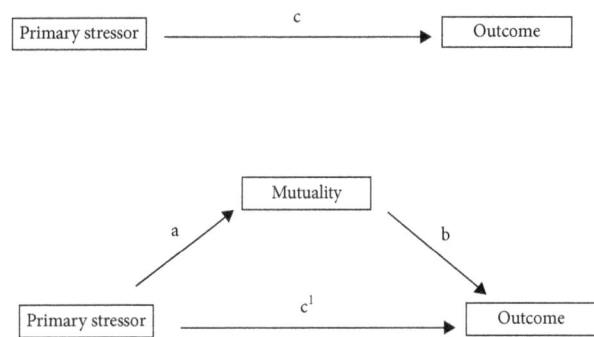

FIGURE 1: Illustration of a simple mediation with total, direct, and indirect effects.

Zhao et al. was used [32]. A complementary mediation is when both indirect and direct effects exist and point in the same direction, similar to what Baron and Kenny referred to as partial mediation [32, 33]. The second type of mediation, named competitive mediation, is when both the indirect and direct effects exist but the effects point in opposite direction, which also has been referred in the literature as inconsistent mediation [32, 34]. The third type of mediation, named as indirect-only mediation, is when indirect effect exists but there is no direct effect, referred to as full mediation by Baron and Kenny [32, 33]. A complementary mediation or a competitive mediation indicates that there may be omitted mediators which coexist with the mediator within the explored model. An indirect-only mediation implies that the mediator fully explains the association between the included variable and the outcome variable. Two types of patterns consistent with non-mediation are also described, namely, direct-only non-mediation when direct effects between the independent variable and the outcome exist but there is no indirect effect and no-effect non-mediation when neither direct nor indirect effects exist [32].

In the whole analysis, the path model was adjusted by age and gender. Based on prior results, gender was chosen to adjust the effect on PD patients' mutuality [21]. A *p* value of 0.05 or less was regarded as statistically significant.

All data analyses were conducted using SPSS Statistics for Windows, version 23 (IBM Corp., Armonk, NY, USA), and AMOS graphics module version 23 (IBM INC).

3. Results

3.1. Participants. The mean age of patients and partners was 70.9 (SD = 8.5) and 70.7 (SD = 9.3) years, respectively. Of the patients, 35/51 (68.6%) needed some form of supervision or help from their partners in daily activities. Other demographic and clinical characteristics are presented in Table 1.

All patients were treated with a combination of antiparkinsonian drugs. Of the 51 patients, four were treated with deep brain stimulation, three with carbidopa-levodopa infusion, and two with infusion of dopamine agonists. Complications were quite common: 33/48 (65%) had experienced dyskinesia and 29/48 (57%) had motor fluctuations. Urinary problems (76%) were the most frequent

TABLE 1: Sociodemographic and clinical features ($n = 51$ dyads).

	Patient	Partner
Female, n (%)	22 (43.1)	29 (56.9)
Retired, n (%)	45 (88.2)	39 (76.5)
Working,* n (%)	10 (19.6)	16 (31.4)
Level of education, n (%)		
Elementary	8 (15.7)	6 (11.8)
Secondary	11 (21.6)	16 (31.4)
University	32 (62.7)	29 (56.9)
Level of income (SEK)		
0–199000	13 (25.5)	13 (25.5)
200000–450000	27 (52.9)	30 (58.8)
>450000	11 (21.6)	8 (15.7)
MS, m (SD)	3.2 (0.65)	2.9 (0.77)
PD duration, m (SD)	8.4 (6.4)	—
UPDRS III, m (SD)	18.1 (5.8)	—
NMSQuest, m (SD)	12.1 (4.6)	—
IQCODE, m (SD)	3.2 (0.53)	—
PDQ8, m (SD)	27.4 (14.6)	—
Dependency in ADL ($n = 35$)		
Shopping, n (%)	32 (91.4)	—
Cooking/cleaning, n (%)	28 (80.0)	—
Walking/transferring, n (%)	23 (65.7)	—
Bath/showering, n (%)	13 (37.1)	—
Grooming/dressing, n (%)	11 (31.4)	—
Toileting, n (%)	9 (25.7)	—
Food intake, n (%)	7 (20.0)	—

Note: PD: Parkinson's disease; MS: mutuality scale; PDQ8: Parkinson's disease questionnaire summary index; IQCODE: informant questionnaire on cognitive decline in the elderly; NMSQuest: non-motor symptoms questionnaire; UPDRS III: unified Parkinson's disease rating scale-part III; ADL: activities of daily life; *some of the study subjects were still working.

reported non-motor domain, and hallucination/delusion (21%) was the least reported domain (Table 2).

3.2. Path Analysis.
Figure 2 illustrates the relationship of the included factors which affects patients' and partners' mutuality and patients' HRQoL.

The first model resulted in acceptable fit. However, several of the path coefficients were small and non-significant including the path between partners' MS score and PDQ8 (beta = −0.027; $p = 0.825$), indicating that partners' mutuality did not act as a mediator on patients' HRQoL. Due to the small sample size, all unrequired and non-significant paths were discarded one by one (Figure 2). The final model resulted in acceptable fit. The fit of the final model and the standardized direct path and coefficients are presented in Figure 2. The final model explained 15.3% of the variance in partners' mutuality, 42.0% in patients' mutuality, and 55.8% in patients' HRQoL.

3.3. Direct Effects.
The significant direct effect of patients' MS score (beta = −0.435; $p < 0.001$) on PDQ8 indicated that patients' mutuality may act as a mediator between the included clinical variables, which were significantly associated with patients' mutuality (Figure 2): UPDRS III (beta = −0.237; $p = 0.037$), NMS (beta = −0.258; $p = 0.035$),

and ADL (beta = 0.276; $p = 0.040$). This means that increasing severity of motor and NMS was associated with a lower level of patients' mutuality. Furthermore, a higher level of patients' mutuality was associated with better HRQoL, and the combined effect of these symptoms and mutuality may influence patients' HRQoL. Patients who had some form of dependency in ADL, assessed by the partners, had higher MS scores compared to the non-dependent patients. Impaired cognition was not associated with the patients' MS scores (beta = 0.060; $p = 0.629$). Instead, worse cognition (beta = −0.391; $p = 0.003$) decreased partners' MS scores. Furthermore, increasing MS scores of partners (beta = 0.509; $p < 0.001$) had a positive direct effect on patients' MS scores. This means that the effect of reduced cognitive function may influence patients' mutuality through partners' mutuality.

3.4. Indirect Effect and Total Effect.
Indirect effects and total effects are presented in Table 3.

The mediating test of indirect effects revealed that the effect of NMS (beta = 0.112; $p = 0.043$) on patients' HRQoL was mediated by patients' mutuality, implying that increasing frequency of NMS leads to a decrease in patients' mutuality, in turn leading to worse HRQoL (increasing PDQ8 score). The significant direct (beta = 0.440; $p = 0.001$) and total effects (beta = 0.552; $p = 0.001$) of NMS on HRQoL indicate a complementary mediation and point to the possibility of omitted mediators.

The effect of increasing UPDRS III scores (beta = 0.103; $p = 0.026$) on patients' HRQoL was also mediated by patients' mutuality. In other words, increasing severity of motor symptoms decreases patients' mutuality resulting in worse HRQoL. There was no significant direct (beta = 0.023; $p = 0.883$) or total effect (beta = 0.126; $p = 0.372$) of increasing UPDRS III scores on patients' HRQoL signaling an indirect-only mediation.

Patients' mutuality did not mediate the effect of impaired cognition. Instead, partners' mutuality mediated the effect of increasing IQCODE scores (beta = −0.199; $p = 0.011$) on patients' mutuality. In other words, worse cognition decreases partners' mutuality, in turn leading to the decreasing level of patients' mutuality. The lack of significant direct effect (beta = 0.060; $p = 0.629$) points to an indirect-only mediation.

4. Discussion

This is, to our knowledge, the first study to explore if mutuality of PD patients and PD partners acts as a mediator between clinical PD features and patients' HRQoL. Our findings suggest that patients' mutuality mediates the effect of motor and NMS on patients' HRQoL. In contrast to our initial hypothesis, partners' mutuality did not act as a mediator on patients' HRQoL. Instead, partners' mutuality mediated the effect of impaired cognition on patients' mutuality.

We explored direct and indirect effects of specific PD symptoms on patients' HRQoL. Consistent with prior

TABLE 2: Frequency of positive answers classified by NMSQuest* domains ($n = 51$).

| NMSQuest* domains | Number of items | Positive answers | | |
		Frequency	Maximum of possible	% of maximum
Urinary	2	78	102	76
Cardiovascular	2	45	102	44
Depression/anxiety	2	44	102	43
Memory	3	65	153	42
Sexual function	2	43	102	42
Sleep disorder	5	100	255	39
Digestive	7	135	357	38
Miscellany	5	88	255	35
Hallucination/delusion	2	21	102	21

*NMSQuest = non-motor symptoms questionnaire.

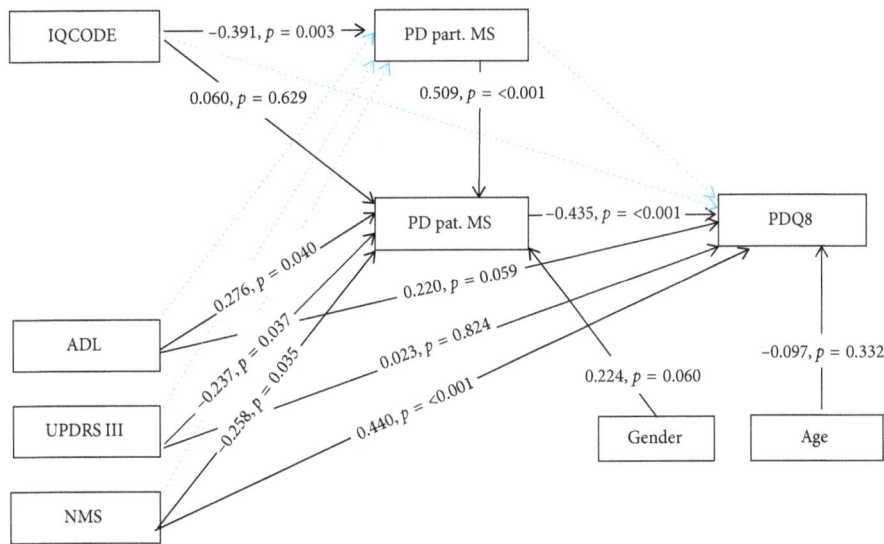

FIGURE 2: Direct effects reported as standardized path coefficients for the final model with HRQoL (PDQ8) as the outcome variable. Dashed lines are nonsignificant direct paths which were removed in the final model. The best fit of the final path model was achieved with $\chi^2 = 7.980$, $df = 9$, CMIN/DF = 0.887, $p = 0.536$, GFI = 0.968, NFI = 0.939, CFI = 1.0, TLI = 1.0, and RMSEA = 0.00 (95% CI = 0.00 − 0.146) ($n = 51$ dyads). Note: PD: Parkinson's disease; Pat. MS: PD patients' mutuality scale; Part. MS: PD partners' mutuality scale; PDQ8: Parkinson's disease questionnaire summary index; IQCODE: informant questionnaire on cognitive decline in the elderly; NMS: non-motor symptoms questionnaire; UPDRS III: unified Parkinson's disease rating scale-part III; ADL: activities of daily life (0 = independent; 1 = dependent); gender: 0 = female; 1 = male; age: PD partners' age.

TABLE 3: Indirect and total effects of disease-related factors on PD patients' health-related quality of life (bootstrap sample = 2000).

Effects	Path	Standardized path coefficient	95% CI bias-corrected percentile		p value
Indirect effect with one mediator	ADL ⟶ Pat. MS ⟶ PDQ8	−0.120	−0.300	— 0.014	0.079
	UPDRS III ⟶ Pat. MS ⟶ PDQ8	0.103	0.010	— 0.239	0.026
	NMS ⟶ Pat. MS ⟶ PDQ8	0.112	0.006	— 0.263	0.043
	IQCODE ⟶ Part. MS ⟶ Pat. MS	−0.199	−0.339	— −0.057	0.011
Total effect	ADL ⟶ PDQ8	0.100	−0.115	— 0.351	0.335
	UPDRS III ⟶ PDQ8	0.126	−0.116	— 0.334	0.372
	NMS ⟶ PDQ8	0.552	0.344	— 0.735	0.001
	IQCODE ⟶ PD-pat. MS	−0.139	−0.343	— 0.157	0.295

Note: PD: Parkinson's disease; ADL: activities of daily life (0 = independent; 1 = dependent); Pat. MS: PD patients' mutuality scale; PDQ8: Parkinson's disease questionnaire summary index; UPDRS III: unified Parkinson's disease rating scale-part III; NMS: non-motor symptoms questionnaire; IQCODE: informant questionnaire on cognitive decline in the elderly; Part. MS: PD partners' mutuality scale.

research studies, NMS had a larger direct negative impact on patients' HRQoL than motor symptoms [2, 3, 21, 35–37]. Our findings suggest that the effect of NMS on HRQoL was also mediated by patients' mutuality, and this type of indirect effect could be classified as a complementary mediation [32]. Although there might be other important mediators such as personality, coping, and perceived external support, the combined effect of NMS and mutuality on HRQoL has an important contribution [16]. The mean frequency of NMS was 12 which is similar to that in other studies [23, 38, 39]. Urinary problems (76%), cardiovascular (44%), depression/anxiety (43%), memory (42%), and sexual dysfunction (42%) were the most frequent reported non-motor domains. Thus, consequences of the wide variety of NMS are likely to influence several domains of mutuality such as love and affection, less-shared leisure activities with the partner, and perhaps disagreement in how to adjust and cope with PD. This can cause tension and result in a less supportive relationship leading to worse HRQoL. This corresponds with results from a qualitative study where PD patients expressed that family members do not understand how anxiety, depression, and apathy influence daily activities [40].

Indirect-only mediation was identified for the effect of motor symptoms on patients' HRQoL and patients' mutuality. The indirect-only mediation indicates that the motor symptoms' influence on HRQoL is only effective through motor symptoms' effect on patients' mutuality. This means that increasing severity of motor symptoms did not directly influence patients' HRQoL, instead, the combination of motor symptoms and mutuality was associated with worse HRQoL. This finding corresponds with results from a qualitative study where motor symptoms and constant struggle with unpredictability made the patients engage in fewer leisure activities and in some cases feel alone and less close to their partner [9]. Similarly, a recent study found that severity of motor features such as UPDRS III, falls, and ADL were mediated by NMS such as depression, psychosocial functioning, and nutritional status which led to worse HRQoL [36].

Impaired cognition has a detrimental effect on patients' HRQoL [3, 6, 41]. However, in the present study, impaired cognition was not significantly associated with patients' mutuality or HRQoL. Instead, an indirect-only mediation of impaired cognition on patients' mutuality was observed through partners' mutuality, indicating that worsening of cognitive function decreases partners' mutuality, which in turn leads to a lower level of patients' mutuality. The non-significant direct and indirect effects of impaired cognition on patients' HRQoL may be explained by the fact that cognitive function was assessed by partners and not the patients themselves. Another explanation may be that the cognitive decline was mild and the decline did not influence patients' appraisal of daily functioning. Thus, patients' perceived cognitive function and its consequences were not in concordance with the assessment done by the partners.

Our findings suggest that patients' mutuality is a mediator between symptoms and HRQoL in PD and that partners' mutuality mediates the relationship between impaired cognition and patients' mutuality.

These findings can be helpful for clinicians. Understanding the complexity and the combined effect that PD symptoms and mutuality have on HRQoL may aid clinicians to identify highrisk dyads. Clinicians should discuss with PD dyads how PD affects different dimensions of mutuality. Setting regular family meetings, improving the knowledge of partners towards the motor and NMS of PD and their progression over time, as well as highlighting the importance of the dyadic relationship should be considered to enhance mutuality and consequently improve patients' quality of life. For example, if the patient no longer is able to engage in earlier joint pleasurable activities with their partner, as a result of either motor or NMS, interventions aiming to find new enjoyable activities may improve the patient's mutuality and HRQoL. Furthermore, changes in cognitive function may negatively affect reciprocity and relational roles. Interventions aiming to understand the others' perspective of how different symptoms influence different dimensions of mutuality may enhance understanding of one another and facilitate coping and adjustment to PD. Not all relational issues can be solved by clinicians, and couple therapy or counseling may be needed for those with low mutuality before the PD diagnosis or for those who are uncertain if they should remain in the relationship. Nevertheless, our results could help clinicians to personalize interventions and improve PD dyads' ability to cope with the challenges they may encounter. Although specific PD symptoms are not often explicitly defined in qualitative studies in general, it seems that PD either brings dyads together or creates a distance between the members of the dyad. Some dyads even seem to have succeeded to move from distance towards a closer relationship by working together and find solution to PD challenges [9, 10, 42].

Our findings should be interpreted with caution. The design was based on a stress process model for persons with dementia rather than PD [16], and the model is based on complex interrelationships between different factors that have not been explored in the present study. Future research should explore other potential mediators such as external support, perceived stress, or perceived dependency. Another limitation is that dependency was assessed by the partners rather than as perceived by the patients, which may contribute to the nonsignificant direct and indirect effects. Other limitations are the cross-sectional design and the relatively small sample size for SEM. Thus, conclusions regarding causality cannot be made. Also, the sample had a predominance of older patients with mild to moderate PD which limits the generalizability. Future research would benefit from using a larger sample consisting of PD patients with different severity stages and using a longitudinal design. Nonetheless, our findings provide novel insights into the association between clinical symptoms and HRQoL in PD and offer a basis for future research to further understand the complexity and experience of living with PD, thus helping health professionals improve the quality of lives of PD patients and their carers.

Acknowledgments

The authors would like to thank all the participants. This study was supported by the Parkinson Foundation in Sweden.

References

[1] P. Martinez-Martin, "What is quality of life and how do we measure it? Relevance to Parkinson's disease and movement disorders," *Movement Disorders*, vol. 32, no. 3, pp. 382–392, 2017.

[2] B. Muller, J. Assmus, K. Herlofson, J. P. Larsen, and O. B. Tysnes, "Importance of motor vs. non-motor symptoms for health-related quality of life in early Parkinson's disease," *Parkinsonism and Related Disorders*, vol. 19, no. 11, pp. 1027–1032, 2013.

[3] G. W. Duncan, T. K. Khoo, A. J. Yarnall et al., "Health-related quality of life in early Parkinson's disease: the impact of nonmotor symptoms," *Movement Disorders*, vol. 29, no. 2, pp. 195–202, 2014.

[4] S. M. Fereshtehnejad, "Strategies to maintain quality of life among people with Parkinson's disease: what works?," *Neurodegenerative Disease Management*, vol. 6, no. 5, pp. 399–415, 2016.

[5] D. Aarsland and M. G. Kramberger, "Neuropsychiatric symptoms in Parkinson's disease," *Journal of Parkinson's Disease*, vol. 5, no. 3, pp. 659–667, 2015.

[6] A. Schrag, M. Jahanshahi, and N. Quinn, "What contributes to quality of life in patients with Parkinson's disease?," *Journal of Neurology, Neurosurgery, and Psychiatry*, vol. 69, no. 3, pp. 308–312, 2000.

[7] R. F. Lyons, M. J. L. Sullivan, and P. G. Ritvo, *Relationships in Chronic Illness and Disability*, Sage Publications, Thousand Oaks, CA, USA, 1995.

[8] M. A. Soleimani, R. Negarandeh, F. Bastani, and R. Greysen, "Disrupted social connectedness in people with Parkinson's disease," *British Journal of Community Nursing*, vol. 19, no. 3, pp. 136–141, 2014.

[9] S. C. Martin, "Relational issues within couples coping with Parkinson's disease: implications and ideas for family-focused care," *Journal of Family Nursing*, vol. 22, no. 2, pp. 224–251, 2016.

[10] L. J. Smit and R. L. Shaw, "Learning to live with Parkinson's disease in the family unit: an interpretative phenomenological analysis of well-being," *Medicine, Health Care, and Philosophy*, vol. 20, no. 1, pp. 13–21, 2017.

[11] P. G. Archbold, B. J. Stewart, M. R. Greenlick, and T. Harvath, "Mutuality and preparedness as predictors of caregiver role strain," *Research in Nursing & Health*, vol. 13, no. 6, pp. 375–384, 1990.

[12] P. Archbold, M. R. Greenlick, and T. A. Harvath, "The clinical assessment of mutuality and preparedness in family caregivers to frail older people," in *Key Aspects of Elder Care: Managing Falls, Incontinence, and Cognitive Impairment*, S. G. Funk, E. M. Tornquist, M. T. Champagne et al., Eds., Springer Publishing Company, New York, NY, USA, 1992.

[13] E. O. Park and K. L. Schumacher, "The state of the science of family caregiver-care receiver mutuality: a systematic review," *Nursing Inquiry*, vol. 21, no. 2, pp. 140–152, 2014.

[14] L. Ricciardi, M. Pomponi, B. Demartini et al., "Emotional awareness, relationship quality, and satisfaction in patients with Parkinson's disease and their spousal caregivers," *Journal of Nervous and Mental Disease*, vol. 203, no. 8, pp. 646–649, 2015.

[15] S. Mavandadi, R. Dobkin, E. Mamikonyan, S. Sayers, T. T. Have, and D. Weintraub, "Benefit finding and relationship quality in Parkinson's disease: a pilot dyadic analysis of husbands and wives," *Journal of Family Psychology*, vol. 28, no. 5, pp. 728–734, 2014.

[16] K. S. Judge, H. L. Menne, and C. J. Whitlatch, "Stress process model for individuals with dementia," *Gerontologist*, vol. 50, no. 3, pp. 294–302, 2010.

[17] D. D. Rucker, K. J. Preacher, Z. L. Tormala, and R. E. Petty, "Mediation analysis in social psychology: current practices and new recommendations: mediation analysis in social psychology," *Social and Personality Psychology Compass*, vol. 5, no. 6, pp. 359–371, 2011.

[18] D. P. MacKinnon, *Introduction to Statistical Mediation Analysis*, Lawrence Erlbaum Associates: Taylor & Francis Group, New York, NY, USA, 2008.

[19] B. Goldsworthy and S. Knowles, "Caregiving for Parkinson's disease patients: an exploration of a stress-appraisal model for quality of life and burden," *Journals of Gerontology Series B, Psychological Sciences and Social Sciences*, vol. 63, no. 6, pp. P372–P376, 2008.

[20] K. Greenwell, W. K. Gray, A. van Wersch, P. van Schai, and R. Walker, "Predictors of the psychosocial impact of being a carer of people living with Parkinson's disease: a systematic review," *Parkinsonism and Related Disorders*, vol. 21, no. 1, pp. 1–11, 2015.

[21] M. Karlstedt, S. M. Fereshtehnejad, D. Aarsland, and J. Lokk, "Determinants of dyadic relationship and its psychosocial impact in patients with Parkinson's disease and their spouses," *Parkinson's Disease*, vol. 2017, Article ID 4697052, 9 pages, 2017.

[22] S. Fahn and R. Elton, "The unified Parkinson's disease rating scale," in *Recent Developments in Parkinson's Disease*, S. Fahn, C. D. Marsden, M. Goldstein et al., Eds., vol. 2, pp. 153–163, Macmillan Health Care Information, Florham Park, NJ, USA, 1987.

[23] K. R. Chaudhuri, P. Martinez-Martin, A. H. Schapira et al., "International multicenter pilot study of the first comprehensive self-completed nonmotor symptoms questionnaire for Parkinson's disease: the NMSQuest study," *Movement Disorders*, vol. 21, no. 7, pp. 916–923, 2006.

[24] P. Martinez-Martin, A. H. Schapira, F. Stocchi et al., "Prevalence of nonmotor symptoms in Parkinson's disease in an international setting; study using nonmotor symptoms questionnaire in 545 patients," *Movement Disorders*, vol. 22, no. 11, pp. 1623–1629, 2007.

[25] A. F. Jorm, "The informant questionnaire on cognitive decline in the elderly (IQCODE): a review," *International Psychogeriatrics*, vol. 16, no. 3, pp. 275–293, 2004.

[26] K. H. Asberg and U. Sonn, "The cumulative structure of personal and instrumental ADL. A study of elderly people in a health service district," *Scandinavian Journal of Rehabilitation Medicine*, vol. 21, no. 4, pp. 171–177, 1989.

[27] C. Jenkinson, R. Fitzpatrick, V. Peto, R. Greenhall, and N. Hyman, "The PDQ-8: development and validation of a short-form Parkinson's disease questionnaire," *Psychology and Health*, vol. 12, no. 6, pp. 805–814, 1997.

[28] M. Karlstedt, S. M. Fereshtehnejad, E. Winnberg, D. Aarsland, and J. Lokk, "Psychometric properties of the mutuality scale in Swedish dyads with Parkinson's disease," *Acta Neurologica Scandinavica*, vol. 136, no. 2, pp. 122–128, 2017.

[29] B. G. Tabachnick, *Using Multivariate Statistics*, Pearson Education, London, UK, 6th edition, 2012.

[30] D. Hooper, J. Coughlan, and M. Mullen, "Structural equation modelling: guidelines for determining model fit," *Electronic Journal of Business Research Methods*, vol. 6, no. 1, pp. 53–60, 2008.

[31] K. J. Preacher and A. F. Hayes, "Asymptotic and resampling strategies for assessing and comparing indirect effects in multiple mediator models," *Behavior Research Methods*, vol. 40, no. 3, pp. 879–891, 2008.

[32] X. S. Zhao, J. G. Lynch, and Q. M. Chen, "Reconsidering Baron and Kenny: myths and truths about mediation analysis," *Journal of Consumer Research*, vol. 37, no. 2, pp. 197–206, 2010.

[33] R. M. Baron and D. A. Kenny, "The moderator-mediator variable distinction in social psychological research: conceptual, strategic, and statistical considerations," *Journal of Personality and Social Psychology*, vol. 51, no. 6, pp. 1173–1182, 1986.

[34] D. P. MacKinnon, J. L. Krull, and C. M. Lockwood, "Equivalence of the mediation, confounding and suppression effect," *Prevention Science*, vol. 1, no. 4, pp. 173–181, 2000.

[35] Z. Qin, L. Zhang, F. Sun et al., "Health related quality of life in early Parkinson's disease: impact of motor and non-motor symptoms, results from Chinese levodopa exposed cohort," *Parkinsonism and Related Disorders*, vol. 15, no. 10, pp. 767–771, 2009.

[36] S. M. Fereshtehnejad, M. Shafieesabet, F. Farhadi et al., "Heterogeneous determinants of quality of life in different phenotypes of Parkinson's disease," *PLoS One*, vol. 10, no. 9, Article ID e0137081, 2015.

[37] C. Hinnell, C. S. Hurt, S. Landau, R. G. Brown, and M. Samuel, "Nonmotor versus motor symptoms: how much do they matter to health status in Parkinson's disease?," *Movement Disorders*, vol. 27, no. 2, pp. 236–241, 2012.

[38] D. A. Gallagher, A. J. Lees, and A. Schrag, "What are the most important nonmotor symptoms in patients with Parkinson's disease and are we missing them?," *Movement Disorders*, vol. 25, no. 15, pp. 2493–2500, 2010.

[39] P. Martinez-Martin, C. Rodriguez-Blazquez, M. M. Kurtis, and K. R. Chaudhuri, "The impact of non-motor symptoms on health-related quality of life of patients with Parkinson's disease," *Movement Disorders*, vol. 26, no. 3, pp. 399–406, 2011.

[40] M. A. Soleimani, F. Bastani, R. Negarandeh, and R. Greysen, "Perceptions of people living with Parkinson's disease: a qualitative study in Iran," *British Journal of Community Nursing*, vol. 21, no. 4, pp. 188–195, 2016.

[41] P. Valkovic, J. Harsany, M. Hanakova, J. Martinkova, and J. Benetin, "Nonmotor symptoms in early- and advanced-stage Parkinson's disease patients on dopaminergic therapy: how do they correlate with quality of life?," *ISRN Neurology*, vol. 2014, Article ID 587302, 4 pages, 2014.

[42] A. M. Birgersson and A. K. Edberg, "Being in the light or in the shade: persons with Parkinson's disease and their partners' experience of support," *International Journal of Nursing Studies*, vol. 41, no. 6, pp. 621–630, 2004.

24

Oral Health of Parkinson's Disease Patients

Marjolein A. E. van Stiphout ⓘ,[1] **Johan Marinus,**[2] **Jacobus J. van Hilten,**[2]
Frank Lobbezoo ⓘ,[3] **and Cees de Baat** ⓘ[1,4]

[1]*Foundation for Oral Health and Parkinson's Disease, P.O. Box 1155, 2340 BD Oegstgeest, Netherlands*
[2]*Department of Neurology, Leiden University Medical Center, Albinusdreef 2, 2333 ZA Leiden, Netherlands*
[3]*Department of Oral Kinesiology, Academic Centre for Dentistry Amsterdam (ACTA),*
 University of Amsterdam and Vrije Universiteit Amsterdam, Gustav Mahlerlaan 3004, 1081 LA Amsterdam, Netherlands
[4]*Department of Dentistry, Radboud university medical center, P.O. Box 9101, 6500 HB Nijmegen, Netherlands*

Correspondence should be addressed to Cees de Baat; debaat_cees@hotmail.com

Academic Editor: Hélio Teive

The aim of the study was to examine the oral health status of Parkinson's disease (PD) patients, to compare their oral health status to that of a control group, and to relate it to the duration and severity of PD. *Materials and Methods.* 74 PD patients and 74 controls were interviewed and orally examined. Among PD patients, the duration and the Hoehn and Yahr stage (HY) of the disease were registered. *Results.* More PD patients than controls reported oral hygiene care support as well as chewing/biting problems, taste disturbance, tooth mobility, and xerostomia, whereas dentate patients had more teeth with carious lesions, tooth root remnants, and biofilm. Both longer duration and higher HY were associated with more chewing problems and, in dentates, more teeth with restorations. In dentates, longer duration of the disease was associated with higher number of mobile teeth. Higher HY was associated with more oral hygiene care support as well as biting problems and, in dentates, more teeth with carious lesions and tooth root remnants. *Conclusions.* Comparatively, PD patients had weakened oral health status and reduced oral hygiene care. Both duration and severity of the disease were associated with more oral health and hygiene care problems.

1. Introduction

Parkinson's disease is a progressive degenerative neurological disorder, characterized by motor and nonmotor symptoms. The motor symptoms include akinesia, bradykinesia, rigidity, and tremor, which remain not restricted to the trunk and extremities, but may also occur in the orofacial system [1–3]. Motor impairments of the orofacial system include dysphagia, masticatory dysfunction, orofacial dyskinesia, and oromandibular dystonia [4–7]. In addition, related to oral health, the potentially impaired dexterity of arms and fingers may hamper the required daily oral hygiene care [8].

Advances in oral health care and treatment during the past few decades have resulted in a reduced number of edentulous individuals. The proportion of adults who retain their teeth until late in life has increased substantially [9]. Consequently, a still increasing number of dentate older people experience oral health problems, such as dental caries,

periodontal disease, and substantial wear of hard tooth tissues (tooth wear). Furthermore, many older people have been treated with oral implants and/or sophisticated tooth- and/or implant-supported fixed and/or removable dental prostheses. Hence, these older people are in continuous need of both preventive and curative oral health care. The complexity of oral health status, the potential presence of systemic diseases, and the use of several medications make older people more vulnerable to oral problems when compared to younger age groups, particularly in those who are cognitively impaired [10, 11]. In addition, weakened oral health due to neglected oral hygiene care and reduced oral health care utilization has previously been found in older people [11–14].

Oral diseases, such as dental caries and periodontal disease, not only have oral effects, for example oral pain and oral functioning problems, but may also impact a number of systemic conditions. Emerging evidence suggests that poor oral health influences the initiation and/or progression of diseases, such as atherosclerosis, diabetes mellitus, Alzheimer's disease, and rheumatoid arthritis [15]. Aspiration of oropharyngeal bacteria may cause pneumonia [15–17]. Concerns were expressed about relationships between older people's poor oral health status and nutrition [18].

Study of the international literature revealed that, when compared to control subjects, Parkinson's disease patients generally had a lower number of teeth, more dental carious lesions, poorer periodontal health, higher objective periodontal treatment needs, more subjective chewing difficulties, more subjective swallowing difficulties, more subjective denture discomfort, more limited active mouth opening, and more negative impact of oral health on daily life (Table 1) [19–28]. However, each of the aforementioned studies investigated only few aspects of oral health; none investigated the whole picture of the oral health status. Furthermore, the relationships between aspects of oral health and the duration and severity of Parkinson's disease have not been addressed.

Therefore, the aim of the current study was to examine the most relevant aspects of the subjective and objective oral health status of Parkinson's disease patients, to compare their oral health status to that of an optimally gender-, age-, social background-, and lifestyle-matched control group, and to relate their oral health status to the duration and severity of Parkinson's disease.

2. Materials and Methods

2.1. Study Population. The current cross-sectional, case-control, optimally gender-, age-, social background-, and lifestyle-matched study was approved by the Medical Ethical Committee of Leiden University Medical Center, Leiden, the Netherlands, approval number P13.079. Assuming a power $(1-\beta)$ of 0.80 and an α of 0.05 and an objective to detect a prevalence difference of 25% between groups across a range of different hypothetical prevalence rates, a sample size calculation indicated that 69 persons per group of Parkinson's disease patients and control subjects would be sufficient.

Patients with Parkinson's disease, without severe comorbidity according to classes III and IV of the Physical Status Classification System of the American Society of Anesthesiologists, were requested to participate when they visited the Department of Neurology of the Leiden University Medical Center, Leiden, the Netherlands, for a routine periodic consultation. The Parkinson's disease patients who agreed to participate, were subsequently requested to identify a control person, for instance a family member or other close relative, who had no Parkinson's disease or other severe systemic diseases according to classes III and IV of the Physical Status Classification System of the American Society of Anesthesiologists, who had approximately the same age (±5 years) as well as a similar social background and lifestyle, and who would likely be prepared to participate. The group of control subjects was also optimally gender matched, meaning that men with Parkinson's disease preferably indicated men and women with Parkinson's disease preferably indicated women. Assuming that not every person proposed by a Parkinson's disease patient as control subject would agree to participate, initially 74

Parkinson's disease patients were included. All Parkinson's disease patients and indicated control subjects were visited at their homes to inform them about the research project. Luckily, all of them provided informed consent and were subsequently interviewed and examined.

After the interview and the examination, every participant received information on his/her actual oral health condition and was recommended consultation with a dentist in case the actual oral health condition required attention and/or treatment.

2.2. Assessments. Using a common history form, data were gathered about educational level (primary, secondary, and tertiary), smoking habits, length of time since the last oral health consultation, number of oral health consultations during the previous five years, daily oral hygiene care (whether or not supported by a professional or voluntary care provider), type of toothbrush used, chewing problems, biting problems, taste disturbance, burning mouth, xerostomia, halitosis, remaining food particles, tooth mobility, toothache, tooth sensitivity, painful gums, and bleeding gums. Persons with an edentulous maxilla/mandible were requested to indicate the duration since the last teeth in the maxilla/mandible had been removed, the number of years during which a current complete maxillary/mandibular removable dental prosthesis was functioning, and their potential experience with a loose coming complete maxillary/mandibular removable dental prosthesis during oral movements.

An experienced dentist performed an oral health examination in all participants, using a common oral screening form. Variables included were edentulousness, soft tissue lesions, complete or partial maxillary/mandibular removable dental prostheses, number of teeth, number of teeth with carious lesions, number of teeth with restorations, number of tooth root remnants, amount of biofilm and food, periodontal health, and number of posterior functional tooth units, including (implant-supported) single- and multiunit fixed dental prostheses.

The amount of biofilm and food on teeth and soft tissues was assessed by a simple 3-points scale: 1 = hardly any biofilm and food; 2 = thin layer of biofilm and food; 3 = thick layer of biofilm and food.

Periodontal health was assessed using the tooth mobility scoring system. This clinically easy-to-determine system differentiates three grades: grade I: mobility in a horizontal direction more than 0.2 mm and less than 1 mm; grade II: mobility in a horizontal direction of 1 mm or more; and grade III: mobility in vertical direction [29].

The number of posterior functional tooth units is an important proxy for masticatory efficiency. One maxillary and one mandibular premolar in occluding contact constitute one posterior functional tooth unit. One occluding maxillary and mandibular molar are equivalent to two posterior functional tooth units [30].

In persons with an edentulous maxilla/mandible, the reduction of the edentulous residual alveolar ridge was clinically classified as moderate reduction, high degree of reduction, or extensive reduction, using a standard set of edentulous alveolar ridge models [31].

TABLE 1: Studies on Parkinson's disease and oral health, available in the international literature.

Publication	Country	Research design	Population	Results of PD patients when compared to controls	OR	95% CI	P
Nakayama et al., 2004 [19]	Japan	Questionnaire survey by mail	104 with PD 191 controls	Gender- and age-adjusted: More chewing difficulties More denture discomfort More edentulousness Less daily denture care 50% swallowing problems	6.0 3.9 3.5 10.5	2.8–12.8 1.9–8.0 1.8–6.8 2.9–37.3	
Schwarz et al., 2006 [20]	Germany	Case-control, age-matched	70 with PD 85 controls	Higher scores on indices of the Community Periodontal Index for Treatment Needs (CPITN)			<0.05
Einarsdóttir et al., 2009 [21]	Iceland	Case-control	67 with PD 55 controls	Lower number of teeth More dental carious lesions More biofilm Poorer periodontal health Greater number of cariogenic bacteria in saliva	3.13 2.28	1.4–6.9 1.0–4.9	<0.036 <0.007 <0.004 0.035 <0.05
Hanaoka and Kashihara, 2009 [22]	Japan	Case-control, age-matched	89 with PD 68 mild cognitively impaired 60 with ischemic stroke	Lower number of teeth More dental carious lesions More deep periodontal pockets			<0.05 <0.001 <0.001
Bakke et al., 2011 [23]	Denmark	Case-control, age-matched, gender-matched	15 with moderate to advanced PD 15 controls	Overall objective orofacial function Poorer subjective masticatory ability Poorer active mouth opening More negative impact of oral health on daily life			<0.001 <0.001 <0.001 <0.001
Müller et al., 2011 [24]	Germany	Case-control	101 with PD 75 controls	Lower gingival index Lower frequency of daily tooth brushing More dental carious lesions Longer time since last dental visit Lower salivary flow rate More gingival recession More tooth mobility			<0.001 <0.01 <0.01 <0.001 <0.001 <0.001 <0.001
Cicciù et al., 2012 [25]	Italy	Case-control, age-matched	45 with mild to moderate PD 45 controls	More dental carious lesions Higher gingival index Higher sulcus bleeding index Higher biofilm index			not reported not reported not reported not reported
Pradeep et al., 2015 [26]	India	Case-control, age-matched	45 with PD 46 controls	More periodontal pockets More periodontal attachment loss Lower gingival index Lower biofilm index			<0.001 <0.001 <0.001 <0.001
Ribeiro et al., 2016 [27]	Brasil	Case-control	Wearers of complete removable dental prostheses 17 with PD 20 controls	Poorer self-perception of oral health			<0.04
Barbe et al., 2017 [28]	Germany	Questionnaire survey	100 with PD Frequencies compared with results of other studies	Poorer oral health impact profile, among others due to complaints of xerostomia, drooling and dysphagia			

For Parkinson's disease patients, the duration of the disease (since the onset of motor symptoms) and the severity of the disease expressed by the Hoehn and Yahr stage were registered from the patients' medical records [32]. The duration of the disease was categorized as less than 5 years, between 5 and 9 years, and 10 years or longer.

2.3. Statistical Analysis. Data were analyzed using SPSS version 22.0 (SPSS, Inc., Chicago, IL). Numbers and percentages were compared between groups using a Chi-square test (χ^2). An independent-samples Student's t-test was only used to compare the age of Parkinson's disease patients and control subjects. Mann–Whitney U test was used to compare

TABLE 2: Frequencies, including percentages, of the general subjective aspects of oral health and the often/occasional oral health complaints of the (dentate) Parkinson's disease patients (PD) and the (dentate) control subjects (control) and the results of the Chi-square test carried out to assess statistically significant differences (∗) between PD and control.

Variables	PD	Control	Chi-square test
All persons: general subjective variables	$n = 74$	$n = 74$	
Educational level			
(i) primary	18 (24%)	12 (16%)	
(ii) secondary	21 (29%)	35 (47%)	
(iii) tertiary	34 (46%)	27 (37%)	
(iv) missing value	1 (1%)	—	$\chi^2_{(7)} = 11.947$; $P = 0.102$
Smoking status	6 (8.1%)	6 (8.1%)	—
Length of time since the last oral health consultation			
(i) less than half a year	52 (70.3%)	49 (66.2%)	
(ii) between a half and two years	15 (20.3%)	22 (29.8%)	$\chi^2_{(5)} = 5.704$; $P = 0.336$
Number of oral health consultations during the previous five years			
(i) 0	4 (5.4%)	2 (2.7%)	
(ii) 1–5	13 (17.6%)	17 (23.0%)	
(iii) 6–10	30 (40.5%)	36 (48.6%)	
(iv) 11 or more	27 (36.5%)	19 (25.7%)	$\chi^2_{(6)} = 6.607$; $P = 0.359$
Daily oral hygiene care supported by a professional or voluntary care provider	11 (14.9%)	1 (1.4%)	$\chi^2_{(1)} = 9.069$; $P = 0.003^*$
Electric toothbrush used	36 (48.6%)	30 (40.5%)	$\chi^2_{(3)} = 3.091$; $P = 0.378$
All persons: oral health complaints	$n = 74$	$n = 74$	
Chewing problems	22 (29.7%)	3 (4.1%)	$\chi^2_{(4)} = 18.973$; $P = 0.001^*$
Biting problems	26 (35.1%)	7 (9.5%)	$\chi^2_{(4)} = 15.047$; $P = 0.005^*$
Taste disturbance	17 (23.0%)	1 (1.4%)	$\chi^2_{(4)} = 19.523$; $P = 0.001^*$
Burning mouth	3 (4.1%)	0	$\chi^2_{(4)} = 8.0290$; $P = 0.091$
Xerostomia	48 (64.9%)	24 (32.4%)	$\chi^2_{(4)} = 19.510$; $P = 0.001^*$
Halitosis	14 (18.9%)	9 (12.2%)	$\chi^2_{(4)} = 7.037$; $P = 0.134$
Remaining food particles	52 (70.3%)	51 (68.9%)	$\chi^2_{(4)} = 2.877$; $P = 0.579$
Dentate persons: oral health complaints	$n = 65$	$n = 65$	
Tooth mobility	12 (18.5%)	2 (3.1%)	$\chi^2_{(3)} = 11.215$; $P = 0.011^*$
Toothache	10 (15.4%)	6 (9.2%)	$\chi^2_{(3)} = 2.000$; $P = 0.572$
Tooth sensitivity	17 (26.2%)	11 (16.9%)	$\chi^2_{(4)} = 4.500$; $P = 0.343$
Painful gums	12 (18.5%)	7 (10.8%)	$\chi^2_{(4)} = 2.810$; $P = 0.590$
Bleeding gums	13 (20.0%)	12 (18.5%)	$\chi^2_{(4)} = 5.826$; $P = 0.213$

ordinal or nonnormally distributed continuous variables between groups. Kruskal–Wallis test was used to examine group differences of nonnormally distributed continuous variables with three or more categories. Statistical significance was accepted at $P < 0.05$. Given the exploratory character of the study, no attempt was made to control for multiple comparisons.

3. Results

3.1. Participants. Interviews and oral health examinations were performed in 26 women and 48 men with Parkinson's disease and in 35 female and 39 male control subjects ($\chi^2_{(1)} = 2.259$, $P = 0.133$). Mean age ± standard deviation was 70.2 ± 8.8 years in the Parkinson's disease patients and 67.9 ± 10.1 years in the control subjects (Student's t-test; $P = 0.641$).

3.2. Subjective Variables. Table 2 presents frequencies and percentages of the subjective variables of the Parkinson's disease patients and the control subjects. When compared to

the control subjects, statistically significantly more Parkinson's disease patients reported daily oral hygiene care support by a professional or voluntary care provider, chewing problems, biting problems, taste disturbance, and xerostomia. When compared to the dentate control subjects, statistically significantly more dentate Parkinson's disease patients reported tooth mobility.

The Parkinson's disease patients and control subjects with an edentulous maxilla (and mandible) showed no statistically significant group differences with regard to length of time since the last teeth had been removed, number of years during which a current complete maxillary/mandibular removable dental prosthesis was functioning, and persons' experiences with a loose coming complete maxillary/mandibular removable dental prosthesis during oral movements.

3.3. Objective Variables. Table 3 presents frequencies and percentages of the objective variables of the Parkinson's disease patients and the control subjects. Statistical analysis of the data of dentate persons did point out that the

TABLE 3: Frequencies, including percentages, of the objective oral health variables of the Parkinson's disease patients (PD) and the control subjects (control) and statistically significant group differences.

Variables	PD	Control	Statistical test
All persons	$n = 74$	$n = 74$	
Number of persons with an edentulous maxilla	14 (18.9%)	14 (18.9%)	
Number of persons with an edentulous maxilla and mandible	9 (12.2%)	9 (12.2%)	
Number of persons with a soft tissue lesion	20 (27.0%)	18 (24.3%)	
Number of complete maxillary removable dental prostheses	14	15	
Number of complete mandibular removable dental prostheses	9	9	
Number of partial maxillary removable dental prostheses	8	7	
Number of partial mandibular removable dental prostheses	10	9	
Dentate persons	$n = 65$	$n = 65$	
Mean number of teeth	21.2	22.5	
Number of teeth with carious lesions	74	12	Mann–Whitney U test; $U = 1526.500$, $P \leq 0.001$
Number of teeth with restorations	466	518	
Number of tooth root remnants	24	5	Mann–Whitney U test; $U = 1818.000$, $P < 0.022$
Amount of biofilm and food (scores 2 and 3)	39 (60%)	20 (31%)	$\chi^2_{(2)} = 18.127$; $P < 0.001$
Mean number of posterior functional tooth units, including (implant-supported) single- and multiunit fixed dental prostheses	3.2	2.8	

Parkinson's disease patients had statistically significantly more teeth with carious lesions, a greater number of tooth root remnants, and a greater amount of biofilm and food when compared to the control subjects.

Only few Parkinson's disease patients and control subjects had teeth with grades II and III of tooth mobility, 11 and 6 persons, respectively. Therefore, comparisons of periodontal health between Parkinson's disease patients and control subjects were not performed.

The persons who had an edentulous maxilla/mandible, showed no statistically significant differences between Parkinson's disease patients and control subjects with regard to grades of reduction of the edentulous residual alveolar ridges.

3.4. Parkinson's Disease Patients. The distribution of the Parkinson's disease patients across duration and Hoehn and Yahr stage of the disease is presented in Table 4.

The mean duration of the disease was 9.1 ± 6.4 years. Reported chewing problems were statistically significantly positively related to the duration of the disease ($\chi^2_{(8)} = 17.690$, $P = 0.024$). In dentate patients, the number of teeth with restorations and the number of teeth with mobility grade II or III were statistically significantly related to the duration of the disease (Kruskal–Wallis test; resp. $H_{(2)} = 6.398$, $P = 0.041$ and $H_{(2)} = 8.058$, $P = 0.018$).

For subsequent statistical analysis, the Hoehn and Yahr stages were dichotomized, resulting in a group of 47 patients with the mild stages 1 and 2 and a group of 27 patients with the moderate/severe stages 3, 4, and 5. The reported chewing and biting problems as well as the reported daily support for oral hygiene care by a professional or voluntary care provider were statistically significantly positively related to the Hoehn and Yahr stage of the disease (resp. $\chi^2_{(4)} = 14.045$, $P = 0.007$; $\chi^2_{(4)} = 10.939$, $P = 0.027$; $\chi^2_{(1)} = 11.457$, $P = 0.001$). Furthermore, the number of teeth with carious lesions, the number of teeth with restorations, and the number of tooth

TABLE 4: Distribution, including percentages, of the Parkinson's disease patients by duration (D) and Hoehn & Yahr stage (HY) of the disease.

D/HY	Number of patients	Percentage
D less than 5 years	20	27
D between 5 and 9 years	19	26
D 10 years or more	35	47
HY1	16	22
HY2	31	42
HY3	11	14
HY4	12	16
HY5	4	6

root remnants appeared statistically significantly higher in dentate patients with the moderate/severe Hoehn and Yahr stages 3–5, when compared to dentate patients with the mild Hoehn and Yahr stages 1-2 (Mann–Whitney U test; resp., $U = 246.500$, $P = 0.001$; $U = 252.500$, $P = 0.004$; $U = 311.000$, $P = 0.002$).

4. Discussion

This is the first study which examined the most relevant aspects of the subjective as well as the objective oral health status of a large group of Parkinson's disease patients, which compared these findings with the same data of an optimally gender-, age-, social background-, and lifestyle-matched control group and which related the oral health status of the Parkinson's disease patients to the duration and severity of the disease. The findings demonstrate that more Parkinson's disease patients than control subjects reported daily oral hygiene care support by a professional or voluntary care provider, as well as chewing problems, biting problems, taste disturbance, tooth mobility, and xerostomia. Objectively, the dentate Parkinson's disease patients had a greater number of teeth with carious lesions, a greater number of tooth root remnants, and a greater amount of biofilm and food, when compared to the dentate control subjects. These findings represent symptoms of weakened oral health and reduced oral hygiene care, probably due to Parkinson's disease impairments. Within the group of Parkinson's disease patients, both longer duration and higher Hoehn and Yahr stage of the disease were associated with more chewing problems and, in dentate persons, with more teeth with restorations. Additionally, in dentate persons, longer duration of the disease was associated with a higher number of teeth with mobility grade II or III, whereas a higher Hoehn and Yahr stage of the disease was associated with more daily oral hygiene care support by a care provider as well as biting problems and, in dentate persons, with more teeth with carious lesions and more tooth root remnants. These findings reflect symptoms of weakening oral health, probably due to the reducing ability to manage oral hygiene care as the disease advances.

Existing data on the oral health of Parkinson's disease patients, as presented in Table 1, are extended by the results of the current study. Novel identified oral health problems include taste disturbance and more oral health problems in advanced stages of the disease. Together, these data indicate that weakening oral health and its potential negative impact on several systemic conditions are serious problems in Parkinson's disease patients, which demand more attention worldwide by the multidisciplinary Parkinson's disease medical management teams as well as standard referrals to oral health-care providers.

Chewing and biting problems, more reported by Parkinson's disease patients than control subjects, predominantly in advanced stages of the disease, may reflect (increasing) motor impairments of the orofacial system. Consequently, it is recommended to consider research of chewing and biting problems in Parkinson's disease patients with the objective to manage or reduce these problems. Other impairments of the orofacial system of Parkinson's disease patients may present as temporomandibular dysfunction. A recent study among a group of Parkinson's disease patients found temporomandibular dysfunction in about one-fifth of the patients [33]. Nevertheless, since diagnosing and classifying temporomandibular dysfunction is a rather complicated and time-consuming activity [34], we decided consciously not to include temporomandibular dysfunction as a research variable in our study. A separate and specific study on this topic is in preparation by the research groups involved in the current study.

When considered in relation to oral health, taste disturbance is certainly a novel finding in Parkinson's disease patients since none of the studies mentioned in Table 1 reported this problem. However, olfactory loss as well as smell and taste loss are well-known neurological problems in Parkinson's disease. Results of a recent (neurological) study suggest that the problems are caused by a decline of central brain networks rather than a damage of the peripheral olfactory system [35]. Previously, the olfactory deficit was demonstrated to be independent of Parkinson's disease severity and duration and preceding clinical motor symptoms by years. For this reason, taste disturbance was even suggested to be used for assessing the risk of Parkinson's disease in otherwise asymptomatic individuals [36]. From an oral health perspective, taste ability may change due to deterioration of oral health status, deficient oral hygiene, and impaired masticatory ability [37]. Additionally, saliva is of great importance since it acts as a solvent of taste substances, affects taste sensitivity, and maintains the health and function of the taste receptors. Consequently, hyposalivation results, among others, in significant altered taste sensation or taste disturbance [38]. Hyposalivation may induce oral health problems, such as tooth wear, oral soft tissue lesions, dental caries, candidiasis, and periodontal disease [39]. Nearly 65% of the Parkinson's disease patients in our study reported xerostomia (Table 2), confirming previous results demonstrating or suggesting that xerostomia and the commonly underlying hyposalivation are prevalent complications of Parkinson's disease [28, 40]. Another saliva complication of Parkinson's disease patients is drooling. Most likely, impaired intraoral saliva clearance is the basis of its pathophysiology. However, research to explore the exact pathophysiology and to develop standard diagnostic criteria and assessment tools are needed [41]. Therefore, taste disturbance, xerostomia, hyposalivation, and drooling are topics challenging collaboration between movement disorders specialists and dentists.

Several results of the current study suggest a reduced ability to manage oral hygiene care due to Parkinson's disease impairments, which increases as the disease advances. This assumption concurs with the finding of impaired dexterity in Parkinson's disease, predominantly in advanced stages of the disease [8]. Furthermore, a recent study proved that fine motor skills in Parkinson's disease patients are impaired, predominantly in patients with mild cognitive impairment [42]. Probably, at a certain, difficult to predict stage of Parkinson's disease, patients become dependent on professional or voluntary care providers for proper daily oral hygiene care. In the current study, 15% of the Parkinson's disease patients reported as such. Unfortunately, oral hygiene care is generally not prioritized, either by the professional care providers, or by the patients themselves. Even providing a guideline to nursing home care providers and supervised implementation of this guideline did not result in a general improvement of oral hygiene of nursing home residents [43]. Subsequently, it was recommended to better integrate professional oral hygiene care into professional general health care (also in Parkinson's disease patients) in order to prevent poor oral health to become a new geriatric syndrome [44].

A retrospectively ascertained weakness of this study is the lack of data on social background and lifestyle of both the Parkinson's disease patients and the control subjects. Although the patients were requested to identify a family member or other close relative who had a similar social background and lifestyle as a control person, these variables were not actually assessed. Therefore, some selection bias cannot be ruled out.

5. Conclusions

The results of the current study reveal that the Parkinson's disease patients had a weakened oral health status and reduced oral hygiene care, when compared to an optimally gender-, age-, social background-, and lifestyle-matched control group. Additionally, both longer duration of the disease and more severe disease were associated with more oral health and oral hygiene care problems, altogether suggesting that their weakened oral health and reduced oral hygiene care are due to Parkinson's disease impairments. The authors recommend worldwide multidisciplinary Parkinson's disease medical management teams to pay more attention to their patients' oral health including standard referrals to oral health-care providers, to establish research of chewing and biting problems, taste disturbance, xerostomia, hyposalivation, and drooling in Parkinson's disease patients through collaboration of movement disorders specialists and dentists, and to integrate professional oral hygiene care into professional general health care for Parkinson's disease patients.

Disclosure

The intention of this research project has been presented at the XX World Congress on Parkinson's Disease and Related Disorders in Geneva, Switzerland, 8–11 December 2013. On 4–7 December 2014, the design of this research project has been presented at the 10th International Congress on Non-Motor Dysfunctions in Parkinson's Disease and Related Disorders in Nice, France. Some preliminary results of the study have been presented at the XXII World Congress on Parkinson's Disease and Related Disorders in Ho Chi Minh City, Vietnam, 12–15 November 2017.

Acknowledgments

The authors thank all research subjects involved in this case-control study and are grateful to Mrs. H. C. Bakker, who did the English editing of the final manuscript and to Dr. W. J. Klüter, Dr. J. A. H. G. Moerenburg, and Miss A. Jonker who were of great assistance in gathering the research data. This work was supported by Parkinson Vereniging (member of the European Parkinson's Disease Association), Bunnik, Netherlands, and by Foundation for Oral Health and Parkinson's Disease, Oegstgeest, Netherlands.

References

[1] K. R. Chaudhuri, D. G. Healy, and A. H. V. Schapira, "Non-motor symptoms of Parkinson's disease: diagnosis and management," *Lancet Neurology*, vol. 5, no. 3, pp. 235–245, 2006.

[2] K. A. Jellinger, "Neurobiology of cognitive impairment in Parkinson's disease," *Expert Review of Neurotherapeutics*, vol. 12, no. 12, pp. 1451–1466, 2012.

[3] A. A. Moustafa, S. Chakravarthy, J. R. Phillips et al., "Motor symptoms in Parkinson's disease: a unified framework," *Neuroscience and Biobehavioral Reviews*, vol. 68, no. 9, pp. 727–740, 2016.

[4] F. Lobbezoo, "Taking up challenges at the interface of wear and tear," *Journal of Dental Research*, vol. 86, no. 2, pp. 101–103, 2007.

[5] F. Lobbezoo and M. Naeije, "Dental implications of some common movement disorders: a concise review," *Archives of Oral Biology*, vol. 52, no. 4, pp. 395–398, 2007.

[6] I. Suttrup and T. Warnecke, "Dysphagia in Parkinson's disease," *Dysphagia*, vol. 31, no. 1, pp. 24–32, 2016.

[7] G. R. Ribeiro, C. H. Campos, and R. C. M. Rodrigues Garcia, "Parkinson's disease impairs masticatory function," *Clinical Oral Investigations*, vol. 21, no. 4, pp. 1149–1156, 2017.

[8] T. Vanbellingen, B. Kersten, M. Bellion et al., "Impaired finger dexterity in Parkinson's disease is associated with praxis function," *Brain and Cognition*, vol. 77, no. 1, pp. 48–52, 2011.

[9] F. Müller, M. Naharro, and G. E. Carlsson, "What are the prevalence and incidence of tooth loss in the adult and elderly population in Europe?," *Clinical Oral Implants Research*, vol. 18, no. 3, pp. 2–14, 2007.

[10] R. L. Ettinger, "Oral health and the aging population," *Journal of the American Dental Association*, vol. 138, pp. 5S-6S, 2007.

[11] B. Wu, B. L. Plassman, R. J. Crout, and J. Liang, "Cognitive function and oral health among community-dwelling older adults," *Journals of Gerontology Series A: Biological Sciences and Medical Sciences*, vol. 63, no. 5, pp. 495–500, 2008.

[12] B. Wu, B. L. Plassman, J. Liang, and L. Wei, "Cognitive function and dental care utilization among community-dwelling older adults," *American Journal of Public Health*, vol. 97, no. 12, pp. 2216–2221, 2007.

[13] P. Holm-Pedersen, M. Vigild, I. Nitschke, and D. B. Berkey, "Dental care for aging populations in Denmark, Sweden, Norway, United Kingdom, and Germany," *Journal of Dental Education*, vol. 69, no. 9, pp. 987–997, 2005.

[14] P. Holm-Pedersen, S. L. Russell, K. Avlund, M. Viitanen, B. Winblad, and R. V. Katz, "Periodontal disease in the oldest-old living in Kungsholmen, Sweden: findings from the KEOHS project," *Journal of Clinical Periodontology*, vol. 33, no. 6, pp. 376–384, 2006.

[15] F. A. Scannapieco and A. Cantos, "Oral inflammation and infection, and chronic medical diseases: implications for the elderly," *Periodontology 2000*, vol. 72, no. 1, pp. 153–175, 2000.

[16] C. D. van der Maarel-Wierink, J. N. O. Vanobbergen, E. M. Bronkhorst, J. M. G. A. Schols, and C. de Baat, "Risk factors for aspiration pneumonia in frail older people: a systematic literature review," *Journal of the American Medical Directors Association*, vol. 12, no. 5, pp. 344–354, 2011.

[17] C. D. van der Maarel-Wierink, J. N. O. Vanobbergen, E. M. Bronkhorst, J. M. G. A. Schols, and C. de Baat, "Meta-analysis of dysphagia and aspiration pneumonia in frail elders," *Journal of Dental Research*, vol. 90, no. 12, pp. 1398–1404, 2011.

[18] A. W. G. Walls and J. G. Steele, "The relationship between oral health and nutrition in older people," *Mechanisms of Ageing and Development*, vol. 125, no. 12, pp. 853–857, 2004.

[19] Y. Nakayama, M. Washio, and M. Mori, "Oral health conditions in patients with Parkinson's disease," *Journal of Epidemiology*, vol. 14, no. 5, pp. 143–150, 2004.

[20] J. Schwarz, E. Heimhilger, and A. Storch, "Increased periodontal pathology in Parkinson's disease," *Journal of Neurology*, vol. 253, no. 5, pp. 608–611, 2006.

[21] E. R. Einarsdóttir, H. Gunnsteinsdóttir, M. H. Hallsdóttir et al., "Dental health of patients with Parkinson's disease in Iceland," *Special Care in Dentistry*, vol. 29, no. 3, pp. 123–127, 2009.

[22] A. Hanaoka and K. Kashihara, "Increased frequencies of caries, periodontal disease and tooth loss in patients with Parkinson's disease," *Journal of Clinical Neuroscience*, vol. 16, no. 10, pp. 1279–1282, 2009.

[23] M. Bakke, S. L. Larsen, C. Lautrup, and M. Karlsborg, "Orofacial function and oral health in patients with Parkinson's disease," *European Journal of Oral Sciences*, vol. 119, no. 1, pp. 27–32, 2011.

[24] T. Müller, R. Palluch, and J. Jackowski, "Caries and periodontal disease in patients with Parkinson's disease," *Special Care in Dentistry*, vol. 31, no. 5, pp. 178–181, 2011.

[25] M. Cicciù, G. Risitano, G. Lo Giudice, and E. Bramanti, "Periodontal health and caries prevalence evaluation in patients affected by Parkinson's disease," *Parkinson's Disease*, vol. 2012, Article ID 541908, 6 pages, 2012.

[26] A. R. Pradeep, S. P. Singh, S. S. Martande et al., "Clinical evaluation of the periodontal health condition and oral health awareness in Parkinson's disease patients," *Gerodontology*, vol. 32, no. 2, pp. 100–106, 2015.

[27] G. R. Ribeiro, C. H. Campos, and R. C. M. Rodrigues Garcia, "Oral health in elders with Parkinson's disease," *Brazilian Dental Journal*, vol. 27, no. 3, pp. 340–344, 2016.

[28] A. G. Barbe, N. Bock, S. H. M. Derman, M. Felsch, L. Timmermann, and M. J. Noack, "Self-assessment of oral health, dental health care and oral health-related quality of life among Parkinson's disease patients," *Gerodontology*, vol. 34, no. 1, pp. 135–143, 2017.

[29] P. M. Preshaw, "Detection and diagnosis of periodontal conditions amenable to prevention," *BMC Oral Health*, vol. 15, no. 1, p. S5, 2015.

[30] A. F. Käyser, "Shortened dental arches and oral function," *Journal of Oral Rehabilitation*, vol. 8, no. 5, pp. 457–462, 1981.

[31] W. Kalk and C. de Baat, "Some factors connected with alveolar bone resorption," *Journal of Dentistry*, vol. 17, no. 4, pp. 162–165, 1989.

[32] M. M. Hoehn and M. D. Yahr, "Parkinsonism: onset, progression and mortality," *Neurology*, vol. 17, no. 5, pp. 427–442, 1967.

[33] P. F. da Costa Silva, D. A. Biasotto-Gonzalez, L. J. Motta et al., "Impact in oral health and the prevalence of temporomandibular disorder in individuals with Parkinson's disease," *Journal of Physical Therapy Science*, vol. 27, no. 3, pp. 887–891, 2015.

[34] E. Schiffman, R. Ohrbach, E. Truelove et al., "Diagnostic criteria for temporomandibular disorders (DC/TMD) for clinical and research applications: recommendations of the International RDC/TMD Consortium Network and Orofacial Pain Special Interest Group," *Journal of Oral & Facial Pain and Headache*, vol. 28, no. 1, pp. 6–27, 2014.

[35] E. Iannilli, L. Stephan, T. Hummel, H. Reichmann, and A. Haehner, "Olfactory impairment in Parkinson's disease is a consequence of central nervous system decline," *Journal of Neurology*, vol. 264, no. 6, pp. 1236–1246, 2017.

[36] A. Haehner, T. Hummel, and H. Reichmann, "A clinical approach towards smell loss in Parkinson's disease," *Journal of Parkinson's Disease*, vol. 4, no. 2, pp. 189–195, 2014.

[37] C. Batisse, G. Bonnet, C. Eschevins, M. Hennequin, and E. Nicolas, "The influence of oral health on patients' food perception: a systematic review," *Journal of Oral Rehabilitation*, vol. 44, no. 12, pp. 996–1003, 2017.

[38] H. Mese and R. Matsuo, "Salivary secretion, taste and hyposalivation," *Journal of Oral Rehabilitation*, vol. 34, no. 10, pp. 711–723, 2007.

[39] G.-J. van der Putten, H. S. Brand, J. M. G. A. Schols, and C. de Baat, "The diagnostic suitability of a xerostomia questionnaire and the association between xerostomia, hyposalivation and medication use in a group of nursing home residents," *Clinical Oral Investigations*, vol. 15, no. 2, pp. 185–192, 2011.

[40] Y. Zlotnik, Y. Balash, A. D. Korczyn, N. Giladi, and T. Gurevich, "Disorders of the oral cavity in Parkinson's disease and parkinsonian syndromes," *Parkinson's Disease*, vol. 2015, Article ID 379482, 6 pages, 2015.

[41] P. Srivanitchapoom, S. Pandey, and M. Hallett, "Drooling in Parkinson's disease: a review," *Parkinsonism and Related Disorders*, vol. 20, no. 11, pp. 1109–1118, 2014.

[42] P. Dahdal, A. Meyer, M. Chaturvedi et al., "Fine motor function skills in patients with Parkinson disease with and without mild cognitive impairment," *Dementia and Geriatric Cognitive Disorders*, vol. 42, no. 3-4, pp. 127–134, 2016.

[43] G.-J. van der Putten, J. Mulder, C. de Baat, L. M. J. De Visschere, J. N. O. Vanobbergen, and J. M. G. A. Schols, "Effectiveness of supervised implementation of an oral health care guideline in care homes; a single-blinded cluster randomized controlled trial," *Clinical Oral Investigations*, vol. 17, no. 4, pp. 1143–1153, 2013.

[44] G.-J. van der Putten, C. de Baat, L. De Visschere, and J. Schols, "Poor oral health, a potential new geriatric syndrome," *Gerodontology*, vol. 31, no. 1, pp. 17–24, 2014.

25

Meta-Analysis of the Relationship between Deep Brain Stimulation in Patients with Parkinson's Disease and Performance in Evaluation Tests for Executive Brain Functions

A. M. Martínez-Martínez,[1] O. M. Aguilar,[2] and C. A. Acevedo-Triana[1]

[1]*Department of Psychology, Pontificia Universidad Javeriana, Bogotá, Colombia*
[2]*Department of Brain Repair and Rehabilitation, University College London, London, UK*

Correspondence should be addressed to C. A. Acevedo-Triana; cesar.acevedo@javeriana.edu.co

Academic Editor: Rajka M. Liscic

Parkinson's disease (PD) is a neurodegenerative condition, which compromises the motor functions and causes the alteration of some executive brain functions. The presence of changes in cognitive symptoms in PD could be due to the procedure of deep brain stimulation (DBS). We searched in several databases for studies that compared performance in executive function tests before and after the DBS procedure in PE and then performed a meta-analysis. After the initial search, there were 15 articles that specifically evaluated the functions of verbal fluency, working memory, cognitive flexibility, abstract thinking, and inhibition. It was found that there were differences in the evaluation of the cognitive functions in terms of the protocols, which generated heterogeneity in the results of the meta-analysis. Likewise, a tendency to diminish functions like verbal fluency and inhibition was found, being this consistent with similar studies. In the other functions evaluated, no difference was found between pre- and postsurgery scores. Monitoring of this type of function is recommended after the procedure.

1. Introduction

Parkinson's disease (PD) is a common, progressive and incurable neurodegenerative disease with an unknown etiology, whose main symptoms include motor alterations such as shaking, an abnormal increase in muscle tone, bradykinesia, postural instability, impaired balance and walking, and emotional inexpressiveness [1–6]. In postmortem studies of patients with PD, these clinical features have been directly related to the reduction of dopamine neurons in the cortical-thalamus-striated loop [1, 4–7], mitochondrial alterations [4], and the presence of clusters of α-synuclein presynaptic protein, known as Lewy bodies [4, 7, 8].

From a neurological perspective, the symptoms of PD have been considered to be the result of alterations in the communication between the direct/indirect motor control pathways of the basal ganglia. According to this "classic" model, this deficiency in communication is given by a reduction in the dopaminergic transmission which in turn results in the diminished inhibition of the indirect pathway, the excitation of the direct pathway, and the excessive activation in the discharge of internal globus pallidus (GPi) and an inhibition of the thalamic cortical motor system [9, 10]. Given the model's limitations in explaining PD systems other than the motor ones, it is recognized that the Cortico-Basal Ganglia-Thalamus loop is implied in eye movement control functions (the oculomotor circuit) [11], memory and spatial orientation (dorsolateral prefrontal circuit) [10], behavioral adjustment and control, and the reward and punishment system (lateral orbitofrontal circuit) [9].

It has been suggested that cognitive [9], emotional [12], and behavioral [13] alterations can be generated in the BG-cortex communication. In this same sense, although it has not been a characteristic present in all the reports, a significant metabolic reduction has been found in patients with Parkinson's disease, predominantly in areas of parietal and medial frontal association [5].

Among the nonmotor clinical symptoms there is a broad spectrum of alterations at cognitive [1, 9, 14], emotional, mood [15], behavioral [16, 17], and psychiatric levels [17,

18]. In some cases, the cognitive deficit is comparable to executive alterations similar to patients with lesions in the frontal lobe, given the reduction of dopaminergic activity in the frontostriatal circuits, but without being considered a "frontal lobe syndrome," leading to episodic alterations and visuospatial and verbal fluency dysfunctions [9, 19]. Previous studies have reported on the appearance of alterations in tasks that assess executive brain functions, such as verbal fluency [20], Trail Making Test (TMT-B), Wisconsin Card Sorting Test (WCST), Stroop [19], Theory of Mind [21, 22], and timing deficits [23].

The treatments reported for PD include dopamine antagonist pharmacological treatments [2, 3, 24], physical therapy [25, 26], genetic therapy [24], transcranial magnetic stimulation [15, 27, 28], injury to the subthalamic nucleus [29], and high frequency deep brain stimulation (DBS) [30–37]. The latter has been proven to reduce the severity of motor symptoms, to reduce pharmacological treatment significantly, and to improve patients' quality of life [1, 31, 32, 35, 36, 38–40]. DBS has been reported in subcortical structures such as the subthalamic nucleus (STN), the internal globus pallidus (GPi), the pedunculopontine nucleus (PPN), and prelemniscal radiation [35, 36, 41–45]. Stimulator frequency depends on the patient's clinical aspects and the location of the electrodes [31, 42].

In the assessment of nonmotor symptoms (disturbed sleep patterns, salivation, mood, cognitive, and executive function), it has been reported that the DBS procedure fosters a number of changes. In DBS of the STN, Bickel et al. [29] found that general performance remained constant in frontal executive function tests [16, 23]. In bilateral DBS of the STN, significant improvement has been reported in the learning of verbal information and visuoconstructive skills when there is increased stimulator amplitude [38, 46]. Inasmuch as the DBS of the PPN, improvements have been reported in terms of tasks related to working memory (MT) [23, 47]. It has also been reported that STN-DBS is involved in the generation of impulse control disorders but that this is not a maintained effect [48].

Some studies have identified metabolic changes associated with execution of tasks, reporting that there is an activity reduction network in PD that includes the supplementary motor area (preSMA), precuneus, the inferior parietal lobe, and the left prefrontal cortex, as well as an increase in the cerebellar vermis and the dentate nucleus, probably due to the cerebellum-BG connections [5, 49]. Changes in the structures of this area can be seen in tasks that involve cognitive performance which may suggest that alterations in the network play a role in other cognitive functions [50].

A central aspect of this study is the DBS procedure and its impact on nonmotor symptoms in PD [40]. Thus, a meta-analysis of 28 studies was carried out of studies by Parsons et al. [51]. The authors analyzed the cognitive consequences of STN-DBS, concluding that the procedure presents a small effect on all the cognitive domains assessed, except on verbal fluency, shedding light on a lower statistically significant performance in phonetic and semantic verbal fluency tests after DBS.

Given the lack of consensus inasmuch as the impact of the DBS procedure on executive brain functions specifically, the aim of this study was to identify changes in the executive brain functions tests after DBS in six months or more, reported in the last ten years. To do this, we used studies that showed results for before and after DBS and analyzed these using meta-analysis.

2. Method

2.1. Study Selection. An information search was carried out in the Scopus databases using the following key words: "deep AND brain AND stimulation AND Parkinson AND executive AND functions." The search yielded 126 articles that covered the 2005–2015 period. Using the same key words, the Pubmed database yielded 39 results; the Web of Science (WOS) database, 104 results; the Sage journals database, 142 results; the Taylor Francis Online database, 125 results; the Wiley Online Library, 1362 results; the Embase database, 149 results; and Proquest, 3295 results. Finally, using the PsychNET database, the search initially gave no results; thus it was modified using the words "Parkinson AND DBS," yielding 6 results. This gave a total of 5348 records in 9 databases. The results were subsequently grouped by year and types of journal articles.

The cleaning process was undertaken in two phases. The first was a selection of articles published in science journals, excluding reviews, meta-analyses, and case studies. The results for this first phase are shown in Figure 1.

2.2. Study Inclusion Criteria. The studies were selected considering the following recommendations: (a) types of design; (b) types of intervention; (c) participant characteristics; (d) statistical data; and (e) the tests used [52]. All the reported studies were written in English and dated between 2005 and 2015. The inclusion criteria for this meta-analysis were the following: (a) pre- and postsurgery testing of stimulator implantation; (b) for the target, the subthalamic nucleus, globus pallidus, and other structures related to movement; (c) sociodemographic variables were not taken into account for participant characteristics (age, how long the patient has had the disease, educational level, and type of medication); (d) studies that reported means, standard deviations, t-tests, significance levels; and (e) only those studies that reported some kind of test that assessed executive brain functions (working memory, verbal fluency, cognitive flexibility, planning, inhibition, and abstract thinking) and processing speed. Figure 1 outlines the search procedure. Nonadditional studies were identified by contacting clinical experts and searching bibliographies in local repositories.

2.3. Codification of the Studies. The studies were codified independently by 4 researchers and the codified information was subsequently corroborated. The following characteristics were taken into account for the codification: (a) identification of the study by the first author's surname and the year of publication; (b) the number of participants; (c) the study design (before and after surgery; only after surgery; cases and controls; and correlational); (d) location of implanted

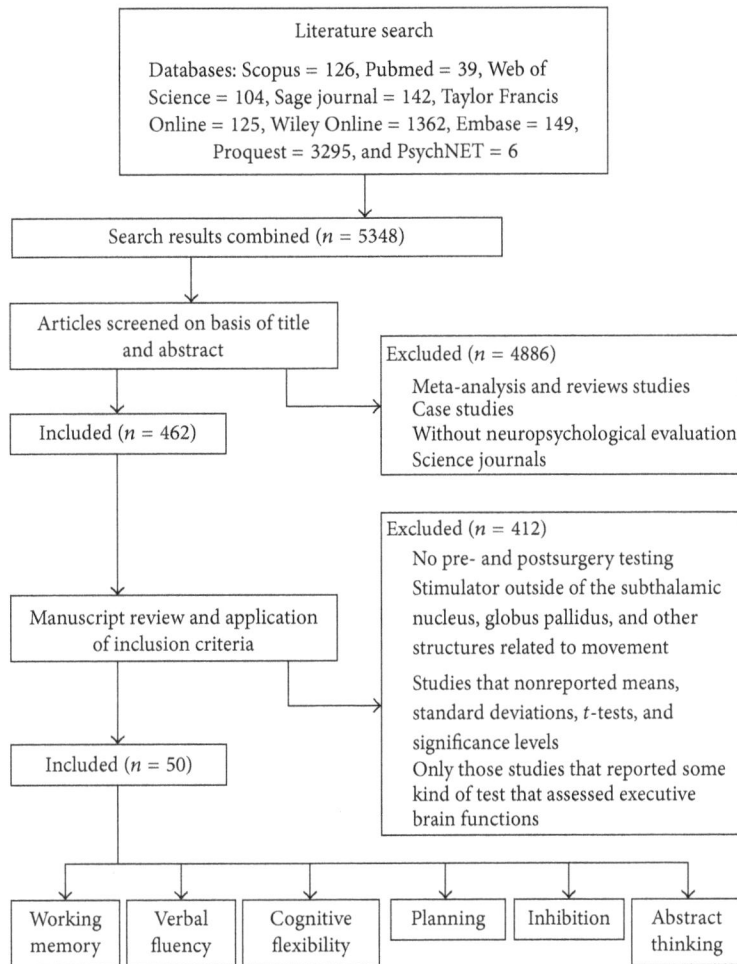

FIGURE 1: Flow diagram of study selection. Adapted from Liberati et al. [53].

deep brain stimulation (subthalamus; globus pallidus; and other); (e) parameter related to the stimulator (pulse, frequency, voltage, and electrode type); (f) schooling (secondary education, university education, graduate studies, none, and not reported); (g) age (under 50, 51–60, 61–70, over 70, and not reported); (h) time of suffering from PD symptoms before brain stimulation surgery (short, less than 5 years; medium, 6–10 years; late, more than 10 years; and not reported); (i) sex (men, women, mixed, and not reported); (j) socioeconomic status (reported, not reported); (k) type of medication; (l) results values associated with the executive brain functions tests undertaken (Table 1); and (m) time before assessment after the stimulator implantation surgery. When the information was codified for the meta-analysis, the time after stimulator implantation variable was not taken as a homogenization criterion for the studies. That is, for those that presented more than one posterior measurement, the measurement closest to 12 months after the surgery was used.

The executive brain functions considered in the study analysis include verbal fluency, cognitive flexibility, working memory, processing speed, behavioral inhibition, and planning (Table 2). Following Parsons et al. [51], the verbal fluency assessment tasks were separated due to the reported systematic reduction of the verbal fluency function in patients with PD with DBS and the difference (category or letters) in terms of task processing.

2.4. Statistical Analysis. The mean scores of the tests undertaken were calculated and Hedges's g values and standard error (SE) for each study are reported together with 95% confidence intervals (CIs). It was assumed that if value I^2 was below 50% of heterogeneity, a meta-analysis with a fixed effects model would be applied; otherwise, a random effects model would be used [57].

To assess the publication bias, a funnel plot was used for each of the meta-analyses [58]. The meta-analysis and funnel plot were carried out using the Comprehensive Meta-analysis 2.0 software. $p < 0.05$ value was considered to have statistical significance.

3. Results

Once the search was refined, 5348 studies were analyzed (Figure 1). Figure 1 shows the results of the initial search.

3.1. Descriptive. The descriptive results are shown in Table 2 which outlines the studies, number of patients, age, time

TABLE 1: Demographic and clinical aspects of patients in studies and frequency of neuropscyhological tests.

Study	N	Country	Design	Target	Age	Education (years)	Onset Parkinson disease	Hoehn & Yahr stage	Time to postevaluation in months	Pulse	Frequency	Voltage	Electrodes
Verb fluency-semantic													
Takehiko-Yamanaka et al. (2012)	30	Japan	Pre-post	STN	61,1 (9,1)	12,5 (4,5)	11,5 (5,7)	—	1, 12	90 μs	130 Hz	2,4	Monopolar
Daniels (2012)	60	Germany	Pre-post + control	STN	60,2 (7,9)	—	13,8 (6,3)	2,29 (0,72)	6	60 μs	130 Hz	—	—
Castelli et al. [54]	19	Italy	Pre-post	STN	62,1 (4,2)	—	14,7 (5)	—	17	Right 61,6 (6,9), left 61,6 (6,9)		Right 3,2 (0,4), left 3,2 (0,5)	Monopolar bilateral
Zangaglia et al. (2009)	65	Italy	Pre-post + control	STN	58,84 (770)	7,31 (3,21)	11,84 (5,07)	2,34 (0,43)	1, 6, 12, 24, 36	—	—	—	Semimicroelectrode
Tang (2015)	27	China	Pre-post	STN					6, 12		—	—	Bilateral
Rothlind (2015)	164	USA	Pre-post + control	STN + GPi	62,3 (8,9)	14,8 (3)	12,8 (5,5)	3,3 (0,9)	6		—	—	Bilateral
Houvenaghel (2015)	26	France	Pre-post + control	STN	55,8 (6,2)	10,1 (2,4)	11,7 (4)	1,8 (0,8)	3		—	—	Bilateral
Tramontana (2015)	30	USA	Pre-post + control	STN + medicine	60 (7)	—	2,2 (1,4)	2	6 y 12		—	—	Bilateral
Verb fluency-phonemic													
Takehiko-Yamanaka (2012)	30	Japan	Pre-post	STN	61,1 (9,1)	12,5 (4,5)	11,5 (5,7)	—	1, 12	90 μs	130 Hz	2,4 V	Monopolar
Merola et al., (2011)	20	Italy	Pre-post + control	STN + OTHER	66,5 (2,5)	—	16,4 (4,3)	—	14	—	—	—	—
Daniels et al., 2010	60	Germany	Pre-post + control	STN	60,2 (7,9)	—	13,8 (6,3)	2,29 (0,72)	6	60 μs	130 Hz	—	—
Castelli et al., [54]	19	Italy	Pre-post	STN	62,1 (4,2)	—	14,7 (5)	—	17	Right 61,6 (6,9), left 61,6 (6,9)	130 Hz	Right 3,2 (0,4), left 3,2 (0,5)	Monopolar bilateral
Le Jeune [55]	13	France	Pre-post + control	STN	57 (7,8)	—	10,9 (2,2)	—	—	64,6	R 135,3 Hz, L 136,5 Hz	Right 2,3 V y, left 2,4 V	Quadripolar
Sáez-Zea, et al. (2012)	9	Spain	Pre-post	STN	54 (14)	—	12 (2)	3	—	—	—	—	—
Castelli et al., (2010)	27	Italy	Pre-post	STN	60,6 (6,7)	8 (4,1)	15,3 (5,1)	—	1	—	—	—	—
Rothlind (2015)	164	USA	Pre-post + control	STN + GPi	62,3 (8,9)	14,8 (3)	12,8 (5,5)	3,3 (0,9)	6	—	—	—	Bilateral
Houvenaghel (2015)	26	France	Pre-post + control	STN	55,8 (6,2)	10,1 (2,4)	11,7 (4)	1,8 (0,8)	3	—	—	—	Bilateral
Tramontana (2015)	30	USA	Pre-post + control	STN + medicine	60 (7)	—	2,2 (1,4)	2	6 y 12	—	—	—	Bilateral

TABLE 1: Continued.

Study	N	Country	Design	Target	Age	Education (years)	Onset Parkinson disease	Hoehn & Yahr stage	Time to postevaluation in months	Pulse	Frequency	Voltage	Electrodes
Wisconsin Card Sorting Test (WCST)													
Zangaglia (2009)	32	Italy	Pre-post + control	STN	58,84 (7,70)	7,31 (3,21)	11,84 (5,07)	2,34 (0,43)	1, 6, 12, 24, 36				Semimicroelectrode
Fraraccio, (2008)	15	Canada	On-off	STN	58,1 (7,46)	11,3 (3,97)	13,6 (4,39)	—	19	Left: 94,0, right: 94,0	Left: 185 Hz, right: 185 Hz	Left: 2,8, right: 2,8	Quadripolar
Williams et al. (2011)	19	USA	Post	STN	62,1 (10,3)	13,6 (1,71)	10,1 (6,24)	1,5–3,0	24	—	—	—	—
Rothlind (2015)	164	USA	Pre-post + control	STN + GPi	62,3 (8,9)	14,8 (3)	12,8 (5,5)	3,3 (0,9)	6	—	—	—	Bilateral
Tramontana (2015)	30	USA	Pre-post + control	STN + medicine	60 (7)	—	2,2 (1,4)	2	6 y 12	—	—	—	Bilateral
Nelson Modified WSCT													
Castelli et al. [54]	19	Italy	Pre-post	STN	62,1 (4,2)	—	14,7 (5)	—	17	Right 61,6 (6,9), left 61,6 (6,9)		right 3,2 (0,4), left 3,2 (0,5)	Monopolar bilateral
Castelli, (2010)	27	Italy	Pre-post	STN	60,6 (6,7)	8 (4,1)	15,3 (5,1)	—	1	—	—	—	—
Fasano 2010	20	Italy	Pre-post	STN	56,9 (7,2)	—	13,7 (4,8)	3	5, 8	60 µs	130 Hz	—	—
Le juene, (2010)	13	France	Pre-post	STN	57 (7,8)	—	10,9 (2,2)	—	3	2,7 (±0,5)	68,7 (±13,9)	38,1 (±17,1)	Quadripolar
Le Jeune et al., [55]	13	France	Pre-post + control	STN	57 (7,8)	—	10,9 (2,2)	—	—	64,6	R 135,3 Hz, L 136,5 Hz	Right 2,3 V, left 2,4 V	Quadripolar
Houvenaghel (2015)	26	France	Pre-post + control	STN	55,8 (6,2)	10,1 (2,4)	11,7 (4)	1,8 (0,8)	3	—	—	—	Bilateral
Trail Making Test (TMT-B)													
Takehiko-Yamanaka (2012)	30	Japan	Pre-post	STN	61,1 (9,1)	12,5 (4,5)	11,5 (5,7)	—	1, 12	90 µs	130 Hz	2,4 V	Monopolar
Merola (2011)	20	Italy	Pre-post + control	STN + OTHER	66,5 (2,5)	—	16,4 (4,3)	—	14	—	—	—	—
Williams (2011)	19	USA	Post	STN	62,1 (10,3)	13,6 (1,71)	10,1 (6,24)	1,5–3,0	24	—	—	—	—
Castelli et al. [54]	19	Italy	Pre-post	STN	62,1 (4,2)	—	14,7 (5)	—	17	Right 61,6 (6,9), left 61,6 (6,9)		Right 3,2 (0,4), left 3,2 (0,5)	Monopolar bilateral
Le juene, (2010)	13	France	Pre-post	STN	57 (7,8)	—	10,9 (2,2)	—	3	2,7 (±0,5)	68,7 (±13,9)	38,1 (±17,1)	Quadripolar
Le Jeune et al. [55]	13	France	Pre-post + control	STN	57 (7,8)	—	10,9 (2,2)	—	—	64,6	R 135,3 Hz, L 136,5 Hz	Right 2,3 V y, left 2,4 V	Quadripolar

TABLE 1: Continued.

Study	N	Country	Design	Target	Age	Education (years)	Onset Parkinson disease	Hoehn & Yahr stage	Time to postevaluation in months	Pulse	Frequency	Voltage	Electrodes
Castelli, (2010)	27	Italy	Pre-post	STN	60,6 (6,7)	8 (4,1)	15,3 (5,1)	—	1	—	—	—	—
Smeding et al. (2005)	20	Netherlands	Pre-post + control	STN + GP	59,2 (8,6)	10,7 (1,9)	12 (3–50)	2,5 (1,0–5,0)	6, 12	—	—	—	—
Rothlind (2015)	164	USA	Pre-post + control	STN + GPi	62,3 (8,9)	14,8 (3)	12,8 (5,5)	3,3 (0,9)	6	—	—	—	Bilateral
Houvenaghel (2015)	26	France	Pre-post + control	STN	55,8 (6,2)	10,1 (2,4)	11,7 (4)	1,8 (0,8)	3	—	—	—	Bilateral
Pan Test Forward													
Takehiko-Yamanaka (2012)	30	Japan	Pre-post	STN	61,1 (9,1)	12,5 (4,5)	11,5 (5,7)		1, 12	90 µs	130 Hz	2,4 V	Monopolar
Corsi Span Backward													
Smeding, (2005)	20	Netherlands	Pre-post + control	STN	59,2 (8,6)	10,7 (1,9)	12 (3–50)	2,5 (1,0–5,0)	6, 12	—	—	—	—
Fasano (2010)	20	Italy	Pre-post	STN	56,9 (7,2)	—	13,7 (4,8)	3	5, 8	60 µs	130 Hz	—	—
Castelli et al. [54]	19	Italy	Pre-post	STN	62,1 (4,2)	—	14,7 (5)	—	17	Right 61,6 (6,9), left 61,6 (6,9)	—	right 3,2 (0,4), left 3,2 (0,5)	Monopolar bilateral
Castelli, (2010)	27	Italy	Pre-post	STN	60,6 (6,7)	8 (4,1)	15,3 (5,1)	—	1	—	—	—	—
Backward digits													
Takehiko-Yamanaka (2012)	30	Japan	Pre-post	STN	61,1 (9,1)	12,5 (4,5)	11,5 (5,7)	—	1, 12	90 µs	130 Hz	2,4 V	Monopolar
Daniels (2010)	60	Germany	Pre-post + control	STN	60,2 (7,9)	—	13,8 (6,3)	2,29 (0,72)	—	60 µs	130 Hz	Adjusted for each one	Bilateral
Fasano (2010)	20	Italy	Pre-post	STN	56,9 (7,2)	—	13,7 (4,8)	3	5, 8	60 µs	130 Hz	—	—
Fraraccio, (2008)	15	Canada	On-off	STN	58,1 (7,46)	11,3 (3,97)	13,6 (4,39)	—	19	Left: 94,0, right: 94,0	Left: 185 Hz, right: 185 Hz	Left: 2,8, right: 2,8	Quadripolar
Witt et al. [56]	60	Germany	Pre-post + control	STN	60,2 (7,9)	—	13,8 (6,3)	3,62 (0,85)	6	—	—	—	—
Rothlind, et al. (2007)	29	USA	On-off	STN + GP	61,4 (10,11)	15,2 (3,21)	12,9 (4,3)	3,3 (0,45)	—	—	—	—	—
Zangaglia (2009)	32	Italy	Pre-post + control	STN	58,84 (7,70)	7,31 (3,21)	11,84 (5,07)	2,34 (0,43)	1, 6, 12, 24, 36	—	—	—	Semimicroelectrode
Rothlind (2015)	164	USA	Pre-post + control	STN + GPi	62,3 (8,9)	14,8 (3)	12,8 (5,5)	3,3 (0,9)	6	—	—	—	Bilateral
Tang (2015)	27	China	Pre-post	STN					6, 12	—	—	—	Bilateral
Trail Making Test (TMT-A)													
Takehiko-Yamanaka (2012)	30	Japan	Pre-post	STN	61,1 (9,1)	12,5 (4,5)	11,5 (5,7)	—	1, 12	90 µs	130 Hz	2,4 V	Monopolar
Smeding, (2005)	20	Netherlands	Pre-post + control	STN + GP	59,2 (8,6)	10,7 (1,9)	12 (3–50)	2,5 (1,0–5,0)	6, 12	—	—	—	—
Williams (2011)	19	USA	Post	STN	62,1 (10,3)	13,6 (1,7)	10,1 (6,24)	1,5–3,0	24	—	—	—	—
Stroop													
Williams (2011)	19	USA	Post	STN	62,1 (10,3)	13,6 (1,7)	10,1 (6,24)	1,5–3,0	24	—	—	—	—
Daniels (2010)	60	Germany	Pre-post + control	STN	60,2 (7,9)	—	13,8 (6,3)	2,29 (0,72)	—	60 µs	130 Hz	Adjusted for each one	Bilateral
Smeding, (2005)	20	Netherlands	Pre-post + control	STN + GP	59,2 (8,6)	10,7 (1,9)	12 (3–50)	2,5 (1,0–5,0)	6, 1	—	—	—	—
Moreines, (2014)	17		Pre-post	OTH	1		2		—	91 µs	130 Hz	—	—

TABLE 1: Continued.

Study	N	Country	Design	Target	Age	Education (years)	Onset Parkinson disease	Hoehn & Yahr stage	Time to postevaluation in months	Pulse	Frequency	Voltage	Electrodes
Fraraccio, (2008)	15	Canada	On-off	STN	58,1 (7,46)	11,3 (3,97)	13,6 (4,39)	—	19	Left: 94,0, right: 94,0	Left: 185 Hz, right: 185 Hz	Left: 2,8, right: 2,8	Quadripolar
Le Jeune et al. [55]	13	France	Pre-post + Control	STN	57 (7,8)	—	10,9 (2,2)	—	—	64,6	R 135,3 Hz, L 136,5 Hz	Right 2,3 V y, left 2,4 V	Quadripolar
Rothlind, (2007)	29	USA	On-off	STN + GP	61,4 (10,11)	15,2 (3,21)	12,9 (4,3)	3,3 (0,45)	—	—	—	—	—
Le juene, (2010)	13	France	Pre-post	STN	57 (7,8)	—	10,9 (2,2)	—	3	2,7 (±0,5)	—	38,1 (±17,1)	Quadripolar
Witt et al. [56]	60	Germany	Pre-post + Control	STN	60,2 (7,9)	—	13,8 (6,3)	3,62 (0,85)	6	—	—	—	—
Rothlind (2015)	164	USA	Pre-post + control	STN + GPi	62,3 (8,9)	14,8 (3)	12,8 (5,5)	3,3 (0,9)	6	—	—	—	Bilateral
Houvenaghel (2015)	26	France	Pre-post + control	STN	55,8 (6,2)	10,1 (2,4)	11,7 (4)	1,8 (0,8)	3	—	—	—	Bilateral
Tramontana (2015)	30	USA	Pre-post + control	STN + medicam	60 (7)		2,2 (1,4)	2	6,12	—	—	—	Bilateral
						Planification							
Zangaglia (2009)	65	Italy	Pre-post + control	STN	58,84 (7,70)	7,31 (3,21)	11,84 (5,07)	2,34 (0,43)	1, 6, 12, 24, 36	—	—		Semimicroelectrode
Castelli, (2010)	27	Italy	Pre-post	STN	60,6 (6,7)	8 (4,1)	15,3 (5,1)	—	1	—	—	—	—
Fasano (2010)	20	Italy	Pre-post	STN	56,9 (7,2)	—	13,7 (4,8)	3	5, 8	60 µs	130 Hz	—	—
Castelli et al. [54]	19	Italy	Pre-post	STN	62,1 (4,2)	—	14,7 (5)	—	17	Right 61,6 (6,9), left 61,6 (6,9)	—	Right 3,2 (0,4), left 3,2 (0,5)	Monopolar bilateral

TABLE 2

Neuropsychological test	k	N	Age	Years PD	DBS	Heterogeneity		
						Q	$p(Q)$	I^2
Verbal fluency-semantic	4	141	60,56	12,96	STN			
Verbal fluency-Phonetic	7	178	60,21	13,51	STN	19,769	0,032	49,41
WSCT	2	51	60,47	10,97	STN			
WSCT-Nelson	5	92	58,72	13,1	STN	34,759	0,021	42,46
Trail Making Test-B	8	161	60,91	12,45	STN	5,26	0,511	0,000
Corsi Span Backward	4	86	59,86	14,56	STN			
Digit Span Test	7	246	59,22	13.06	STN-GPi	3,088	0,686	0,000
Trail Making Test-A	3	69	61,6	10,8	STN	0,581	0,748	0,000
Stroop	9	246	65,2	12,18	STN-Cingulate (1)-GPi (1)	102,7	0,001	77,6
Planning	4	98	59,61	13.85	STN			

Note: k, number of studies; N, number of patients, DBS (deep brain stimulation); Q, heterogeneity intradomain; $p(Q)$ p value of Q statistic; I^2, percent of heterogeneity from difference.

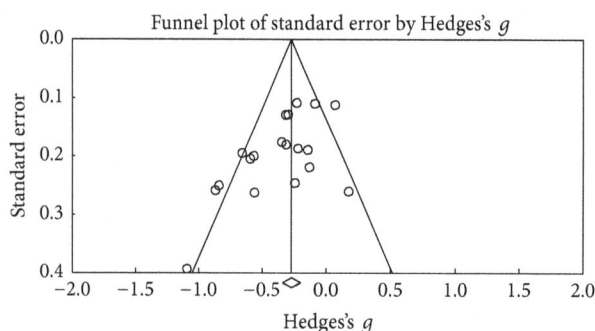

FIGURE 2: Funnel plot for standard error in publications of verbal fluency.

of illness, schooling, PD alteration scores, and other values reported for the studies.

3.2. Meta-Analysis. For this study, a fixed effects model was used due to two conditions. First, the conditions of the participants and characteristics of the disease are similar among the studies and with this a population effect size is theoretically assumed [52, 59]. On the other hand, given that it was previously assumed that the percentage of heterogeneity exceeded 50% measured by coefficient I^2, a random effects model was used [57]. It is important to signal that only one study has results of GPi stimulation (Rothlind, 2015) and because of this the results and figures were not separate.

3.3. Verbal Fluency. Figure 2 outlines the funnel plot of the SE for studies of verbal fluency and there is no bias in the studies reported [58]. In this category, we obtained 21 studies that were clustered depending on the evaluation modality (semantic or phonetic), Hedges's g was used to determine the size of the effect, obtaining a medium effect size (Hedges's g = −0.266; SE = 0.036; CI −0.337 to −0.195), which showed heterogeneity ($Q_{(20)}$ = 42,911; p = 0.002) within an average percentage (I^2 = 53,39%), which, when in excess of 50%, led to the application of a random model [60]. The results also showed a significant reduction in performance in the test after the DBS procedure (Z value = −5,607; p < 0.001) (Figure 3).

3.4. Cognitive Flexibility. This function was assessed based on the Wisconsin Shorting Card Test (WSCT) and Trail Making Test (TMT) in its B and B-A versions. Figure 4 shows the funnel plot used for the SE in WSCT; the figure shows three points outside the projection in the upper threshold, but these are shown as equivalents to the points on the lower threshold. The meta-analysis obtained 27 results in which the Wisconsin Shorting Card Test (WSCT) in its different versions (Nelson or Modified) was assessed, bearing in mind the different types of scores (errors, perseverations, or categories). A small effect size was found (Hedges's g = 0.064; SE = 0.053; CI −0.04 to 0.167), showing heterogeneity ($Q_{(26)}$ = 44,94; p = 0.012) within an average percentage (I^2 = 42,14%), but without exceeding 50% [43, 60]. There seems to be no significant change in the test scores after the DBS procedure (Z value = 1,656; p = 0.098) (Figure 5).

Using the Trail Making Test (TMT-A), 6 results were obtained; Figure 6 shows the funnel plot for the SE of the test, and no biases are observed. The studies in the meta-analysis reveal no differences in terms of execution (Z value = −0.328; p = 0.743), the effect detected was small (Hedges's g = −0.02; SE = 0.061; CI −0.14 to 0.1), and the results showed homogeneity ($Q_{(5)}$ = 3,202; p = 0.669) within the 0% value (I^2 = 0%) (Figure 7). With respect to the other tests for the same function such as version B of the TMT, 10 of the results found did not reveal an important change between the applications (Z value = 0.912; p = 0.362), the effect detected was small

Study name	Subgroup within study	Statistics for each study							Hedges's g and 95% CI
		Hedges's g	Variance	Standard error	Lower limit	Upper limit	Z value	p value	
Rothlind et al., 2015 (STN)	Phonetic	−0.216	0.012	0.110	−0.432	−0.001	−1.966	0.049	
Rothlind et al., 2015 (GPi)	Phonetic	−0.076	0.012	0.112	−0.294	0.143	−0.677	0.499	
Tramontana et al., 2015	Phonetic	−0.553	0.070	0.264	−1.070	−0.035	−2.092	0.036	
Houvenaghel et al., 2015	Phonetic	−0.585	0.043	0.207	−0.991	−0.180	−2.831	0.005	
Takehiko. Y et al. 2012	Phonetic	−0.302	0.033	0.182	−0.659	0.055	−1.660	0.097	
Sáez-Zea C. et al., 2012	Phonetic	−1.083	0.156	0.395	−1.857	−0.310	−2.744	0.006	
Merola et al. 2011	Phonetic	−0.834	0.063	0.252	−1.327	−0.340	−3.309	0.001	
Le Jeune et al., 2008	Phonetic	0.181	0.069	0.262	−0.333	0.694	0.689	0.491	
Daniels et al. 2012	Phonetic	−0.305	0.017	0.130	−0.560	−0.049	−2.336	0.019	
Castelli et al., 2010	Phonetic	−0.206	0.036	0.189	−0.576	0.164	−1.091	0.275	
Castelli et al. 2007	Phonetic	−0.862	0.068	0.260	−1.372	−0.351	−3.309	0.001	
Rothlind et al., 2015 (STN)	Semantic	−0.216	0.012	0.110	−0.432	−0.001	−1.966	0.049	
Rothlind et al., 2015 (GPi)	Semantic	0.077	0.013	0.114	−0.146	0.300	0.677	0.499	
Tramontana et al., 2015	Semantic	−0.231	0.061	0.248	−0.717	0.255	−0.933	0.351	
Houvenaghel et al., 2015	Semantic	−0.130	0.036	0.191	−0.505	0.244	−0.681	0.496	
Takehiko. Y et al. 2012	Semantic	−0.651	0.039	0.197	−1.036	−0.265	−3.309	0.001	
Daniels et al. 2012	Semantic	−0.283	0.017	0.130	−0.538	−0.029	−2.179	0.029	
Zangaglia, R., et al. 2009	Semantic	−0.337	0.032	0.178	−0.685	0.011	−1.897	0.058	
Bergamasco et al 2007	Semantic	−0.117	0.049	0.221	−0.550	0.315	−0.532	0.595	
Tang et al, 2015 (STN)	Semantic	−0.559	0.041	0.202	−0.954	−0.164	−2.771	0.006	
Tang et al, 2015	Semantic	−0.559	0.041	0.202	−0.954	−0.164	−2.771	0.006	
		−0.266	0.001	0.036	−0.337	−0.195	−7.328	0.000	

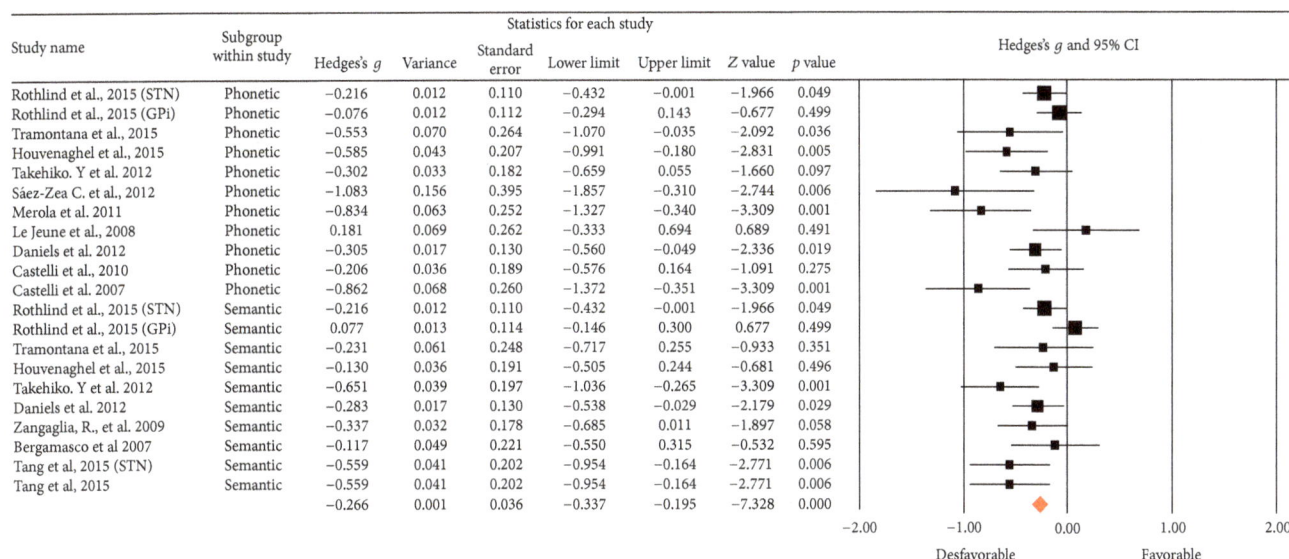

FIGURE 3: Meta-analysis of verbal fluency comparing before and after DBS surgery. Verbal fluency was separated in phonetic and semantic parts. STN = subthalamic nucleus; GPi = internal globus pallidus.

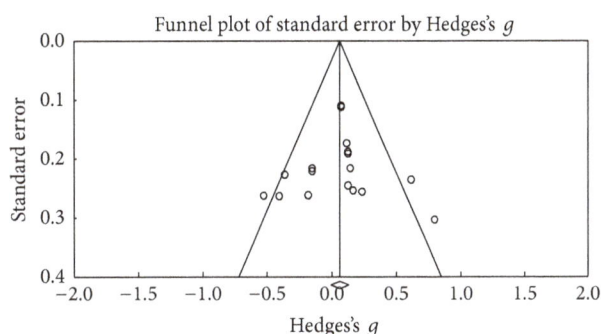

FIGURE 4: Funnel plot for standard error in publications of cognitive flexibility (WSCT).

(Hedges's g = −0.02; SE = 0.053; CI −0.056 to 0.153), and the results showed homogeneity ($Q_{(9)}$ = 6,973; p = 0.64) at a very low percentage (I^2 = 0%) (Figure 9). Figure 8 presents the funnel plot for the SE of the TMT-B. Finally, for the TMT-B-A version (5 results) the funnel plot is presented in Figure 10 and no differences were found between applications before and after the DBS procedure (Z value = −0.404; p = 0.686). The effect detected was small (Hedges's g = −0.04; SE = 0.099; CI −0.234 to 0.154), and the results showed homogeneity ($Q_{(4)}$ = 2,251; p = 0.69) at a very low percentage (I^2 = 0%) (Figure 11).

3.5. Abstract Thinking.
Figure 12 shows the funnel plot and no bias among the studies was observed. In this category, 6 studies were obtained, and no changes in test performance were observed after the DBS procedure (Z value = 0.722; p = 0.471) (Figure 13). A small effect size was obtained (Hedges's g = 0.058; SE = 0.080; CI −0.099 to 0.215), and the result showed homogeneity ($Q_{(5)}$ = 3,088; p = 0.686) within a low percentage (I^2 = 0%).

3.6. Working Memory.
Figure 14 shows the funnel plot and no bias among the studies is observed. In this category, 22 results were obtained, and no changes in test performance were observed after the DBS procedure (Z value = −1,533; p = 0.125) (Figure 15). A small effect size was obtained (Hedges's g = −0.051; SE = 0.033; CI −0.115 to 0.014), and the result showed homogeneity ($Q_{(21)}$ = 13,682; p = 0.883) at a low percentage (I^2 = 0%).

3.7. Inhibition.
Figure 16 shows the funnel plot for inhibition; a number of scores outside the lower and upper thresholds were obtained suggesting a bias in the studies. However, when visual criteria were applied, the bias does not present itself fully, and there are a number of points close to the upper threshold. What does result from this analysis is a high degree of heterogeneity between the studies ($Q_{(40)}$ = 88,95; p < 0.001) corresponding to over 89% of the variability among them (I^2 = 55,03%). In this category, 41 results were obtained.

Given this heterogeneity, a random model meta-analysis was applied and a change in the execution of the test was observed as it significantly reduced after the DBS procedure (Z value = −0.406; p < 0.001) (Figure 17). A small effect size was found (Hedges's g = −0.211; SE = 0.039; CI −0.268 to −0.135).

Study name	Subgroup within study	Statistics for each study							Hedges's g and 95% CI
		Hedges's g	Standard error	Variance	Lower limit	Upper limit	Z value	p value	
Fasano et al., 2010, CAT	MWCST	−0.148	0.216	0.047	−0.571	0.276	−0.684	0.494	
Le Jeune et al., 2010, CAT	MWCST	0.148	0.216	0.047	−0.276	0.571	0.684	0.494	
Fasano et al., 2010, E	MWCST	−0.148	0.216	0.047	−0.571	0.276	−0.684	0.494	
Le Jeune et al., 2010, E	MWCST	0.614	0.236	0.056	0.152	1.076	2.607	0.009	
Fasano et al., 2010, P	MWCST	0.148	0.216	0.047	−0.276	0.571	0.684	0.494	
Le Jeune et al., 2010, P	MWCST	0.614	0.236	0.056	0.152	1.076	2.607	0.009	
Houvenaghel et al., 2015, CAT	MWCST	0.130	0.191	0.036	−0.244	0.505	0.681	0.496	
Houvenaghel et al., 2015, E	MWCST	0.130	0.191	0.036	−0.244	0.505	0.681	0.496	
Zangaglia, R., et al. 2009, E	WSCT	0.118	0.173	0.030	−0.222	0.457	0.680	0.496	
Williams et al., 2011, E	WSCT	−0.359	0.227	0.052	−0.804	0.087	−1.578	0.115	
Fraraccio et al., 2008, EP	WSCT	0.238	0.256	0.065	−0.263	0.738	0.930	0.352	
Rothlind et al., 2015 (GPi) E	WSCT	0.075	0.110	0.012	−0.141	0.291	0.677	0.499	
Rothlind et al., 2015 (STN), P	WSCT	0.076	0.112	0.012	−0.143	0.294	0.677	0.499	
Tramontana et al., 2015, E	WSCT	0.131	0.245	0.060	−0.350	0.612	0.534	0.593	
Tramontana et al., 2015, EP	WSCT	−0.524	0.262	0.069	−1.037	−0.010	−1.997	0.046	
Fraraccio et al., 2008, CAT	WSCT	0.169	0.254	0.064	−0.328	0.666	0.667	0.505	
Fraraccio et al., 2008, NPE	WSCT	−0.403	0.263	0.069	−0.918	0.112	−1.534	0.125	
Castelli et al. 2007, CAT	WSCT Nelson	−0.151	0.221	0.049	−0.585	0.282	−0.684	0.494	
Castelli et al. 2010, CAT	WSCT Nelson	0.128	0.188	0.035	−0.240	0.496	0.681	0.496	
Le Jeune et al., 2010, CAT	WSCT Nelson	−0.181	0.262	0.069	−0.694	0.333	−0.689	0.491	
Castelli et al. 2007, E	WSCT Nelson	−0.151	0.221	0.049	−0.585	0.282	−0.684	0.494	
Castelli et al. 2010, E	WSCT Nelson	0.128	0.188	0.035	−0.240	0.496	0.681	0.496	
Le Jeune et al., 2010, E	WSCT Nelson	0.793	0.303	0.092	0.200	1.386	2.620	0.009	
Castelli et al. 2007, P	WSCT Nelson	−0.151	0.221	0.049	−0.585	0.282	−0.684	0.494	
Castelli et al. 2010, P	WSCT Nelson	0.128	0.188	0.035	−0.240	0.496	0.681	0.496	
Le Jeune et al., 2010, P	WSCT Nelson	0.793	0.303	0.092	0.200	1.386	2.620	0.009	
Williams et al., 2011, P	WSCT Nelson	−0.359	0.227	0.052	−0.804	0.087	−1.578	0.115	
		0.064	0.053	0.003	−0.040	0.167	1.203	0.229	

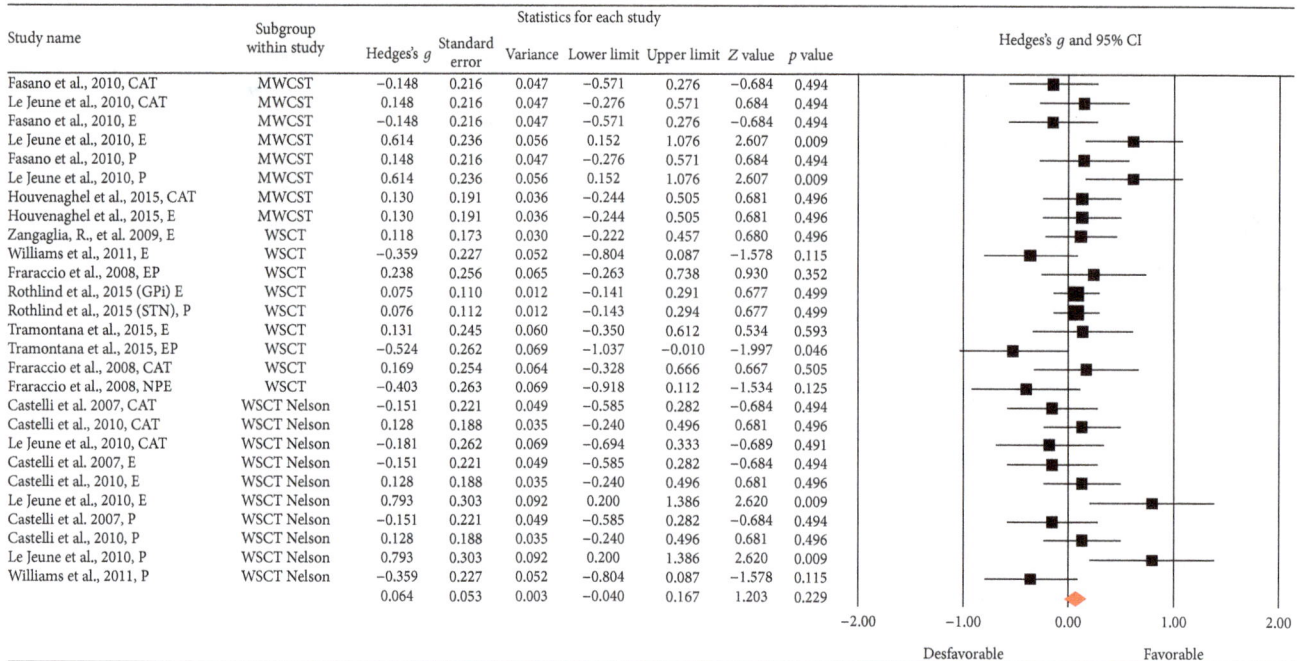

FIGURE 5: Meta-analysis of WSCT comparing before and after DBS surgery. The Wisconsin Short Card Test had three versions. Version one: MWCST = modified WCST; version two: WSCT; and version three: WSCT Nelson version.

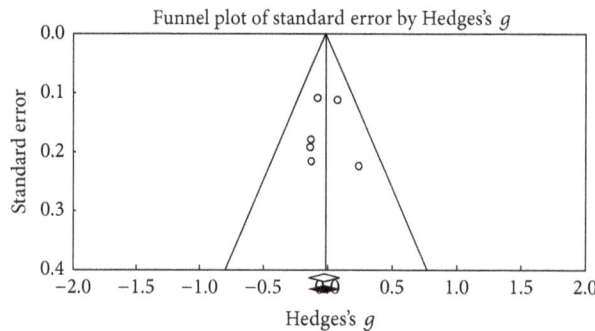

FIGURE 6: Funnel plot for standard error in publications of Trail Making Test (TMT-A).

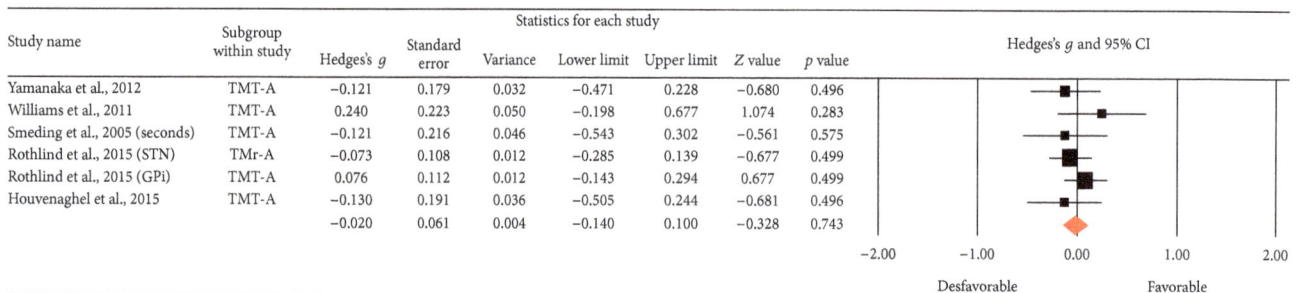

Study name	Subgroup within study	Statistics for each study							Hedges's g and 95% CI
		Hedges's g	Standard error	Variance	Lower limit	Upper limit	Z value	p value	
Yamanaka et al., 2012	TMT-A	−0.121	0.179	0.032	−0.471	0.228	−0.680	0.496	
Williams et al., 2011	TMT-A	0.240	0.223	0.050	−0.198	0.677	1.074	0.283	
Smeding et al., 2005 (seconds)	TMT-A	−0.121	0.216	0.046	−0.543	0.302	−0.561	0.575	
Rothlind et al., 2015 (STN)	TMr-A	−0.073	0.108	0.012	−0.285	0.139	−0.677	0.499	
Rothlind et al., 2015 (GPi)	TMT-A	0.076	0.112	0.012	−0.143	0.294	0.677	0.499	
Houvenaghel et al., 2015	TMT-A	−0.130	0.191	0.036	−0.505	0.244	−0.681	0.496	
		−0.020	0.061	0.004	−0.140	0.100	−0.328	0.743	

FIGURE 7: Meta-analysis of TMT-A comparing before and after DBS surgery.

4. Discussion

The results of this study were found to correspond to similar studies in which there is a general reduction of executive brain functions after the DBS procedure. This does not seem to have an impact on quality of life given the improvement of motor symptoms [19, 51, 61]. It is worth highlighting that the study of EF has shown a reduction in tasks such as WCST, verbal fluency, and Stroop in patients with PD before the DBS procedure. This could be explained by alterations in the BG-dorsolateral prefrontal cortex loop in relation to the reduction

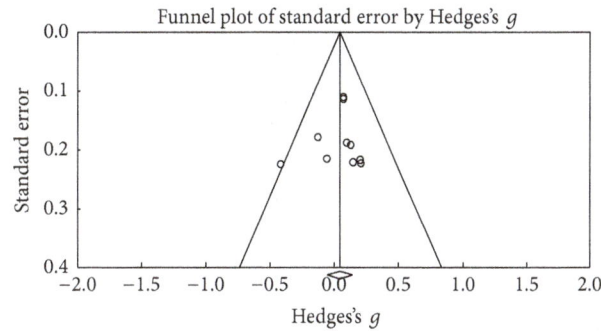

FIGURE 8: Funnel plot for standard error in publications of Trail Making Test (TMT-B).

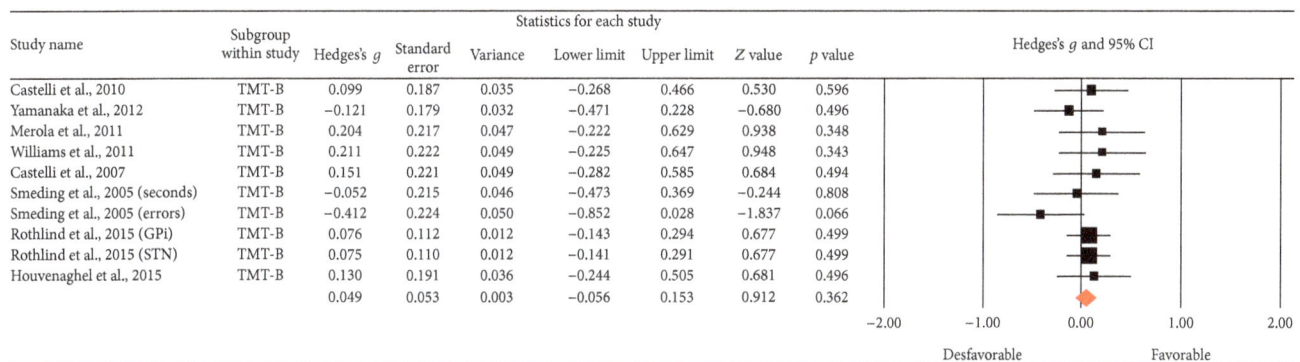

| Study name | Subgroup within study | Statistics for each study | | | | | | | Hedges's *g* and 95% CI |
		Hedges's *g*	Standard error	Variance	Lower limit	Upper limit	*Z* value	*p* value	
Castelli et al., 2010	TMT-B	0.099	0.187	0.035	−0.268	0.466	0.530	0.596	
Yamanaka et al., 2012	TMT-B	−0.121	0.179	0.032	−0.471	0.228	−0.680	0.496	
Merola et al., 2011	TMT-B	0.204	0.217	0.047	−0.222	0.629	0.938	0.348	
Williams et al., 2011	TMT-B	0.211	0.222	0.049	−0.225	0.647	0.948	0.343	
Castelli et al., 2007	TMT-B	0.151	0.221	0.049	−0.282	0.585	0.684	0.494	
Smeding et al., 2005 (seconds)	TMT-B	−0.052	0.215	0.046	−0.473	0.369	−0.244	0.808	
Smeding et al., 2005 (errors)	TMT-B	−0.412	0.224	0.050	−0.852	0.028	−1.837	0.066	
Rothlind et al., 2015 (GPi)	TMT-B	0.076	0.112	0.012	−0.143	0.294	0.677	0.499	
Rothlind et al., 2015 (STN)	TMT-B	0.075	0.110	0.012	−0.141	0.291	0.677	0.499	
Houvenaghel et al., 2015	TMT-B	0.130	0.191	0.036	−0.244	0.505	0.681	0.496	
		0.049	0.053	0.003	−0.056	0.153	0.912	0.362	

FIGURE 9: Meta-analysis of TMT-B comparing before and after DBS surgery.

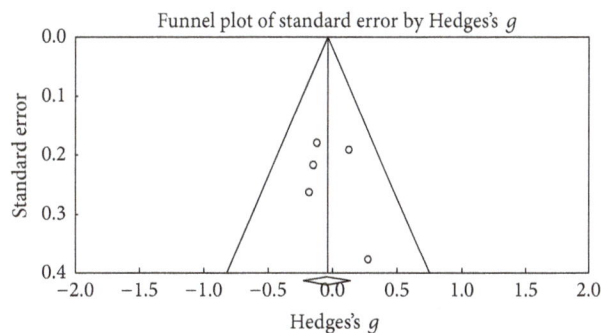

FIGURE 10: Funnel plot for standard error in publications of Trail Making Test (TMT-AB).

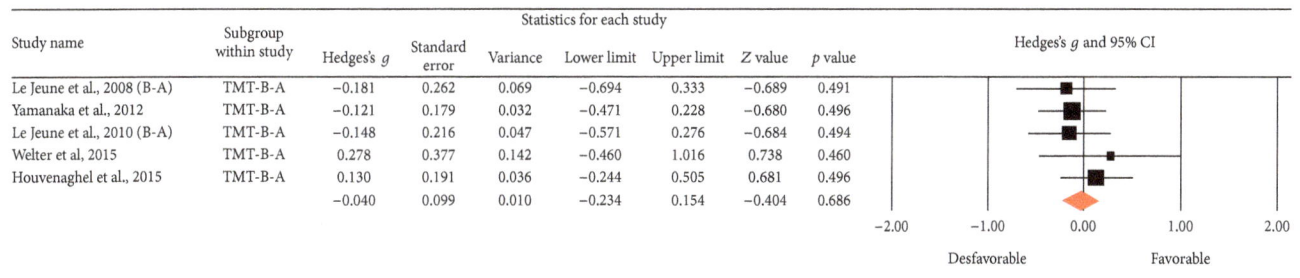

| Study name | Subgroup within study | Statistics for each study | | | | | | | Hedges's *g* and 95% CI |
		Hedges's *g*	Standard error	Variance	Lower limit	Upper limit	*Z* value	*p* value	
Le Jeune et al., 2008 (B-A)	TMT-B-A	−0.181	0.262	0.069	−0.694	0.333	−0.689	0.491	
Yamanaka et al., 2012	TMT-B-A	−0.121	0.179	0.032	−0.471	0.228	−0.680	0.496	
Le Jeune et al., 2010 (B-A)	TMT-B-A	−0.148	0.216	0.047	−0.571	0.276	−0.684	0.494	
Welter et al, 2015	TMT-B-A	0.278	0.377	0.142	−0.460	1.016	0.738	0.460	
Houvenaghel et al., 2015	TMT-B-A	0.130	0.191	0.036	−0.244	0.505	0.681	0.496	
		−0.040	0.099	0.010	−0.234	0.154	−0.404	0.686	

FIGURE 11: Meta-analysis of TMT-AB comparing before and after DBS surgery.

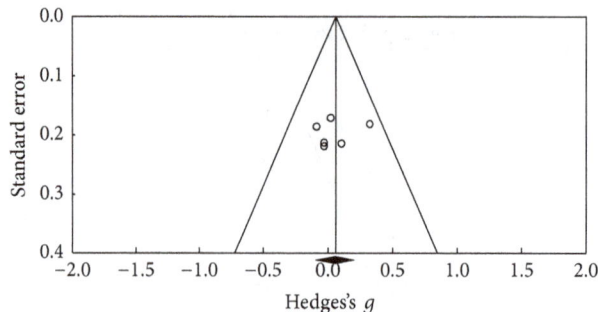

FIGURE 12: Funnel plot for standard error in publications of Raven Matrix.

		Statistics for each study							Hedges's g	
Study name	Subgroup within study	Hedges's g	Standard error	Variance	Lower limit	Upper limit	Z value	p value		
Fasano et al., 2010	Raven's Progressive Matrices (RPM'47)	−0.028	0.224	0.050	−0.467	0.410	−0.127	0.899		
Castelli et al, 2007	Raven's Progressive Matrices (RPM'47)	−0.029	0.229	0.053	−0.479	0.421	−0.127	0.899		
Zangaglia et al., 2009	Raven's Progressive Matrices (RPM'47)	0.022	0.177	0.031	−0.324	0.369	0.127	0.899		
Yamanaka et al., 2012	Raven's Colored Progressive Matrices	0.331	0.188	0.035	−0.036	0.669	1.766	0.077		
Merola et al., 2011	Raven's Colored Progressive Matrices	0.108	0.224	0.050	−0.332	0.547	0.480	0.631		
Castelli et al., 2010	Raven's Colored Progressive Matrices	−0.088	0.193	0.037	−0.466	0.290	−0.458	0.647		
		0.060	0.083	0.007	−0.102	0.222	0.726	0.468		

The thinking abstract function was evaluated with Raven Matrix in two versions: Progressive (RPM'47) and Colored.

FIGURE 13: Meta-analysis of Raven Matrix comparing before and after DBS surgery.

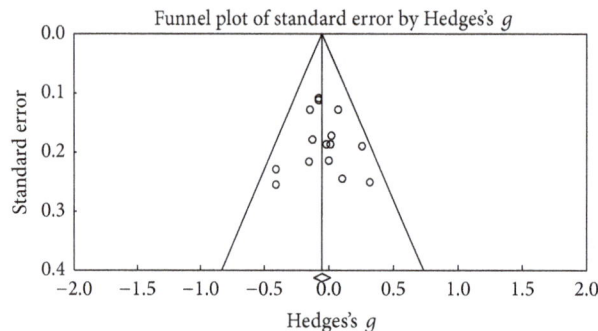

FIGURE 14: Funnel plot for standard error in publications of Digit Span Test (DST).

of dopamine in the nigrostriatal and mesocortical pathways [10].

In general, the study of EF presents a difficulty in terms of the unification of concepts. It has been recognized that the lack of unity in the measurements and significance makes it difficult to establish the relationship with clinical aspects and to explain the improvement or reduction of the functions tested [19]. Following Kudlicka et al. [19], the conclusions are due to the performance in the tests presented without this being an exhaustive analysis of EF. With this, it was found in a number of studies that the same test was used to assess various functions. The lack of representation of Latin American individuals and the lack of studies carried out in Latin America are notable.

The meta-analysis studies and systematic reviews have identified important aspects of PD that could explain part of the emotional functioning, that is, a deficit of emotional

recognition which, although not reported in other clinical studies of PD, could help improve communication processes and mood alterations [62]. Such studies can also help us understand the possible relationship between structures such as STN and the structures involved in emotional and cognitive processes [55] and, as such, better understand the disease as a whole.

In the case of the verbal fluency tests, a deterioration has been reported for PD both with pharmacological treatment and with DBS [54]. There is a change in verbal fluency performance with DBS, and this is coherent with other studies and meta-analyses in which a reduction in performance is reported [46, 51, 56]. This alteration has been related to the position of the electrodes on the STN in the left hemisphere [63]. In neuroimaging studies of patients with PD, an associative-type reduction of the metabolic function of the frontal and parietal areas has been found [5], and other

Study name	Subgroup within study	Statistics for each study							Hedges's g and 95% CI
		Hedges's g	Standard error	Variance	Lower limit	Upper limit	Z value	p value	
Fasano et al., 2010	Forward	−0.148	0.216	0.047	−0.571	0.276	−0.684	0.494	
Tang et al, 2015, 12 months	Forward	0.017	0.187	0.035	−0.350	0.383	0.089	0.929	
Rothlind et al., 2015 (GPi)	Forward	−0.076	0.112	0.012	−0.294	0.143	−0.677	0.499	
Rothlind et al., 2015 (STN)	Forward	−0.073	0.108	0.012	−0.285	0.139	−0.677	0.499	
Yamanaka et al., 2012	Forward	−0.121	0.179	0.032	−0.471	0.228	−0.680	0.496	
Merola et al. 2011	Forward	0.003	0.215	0.046	−0.418	0.424	0.014	0.989	
Williams et al., 2011	Forward	−0.408	0.229	0.053	−0.857	0.042	−1.777	0.076	
Daniels et al., 2010	Forward	0.073	0.128	0.016	−0.177	0.323	0.570	0.568	
Fraraccio et al., 2008	Forward	0.104	0.245	0.060	−0.376	0.583	0.423	0.672	
Will et al, 2008	Forward	0.073	0.128	0.016	−0.177	0.323	0.570	0.568	
Rothlind et al., 2007	Forward	−0.408	0.255	0.065	−0.908	0.092	−1.598	0.110	
Tang et al, 2015, 6 months	Forward	−0.017	0.187	0.035	−0.383	0.350	−0.089	0.929	
Fasano et al., 2010	Backward	−0.148	0.216	0.047	−0.571	0.276	−0.684	0.494	
Yamanaka et al., 2012	Backward	−0.121	0.179	0.032	−0.471	0.228	−0.680	0.496	
Daniels et al., 2010	Backward	−0.139	0.128	0.016	−0.390	0.112	−1.085	0.278	
Will et al, 2008	Backward	−0.139	0.128	0.016	−0.390	0.112	−1.085	0.278	
Rothlind et al., 2007	Backward	0.317	0.251	0.063	−0.175	0.809	1.264	0.206	
Tang et al, 2015, 6 months	Backward	−0.017	0.187	0.035	−0.383	0.350	−0.089	0.929	
Tang et al, 2015, 12 months	Backward	0.256	0.190	0.036	−0.117	0.628	1.345	0.179	
Rothlind et al., 2015 (GPi)	Backward	−0.076	0.112	0.012	−0.294	0.143	−0.677	0.499	
Rothlind et al., 2015 (STN)	Backward	−0.073	0.108	0.012	−0.285	0.139	−0.677	0.499	
Zangaglia et al., 2009	Backward	0.022	0.172	0.030	−0.316	0.360	0.127	0.899	
		−0.051	0.033	0.001	−0.115	0.014	−1.533	0.125	

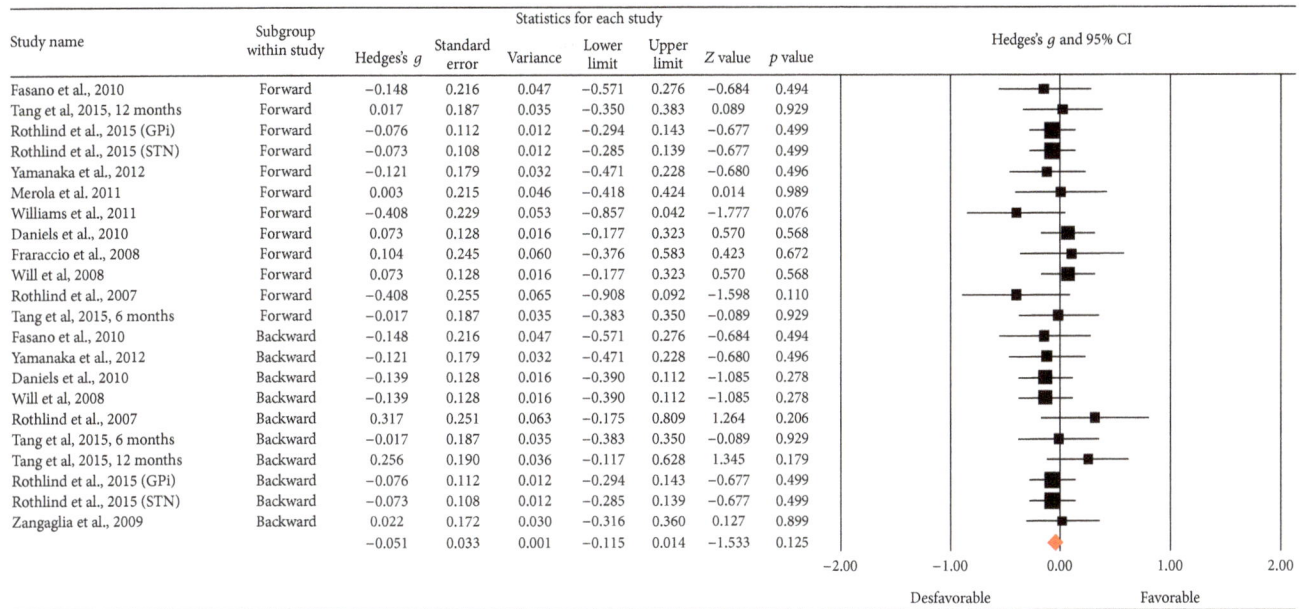

FIGURE 15: Meta-analysis of DST comparing before and after DBS surgery.

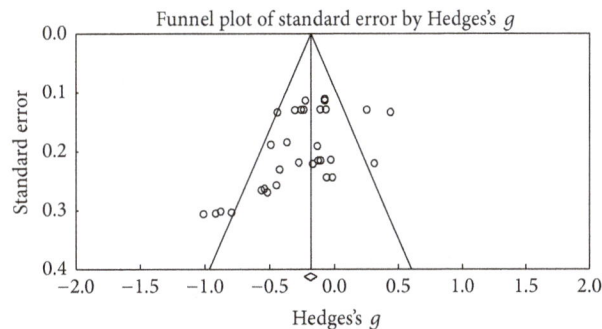

FIGURE 16: Funnel plot for standard error in publications of Stroop Test.

studies suggest that the striate nucleus may play a dissociable role in motor control and language cognitive processes, which would mean that different patterns of stimulation would affect the structures of the basal ganglia and cortical regions in different ways. This, in turn, explains why some patients improve in terms of their language articulation and at the same time present a reduction in their verbal fluency after DBS [51]. It has also been reported that the stimulation may cause a decrease of activity in the temporal cortex and inferior frontal areas in the left hemisphere, which would decrease verbal fluency, especially of the phonological kind [64]. Nevertheless, it is necessary to highlight that these hypotheses are still under study.

Inasmuch as heterogeneity, this can be explained based on the variability in the rigorousness of the application and the standardized test to assess it. Given that the reported heterogeneity is close to 45%, it is proposed that the effect detected cannot necessarily be attributed to the DBS procedure.

Inasmuch as cognitive flexibility, the tests assessed do not show a significant change, despite being one of the functions which in other studies is reported as favorable [56]. Similarly,

the working memory function has been proposed as one of the aspects that becomes altered in PD. More alterations have been identified in the visuospatial modality than the verbal modality [47, 65], and no significant changes are reported in this study for after DBS.

Inasmuch as the Stroop, no clear effect was identified perhaps due to the high heterogeneity of the studies that may be assumed as being derived from the alternative forms of the test [56].

On the other hand, another type of meta-analysis in PD has been carried out, linking the disease to different levels; for example, a genetic level which shows susceptibility to PD depending on polymorphisms in monoamine oxidase genes (MAO) [66], with other diseases or effects of the transcranial magnetic stimulation [15, 27]. This sheds light on the fact that there is a variety of studies that attempt to explain specific aspects of PD, but, as yet, with no unity of analysis that allows us to understand the diversity of the symptoms of patients with PD.

One of the difficulties reported in establishing a STN-DBS effect in systematic changes in the patients and that explains

Study name								Hedges's g and 95% CI
			Statistics for each study					
	Hedges's g	Standard error	Variance	Lower limit	Upper limit	Z value	p value	
Le Jeune et al., 2008	−0.793	0.303	0.092	−1.386	−0.200	−2.620	0.009	
Rothlind et al., 2007 (Stroop word)	−0.448	0.257	0.066	−0.952	0.057	−1.739	0.082	
Rothlind et al., 2007 (Stroop colour)	−0.566	0.265	0.070	−1.086	−0.047	−2.136	0.033	
Rothlind et al., 2007 (Stroop colour-word)	−0.537	0.263	0.069	−1.053	−0.022	−2.042	0.041	
Williams et al., 2011 (Stroop word)	−0.166	0.221	0.049	−0.600	0.268	−0.749	0.454	
Williams et al., 2011 (Stroop colour-word)	−0.423	0.230	0.053	−0.874	0.028	−1.839	0.066	
Le Jeune et al., 2010	−0.027	0.215	0.046	−0.448	0.393	−0.127	0.899	
Fraraccio et al., 2008 (colour naming (# in 45 s))	−0.516	0.270	0.073	−1.045	0.013	−1.912	0.056	
Fraraccio et al., 2008 (word reading (# in 45 s))	−0.878	0.301	0.091	−1.468	−0.287	−2.913	0.004	
Fraraccio et al., 2008 (interference index (c/w) (# in 45 s))	−0.915	0.305	0.093	−1.514	−0.317	−2.998	0.003	
Rothlind et al., 2015 (GPi), word reading	−0.077	0.114	0.013	−0.300	0.146	−0.677	0.499	
Rothlind et al., 2015 (STN), word reading	−0.076	0.112	0.013	−0.296	0.144	−0.677	0.499	
Rothlind et al., 2015 (GPi), colour naming	−0.077	0.114	0.013	−0.300	0.146	−0.677	0.499	
Rothlind et al., 2015 (STN), colour naming	−0.223	0.114	0.013	−0.446	−0.001	−1.966	0.049	
Rothlind et al., 2015 (GPi), colour word	−0.077	0.114	0.013	−0.300	0.146	−0.677	0.499	
Tramontana et al., 2015 (palabra)	−0.060	0.244	0.060	−0.539	0.419	−0.245	0.807	
Tramontana et al., 2015 (colour)	−0.016	0.244	0.060	−0.494	0.463	−0.064	0.949	
Tramontana et al., 2015 (colour-palabra)	−1.011	0.306	0.094	−1.611	−0.411	−3.303	0.001	
Rothlind et al., 2015 (STN), colour word	−0.223	0.114	0.013	−0.446	−0.001	−1.966	0.049	
Houvenaghel et al., 2015, colour	−0.130	0.191	0.036	−0.505	0.244	−0.681	0.496	
Houvenaghel et al., 2015, word	−0.130	0.191	0.036	−0.505	0.244	−0.681	0.496	
Houvenaghel et al., 2015, colour-word	−0.130	0.191	0.036	−0.505	0.244	−0.681	0.496	
Houvenaghel et al., 2015, interference	−0.130	0.191	0.036	−0.505	0.244	−0.681	0.496	
Smeding et al., 2005 (Stroop word seconds)	−0.105	0.215	0.046	−0.527	0.317	−0.488	0.625	
Smeding et al., 2005 (Stroop colour seconds)	0.314	0.220	0.049	−0.118	0.746	1.425	0.154	
Smeding et al., 2005 (Stroop colour word seconds)	−0.124	0.216	0.046	−0.547	0.298	−0.576	0.565	
Smeding et al., 2005 (Stroop colour word errors)	−0.272	0.219	0.048	−0.701	0.157	−1.244	0.214	
Daniels et al., 2010 (Stroop word seconds)	−0.235	0.129	0.017	−0.489	0.018	−1.820	0.069	
Daniels et al., 2010 (Stroop colour seconds)	−0.255	0.130	0.017	−0.509	−0.001	−1.968	0.049	
Daniels et al., 2010 (Stroop interference condition/word reading)	−0.441	0.134	0.018	−0.703	−0.179	−3.302	0.001	
Daniels et al., 2010 (Stroop interference condition/colour naming)	−0.305	0.130	0.017	−0.560	−0.049	−2.336	0.019	
Wills et al., 2008 (Stroop 1 word reading time in black, seconds)	−0.235	0.129	0.017	−0.489	0.018	−1.820	0.069	
Wills et al., 2008 (Stroop 1 word reading time in black, error rates)	0.255	0.130	0.017	0.001	0.509	1.968	0.049	
Wills et al., 2008 (Stroop 2 word reading time naming colour dots for simple colour naming)	−0.255	0.130	0.017	−0.509	−0.001	−1.968	0.049	
Wills et al., 2008 (Stroop 2 naming colour dots for simple colour naming, error rates)	0.441	0.134	0.018	0.179	0.703	3.302	0.001	
Wills et al., 2008 (Stroop 3: interference condition reading words, seconds)	−0.441	0.134	0.018	−0.703	−0.179	−3.302	0.001	
Wills et al., 2008 (Stroop 3: interference condition reading words, error rates)	−0.067	0.128	0.016	−0.317	0.183	−0.527	0.598	
Wills et al., 2008 (Stroop 4 interference condition, seconds)	−0.305	0.130	0.017	−0.560	−0.049	−2.336	0.019	
Wills et al., 2008 (Stroop 4 interference condition, error rates)	−0.113	0.128	0.016	−0.363	0.138	−0.882	0.378	
Yamanaka et al., 2012, MST-A	−0.364	0.184	0.034	−0.724	−0.003	−1.977	0.048	
Yamanaka et al., 2012, MST-B	−0.490	0.189	0.036	−0.860	−0.120	−2.597	0.009	
	−0.211	0.039	0.002	−0.288	−0.135	−5.406	0.000	

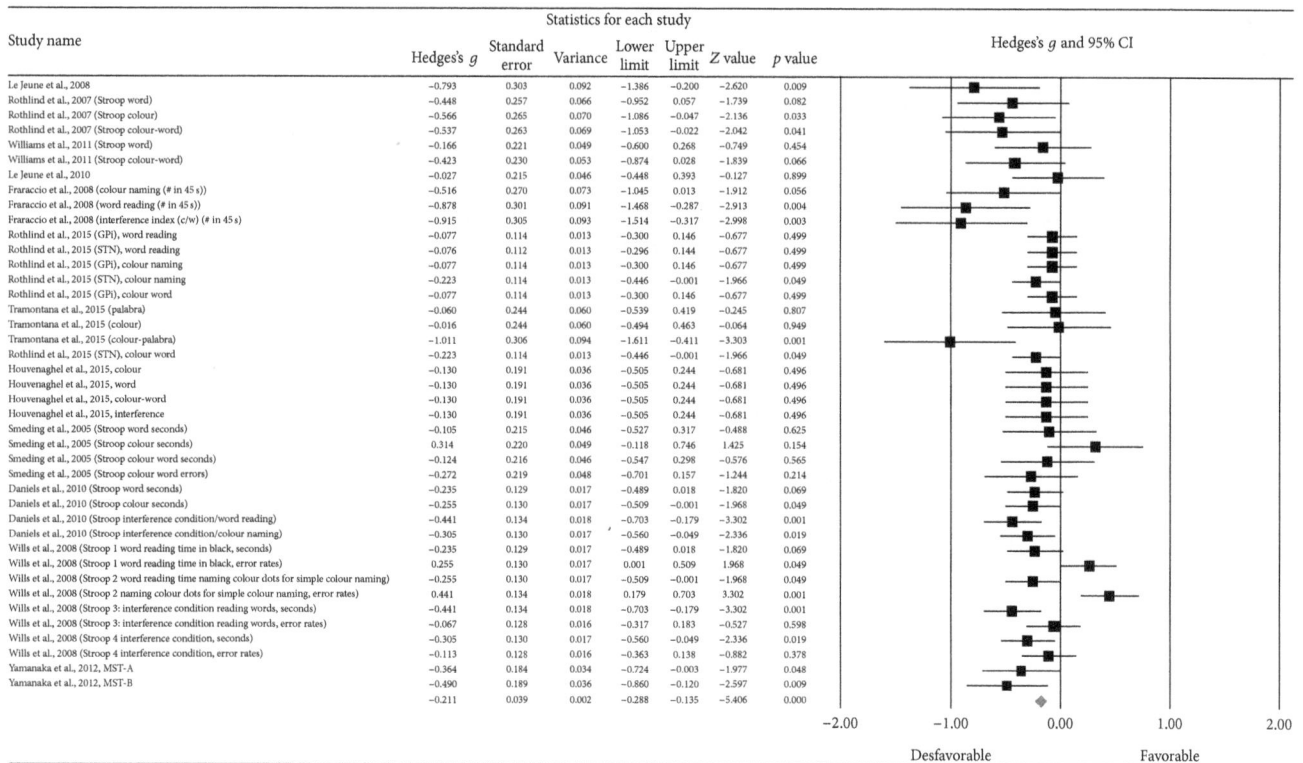

Axis: −2.00   −1.00   0.00   1.00   2.00

Desfavorable   Favorable

FIGURE 17: Meta-analysis of Stroop Test comparing before and after DBS surgery.

the variability of the effects, as well as the tasks, is the exact location of the electrodes. In this respect, it has been found that although the procedure is carried out in STN, the area of location, the area of active stimulation, or the volume of electrode contact is not always homogeneous [6, 63, 67].

Another of the major difficulties in the systematic assessment of the changes realized by the DBS procedure is the lack of standardized tests to measure the functions [16]. In this study, high variability was found in the versions of some of the tests which could be a factor that contributes to the heterogeneity. On the other hand, it has also been proposed that the alterations presented in PD do not always correlate with the specific alterations related to the treatment (e.g., pharmacological). Thus, the alterations in the different domains and the lack of EF improvement after DBS treatment may respond to a nonlinear model that involves different and complex circuits that are not necessarily modified by STN-DBS [68].

Finally, one of the important limitations to detecting of the effects of the procedure is the lack of control or placebo groups that would allow the identification of DBS [56].

Acknowledgments

This paper was made possible thanks to funding of Vicerrectoría de Investigación of the Pontificia Universidad Javeriana with ID Project: 00006578, titled "Effects of Deep Brain Stimulation (DBS) on Performance of Executive Function Test in Patients with Parkinson's Disease."

References

[1] O. M. Aguilar, C. A. Soto, and M. Esguerra, "Cambios neuropsicológicos asociados a estimulación cerebral profunda en enfermedad de Parkinson: revisión teórica," *Suma Psicológica*, vol. 18, no. 2, pp. 89–98, 2011.

[2] G. J. Demakis, "The neuropsychology of Parkinson's disease," *Disease-a-Month: DM*, vol. 53, no. 3, pp. 152–155, 2007.

[3] S. Factor and W. Weiner, *Parkinson's Disease: Diagnosis & Clinical Management?* Demos Medical, 2nd edition, 2007.

[4] N. A. Haelterman, W. H. Yoon, H. Sandoval, M. Jaiswal, J. M. Shulman, and H. J. Bellen, "A mitocentric view of Parkinson's disease," *Annual Review of Neuroscience*, vol. 37, pp. 137–159, 2014.

[5] C. Huang, P. Mattis, C. Tang, K. Perrine, M. Carbon, and D. Eidelberg, "Metabolic brain networks associated with cognitive function in Parkinson's disease," *NeuroImage*, vol. 34, no. 2, pp. 714–723, 2007.

[6] Y. Liu, W. Li, C. Tan et al., "Meta-analysis comparing deep brain stimulation of the globus pallidus and subthalamic nucleus to treat advanced Parkinson disease," *Journal of Neurosurgery*, vol. 121, no. 3, pp. 709–718, 2014.

[7] A. J. Lees, J. Hardy, and T. Revesz, "Parkinson's disease," *The Lancet*, vol. 373, no. 9680, pp. 2055–2066, 2009.

[8] K. Wakabayashi, F. Mori, and H. Takahashi, "Progression patterns of neuronal loss and Lewy body pathology in the substantia nigra in Parkinson's disease," *Parkinsonism & Related Disorders*, vol. 12, no. 2, pp. S92–S98, 2006.

[9] A. L. Bartels and K. L. Leenders, "Parkinson's disease: the syndrome, the pathogenesis and pathophysiology," *Cortex*, vol. 45, no. 8, pp. 915–921, 2009.

[10] M. C. Rodriguez-Oroz, M. Jahanshahi, P. Krack et al., "Initial clinical manifestations of Parkinson's disease: features and pathophysiological mechanisms," *The Lancet Neurology*, vol. 8, no. 12, pp. 1128–1139, 2009.

[11] J. M. Chambers and T. J. Prescott, "Response times for visually guided saccades in persons with Parkinson's disease: a meta-analytic review," *Neuropsychologia*, vol. 48, no. 4, pp. 887–899, 2010.

[12] M. E. Bodden, R. Dodel, and E. Kalbe, "Theory of mind in Parkinson's disease and related basal ganglia disorders: a systematic review," *Movement Disorders*, vol. 25, no. 1, pp. 13–27, 2010.

[13] T. A. Mestre, A. P. Strafella, T. Thomsen, V. Voon, and J. Miyasaki, "Diagnosis and treatment of impulse control disorders in patients with movement disorders," *Therapeutic Advances in Neurological Disorders*, vol. 6, no. 3, pp. 175–188, 2013.

[14] J. V. Hindle, A. Martyr, and L. Clare, "Cognitive reserve in Parkinson's disease: a systematic review and meta-analysis," *Parkinsonism & Related Disorders*, vol. 20, no. 1, pp. 1–7, 2014.

[15] C.-L. Xie, J. Chen, X.-D. Wang et al., "Repetitive transcranial magnetic stimulation (rTMS) for the treatment of depression in Parkinson disease: a meta-analysis of randomized controlled clinical trials," *Neurological Sciences*, vol. 36, no. 10, pp. 1751–1761, 2015.

[16] M. Denheyer, Z. H. Kiss, and A. M. Haffenden, "Behavioral effects of subthalamic deep brain stimulation in Parkinson's disease," *Neuropsychologia*, vol. 47, no. 14, pp. 3203–3209, 2009.

[17] V. Voon, K. Hassan, M. Zurowski et al., "Prevalence of repetitive and reward-seeking behaviors in Parkinson disease," *Neurology*, vol. 67, no. 7, pp. 1254–1257, 2006.

[18] V. Voon, C. Kubu, P. Krack, J.-L. Houeto, and A. I. Tröster, "Deep brain stimulation: neuropsychological and neuropsychiatric issues," *Movement Disorders*, vol. 21, no. S14, pp. S305–S327, 2006.

[19] A. Kudlicka, L. Clare, and J. V. Hindle, "Executive functions in Parkinson's disease: systematic review and meta-analysis," *Movement Disorders*, vol. 26, no. 13, pp. 2305–2315, 2011.

[20] D. Zgaljardic, J. Borod, N. Foldi et al., "An examination of executive dysfunction associated with frontostriatal circuitry in Parkinson's disease," *Journal of Clinical and Experimental Neuropsychology*, vol. 28, no. 7, pp. 1127–1144, 2006.

[21] M. E. Bodden, B. Mollenhauer, C. Trenkwalder et al., "Affective and cognitive theory of mind in patients with Parkinson's disease," *Parkinsonism & Related Disorders*, vol. 16, no. 7, pp. 466–470, 2010.

[22] M. Poletti, I. Enrici, and M. Adenzato, "Cognitive and affective Theory of Mind in neurodegenerative diseases: neuropsychological, neuroanatomical and neurochemical levels," *Neuroscience and Biobehavioral Reviews*, vol. 36, no. 9, pp. 2147–2164, 2012.

[23] K. L. Parker, D. Lamichhane, M. S. Caetano, and N. S. Narayanan, "Executive dysfunction in Parkinson's disease and timing deficits," *Frontiers in Integrative Neuroscience*, vol. 7, article 75, 2013.

[24] Y. Smith, T. Wichmann, S. A. Factor, and M. R. Delong, "Parkinson's disease therapeutics: new developments and challenges since the introduction of levodopa," *Neuropsychopharmacology*, vol. 37, no. 1, pp. 213–246, 2012.

[25] T. M. Cruickshank, A. R. Reyes, and M. R. Ziman, "A systematic review and meta-analysis of strength training in individuals with multiple sclerosis or Parkinson disease," *Medicine*, vol. 94, no. 4, article e411, 2015.

[26] F. M. Weaver, K. Follett, M. Stern et al., "Bilateral deep brain stimulation vs best medical therapy for patients with advanced parkinson disease: a randomized controlled trial," *JAMA-Journal of the American Medical Association*, vol. 301, no. 1, pp. 63–73, 2009.

[27] Y.-H. Chou, P. T. Hickey, M. Sundman, A. W. Song, and N.-K. Chen, "Effects of repetitive transcranial magnetic stimulation on motor symptoms in parkinson disease: a systematic review and meta-analysis," *JAMA Neurology*, vol. 72, no. 4, pp. 432–440, 2015.

[28] H. Zhu, Z. Lu, Y. Jin, X. Duan, J. Teng, and D. Duan, "Low-frequency repetitive transcranial magnetic stimulation on Parkinson motor function: a meta-analysis of randomised controlled trials," *Acta Neuropsychiatrica*, vol. 27, no. 2, pp. 82–89, 2015.

[29] S. Bickel, L. Alvarez, R. Macias et al., "Cognitive and neuropsychiatric effects of subthalamotomy for Parkinson's disease," *Parkinsonism and Related Disorders*, vol. 16, no. 8, pp. 535–539, 2010.

[30] F. Agnesi, M. D. Johnson, and J. L. Vitek, "Deep brain stimulation: how does it work?" in *Handbook of Clinical Neurology*, vol. 116, pp. 39–54, Elsevier, 2013.

[31] A. L. Benabid, S. Chabardes, J. Mitrofanis, and P. Pollak, "Deep brain stimulation of the subthalamic nucleus for the treatment of Parkinson's disease," *The Lancet Neurology*, vol. 8, no. 1, pp. 67–81, 2009.

[32] G. Giannicola, S. Marceglia, L. Rossi et al., "The effects of levodopa and ongoing deep brain stimulation on subthalamic beta oscillations in Parkinson's disease," *Experimental Neurology*, vol. 226, no. 1, pp. 120–127, 2010.

[33] M. Jahanshahi, C. R. G. Jones, J. Zijlmans et al., "Dopaminergic modulation of striato-frontal connectivity during motor timing in Parkinson's disease," *Brain*, vol. 133, part 3, pp. 727–745, 2010.

[34] C. Juri, M. Rodriguez-Oroz, and J. A. Obeso, "The pathophysiological basis of sensory disturbances in Parkinson's disease," *Journal of the Neurological Sciences*, vol. 289, no. 1-2, pp. 60–65, 2010.

[35] G. Kleiner-Fisman, J. Herzog, D. N. Fisman et al., "Subthalamic nucleus deep brain stimulation: summary and meta-analysis of outcomes," *Movement Disorders*, vol. 21, supplement 1, pp. S290–304, 2006.

[36] M. K. Lyons, "Deep brain stimulation: current and future clinical applications," *Mayo Clinic Proceedings*, vol. 86, no. 7, pp. 662–672, 2011.

[37] J. A. Obeso, M. C. Rodríguez-Oroz, M. Rodríguez et al., "Pathophysiology of the basal ganglia in Parkinson's disease," *Trends in Neurosciences*, vol. 23, no. 10, pp. S8–S19, 2000.

[38] D. Cyron, M. Funk, M.-A. Deletter, and K. Scheufler, "Preserved cognition after deep brain stimulation (DBS) in the subthalamic area for Parkinson's disease: a case report," *Acta Neurochirurgica*, vol. 152, no. 12, pp. 2097–2100, 2010.

[39] P. Dowsey-Limousin and P. Pollak, "Deep brain stimulation in the treatment of Parkinson's disease: a review and update," *Clinical Neuroscience Research*, vol. 1, no. 6, pp. 521–526, 2001.

[40] J. M. Nazzaro, R. Pahwa, and K. E. Lyons, "The impact of bilateral subthalamic stimulation on non-motor symptoms of Parkinson's disease," *Parkinsonism & Related Disorders*, vol. 17, no. 8, pp. 606–609, 2011.

[41] M. Deogaonkar, G. A. Monsalve, J. Scott, A. Ahmed, and A. Rezai, "Bilateral subthalamic deep brain stimulation after bilateral pallidal deep brain stimulation for Parkinson's disease," *Stereotactic and Functional Neurosurgery*, vol. 89, no. 2, pp. 123–127, 2011.

[42] A. Franzini, R. Cordella, G. Messina et al., "Deep brain stimulation for movement disorders. Considerations on 276 consecutive patients," *Journal of Neural Transmission*, vol. 118, no. 10, pp. 1497–1510, 2011.

[43] M. D. Johnson, S. Miocinovic, C. C. McIntyre, and J. L. Vitek, "Mechanisms and targets of deep brain stimulation in movement disorders," *Neurotherapeutics*, vol. 5, no. 2, pp. 294–308, 2008.

[44] P. Limousin and I. Martinez-Torres, "Deep brain stimulation for Parkinson's disease," *Neurotherapeutics*, vol. 5, no. 2, pp. 309–319, 2008.

[45] F. Weaver, K. Follett, K. Hur, D. Ippolito, and M. Stern, "Deep brain stimulation in Parkinson disease: a metaanalysis of patient outcomes," *Journal of Neurosurgery*, vol. 103, no. 6, pp. 956–967, 2005.

[46] M. R. Schoenberg, K. M. Mash, K. J. Bharucha, P. C. Francel, and J. G. Scott, "Deep brain stimulation parameters associated with neuropsychological changes in subthalamic nucleus stimulation for refractory Parkinson's disease," *Stereotactic and Functional Neurosurgery*, vol. 86, no. 6, pp. 337–344, 2008.

[47] R. J. Siegert, M. Weatherall, K. D. Taylor, and D. A. Abernethy, "A meta-analysis of performance on simple span and more complex working memory tasks in Parkinson's disease," *Neuropsychology*, vol. 22, no. 4, pp. 450–461, 2008.

[48] M. Broen, A. Duits, V. Visser-Vandewalle, Y. Temel, and A. Winogrodzka, "Impulse control and related disorders in Parkinson's disease patients treated with bilateral subthalamic nucleus stimulation: a review," *Parkinsonism and Related Disorders*, vol. 17, no. 6, pp. 413–417, 2011.

[49] T. Wu and M. Hallett, "The cerebellum in Parkinson's disease," *Brain*, vol. 136, no. 3, pp. 696–709, 2013.

[50] M. C. Keuken, L. Van Maanen, R. Bogacz et al., "The subthalamic nucleus during decision-making with multiple alternatives," *Human Brain Mapping*, vol. 36, no. 10, pp. 4041–4052, 2015.

[51] T. D. Parsons, S. A. Rogers, A. J. Braaten, S. P. Woods, and A. I. Tröster, "Cognitive sequelae of subthalamic nucleus deep brain stimulation in Parkinson's disease: a meta-analysis," *The Lancet Neurology*, vol. 5, no. 7, pp. 578–588, 2006.

[52] J. Sánchez-Meca, "Cómo realizar una revisión sistemática y un meta-análisis," *Aula Abierta*, vol. 38, pp. 53–63, 2010.

[53] A. Liberati, D. G. Altman, J. Tetzlaff et al., "The PRISMA statement for reporting systematic reviews and meta-analyses of studies that evaluate health care interventions: explanation and elaboration," *PLoS Medicine*, vol. 6, no. 7, Article ID e1000100, 2009.

[54] L. Castelli, M. Lanotte, M. Zibetti et al., "Apathy and verbal fluency in STN-stimulated PD patients: An Observational Follow-up Study," *Journal of Neurology*, vol. 254, no. 9, pp. 1238–1243, 2007.

[55] F. Le Jeune, J. Péron, I. Biseul et al., "Subthalamic nucleus stimulation affects orbitofrontal cortex in facial emotion recognition: A Pet Study," *Brain*, vol. 131, no. 6, pp. 1599–1608, 2008.

[56] K. Witt, C. Daniels, J. Reiff et al., "Neuropsychological and psychiatric changes after deep brain stimulation for Parkinson's disease: a randomised, multicentre study," *The Lancet Neurology*, vol. 7, no. 7, pp. 605–614, 2008.

[57] L. Yang, G.-D. Zhan, J.-J. Ding et al., "Psychiatric illness and intellectual disability in the prader-willi syndrome with different molecular defects—a meta analysis," *PLoS ONE*, vol. 8, no. 8, Article ID e72640, 2013.

[58] J. A. C. Sterne and M. Egger, "Funnel plots for detecting bias in meta-analysis: guidelines on choice of axis," *Journal of Clinical Epidemiology*, vol. 54, no. 10, pp. 1046–1055, 2001.

[59] M. Borenstein, L. V. Hedges, J. P. T. Higgins, and H. R. Rothstein, "A basic introduction to fixed- effect and random-effects models for meta-analysis," *Research Synthesis Methods*, vol. 1, no. 2, pp. 97–111, 2010.

[60] B. T. Johnson, L. A. J. Scott-Sheldon, L. B. Snyder, S. M. Noar, and T. B. Huedo-Medina, "Contemporary approaches to meta-analysis in communication research: SAGE research methods," in *The SAGE Sourcebook of Advanced Data Analysis Methods for Communication Research*, A. F. Hayes, M. D. Slater, and L. B. Snyder, Eds., SAGE, Los Angeles, Calif, USA, 2008.

[61] B. Wu, L. Han, B.-M. Sun, X.-W. Hu, and X.-P. Wang, "Influence of deep brain stimulation of the subthalamic nucleus on cognitive function in patients with Parkinson's disease," *Neuroscience Bulletin*, vol. 30, no. 1, pp. 153–161, 2014.

[62] H. M. Gray and L. Tickle-Degnen, "A meta-analysis of performance on emotion recognition tasks in Parkinson's disease," *Neuropsychology*, vol. 24, no. 2, pp. 176–191, 2010.

[63] M. K. York, E. A. Wilde, R. Simpson, and J. Jankovic, "Relationship between neuropsychological outcome and DBS surgical trajectory and electrode location," *Journal of the Neurological Sciences*, vol. 287, no. 1-2, pp. 159–171, 2009.

[64] A. Fasano, A. Daniele, and A. Albanese, "Treatment of motor and non-motor features of Parkinson's disease with deep brain stimulation," *The Lancet Neurology*, vol. 11, no. 5, pp. 429–442, 2012.

[65] M. L. Waterfall and S. F. Crowe, "Meta-analytic comparison of the components of visual cognition in Parkinson's disease," *Journal of Clinical and Experimental Neuropsychology*, vol. 17, no. 5, pp. 759–772, 1995.

[66] Y.-X. Sun, X.-H. Wang, A.-H. Xu, and J.-H. Zhao, "Functional polymorphisms of the MAO gene with Parkinson disease susceptibility: a meta-analysis," *Journal of the Neurological Sciences*, vol. 345, no. 1, pp. 97–105, 2014.

[67] F. Caire, D. Ranoux, D. Guehl, P. Burbaud, and E. Cuny, "A systematic review of studies on anatomical position of electrode contacts used for chronic subthalamic stimulation in Parkinson's disease," *Acta Neurochirurgica*, vol. 155, no. 9, pp. 1647–1654, 2013.

[68] R. Pavão, A. F. Helene, and G. F. Xavier, "Parkinson's disease progression: implicit acquisition, cognitive and motor impairments, and medication effects," *Frontiers in Integrative Neuroscience*, vol. 6, article 56, 2012.

26

Depression in Parkinson's Disease: The Contribution from Animal Studies

Jéssica Lopes Fontoura,[1] Camila Baptista,[1] Flávia de Brito Pedroso,[2]
José Augusto Pochapski,[2] Edmar Miyoshi,[2] and Marcelo Machado Ferro[1]

[1]*Department of Biology, Universidade Estadual de Ponta Grossa, Ponta Grossa, PR, Brazil*
[2]*Department of Pharmaceutical Sciences, Universidade Estadual de Ponta Grossa, Ponta Grossa, PR, Brazil*

Correspondence should be addressed to Marcelo Machado Ferro; mferro@uepg.br

Academic Editor: Daniel Martínez-Ramírez

Besides being better known for causing motor impairments, Parkinson's disease (PD) can also cause many nonmotor symptoms, like depression and anxiety, which can cause significant loss of life quality and may not respond to regular drugs treatment. In this review, we discuss the depression in PD, based on data from studies in humans and rodents. Depression frequency seems higher in PD patients than in general population, despite high variation in data due to diagnosis disparities. Development of depression in PD seems more likely to be caused by the nigrostriatal pathway degeneration than as a consequence of the awareness of disease prognostic, and it seems to be related to dopaminergic, noradrenergic, and serotoninergic synapses deficits. The dopaminergic role could be more significant, since it can modulate the release of the others, and its depletion is progressive, due to the degenerative feature of PD. Highly regarded in major depression, serotonin can be depleted in rats after nigrostriatal damage, but data from human patients are more conflicting. Animal studies can help in understanding the neurobiological mechanisms of depression in PD and the pursuit for more effective drugs for its treatment, but they lack the complexity of the disease progression, especially the nondopaminergic degeneration.

1. Introduction

Parkinson's disease (PD) is a progressively debilitating neurologic disorder that affects about 6 million people around the world [1]. The disease is mainly characterized by the progressive and irreversible degeneration of dopaminergic neurons localized at the substantia nigra pars compacta (SNc), on the mesencephalon, causing reduction in the striatal dopamine (DA) release [2–5].

The striatal DA deficit interferes directly in the basal nuclei's motor control circuitry, causing the most known PD symptoms: resting tremor, muscular rigidity, postural instability, and bradykinesia [3, 6, 7]. These symptoms and the consequent PD diagnosis occur when about 50% of the dopaminergic neurons at the SNc are already degenerated and striatal dopamine has been reduced in 80%. It must be considered that several other brain areas are also affected,

some even before the mesencephalon. Among those structures, the mesolimbic pathway, the locus coeruleus, and the raphe nuclei can be damaged. This feature may be related to PD nonmotor symptoms [2].

Most PD patients can also present a series of nonmotor symptoms, sometimes even before the onset of the motor ones [8]. They significantly affect patient's life quality and many times do not respond to motor symptom treatments [9].

Nonmotor symptoms can include olfactive deficits, sleep disorders, autonomic disturbances, fatigue, pain, depression, and anxiety [1, 8, 10]. Additionally, patients may present cognitive dysfunction, which can evolve to dementia with compromised memory, thinking, and language [11]. PD patients suffer mostly from working memory and executive functions impairments, due to the dopaminergic nigrostriatal and mesocortical depletion, while the episodic memory and language are better preserved [12, 13]. This is confirmed by animal studies in which the nigrostriatal lesion affects cued and very short-term memory tests, while long-term spatial memory seems to be more dependent on the hippocampus integrity [14, 15].

Depression or anxiety symptoms are common in PD patients and are frequently associated [16]. Menza and coworkers reported depressive behavior in 92% of PD patients diagnosed with anxiety, as well as anxious behavior in 67% of PD depressed patients [17]. Those symptoms are implicated as the highest causes of poor life quality among PD patients, affecting their daily activities and increasing incapability more severely than the motor symptoms, even when in their advanced stage [18–20].

2. Depression in Parkinson's Disease

Depression is more frequent in PD patients than in general population [21, 22]. Incidence (4 to 75%) and prevalence (2.7 to 90%) of depression in PD patients in published studies vary substantially due to differences in depression definition or diagnostic criteria (i.e., a patient diagnosed with minor depressive symptoms or dysthymia by some authors and not included in the prevalence rates could be classified as depressed by others) [22]. Most of those studies do not correlate the depression prevalence with period of life of PD patients [22, 23]. In one study, patients with PD onset before 50 years of age presented higher frequency of depression than older-onset patients [23]. Despite its known high incidence and impact on life quality, there are no specific diagnostic criteria for depression in PD. Most diagnoses are based on the major depression criteria of the Diagnostic and Statistical Manual of Mental Disorders (DSM-V) [24, 25]. Besides, the difficulty in making a proper diagnosis due to symptom overlapping must be pointed out, since depression, sleep disturbances, and cognitive deficits are also seen in nondepressed PD patients [26].

Studies report an increase in depression prevalence in PD patients even before the onset of motor symptoms, indicating that the depression cannot be explained by a behavioral reaction to the PD diagnosis but more probably as a direct consequence of the degenerative process [27–29]. Furthermore, around 20% of the patients are already suffering from depression when diagnosed with PD [30]. In a 25-year-long study, it was concluded that the risk for the development of PD was higher among depressed patients, considering then depression as a risk factor to the development of PD [31]. Other depression risk factors in PD have been proposed, like severe cognitive impairment, female gender, and motor symptoms onset before the age of 40 years [32].

Depression in PD shows distinct characteristics from major depression not related to PD. Symptoms as irritability, sadness, dysphoria, pessimism, and suicidal ideation (to consider suicide without necessarily trying) are more frequent in PD depressed patients, while guilt, self-blame, feelings of failure, and suicide attempts are less usual [33]. In fact, it is reported that only a small percentage of PD patients are afflicted with major depression (2–7%); most of them present light depression or only a few depressive symptoms [34]. These symptoms receive less attention than the motor disturbances and often are not properly treated, increasing the risk for greater morbidity, disability, and lower quality of life [9, 35, 36].

3. Biochemical Theory of Depression

Much is discussed about the probable mechanism that leads to depression in PD and whether it is related to other psychiatric symptoms like apathy and anxiety. Among the more accepted theories, Schildkraut proposed that depression is linked to a deficit in monoaminergic neurotransmitters in specific brain regions [37]. This is based mostly on the mechanism of action of the first and second generations of antidepressants, which is the block of norepinephrine and/or serotonin presynaptic reuptake, enhancing their transmission [38–40].

Apart from their action on reuptake transporters, some antidepressants act on serotoninergic receptors, reinforcing the importance of this neurotransmitter in behavior. Serotonin acts by activating 5-HT receptors, a family with 14 identified subtypes. Besides the well-studied 5-HT$_{1A}$, 5-HT$_7$ have been indicated to be involved in depressive behavior, and 5-HT$_{2C}$ antagonists can be used to treat both PD and depression. Since those receptors modulate dopamine release in distinct brain regions, this neurotransmitter also can be considered to be related to depressive behavior [41, 42].

Besides noradrenaline and serotonin, dopamine may also be involved in depression pathophysiology. Dopaminergic agonists, like pramipexole, efficiently improve depressive behavior in PD patients. It is suggested that this improvement is related to the D3 receptors stimulation, present on the mesolimbic system and participating in mood and behavior modulation [34]. The dopaminergic influence on depression is also suggested by the high therapeutic effectiveness of bupropion, a dopamine and noradrenalin reuptake inhibitor, useful regardless of whether it is prescribed alone or with other antidepressants [43].

A curious find is that high-frequency stimulation (HFS) of the subthalamic nucleus (STN), which is successfully used to treat movement disability in advanced Parkinson's disease, can cause or worsen depression and other psychiatric effects on patients [44].

4. Animal Models of PD

Since PD neurobiology is not fully understood, the use of animal models to improve the understanding of its etiology, pathophysiology, and molecular mechanisms is still of significant importance [45]. Also, these models became very useful to evaluate the efficacy of potential treatments in preclinical studies [46].

There are many forms of PD animal models, but, basically, they can be divided into two groups: models in which a neurotoxin (natural or synthetic) is used to kill dopaminergic neurons and the genetic models in which mutations in PD-related genes are induced [47]. Among the neurotoxins used, they can be either reversible, like reserpine, or irreversible, as 1-methyl-4-phenyl-1,2,3,6-tetrahydropyridine (MPTP), 6-hydroxydopamine (6-OHDA), paraquat, and rotenone. Irreversible toxins are usually preferred [45, 48–50].

Neurotoxin-based models provoke the degeneration of striatal pathway [51]. The infusion of different toxins on the same site may cause different responses. As an example, MPTP causes less dopaminergic cell death than 6-OHDA in rats [14, 52]. On the other hand, it is suggested that these toxins have different mechanisms of action, since MPTP causes a significant lesion only when infused at the SNc, a region rich in dopaminergic cell bodies, while 6-OHDA causes neuron degeneration when infused on cell bodies, axons (at the medial forebrain bundle), and even terminals (at the striatum) [50–53]. This reinforces the idea that 6-OHDA and MPTP can be taken by DA terminals, but 6-OHDA can damage DA neurons by other mechanisms, like extracellular oxidative stress generation [14, 52, 53].

6-OHDA lesions in the medial forebrain bundle, either unilateral or bilateral, promote the degeneration of the SNc and ventral tegmental area [54, 55]. On the other hand, lesions at the SNc are more selective to this region and therefore cause more modest dopaminergic depletion, affecting the nigrostriatal pathway without significantly damaging the mesolimbic pathway [56, 57]. A study using bilateral lesions suggested, based on forced swim test and elevated plus maze results, that SNc lesions caused more depressive and anxious behavior than ventral tegmental area lesions [58].

In addition, some works indicate that the bilateral lesion at the medial forebrain bundle can provoke severe motor impairment on rats, similar to the akinesia seen in more advanced stages of PD [59], while the SNc lesion is less severe and would mimic early stages of PD, when nonmotor symptoms are more evident [60]. Also, rats with severe motor deficit should not be used to study behavior, since their performance on swimming, drinking water, or walking through a maze will be compromised [61].

Genetic models often involve mice depleted from dopaminergic synapse-related genes. Although several genes have been related to the development of nonmotor signs of PD in humans (e.g., SNCA, LRRK2, VPS35, and Parkin), only a few studies have explored the influence of these mutations on depressive-like behavior in mice [62].

5. Behavioral Tests

To measure the behavioral alterations caused by the toxins or mutations, animal models are usually submitted to tests designed to evaluate depressive behavior in rats and mice [63].

In sucrose preference test, two bottles are offered to the animals: one containing water and the other containing 0,5 to 4% sucrose in water. Consumption of both is computed and two parameters are measured: total liquid consumption and preference for sweetened water over pure water. Reduction in the first is mostly related to motor disturbances or hypothalamic lesion, while the latter is related to anhedonia or loss of pleasure for formerly pleasant activities, which is a major depressive symptom and one of the few that can

be evaluated in animals and related to what is reported by patients on questionnaires [63–65].

Another usual test for depressive behavior is the forced swimming test. Known as a behavioral despair test, it was developed by Porsolt et al. (1978) to evaluate antidepressant drugs [66]. Rats or mice are put in water in a cylinder with no chance to escape and tend to stop swimming after a while. A 15-minute-long pretest phase (stress generator) precedes the 5-minute-long test phase that happens 24 hours later. During the test, time spent on immobility over trying to escape is compared, and it is validated that antidepressant drugs reduce immobility and increase either swimming over water or climbing attempts on the cylinder walls. Based on that, it is considered that immobility mimics the giving up behavior seen in depressive patients [67, 68]. Also, it is proposed that serotoninergic antidepressant drugs are more prone to increase swimming, while noradrenergic drugs tend to promote climbing [69].

The tail suspension test is one of the most used tests to evaluate depressive behavior in mice. The test consists in suspending a mouse by its tail for 6 minutes. Similar to the forced swimming test, the animals tend to move and try to escape at first but later quit and stand immobile. Clinically effective antidepressant drugs promote an increase in the time spent trying to escape [70, 71].

6. Data from Animal Studies

A considerable amount of studies indicates that PD animal models present depressive behavior. Both unilateral and bilateral infusions of 6-OHDA on the SNc lead to a significant increase in immobility time on the forced swimming test and a decrease of sucrose consumption but not in total liquid consumption in rats when compared to control groups, characterizing a depressive-like behavior [72–75]. Santiago and coworkers (2014) [73] also reported a significant reduction in hippocampal serotonin, while Tadaiesky and coworkers (2008) showed a striatal serotonin reduction after a bilateral SNc 6-OHDA infusion, a toxin which is supposed to affect only catecholaminergic neurons [76]. Premotor symptoms of PD were also observed in a model generated by intrastriatal injection of 6-OHDA. The depressive-like behavior, observed in the sucrose preference test, was accompanied by a reduction in DA content in the dorsal striatum, indicating that dopaminergic deficit may be related to this behavior [77].

These data reinforce the cross-effect of the lesion on different neurotransmitters and the theory that depression in PD patients may be linked to alterations in serotoninergic systems and therefore is not strictly related to the dopaminergic degeneration. In addition, a study demonstrated reduced expression of tryptophan hydroxylase (TPH) and 5-HT$_{1A}$ receptors in the dorsal raphe after rotenone injection, leading to a depressive-like behavior; this effect was improved with treadmill exercise [78].

In a study with noradrenergic drugs, pretreatment with desipramine minutes before the 6-OHDA infusion in mice did not prevent depressive behavior. On the other hand, reboxetine reduced lesion-induced depressive behavior on the forced swimming test [79].

A smaller variety of studies with lesion on the medial forebrain bundle are available. Carvalho and coworkers (2013) reported depressive behavior in rats by lesion on this site, indicated by reduced sucrose consumption similar to SNc lesion studies. However, they also stressed that both bupropion, a dopamine and noradrenaline reuptake inhibitor, and paroxetine, a serotonin reuptake inhibitor, were not able to reverse the depressive-like state, differently from other studies [80].

When tested in rats, STN HFS reduces both dorsal and medial raphe nuclei stimulation, which in turn reduces serotonin release [81]. On the other hand, Faggianni et al. showed that STN HFS was able to reduce immobility time in dopamine depleted rats but was less effective when applied in dopamine, noradrenaline, and serotonin depleted rats. These data support the idea that PD patients suffer a multineurotransmitter depletion, not restricted to dopamine [82].

Recently, cannabinoid receptors activation has been reported to have neuroprotective and antidyskinetic effects on animal models [83–85]. In humans, polymorphisms of CB1 have been related to signs of depression in PD patients [86]. However, to the authors' knowledge, no study has showed the effects of CB1 modulators on mood alterations seen in either PD rats or mice models.

In addition to studies that use lesions, studies using genetic models of Parkinson's disease have also indicated the involvement of neurotransmitter deficits in depressive behavior. Signs of apathy were observed in mice with deficiency of vesicular monoamine transporter 2 (VMAT2) by reducing sucrose preference, becoming a potential study model for investigation of the neurobiology of depression in PD [87].

A recent study used CD157 KO mice, a PD genetic model displaying depression- and anxiety-like behaviors, to explore the antidepressant and anxiolytic effects of selegiline, an irreversible monoamine oxidase-B (MAO-B) inhibitor. The administration of selegiline reduced immobility time and increased climbing time in the FST in mice with depressive-like behavior. The mice with depressive-like behavior showed decreases in striatal and hippocampal serotonin. The levels of striatal serotonin returned after single administration of selegiline [88].

In mice, Pitx3 depletion has presented both depressive behavior and motor dysfunction [89]. PINK1 knockout mice have been shown to develop cannabinoid CB1 receptor dysfunction, which could play a role in the development of familiar PD [90].

7. Data from Human Studies

It is suggested that dopamine may have a role in the development of depression in PD patients, due to its association with the dopaminergic denervation in regions like the ventral striatum and prefrontal cortex [91]. These data are reinforced by the fact that dopaminergic agonists like rotigotine and pramipexole, used to treat PD, reduce depression symptoms [92].

Histologic studies in PD patients also reported a loss of nondopaminergic neurons in structures that do not compose the nigrostriatal pathway, including locus coeruleus and the dorsal vagal nucleus noradrenergic neurons or raphe serotoninergic neurons [93, 94]. Considering this, nonmotor symptoms of PD as depression and cognitive dysfunction could be related either to dopaminergic deficits in mesolimbic or mesocortical pathways or to other neurotransmitter areas in other regions [10].

Through positrons and single-photon emission computed tomography (PET and SPECT, resp.), loss in the integrity of dopaminergic, noradrenergic, serotoninergic, and cholinergic systems has been demonstrated in the brains of PD patients [95]. While striatal dopamine depletion in striatal pathway was considered responsible for the motor alterations, reduced binding to noradrenaline and dopamine transporters at locus coeruleus and several limbic system regions like thalamus, amygdala, and the ventral striatum of depressing patients was associated with depressive behavior [96].

Considering the serotonin role in PD, results in human studies are less certain. On one hand, some studies showed a correlation between degeneration of serotoninergic neurons and depression in PD patients [97–99]. On the other hand, a recent study did not suggest this correlation, based on the lack of neuropathological differences between depressed and nondepressed PD patients at the dorsal raphe nuclei, amygdala, and cortical regions, proposing that depression in PD is related more to dopamine and noradrenaline than to serotoninergic system dysfunction [100]. There is also contradiction among neurochemical studies, existing studies showing a reduction in serotoninergic metabolites like 5-hydroxyindoleacetic acid (5-HIAA) in the cerebrospinal fluid of depressed patients [101, 102], while others indicate no difference between depressed and nondepressed patients [34].

Other studies report an impairment in the cholinergic system. A reduction of acetylcholinesterase activity in the cortex of PD depressed patients has been shown [103], and PD depressed patients presented a reduction in acetylcholine receptor binding in the cingulate cortex and fronto-parieto-occipital cortex [104].

In addition to neurotransmitters, a recent study has indicated that neuropeptides may be involved in the pathophysiology of depression in Parkinson's disease. Neuropeptide Y (NPY) and calcitonin gene-related peptide (CGRP) are neuropeptides abundantly present in brain and may have their expression altered in several affective disorders. Svenningsson and coworkers examined the levels of NPY, CGRP, and 5-hydroxyindoleacetic acid (5-HIAA), the major serotonin metabolite, in cerebrospinal fluid (CSF) from PD patients, with or without comorbid depression, and compared them to the levels in patients with major depressive disorder. The levels of NPY and CGRP were higher in PD patients with depression compared to major depressive disorder patients. However, there was no difference in 5-HIAA levels between groups, indicating that depression in Parkinson's disease and the major depressive disorder can be generated by different processes [105].

8. Concluding Remarks

The development of depression in PD patients is linked to neurodegeneration and is not only a consequence of the realization of the disease prognostic. This is supported by the number of DP patients who present depressive behavior before the motor symptoms onset and by the depressive-like behavior shown by rats lesioned in the nigrostriatal pathway.

Depression in PD is at least partly dopaminergic, since lesions specific to these neurons cause this behavioral alteration and it is reversed or even protected by dopamine reuptake inhibitors.

Other neurotransmitters like acetylcholine, noradrenalin, and serotonin could also be implicated, just like the case in major depression. In rats, their release can be modulated by dopamine and influenced by this system depletion. However, in humans, the degeneration of other brain areas and consequent deficit in these neurotransmitters could happen at the same speed or even before the dopaminergic neurons.

Taken altogether, animal studies are very useful to study the neurobiological mechanisms of depression in PD, but with the fact that most of them fail to mimic the neurodegeneration observed in the PD patients, there are still many gaps to be filled by future investigations.

Acknowledgments

The authors wish to acknowledge Coordenação de Aperfeiçoamento de Pessoal de Nível Superior (CAPES, Brazil) for the financial support.

References

[1] K. R. Chaudhuri, D. G. Healy, and A. H. V. Schapira, "Non-motor symptoms of Parkinson's disease: diagnosis and management," *The Lancet Neurology*, vol. 5, no. 3, pp. 235–245, 2006.

[2] H. Braak, K. del Tredici, U. Rüb, R. A. I. de Vos, E. N. H. Jansen Steur, and E. Braak, "Staging of brain pathology related to sporadic Parkinson's disease," *Neurobiology of Aging*, vol. 24, no. 2, pp. 197–211, 2003.

[3] J. Hardy, H. Cai, M. R. Cookson, K. Gwinn-Hardy, and A. Singleton, "Genetics of Parkinson's disease and parkinsonism," *Annals of Neurology*, vol. 60, no. 4, pp. 389–398, 2006.

[4] M. T. Herrero, J. Pagonabarraga, and G. Linazasoro, "Neuroprotective role of dopamine agonists: Evidence from animal models and clinical studies," *The Neurologist*, vol. 17, no. 6, pp. S54–S66, 2011.

[5] K. Wirdefeldt, H. Adami, P. Cole, D. Trichopoulos, and J. Mandel, "Epidemiology and etiology of Parkinson's disease: a review of the evidence," *European Journal of Epidemiology*, vol. 26, no. 1, supplement, pp. S1–S58, 2011.

[6] J. A. Obeso, M. C. Rodríguez-Oroz, M. Rodríguez, J. Arbizu, and J. M. Giménez-Amaya, "The basal ganglia and disorders of movement: Pathophysiological mechanisms," *News in Physiological Sciences*, vol. 17, no. 2, pp. 51–55, 2002.

[7] A. Berardelli, J. C. Rothwell, P. D. Thompson, and M. Hallett, "Pathophysiology of bradykinesia in Parkinson's disease," *Brain*, vol. 124, part 11, pp. 2131–2146, 2001.

[8] E. C. Wolters, "Variability in the clinical expression of Parkinson's disease," *Journal of the Neurological Sciences*, vol. 266, no. 1-2, pp. 197–203, 2008.

[9] K. R. Chaudhuri and A. H. Schapira, "Non-motor symptoms of Parkinson's disease: dopaminergic pathophysiology and treatment," *The Lancet Neurology*, vol. 8, no. 5, pp. 464–474, 2009.

[10] H. Braak, E. Ghebremedhin, U. Rüb, H. Bratzke, and K. del Tredici, "Stages in the development of Parkinson's disease-related pathology," *Cell and Tissue Research*, vol. 318, no. 1, pp. 121–134, 2004.

[11] J. L. Cummings, "Depression and parkinson's disease: a review," *The American Journal of Psychiatry*, vol. 149, no. 4, pp. 443–454, 1992.

[12] H. A. Hanagasi, Z. Tufekcioglu, and M. Emre, "Dementia in Parkinson's disease," *Journal of the Neurological Sciences*, vol. 374, pp. 26–31, 2017.

[13] M. Petrova, M. Raycheva, and L. Traykov, "Cognitive profile of the earliest stage of dementia in Parkinson's disease," *American Journal of Alzheimer's Disease & Other Dementias*, vol. 27, no. 8, pp. 614–619, 2012.

[14] M. M. Ferro, M. I. Bellissimo, J. A. Anselmo-Franci, M. E. M. Angellucci, N. S. Canteras, and C. Da Cunha, "Comparison of bilaterally 6-OHDA- and MPTP-lesioned rats as models of the early phase of Parkinson's disease: histological, neurochemical, motor and memory alterations," *Journal of Neuroscience Methods*, vol. 148, no. 1, pp. 78–87, 2005.

[15] E. Miyoshi, S. Wietzikoski, M. Camplessei, R. Silveira, R. N. Takahashi, and C. Da Cunha, "Impaired learning in a spatial working memory version and in a cued version of the water maze in rats with MPTP-induced mesencephalic dopaminergic lesions," *Brain Research Bulletin*, vol. 58, no. 1, pp. 41–47, 2002.

[16] O. Kano, K. Ikeda, D. Cridebring, T. Takazawa, Y. Yoshii, and Y. Iwasaki, "Neurobiology of depression and anxiety in parkinson's disease," *Parkinson's Disease*, Article ID 143547, 2011.

[17] M. A. Menza, D. E. Robertson-Hoffman, and A. S. Bonapace, "Parkinson's disease and anxiety: Comorbidity with depression," *Biological Psychiatry*, vol. 34, no. 7, pp. 465–470, 1993.

[18] F. J. Carod-Artal, S. Ziomkowski, H. Mourão Mesquita, and P. Martínez-Martin, "Anxiety and depression: Main determinants of health-related quality of life in Brazilian patients with Parkinson's disease," *Parkinsonism & Related Disorders*, vol. 14, no. 2, pp. 102–108, 2008.

[19] M. A. Hely, J. G. L. Morris, W. G. J. Reid, and R. Trafficante, "Sydney Multicenter Study of Parkinson's disease: non-L-dopa-responsive problems dominate at 15 years," *Movement Disorders*, vol. 20, no. 2, pp. 190–199, 2005.

[20] B. Ravina, R. Camicioli, P. G. Como et al., "The impact of depressive symptoms in early Parkinson disease," *Neurology*, vol. 69, no. 4, pp. 342–347, 2007.

[21] A. Lieberman, "Depression in Parkinson's disease—a review," *Acta Neurologica Scandinavica*, vol. 113, no. 1, pp. 1–8, 2006.

[22] J. S. A. M. Reijnders, U. Ehrt, W. E. J. Weber, D. Aarsland, and A. F. G. Leentjens, "A systematic review of prevalence studies of depression in Parkinson's disease," *Movement Disorders*, vol. 23, no. 2, pp. 183–189, 2008.

[23] A. Schrag, A. Hovris, D. Morley, N. Quinn, and M. Jahanshahi, "Young- versus older-onset Parkinson's disease: impact of disease and psychosocial consequences," *Movement Disorders*, vol. 18, no. 11, pp. 1250–1256, 2003.

[24] L. Marsh, W. M. McDonald, J. Cummings et al., "Provisional diagnostic criteria for depression in Parkinson's disease: report of an NINDS/NIMH Work Group," *Movement Disorders*, vol. 21, no. 2, pp. 148–158, 2006.

[25] M. Fernández-Prieto, A. Lens, A. López-Real et al., "Alteraciones de la esfera emocional y el control de los impulsos em la enfermedad de Parkinson," *Revista Neurologia*, vol. 50, pp. 41–49, 2010.

[26] N. Schintu, X. Zhang, and P. Svenningsson, "Studies of Depression-Related States in Animal Models of Parkinsonism," *Journal of Parkinsons Disease*, vol. 2, no. 2012, p. 87106, 2012.

[27] L. Ishihara and C. Brayne, "A systematic review of depression and mental illness preceding Parkinson's disease," *Acta Neurologica Scandinavica*, vol. 113, no. 4, pp. 211–220, 2006.

[28] E. L. Jacob, N. M. Gatto, A. Thompson, Y. Bordelon, and B. Ritz, "Occurrence of depression and anxiety prior to Parkinson's disease," *Parkinsonism & Related Disorders*, vol. 16, no. 9, pp. 576–581, 2010.

[29] D. Aarsland, K. Brønnick, U. Ehrt et al., "Neuropsychiatric symptoms in patients with Parkinson's disease and dementia: frequency, profile and associated care giver stress," *Journal of Neurology, Neurosurgery & Psychiatry*, vol. 78, no. 1, pp. 36–42, 2007.

[30] M. Shiba, J. H. Bower, D. M. Maraganore et al., "Anxiety disorders and depressive disorders preceding Parkinson's disease: A case-control study," *Movement Disorders*, vol. 15, no. 4, pp. 669–677, 2000.

[31] H. Gustafsson, A. Nordström, and P. Nordström, "Depression and subsequent risk of Parkinson disease A nationwide cohort study," *Neurology*, vol. 84, no. 24, pp. 2422–2429, 2015.

[32] F. H. D. R. Costa, A. L. Z. Rosso, H. Maultasch, D. H. Nicaretta, and M. B. Vincent, "Depression in Parkinson's disease: Diagnosis and treatment," *Arquivos de Neuro-Psiquiatria*, vol. 70, no. 8, pp. 617–620, 2012.

[33] D. J. Burn, "Beyond the iron mask: Towards better recognition and treatment of depression associated with Parkinson's disease," *Movement Disorders*, vol. 17, no. 3, pp. 445–454, 2002.

[34] M. Baquero and N. Martín, "Depressive symptoms in neurodegenerative diseases," *World Journal of Clinical Cases*, vol. 3, no. 8, pp. 682–693, 2015.

[35] K. D'Ostilio and G. Garraux, "The network model of depression as a basis for new therapeutic strategies for treating major depressive disorder in Parkinson's disease," *Frontiers in Human Neuroscience*, vol. 10, no. 2016, pp. 1–10, 2016.

[36] P. G. Frisina, J. C. Borod, N. S. Foldi, and H. R. Tenenbaum, "Depression in Parkinson's disease: Health risks, etiology, and treatment options," *Neuropsychiatric Disease and Treatment*, vol. 4, no. 1 A, pp. 81–91, 2008.

[37] J. J. Schildkraut, "The catecholamine hypothesis of affective disorders: a review of supporting evidence. 1965.," *The Journal of Neuropsychiatry and Clinical Neurosciences*, vol. 7, no. 4, pp. 524-524, 1995.

[38] D. A. Slattery, A. L. Hudson, and D. J. Nutt, "Invited review: The evolution of antidepressant mechanisms," *Fundamental & Clinical Pharmacology*, vol. 18, no. 1, pp. 1–21, 2004.

[39] R. Massart, R. Mongeau, and L. Lanfumey, "Beyond the monoaminergic hypothesis: neuroplasticity and epigenetic changes in a transgenic mouse model of depression," *Philosophical Transactions of the Royal Society B: Biological Sciences*, vol. 367, no. 1601, pp. 2485–2494, 2012.

[40] N. Haddjeri, E. Abrial, S. Bahri, and O. Mnie-Filali, "Neuroadaptations of the 5-HT system induced by antidepressant treatments: Old and new strategies," *Journal of allergy disorders and therapy*, vol. 1, no. 1, pp. 1–11, 2014.

[41] M. V. Burke, C. Nocjar, A. J. Sonneborn, A. C. McCreary, and E. A. Pehek, "Striatal serotonin 2C receptors decrease nigrostriatal dopamine release by increasing GABA-A receptor tone in the substantia nigra," *Journal of Neurochemistry*, vol. 131, no. 4, pp. 432–443, 2014.

[42] O. Stiedl, E. Pappa, Å. Konradsson-Geuken, and S. O. Ögren, "The role of the serotonin receptor subtypes 5-HT1A and 5-HT7 and its interaction in emotional learning and memory," *Frontiers in Pharmacology*, vol. 6, article 162, 2015.

[43] K. Patel, S. Allen, M. N. Haque, I. Angelescu, D. Baumeister, and D. K. Tracy, "Bupropion: a systematic review and meta-analysis of effectiveness as an antidepressant," *Therapeutic Advances in Psychopharmacology*, vol. 6, no. 2, pp. 99–144, 2016.

[44] H. Hartung, S. K. H. Tan, Y. Temel, and T. Sharp, "High-frequency stimulation of the subthalamic nucleus modulates neuronal activity in the lateral habenula nucleus," *European Journal of Neuroscience*, vol. 44, no. 9, pp. 2698–2707, 2016.

[45] W. Dauer and S. Przedborski, "Parkinson's disease: mechanisms and models," *Neuron*, vol. 39, no. 6, pp. 889–909, 2003.

[46] F. M. Ribeiro, E. R. D. S. Camargos, L. C. De Souza, and A. L. Teixeira, "Animal models of neurodegenerative diseases," *Revista Brasileira de Psiquiatria*, vol. 35, no. 2, pp. S82–S91, 2013.

[47] J. Blesa, S. Phani, V. Jackson-Lewis, and S. Przedborski, "Classic and new animal models of Parkinson's disease," *Journal of Biomedicine and Biotechnology*, vol. 2012, Article ID 845618, 10 pages, 2012.

[48] A. Carlsson, M. Lindqvist, and T. Magnusson, "3,4-Dihydroxyphenylalanine and 5-hydroxytryptophan as reserpine antagonists," *Nature*, vol. 180, no. 4596, p. 1200, 1957.

[49] A. Carlsson, "The occurrence, distribution and physiological role of catecholamines in the nervous system," *Pharmacological Reviews*, vol. 11, no. 2, pp. 490–493, 1959.

[50] R. Betarbet, T. B. Sherer, and J. T. Greenamyre, "Animal models of Parkinson's disease," *BioEssays*, vol. 24, no. 4, pp. 308–318, 2002.

[51] S. A. Jagmag, N. Tripathi, S. D. Shukla, S. Maiti, and S. Khurana, "Evaluation of models of Parkinson's disease," *Frontiers in Neuroscience*, vol. 9, article no. 503, 2016.

[52] C. Da Cunha, E. C. Wietzikoski, M. M. Ferro et al., "Hemiparkinsonian rats rotate toward the side with the weaker dopaminergic neurotransmission," *Behavioural Brain Research*, vol. 189, no. 2, pp. 364–372, 2008.

[53] K. Hanrott, L. Gudmunsen, M. J. O'Neill, and S. Wonnacott, "6-Hydroxydopamine-induced apoptosis is mediated via extracellular auto-oxidation and caspase 3-dependent activation of protein kinase Cδ," *The Journal of Biological Chemistry*, vol. 281, no. 9, pp. 5373–5382, 2006.

[54] I. Q. Whishaw and S. B. Dunnett, "Dopamine depletion, stimulation or blockade in the rat disrupts spatial navigation and locomotion dependent upon beacon or distal cues," *Behavioural Brain Research*, vol. 18, no. 1, pp. 11–29, 1985.

[55] D. A. Perese, J. Ulman, J. Viola, S. E. Ewing, and K. S. Bankiewicz, "A 6-hydroxydopamine-induced selective parkinsonian rat model," *Brain Research*, vol. 494, no. 2, pp. 285–293, 1989.

[56] L. S. Carman, F. H. Gage, and C. W. Shults, "Partial lesion of the substantia nigra: relation between extent of lesion and

rotational behavior," *Brain Research*, vol. 553, no. 2, pp. 275–283, 1991.

[57] R. V. Van Oosten and A. R. Cools, "Functional updating of the bilateral 6-OHDA rat model for Parkinsons disease," *Society Neuroscience*, vol. 25, p. 1599, 1999.

[58] G. Drui, S. Carnicella, C. Carcenac et al., "Loss of dopaminergic nigrostriatal neurons accounts for the motivational and affective deficits in Parkinson's disease," *Molecular Psychiatry*, vol. 19, no. 3, pp. 358–367, 2014.

[59] U. Ungerstedt, "Adipsia and Aphagia after 6-Hydroxydopamine Induced Degeneration of the Nigro-striatal Dopamine System," *Acta Physiologica Scandinavica*, vol. 82, no. 367 S, pp. 95–122, 1971.

[60] D. Kirik, C. Rosenblad, and A. Björklund, "Characterization of behavioral and neurodegenerative changes following partial lesions of the nigrostriatal dopamine system induced by intrastriatal 6-hydroxydopamine in the rat," *Experimental Neurology*, vol. 152, no. 2, pp. 259–277, 1998.

[61] R. Deumens, A. Blokland, and J. Prickaerts, "Modeling Parkinson's disease in rats: an evaluation of 6-OHDA lesions of the nigrostriatal pathway," *Experimental Neurology*, vol. 175, no. 2, pp. 303–317, 2002.

[62] M. Kasten, C. Marras, and C. Klein, "Nonmotor signs in genetic forms of parkinson's disease," in *Nonmotor Parkinson's: The Hidden Face—The Many Hidden Faces*, vol. 133 of *International Review of Neurobiology*, pp. 129–178, Elsevier, 2017.

[63] D. H. Overstreet, "Modeling depression in animal models," *Methods in Molecular Biology*, vol. 829, pp. 125–144, 2012.

[64] D. A. Slattery, A. Markou, and J. F. Cryan, "Evaluation of reward processes in an animal model of depression," *Psychopharmacology*, vol. 190, no. 4, pp. 555–568, 2007.

[65] C. A. Hales, S. A. Stuart, M. H. Anderson, and E. S. J. Robinson, "Modelling cognitive affective biases in major depressive disorder using rodents," *British Journal of Pharmacology*, vol. 171, no. 20, pp. 4524–4538, 2014.

[66] R. D. Porsolt, A. Bertin, and M. Jalfre, "'Behavioural despair' in rats and mice: strain differences and the effects of imipramine," *European Journal of Pharmacology*, vol. 51, no. 3, pp. 291–294, 1978.

[67] V. Castagné, R. D. Porsolt, and P. Moser, "Use of latency to immobility improves detection of antidepressant-like activity in the behavioral despair test in the mouse," *European Journal of Pharmacology*, vol. 616, no. 1-3, pp. 128–133, 2009.

[68] J. F. Cryan, R. J. Valentino, and I. Lucki, "Assessing substrates underlying the behavioral effects of antidepressants using the modified rat forced swimming test," *Neuroscience & Biobehavioral Reviews*, vol. 29, no. 4-5, pp. 547–569, 2005.

[69] O. V. Bogdanova, S. Kanekar, K. E. D'Anci, and P. F. Renshaw, "Factors influencing behavior in the forced swim test," *Physiology & Behavior*, vol. 118, no. 13, pp. 227–239, 2013.

[70] L. Steru, R. Chermat, B. Thierry, and P. Simon, "The tail suspension test: a new method for screening antidepressants in mice," *Psychopharmacology*, vol. 85, no. 3, pp. 367–370, 1985.

[71] J. F. Cryan, C. Mombereau, and A. Vassout, "The tail suspension test as a model for assessing antidepressant activity: Review of pharmacological and genetic studies in mice," *Neuroscience & Biobehavioral Reviews*, vol. 29, no. 4-5, pp. 571–625, 2005.

[72] R. M. Santiago, J. Barbieiro, M. M. S. Lima, P. A. Dombrowski, R. Andreatini, and M. A. B. F. Vital, "Depressive-like behaviors alterations induced by intranigral MPTP, 6-OHDA, LPS and rotenone models of Parkinson's disease are predominantly

associated with serotonin and dopamine," *Progress in Neuro-Psychopharmacology & Biological Psychiatry*, vol. 34, no. 6, pp. 1104–1114, 2010.

[73] R. M. Santiago, J. Barbiero, R. W. Gradowski et al., "Induction of depressive-like behavior by intranigral 6-OHDA is directly correlated with deficits in striatal dopamine and hippocampal serotonin," *Behavioural Brain Research*, vol. 259, pp. 70–77, 2014.

[74] R. M. Santiago, F. S. Tonin, J. Barbiero et al., "The nonsteroidal antiinflammatory drug piroxicam reverses the onset of depressive-like behavior in 6-OHDA animal model of Parkinson's disease," *Neuroscience*, vol. 300, pp. 246–253, 2015.

[75] G. J. Beppe, A. B. Dongmo, H. S. Foyet, T. Dimo, M. Mihasan, and L. Hritcu, "The aqueous extract of Albizia adianthifolia leaves attenuates 6-hydroxydopamine-induced anxiety, depression and oxidative stress in rat amygdala," *BMC Complementary and Alternative Medicine*, vol. 15, no. 1, article no. 374, 2015.

[76] M. T. Tadaiesky, P. A. Dombrowski, C. P. Figueiredo, E. Cargnin-Ferreira, C. Da Cunha, and R. N. Takahashi, "Emotional, cognitive and neurochemical alterations in a premotor stage model of Parkinson's disease," *Neuroscience*, vol. 156, no. 4, pp. 830–840, 2008.

[77] T. P. D. Silva, A. Poli, D. B. Hara, and R. N. Takahashi, "Time course study of microglial and behavioral alterations induced by 6-hydroxydopamine in rats," *Neuroscience Letters*, vol. 622, pp. 83–87, 2016.

[78] M. Shin, T. Kim, J. Lee, Y. Sung, and B. Lim, "Treadmill exercise alleviates depressive symptoms in rotenone-induced Parkinson disease rats," *Journal of Exercise Rehabilitation*, vol. 13, no. 2, pp. 124–129, 2017.

[79] A. Bonito-Oliva, D. Masini, and G. Fisone, "A mouse model of non-motor symptoms in Parkinson's disease: focus on pharmacological interventions targeting affective dysfunctions," *Frontiers in Behavioral Neuroscience*, vol. 8, article 290, 2014.

[80] M. M. Carvalho, F. L. Campos, B. Coimbra et al., "Behavioral characterization of the 6-hydroxidopamine model of Parkinson's disease and pharmacological rescuing of non-motor deficits," *Molecular Neurodegeneration*, vol. 8, no. 1, article 14, 2013.

[81] E. Kocabicak, A. Jahanshahi, L. Schonfeld, S.-A. Hescham, Y. Temel, and S. Tan, "Deep brain stimulation of the rat subthalamic nucleus induced inhibition of median raphe serotonergic and dopaminergic neurotransmission," *Turkish Neurosurgery*, vol. 25, no. 5, pp. 721–727, 2015.

[82] E. Faggiani, C. Delaville, and A. Benazzouz, "The combined depletion of monoamines alters the effectiveness of subthalamic deep brain stimulation," *Neurobiology of Disease*, vol. 82, pp. 342–348, 2015.

[83] M. Celorrio, E. Rojo-Bustamante, D. Fernández-Suárez et al., "GPR55: A therapeutic target for Parkinson's disease?" *Neuropharmacology*, vol. 125, pp. 319–332, 2017.

[84] S. Ojha, H. Javed, S. Azimullah, and M. E. Haque, "β-Caryophyllene, a phytocannabinoid attenuates oxidative stress, neuroinflammation, glial activation, and salvages dopaminergic neurons in a rat model of Parkinson disease," *Molecular and Cellular Biochemistry*, vol. 418, no. 1-2, pp. 59–70, 2016.

[85] Y. Gómez-Gálvez, C. Palomo-Garo, J. Fernández-Ruiz, and C. García, "Potential of the cannabinoid CB(2) receptor as a pharmacological target against inflammation in Parkinson's disease," *Progress in Neuro-Psychopharmacology & Biological Psychiatry*, vol. 64, pp. 200–208, 2016.

[86] F. J. Barrero, I. Ampuero, B. Morales et al., "Depression in Parkinson's disease is related to a genetic polymorphism of

the cannabinoid receptor gene (CNR1)," *The Pharmacogenomics Journal*, vol. 5, no. 2, pp. 135–141, 2005.

[87] A. Baumann, C. G. Moreira, M. M. Morawska, S. Masneuf, C. R. Baumann, and D. Noain, "Preliminary evidence of apathetic-like behavior in aged vesicular monoamine transporter 2 deficient mice," *Frontiers in Human Neuroscience*, vol. 10, no. 2016, article no. 587, 2016.

[88] S. Kasai, T. Yoshihara, O. Lopatina, K. Ishihara, and H. Higashida, "Selegiline Ameliorates Depression-Like Behavior in Mice Lacking the CD157/BST1 Gene, a Risk Factor for Parkinson's Disease," *Frontiers in Behavioral Neuroscience*, vol. 11, 2017.

[89] K.-S. Kim, Y.-M. Kang, T.-S. Park et al., "Pitx3 deficient mice as a genetic animal model of co-morbid depressive disorder and parkinsonism," *Brain Research*, vol. 1552, pp. 72–81, 2014.

[90] G. Madeo, T. Schirinzi, M. Maltese et al., "Dopamine-dependent CB1 receptor dysfunction at corticostriatal synapses in homozygous PINK1 knockout mice," *Neuropharmacology*, vol. 101, pp. 460–470, 2016.

[91] J. Pagonabarraga, J. Kulisevsky, A. P. Strafella, and P. Krack, "Apathy in Parkinson's disease: clinical features, neural substrates, diagnosis, and treatment," *The Lancet Neurology*, vol. 14, no. 5, pp. 518–531, 2015.

[92] K. R. Chaudhuri, P. Martinez-Martin, A. Antonini et al., "Rotigotine and specific non-motor symptoms of Parkinson's disease: post hoc analysis of RECOVER," *Parkinsonism & Related Disorders*, vol. 19, no. 7, pp. 660–665, 2013.

[93] K. Jellinger, "The pathology of parkinsonism," in *Movement Disorders*, vol. 2, pp. 124–165, 1987.

[94] K. Jellinger, "New developments in the pathology of Parkinsons disease," *Advances in Neurology*, vol. 53, pp. 1–16, 1990.

[95] M. Doder, E. A. Rabiner, N. Turjanski, A. J. Lees, and D. J. Brooks, "Tremor in Parkinson's disease and serotonergic dysfunction: an 11C-WAY 100635 PET study," *Neurology*, vol. 60, no. 4, pp. 601–605, 2003.

[96] P. Remy, M. Doder, A. Lees, N. Turjanski, and D. Brooks, "Depression in Parkinson's disease: loss of dopamine and noradrenaline innervation in the limbic system," *Brain*, vol. 128, no. 6, pp. 1314–1322, 2005.

[97] W. Paulus and K. Jellinger, "The neuropathologic basis of different clinical subgroups of parkinson's disease," *Journal of Neuropathology & Experimental Neurology*, vol. 50, no. 6, pp. 743–755, 1991.

[98] T. Becker, G. Becker, J. Seufert et al., "Parkinson's disease and depression: evidence for an alteration of the basal limbic system detected by transcranial sonography," *Journal of Neurology, Neurosurgery & Psychiatry*, vol. 63, no. 5, pp. 590–595, 1997.

[99] T. Murai, U. Müller, K. Werheid et al., "In vivo evidence for differential association of striatal dopamine and midbrain serotonin systems with neuropsychiatric symptoms in Parkinson's disease," *The Journal of Neuropsychiatry and Clinical Neurosciences*, vol. 13, no. 2, pp. 222–228, 2001.

[100] P. G. Frisina, V. Haroutunian, and L. S. Libow, "The neuropathological basis for depression in Parkinson's disease," *Parkinsonism & Related Disorders*, vol. 15, no. 2, pp. 144–148, 2009.

[101] R. Mayeux, Y. Stern, L. Cote, and J. B. W. Williams, "Altered serotonin metabolism in depressed patients with parkinson's disease," *Neurology*, vol. 34, no. 5, pp. 642–646, 1984.

[102] V. S. Kostic, B. M. Djuricic, N. Covickovic-Sternic et al., "Depression and Parkinsons disease: Possible role of serotonergic mechanisms," *Journal of Neurology*, vol. 234, no. 2, pp. 94–96, 1987.

[103] N. I. Bohnen, D. I. Kaufer, R. Hendrickson, G. M. Constantine, C. A. Mathis, and R. Y. Moore, "Cortical cholinergic denervation is associated with depressive symptoms in Parkinson's disease and parkinsonian dementia," *Journal of Neurology, Neurosurgery & Psychiatry*, vol. 78, no. 6, pp. 641–643, 2007.

[104] P. M. Meyer, K. Strecker, K. Kendziorra et al., "Reduced $\alpha 4\beta 2^*$-nicotinic acetylcholine receptor binding and its relationship to mild cognitive and depressive symptoms in Parkinson disease," *Archives of General Psychiatry*, vol. 66, no. 8, pp. 866–877, 2009.

[105] P. Svenningsson, S. Pålhagen, and A. A. Mathé, "Neuropeptide Y and Calcitonin Gene-Related Peptide in Cerebrospinal Fluid in Parkinson's Disease with Comorbid Depression versus Patients with Major Depressive Disorder," *Frontiers in Psychiatry*, vol. 8, no. 102, pp. 1–5, 2017.

27

Twice-Daily versus Once-Daily Pramipexole Extended Release Dosage Regimens in Parkinson's Disease

Ji Young Yun,[1] Young Eun Kim,[2] Hui-Jun Yang,[3] Han-Joon Kim,[4] and Beomseok Jeon[4]

[1]Department of Neurology, Ewha Womans University Mokdong Hospital, Ewha Womans University College of Medicine, Seoul, Republic of Korea

[2]Department of Neurology, Hallym University Sacred Heart Hospital, Hallym University College of Medicine, Anyang, Republic of Korea

[3]Department of Neurology, Ulsan University Hospital, Ulsan, Republic of Korea

[4]Department of Neurology and Movement Disorder Center, Seoul National University Hospital, Seoul National University College of Medicine, Seoul, Republic of Korea

Correspondence should be addressed to Beomseok Jeon; brain@snu.ac.kr

Academic Editor: Antonio Pisani

This open-label study aimed to compare once-daily and twice-daily pramipexole extended release (PER) treatment in Parkinson's disease (PD). PD patients on dopamine agonist therapy, but with unsatisfactory control, were enrolled. Existing agonist doses were switched into equivalent PER doses. Subjects were consecutively enrolled into either once-daily-first or twice-daily-first groups and received the prescribed amount in one or two, respectively, daily doses for 8 weeks. For the second period, subjects switched regimens in a crossover manner. The forty-four patients completed a questionnaire requesting preference during their last visit. We measured the UPDRS-III, Hoehn and Yahr stages (H&Y) in medication-on state, Parkinson's disease sleep scale (PDSS), and Epworth Sleepiness Scale. Eighteen patients preferred a twice-daily regimen, 12 preferred a once-daily regimen, and 14 had no preference. After the trial, 14 subjects wanted to be on a once-daily regimen, 25 chose a twice-daily regimen, and 5 wanted to maintain the prestudy regimen. Main reasons for choosing the twice-daily regimen were decreased off-duration, more tolerable off-symptoms, and psychological stability. The mean UPDRS-III, H&Y, and PDSS were not different. Daytime sleepiness was significantly high in the once-daily regimen, whereas nocturnal hallucinations were more common in the twice-daily. Multiple dosing should be considered if once-daily dosing is unsatisfactory. This study is registered as NCT01515774 at ClinicalTrials.gov.

1. Introduction

The dopamine agonist pramipexole is an effective option for treatment of Parkinson's disease (PD) treatment [1, 2]. Pramipexole, when given in the immediate-release (IR) form, is taken orally three times a day. At a theoretical level, motor fluctuation risks can be reduced by continuous stimulation of the dopamine receptors [3, 4]. However, once-daily dosing has shown improved medication compliance [5] and less off-time [6]. To encourage stable dopaminergic delivery and compliance, an extended-release (ER) formulation of pramipexole was introduced.

The pramipexole extended-release (PER) formulation can be taken once daily and is reportedly not inferior to the IR formulation for efficacy, safety, and tolerability in early and advanced PD patients [7–9]. A once-daily PER dosage regimen permits smaller plasma concentration fluctuation and better convenience of use compared to those from a thrice-daily pramipexole IR (PIR) regimen [10].

However, we have met patients who express dissatisfaction with their motor fluctuations and adverse events (AEs) when taking once-daily PER, and some patients have asked for multiple daily dosing. In a previous study of a prolonged release form of ropinirole, we reported that multiple dosing might be a therapeutic option if once-daily dosing is unsatisfactory [11]. In this study, we evaluated preferences for dosing frequency in PER treatment and compared once-daily and twice-daily regimens by assessing a variety of measures of parkinsonism and sleepiness in patients with PD.

2. Methods

2.1. Patients. Inclusion criteria were patients with idiopathic PD, according to the United Kingdom Parkinson's Disease Society brain bank criteria [12], aged between 30 and 80 years old. All patients were on a dopamine agonist (PIR, ropinirole IR (RIR), or ropinirole ER (RER)) and were considering changing to PER due to suboptimal control with their current levodopa or dopamine agonist therapy. Reasons for changing to PER included subjective complaints of hypersomnolence, hallucination, motor fluctuation, drug-induced dyskinesia, and gastrointestinal discomfort. All patients were taking stable doses of antiparkinsonian medications including levodopa and dopamine agonist for at least 4 weeks prior to screening for inclusion in the study.

Patients with a history of significant or uncontrolled cognitive, neurologic, or other medical disorders; a history of impulsive compulsive disorder (ICD), depression, and apathy; a recent history or current evidence of drug abuse or alcoholism; severe dizziness or fainting due to orthostatic hypotension; a history of severe AEs related to dopaminergic agents; a history of allergic reaction to similar medications; or a history of heavy metal poisoning were eligible for enrollment. Patients were excluded if they were taking neuroleptics at the baseline visit. Patients were also excluded from the study if they had used PER or an investigational medication within the 4 weeks prior to study initiation. In addition, because a twice-daily dose could not be prescribed without splitting the tablet, patients who were on less than 0.7 mg of PIR or less than 3.0 mg of ropinirole were ineligible (Table 2).

2.2. Study Design. The investigation was designed as a 16-week, two-period, open-label crossover study to compare once-daily and twice-daily dosing of PER. The two 8-week crossover treatment periods were separated without a washout phase. The study protocol was approved by the Institutional Review Board of the Seoul National University Hospital (SNUH) and conformed to the principles of the Declaration of Helsinki. All patients signed an informed consent before participation in the study.

Patients were arranged sequentially to once-daily dosing first or twice-daily dosing first groups in an open-label trial. Each group initially received 8 weeks of PER once daily or twice daily for 8 weeks and then switched to twice-daily or once-daily, respectively, for the final dosing schedule of 8 weeks. Crossover occurred without a washout period (Figure 1).

The conversion ratios between PIR to PER and RIR to PER were 1 : 1 and 5 : 1, respectively. Tablets of PER were available only in 0.375, 0.75, and 1.5 sizes; therefore, conversion from PIR or RIR to the PER dose was upwardly adjusted, if needed, to avoid breaking the PER tablets. For example, when PIR was being given at 1.1 mg/d, the PER dosage was 1.5 mg/d. In twice-daily dosing, we split the daily PER dose into two doses. If possible, the split doses were equal; however, unequal doses were used when necessary to avoid breaking PER (e.g.,

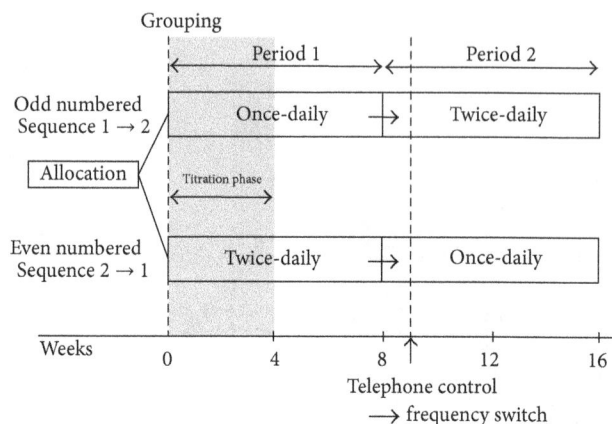

FIGURE 1: Study design.

a 2.625 mg dose was converted to 1.5 mg and 1.125 mg doses, Table 2). First dosing of PER was given with the first dosing of the patient's other antiparkinsonian medications. The timing and dose of the second PER dosing was based on criteria they used to take dopaminergic agent prior to this study. Therefore, the second PER dosing occurred in the evening or the late afternoon and at an equal or lower dosage than the first PER dosing.

Titration of PER was undertaken only in the initial 4 weeks of the first period of the crossover sequence. The dose was titrated until an optimal therapeutic response was achieved or intolerable adverse effects disappeared. Dosing frequency was maintained during the titration phase. Once an optimal dose was achieved, the subject was maintained on that dose for the remainder of the study. Changes in dosage of other antiparkinsonian medications and sedatives were not allowed. In the second period of the crossover sequence, titration of PER was not allowed. However, if the subject complained of intolerable off-symptoms, dyskinesia, or adverse effects in the second period, early completion was accepted at a patient visit earlier than that at 16 weeks.

Patient visits to the clinic were scheduled to occur at baseline at weeks 1, 8, and 16. Telephone control was scheduled in week 9 (1 week after crossing over to second period) to check for AEs. Patients were allowed to make nonscheduled clinic visits when needed. At the baseline visit, all subjects were assessed by using the Unified Parkinson's Disease Rating Scale part 3 (mUPDRS) [13] and the Hoehn and Yahr stage (H&Y) [14] in the medication-on state, the Parkinson's Disease Sleep Questionnaire (PDSS) [15, 16], and the Epworth Sleepiness Scale (ESS) [17, 18].

At 8 and 16 weeks, or at last visit for early completion, all assessments were repeated and the Patient's Global Impressions (PGI) and compliance, including medication compliance, for each treatment period were determined. For each period, mean compliance rates were calculated based on the total prescribed doses and total actually taken doses for all subjects. In addition, AEs and changes in wearing-off and dyskinesia were recorded throughout the study.

At the completion of the second period, patients' dosage regimen preference was assessed by asking the following question: "Which regimen do you prefer?" The possible answers were "I prefer the once-daily dosing," "I prefer the twice-daily dosing," and "I do not prefer one regimen over the other." If subjects completed the study earlier than the end of the second treatment period, they were still asked for their preferences. Patients who did not complete the first treatment period or did not complete the preference questionnaire were excluded from the analysis.

In addition, patients' medication choices after completing this trial were also determined by asking the question: "Which regimen will you choose after this trial?" Possible choices were "PER" and "other dopamine agonists." If they chose "PER," we asked them "which PER regimen will you choose between once-daily and twice-daily dosing?" In addition, we asked for their reasons for their choices.

2.3. Outcome Measures. The primary outcome measure was the preference of the subjects for once-daily or twice-daily PER treatment as reported at study completion or at early completion after crossover. Secondary outcome measures included the mUPDRS [13], H&Y [14] in the medication-on state, PDSS [15, 16], ESS [17, 18], compliance, and the proportion of PGI of improvement (PGI-I). In addition, the duration and severity of motor complication were evaluated by using visual rating scales for wearing-off and dyskinesia, respectively.

To monitor patient safety, AEs were recorded throughout the study. We assessed the occurrence, type, and intensity of AEs. The intensity of AEs was categorized by severity as mild (causing minimal discomfort and not interfering with everyday activities), moderate (sufficiently discomforting to interfere with normal daily activities), or severe (incapacitating or causing inability to undertake usual activities). A serious AE was defined as fatal, life-threatening, required or prolonging hospitalization, or leading to significant disability.

2.4. Statistical Analyses. Comparisons of the once-daily to twice-daily ($1 \rightarrow 2$) and twice-daily to once-daily ($2 \rightarrow 1$) crossover groups at baseline were performed by using Mann-Whitney tests. The primary analysis was based on descriptive statistics to determine subject preferences. Comparisons of the groups that preferred once-daily or twice-daily were analyzed by applying Mann-Whitney tests. Comparisons of mUPDRS, H&Y, PGI-I, PDSS, ESS, compliance, and visual analogue scale (VAS) for wearing-off and dyskinesia values for the once-daily and twice-daily periods were analyzed by performing Wilcoxon signed rank tests. McNemar tests were used to evaluate differences in AE occurrence in the once-daily and twice-daily periods. Statistical analyses were done by using SPSS statistical package version 21 (SPSS Inc., Chicago, IL, USA).

3. Results

3.1. Subjects and Subject Discontinuations. Forty-eight patients with PD were enrolled in this study. Of those, 24 patients started the once-daily regimen and another 24 patients the twice-a-day regimen. Four subjects (8.3%) did

not complete the study (Figure 2). Three patients discontinued the study during sequence $1 \rightarrow 2$ and one patient discontinued during sequence $2 \rightarrow 1$. One patient was excluded after self-titrating her levodopa dose without noticing in the once-daily regimen. According to dosing frequency, two subjects discontinued in each dosing regimen. According to treatment period, three patients dropped out during the first period and one patient discontinued during the second period. As a result, 44 subjects (91.7% of those enrolled) were included in the final analysis (Figure 2). Baseline demographics characteristics were not significantly different between those two treatment groups (Table 1).

At the baseline visit, one patient was on RIR (6 mg/day), 20 patients on RER (10.6 ± 6.4 mg/day), and 27 on PIR (2.2 ± 1.1 mg/day). Based on the study's conversion ratios, the dose levels of RIR, RER, and PIR averaged 2.2 ± 1.2 mg/day of PER. To avoid breaking the PER tablets, the average actual converted dose of PER was 2.4 ± 1.2 mg/day before titration (Table 2). After the titration, the average dose of PER was 2.5 ± 1.2 mg/day.

3.2. Primary and Secondary Outcomes. Analysis of responses to the preference questionnaire showed that 27% ($n = 12$) of the patients preferred the once-daily regimens, 41% ($n = 18$) preferred the twice-daily regimens, and 32% ($n = 14$) did not express a preference for either regimen (Figure 3(a)).

Their mean ESS was higher in once-daily group than in the twice-daily group (4.8 ± 2.9 versus 4.3 ± 2.8, $P = 0.040$). However, the mean mUPDRS, H&Y, PGI-I, compliance, and AE values were not significantly different between the two regimens (Table 3). Total PDSS tended to be higher in twice-daily group; however the difference was not significant ($P = 0.082$). With regard to PDSS subscores, the night hallucinations were more common in the twice-daily group ($P = 0.008$). At the end of each period, the proportions of PGI-I were not significantly different between the two regimens ($P = 0.279$, Table 3).

With regard to wearing-off and dyskinesia, the VAS scores for duration and severity were not significantly different between the once-daily and twice-daily regimens ($P = 0.872$ and $P = 0.284$, resp., for wearing-off; $P = 0.690$ and $P = 0.472$, resp., for dyskinesia). Although the PGI-I tended to be higher in twice-daily group than the once-daily group, there was no significant difference between PGI-I values ($P = 0.109$).

3.3. Patients' Choices at Completion. Analysis of the responses to the questionnaire about patients' choices at completion of the clinical trial showed that 39 patients chose to remain on PER; five patients chose to revert to the other dopamine agonists that they had taken previous to the trial. Among patients whose choice was to continue with PER, 32% ($n = 14$) wanted to follow a once-daily regimen, whereas 57% ($n = 25$) chose the twice-daily regimens (Figure 3(b)).

Among the patients that chose the once-daily regimen, the reasons provided were convenience ($n = 7$), decreased off-duration ($n = 6$), more tolerable off-symptoms ($n = 6$), better on-quality ($n = 5$), and less intolerable dyskinesia ($n = 1$). The reasons for choosing the twice-daily regimen were decreased off-duration ($n = 15$), more tolerable off-symptoms ($n = 13$),

TABLE 1: Baseline characteristics in the per-protocol population.

	QD → BID (N = 21)	BID → QD (N = 23)	P Value	Overall (N = 44)
Age (years)	62.3 ± 8.7	58.4 ± 8.8	0.095	60.3 ± 8.9
Disease duration	8.9 ± 5.0	10.7 ± 5.4	0.187	9.8 ± 5.3
Sex (M : F)	10 : 11	9 : 14	0.570	19 : 25
mUPDRS	19.7 ± 7.6	17.3 ± 7.9	0.365	18.5 ± 7.7
Hoehn and Yahr stage	2.1 ± 0.4	2.0 ± 0.5	0.728	2.0 ± 0.4
Pramipexole ER dose before titration	2.4 ± 1.2	2.3 ± 1.2	0.943	2.4 ± 1.2
Pramipexole ER dose after titration	2.5 ± 1.3	2.4 ± 1.2	0.925	2.5 ± 1.2
LEDD	937.5 ± 323.8	1036.1 ± 252.3	0.455	989.0 ± 289.5
Epworth Sleep Scale	4.5 ± 3.3	5.0 ± 2.7	0.463	4.8 ± 3.0
PDSS				
Overall sleep quality	7.7 ± 2.3	7.2 ± 2.0	0.331	7.5 ± 2.2
Falling in sleep	8.5 ± 2.9	8.2 ± 2.3	0.348	8.3 ± 2.6
Staying asleep	5.5 ± 4.6	4.7 ± 4.1	0.457	5.1 ± 4.3
Sleep disruption due to restlessness of limbs at night or evening	8.8 ± 2.2	8.3 ± 3.2	0.749	8.5 ± 2.7
Fidget in bed	7.9 ± 3.5	8.7 ± 2.0	0.728	8.3 ± 2.8
Distressing dreams at night	8.1 ± 3.6	8.2 ± 2.9	0.668	8.2 ± 3.2
Distressing hallucination at night	9.0 ± 2.4	9.1 ± 2.5	0.641	9.0 ± 2.4
Getting up at night to pass urine	4.1 ± 4.7	4.2 ± 4.3	0.930	4.2 ± 4.5
Incontinence due to off-symptoms	10.0 ± 0.0	10.0 ± 0.0	1.000	10.0 ± 0.0
Numbness or tingling of limbs	8.3 ± 3.1	8.8 ± 2.3	0.945	8.6 ± 2.7
Painful muscle cramps	8.3 ± 2.8	9.0 ± 2.2	0.680	8.7 ± 2.5
Wake early in the morning with painful posturing of limbs	9.6 ± 1.7	9.6 ± 0.9	0.224	9.6 ± 1.4
On waking tremor	8.9 ± 2.8	8.8 ± 3.1	0.958	8.8 ± 2.9
Morning tiredness or sleepiness	7.9 ± 3.8	8.4 ± 3.0	0.932	8.2 ± 3.4
Unexpected falling asleep in the day	8.4 ± 2.6	8.6 ± 2.7	0.785	8.5 ± 2.6
Total PDSS	121.0 ± 24.4	121.9 ± 16.1	0.589	121.5 ± 20.2
VAS for wearing off-duration	7.8 ± 1.5	7.6 ± 1.3	0.524	7.7 ± 1.4
VAS for wearing off-severity	6.2 ± 2.6	6.0 ± 1.5	0.569	6.1 ± 2.1
VAS for dyskinesia-duration	9.1 ± 1.1	8.5 ± 2.2	0.500	8.8 ± 1.8
VAS for dyskinesia-severity	8.3 ± 2.2	8.6 ± 1.7	0.941	8.4 ± 2.0

QD, once-daily; BID, twice-daily; mUPDRS, Unified Parkinson's Disease Rating Scale part 3; ER, extended-release; LEDD, levodopa equivalent dose; VAS, visual analogue scale; PDSS, Parkinson's disease sleep scale.

TABLE 2: Dose switches from conventional dopaminergic agonist to pramipexole ER.

Pramipexole IR → pramipexole ER			Ropinirole → pramipexole ER		
Pramipexole IR daily dose, mg	Pramipexole ER, mg		Ropinirole daily dose, mg	Pramipexole ER, mg	
	Once-daily	Twice-daily		Once-daily	Twice-daily
0.7 ≤ pramipexole < 0.8	0.75	0.375-0.375	3.0 ≤ ropinirole < 4.0	0.75	0.375-0.375
0.8 ≤ pramipexole < 1.1	1.125	0.75-0.375	4.0 ≤ ropinirole < 7.0	1.125	0.75-0.375
1.1 ≤ pramipexole < 1.6	1.5	0.75-0.75	7.0 ≤ ropinirole < 8.0	1.5	0.75-0.75
1.6 ≤ pramipexole < 1.9	1.875	1.125-0.75	8.0 ≤ ropinirole < 10.0	1.875	1.125-0.75
1.9 ≤ pramipexole < 2.3	2.25	1.125-1.125	10.0 ≤ ropinirole < 12.0	2.25	1.125-1.125
2.3 ≤ pramipexole < 2.7	2.625	1.5-1.125	12.0 ≤ ropinirole < 14.0	2.625	1.5-1.125
2.7 ≤ pramipexole < 3.1	3.0	1.5-1.5	14.0 ≤ ropinirole < 16.0	3.0	1.5-1.5
3.1 ≤ pramipexole < 3.4	3.375	1.875-1.5	16.0 ≤ ropinirole < 17.0	3.375	1.875-1.5
3.4 ≤ pramipexole < 3.8	3.75	1.875-1.875	17.0 ≤ ropinirole < 19.0	3.75	1.875-1.875
3.8 ≤ pramipexole < 4.2	4.125	2.25-1.875	19.0 ≤ ropinirole < 21.0	4.125	2.25-1.875
4.2 ≤ pramipexole < 4.6	4.5	2.25-2.25	21.0 ≤ ropinirole < 23.0	4.5	2.25-2.25
4.6 ≤ pramipexole < 4.9	4.875	2.625-2.25	23.0 ≤ ropinirole < 25.0	4.875	2.625-2.25

IR, immediate-release; ER, extended-release.

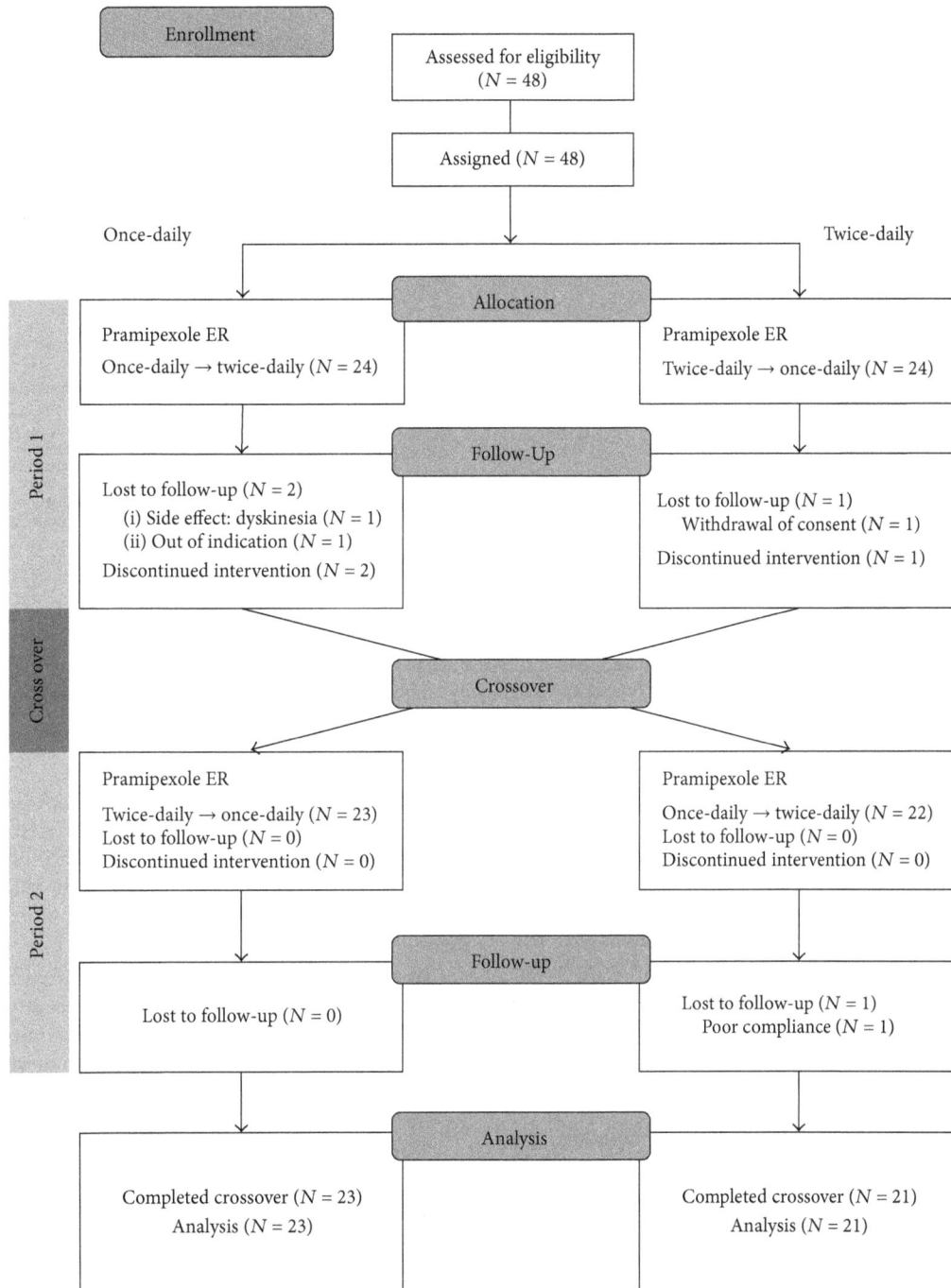

FIGURE 2: Subject flow chart.

psychological stability ($n = 10$), less intolerable dyskinesia ($n = 5$), better on-quality ($n = 3$), decreased dyskinesia duration ($n = 3$), and decreased AEs ($n = 1$).

Among the 5 patients who choose to revert to the previous dopamine agonist treatment, 3 patients had taken PIR thrice-daily and 2 patients took RER twice-daily. The reasons for their choices were more tolerable off-symptoms ($n = 3$, two of RER and one PIR patients), more tolerable dyskinesia (1 PIR patient), and psychological stability due to thrice-daily dosing (1 PIR patient).

Additionally, we compared baseline characteristics between the groups who wanted to be on the once-daily regimen and those who wanted to follow the twice-daily regimen after completing the trial (Table e-1 in Supplementary Material available online at https://doi.org/10.1155/2017/8518929). The patients who chose the twice-daily regimen had longer disease duration ($P = 0.005$) and a longer wearing-off duration ($P = 0.047$). In addition, they had more severe difficulty in staying asleep, more frequent getting-up related to voiding, and more severe daytime sleepiness

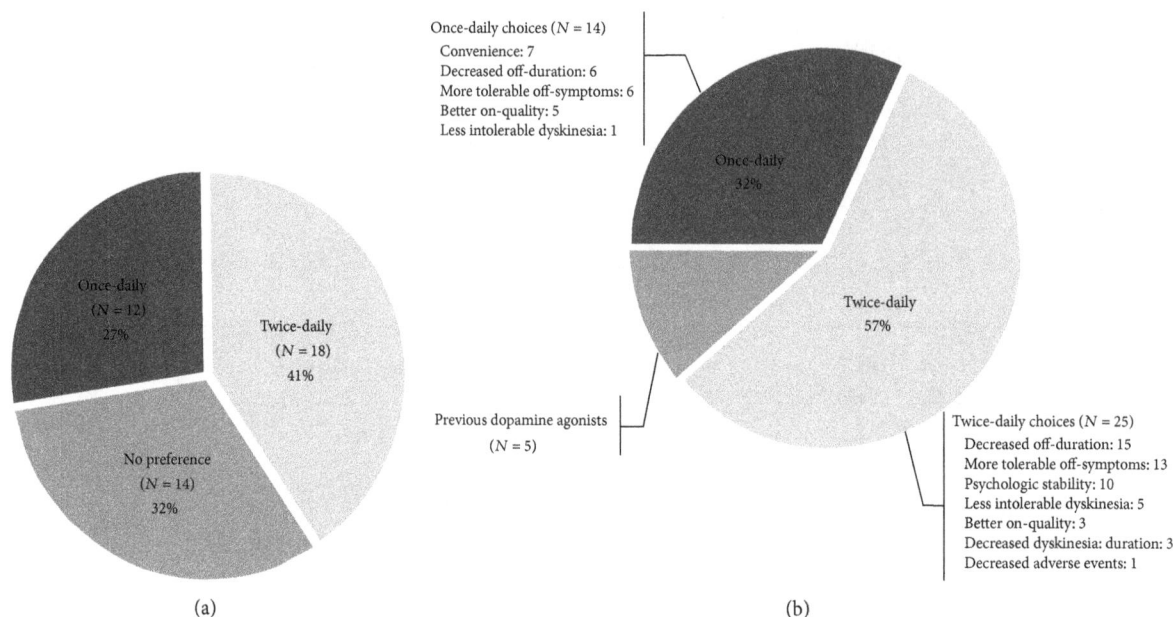

FIGURE 3: Patient's preferences and choices in the end of the trial. (a) Preferences: in response to the final preference questionnaire, 27% (n = 12) of the patients preferred the once-daily regimen, 41% (n = 18) preferred the twice-daily regimen, and 32% (n = 14) did not have a preference. (b) Patient's choices in the end of the trial and reasons. In response to the final choices questionnaire, 32% (n = 14) of the patients wanted to take the once-daily regimen, 57% (n = 25) chose the twice-daily regimen, and 11% (n = 5) wanted to revert to previous dopamine agonists.

(P = 0.047, P = 0.035, and P = 0.039, resp.). There was no statistically significant difference between the baseline nocturnal hallucination values between those who chose once-daily and twice-daily regimens.

3.4. Adverse Events. The incidence of drug-related AEs did not differ significantly between the once-daily (81.8%, 36/44) and twice-daily (84.1%, 37/44) regimens (P = 1.000, Table 4). The most common drug-related AE in both regimens was constipation. Impulsive compulsive behavior, depression, and apathy related to dopamine agonist were not reported in our study.

In the twice-daily regimen, five patients complained the nocturnal visual hallucinations as AEs. Two patients had the visual hallucinations with both regimens. Their intensity of hallucination was mild; however, they complained the hallucinations were more vivid with the twice-daily regimen.

4. Discussion

Generally, PER is prescribed for use in a once-daily regimen. In our assessment of PER in once-daily and twice-daily regimens, when patients switched from once-daily to twice-daily or twice-daily to once-daily regimens their mean mUPDRS, H&Y, ESS, and PDSS and AEs values did not change significantly. Despite the different dosing frequency, the results indicate that whether the daily dosage of PER is provided as one dose or split into two doses, the two treatment regimens have similar efficacy and no difference in the incidences of AEs.

In a previous study, patients had a preference for once-daily PER rather than thrice-daily PIR [19]. In our study, 27%

(n = 12) of the patients preferred the once-daily regimens, and 32% (n = 14) of the patients preferred a once-daily regimen. Among the patients that chose to follow the once-daily regimen, the commonest reasons for that choice were convenience, decreased off-duration, and more tolerable off-symptoms in our study.

In this study, a greater percentage of patients chose to adopt a twice-daily regimen rather than a once-daily regimen after the trial (57 % and 32%, resp.). Among patients who chose the twice-daily regimen, the commonest reasons were decreased off-duration, more tolerable off-symptoms, and psychological stability.

Among the 5 patients that chose to revert to their previous dopaminergic therapy with multiple dosing, the commonest reason for that choice was also more tolerable off-symptoms (n = 3). In addition, one patient chose thrice-daily dosing to achieve psychological comfort. The results indicate that anxiety about off-symptoms may contribute to a patient's dosage regiment reference.

Sleepiness and hallucination are recognized adverse effects of dopamine agonists, including PER [20–22]. In our study, daytime sleepiness was significantly severe in the once-daily group compared to that in the twice-daily group, whereas nocturnal hallucinations were more common in the twice-daily group than in the once-daily group. Thus, clinicians should consider a twice-daily regimen for patients who complain of daytime sleepiness and a once-daily regimen for patients with nocturnal hallucinations.

Among patients taking antiparkinsonian medication, once-daily dosing may improve compliance [23]. In our study, there was no significant difference in compliance

TABLE 3: Secondary outcomes in the per-protocol population.

	Once-daily	Twice-daily	P value
mUPDRS	18.1 ± 8.2	17.8 ± 7.8	0.830
Hoehn and Yahr stage	2.0 ± 0.5	2.0 ± 0.4	0.655
Compliance (%)	99.4 ± 1.6	99.7 ± 0.9	0.182
Total sleep time (hours)	5.5 ± 1.3	5.6 ± 1.4	0.134
Epworth Sleep Scale	4.8 ± 2.9	4.3 ± 2.8	0.040[a]
PDSS			
Overall sleep quality	7.6 ± 2.1	8.2 ± 1.6	0.061
Falling in sleep	8.4 ± 2.5	8.8 ± 2.1	0.234
Staying asleep	5.4 ± 4.3	5.9 ± 4.0	0.347
Sleep disruption due to restlessness of limbs at night or evening	8.4 ± 2.9	8.7 ± 2.9	0.100
Fidget in bed	8.6 ± 2.9	9.0 ± 2.5	0.504
Distressing dreams at night	8.6 ± 2.9	8.7 ± 2.6	0.550
Distressing hallucination at night	9.6 ± 1.4	8.6 ± 3.0	0.008[a]
Getting up at night to pass urine	3.4 ± 4.5	3.9 ± 4.3	0.314
Incontinence due to off-symptoms	9.8 ± 1.5	10.0 ± 0.0	0.317
Numbness or tingling of limbs	8.8 ± 2.2	8.7 ± 2.7	0.555
Painful muscle cramps	8.7 ± 2.3	8.8 ± 2.2	0.825
Wake early in the morning with painful posturing of limbs	9.2 ± 2.2	9.3 ± 2.2	0.859
On waking tremor	9.4 ± 2.1	9.2 ± 2.3	0.285
Morning tiredness or sleepiness	7.8 ± 3.6	8.0 ± 3.1	0.875
Unexpected falling asleep in the day	8.5 ± 2.3	8.7 ± 2.2	0.281
Total PDSS	122.3 ± 18.1	124.4 ± 19.1	0.082
VAS for wearing off-duration	8.1 ± 1.3	8.1 ± 1.3	0.872
VAS for wearing off-severity	6.2 ± 2.2	6.3 ± 2.2	0.284
VAS for dyskinesia-duration	9.1 ± 1.7	9.1 ± 1.6	0.690
VAS for dyskinesia-severity	8.6 ± 2.0	8.6 ± 1.9	0.472
PGI-I, no (%)	17 (38.6)	23 (52.3)	0.180

[a] $P < 0.05$.
mUPDRS, Unified Parkinson's Disease Rating Scale part 3; VAS, visual analogue scale; PDSS, Parkinson's disease sleep scale; PGI-I, patient global impressions of improvement.

TABLE 4: Adverse events.

	Baseline	Once-daily	Twice-daily
Adverse events (%)	36 (81.8)	36 (81.8)	37 (84.1)
Constipation	23 (52.3)	24 (54.5)	20 (45.5)
Dry mouth	19 (43.2)	20 (45.5)	22 (50.0)
Somnolence	11 (25.0)	12 (27.3)	11 (25.0)
Dizziness	9 (20.5)	8 (18.2)	8 (18.2)
Fatigue	8 (18.2)	8 (18.2)	9 (20.5)
Dyspepsia	7 (15.9)	8 (18.2)	10 (22.7)
Nausea	7 (15.9)	6 (13.6)	7 (15.9)
Edema	5 (11.4)	7 (15.9)	9 (20.5)
Hallucination	3 (6.8)	2 (4.5)	5 (11.4)
Headache	2 (4.5)	2 (4.5)	1 (2.3)
Others	2 (4.5)	0 (0.0)	0 (0.0)

levels between once-daily and twice-daily regimens. Because many PD patients are taking multiple antiparkinsonian medications many times a day already, compliance may not be a critical issue, especially for patients with advanced PD.

This study was an open-label study, and there were few statistically significant differences between the once-daily and twice-daily dosage regimen group. Therefore, if patients currently on once-daily PER are not satisfied with that regimen, due to off-symptoms, AEs, sleep-related symptoms, or anxiety related to off-symptoms, clinicians should consider trying a twice-daily dosage regimen.

Acknowledgments

This study was also supported by Republic of Korea and Basic Science Research Program through the National Research Foundation of Korea (NRF) funded by the Ministry of Education, Science and Technology (2010-0021653, BSJ).

References

[1] C. G. Goetz, W. Poewe, O. Rascol, and C. Sampaio, "Evidence-based medical review update: pharmacological and surgical treatments of Parkinson's disease: 2001 to 2004," *Movement Disorders*, vol. 20, no. 5, pp. 523–539, 2005.

[2] R. Pahwa, S. A. Factor, K. E. Lyons et al., "Practice parameter: treatment of Parkinson disease with motor fluctuations and dyskinesia (an evidence-based review): report of the Quality Standards Subcommittee of the American Academy of Neurology," *Neurology*, vol. 66, no. 7, pp. 983–995, 2006.

[3] C. W. Olanow, A. H. V. Schapira, and O. Rascol, "Continuous dopamine-receptor stimulation in early Parkinson's disease," *Trends in Neurosciences*, vol. 23, no. 10, pp. S117–S126, 2000.

[4] J. A. Obeso, M. C. Rodriguez-Oroz, P. Chana et al., "The evolution and origin of motor complications in Parkinson's disease," *Neurology*, vol. 55, no. 11, supplement 4, pp. S13–S23, 2000.

[5] D. Grosset, A. Antonini, M. Canesi et al., "Adherence to Antiparkinson medication in a Multicenter European study," *Movement Disorders*, vol. 24, no. 6, pp. 826–832, 2009.

[6] R. Pahwa, M. A. Stacy, S. A. Factor et al., "Ropinirole 24-hour prolonged release: randomized, controlled study in advanced Parkinson disease," *Neurology*, vol. 68, no. 14, pp. 1108–1115, 2007.

[7] W. Poewe, O. Rascol, P. Barone et al., "Extended-release pramipexole in early Parkinson disease: a 33-week randomized controlled trial," *Neurology*, vol. 77, no. 8, pp. 759–766, 2011.

[8] A. H. V. Schapira, P. Barone, R. A. Hauser et al., "Extended-release pramipexole in advanced Parkinson disease: a randomized controlled trial," *Neurology*, vol. 77, no. 8, pp. 767–774, 2011.

[9] R. A. Hauser, A. H. V. Schapira, O. Rascol et al., "Randomized, double-blind, multicenter evaluation of pramipexole extended release once daily in early Parkinson's disease," *Movement Disorders*, vol. 25, no. 15, pp. 2542–2549, 2010.

[10] A. Antonini and D. Calandrella, "Once-daily pramipexole for the treatment of early and advanced idiopathic Parkinson's disease: implications for patients," *Neuropsychiatric Disease and Treatment*, vol. 7, no. 1, pp. 297–302, 2011.

[11] J. Y. Yun, H.-J. Kim, J.-Y. Lee et al., "Comparison of once-daily versus twice-daily combination of Ropinirole prolonged release in Parkinson's disease," *BMC Neurology*, vol. 13, article 113, 2013.

[12] A. J. Hughes, S. E. Daniel, L. Kilford, and A. J. Lees, "Accuracy of clinical diagnosis of idiopathic Parkinson's disease: a clinico-pathological study of 100 cases," *Journal of Neurology Neurosurgery and Psychiatry*, vol. 55, no. 3, pp. 181–184, 1992.

[13] P. Martinez-Martin, A. Gil-Nagel, L. M. Gracia et al., "Unified Parkinson's disease rating scale characteristics and structure," *Movement Disorders*, vol. 9, no. 1, pp. 76–83, 1994.

[14] C. G. Goetz, W. Poewe, O. Rascol et al., "Movement disorder society task force report on the Hoehn and Yahr staging scale: status and recommendations," *Movement Disorders*, vol. 19, no. 9, pp. 1020–1028, 2004.

[15] J. S. Baik, J. Y. Kim, and J. H. Park, "Parkinson's disease sleep scale in Korea," *Journal of the Korean Neurological Association*, vol. 23, no. 1, pp. 41–48, 2005.

[16] K. R. Chaudhuri and P. Martinez-Martin, "Clinical assessment of nocturnal disability in Parkinson's disease: the Parkinson's Disease Sleep Scale," *Neurology*, vol. 63, no. 8, supplement 3, pp. S17–S20, 2004.

[17] M. W. Johns, "A new method for measuring daytime sleepiness: the epworth sleepiness scale," *Sleep*, vol. 14, no. 6, pp. 540–545, 1991.

[18] Y. W. Cho, J. H. Lee, H. K. Son, S. H. Lee, C. Shin, and M. W. Johns, "The reliability and validity of the Korean version of the Epworth sleepiness scale," *Sleep and Breathing*, vol. 15, no. 3, pp. 377–384, 2011.

[19] A. H. V. Schapira, P. Barone, R. A. Hauser et al., "Patient-reported convenience of once-daily versus three-times-daily dosing during long-term studies of pramipexole in early and advanced Parkinson's disease," *European Journal of Neurology*, vol. 20, no. 1, pp. 50–56, 2013.

[20] R. A. Hauser, L. Gauger, W. M. Anderson, and T. A. Zesiewicz, "Pramipexole-induced somnolence and episodes of daytime sleep," *Movement Disorders*, vol. 15, no. 4, pp. 658–663, 2000.

[21] S. Paus, H. M. Brecht, J. Köster, G. Seeger, T. Klockgether, and U. Wüllner, "Sleep attacks, daytime sleepiness, and dopamine agonists in Parkinson's disease," *Movement Disorders*, vol. 18, no. 6, pp. 659–667, 2003.

[22] M. Ryan, J. T. Slevin, and A. Wells, "Non-ergot dopamine agonist-induced sleep attacks," *Pharmacotherapy*, vol. 20, no. 6, pp. 724–726, 2000.

[23] D. J. Tompson and D. Vearer, "Steady-state pharmacokinetic properties of a 24-hour prolonged-release formulation of ropinirole: results of two randomized studies in patients with Parkinson's disease," *Clinical Therapeutics*, vol. 29, no. 12, pp. 2654–2666, 2007.

28

Outlining a Population "at Risk" of Parkinson's Disease

Tommaso Schirinzi,[1] Giuseppina Martella,[1,2] Alessio D'Elia,[1]
Giulia Di Lazzaro,[1] Paola Imbriani,[1] Graziella Madeo,[1] Leonardo Monaco,[3]
Marta Maltese,[1] and Antonio Pisani[1,2]

[1]Neurology, Department of Systems Medicine, University of Rome Tor Vergata, Via Montpellier 1, 00133 Rome, Italy
[2]IRCCS Fondazione Santa Lucia, Via del Fosso di Fiorano, Rome, Italy
[3]Psychiatry, Department of Systems Medicine, University of Rome Tor Vergata, Via Montpellier 1, 00133 Rome, Italy

Correspondence should be addressed to Antonio Pisani; pisani@uniroma2.it

Academic Editor: Jan Aasly

The multifactorial pathogenesis of Parkinson's Disease (PD) requires a careful identification of populations "at risk" of developing the disease. In this case-control study we analyzed a large Italian population, in an attempt to outline general criteria to define a population "at risk" of PD. We enrolled 300 PD patients and 300 controls, gender and age matched, from the same urban geographical area. All subjects were interviewed on demographics, family history of PD, occupational and environmental toxicants exposure, smoking status, and alcohol consumption. A sample of 65 patients and 65 controls also underwent serum dosing of iron, copper, mercury, and manganese by means of Inductively Coupled-Plasma-Mass-Spectrometry (ICP-MS). Positive family history, toxicants exposure, non-current-smoker, and alcohol nonconsumer status occurred as significant risk factors in our population. The number of concurring risk factors overlapping in the same subject impressively increased the overall risk. No significant differences were measured in the metal serum levels. Our findings indicate that combination of three to four concurrent PD-risk factors defines a condition "at risk" of PD. A simple stratification, based on these questionnaires, might be of help in identifying subjects suitable for neuroprotective strategies.

1. Introduction

Parkinson's Disease (PD) is a common neurodegenerative disorder with progressive disabling motor and nonmotor features. A number of therapeutic interventions allow symptomatic relief, but none of them is able to prevent or halt neurodegeneration. In the recent past, through a better comprehension of PD pathogenesis, several molecular pathways have been identified as potential targets of neuroprotection. Unfortunately, clinical trials often failed in translating the encouraging results obtained from *in vitro* and *in vivo* experimental findings. To some extent, the suboptimal selection of enrolled patients and the lack of measurable biomarkers or reliable outcomes account for such failures [1–3]. Genetically defined populations (LRRK2 or GBA mutations) seem to be suitable candidates for neuroprotection [2], but it is well known that less than 10% of PD cases can be ascribed to a monogenic mutation [4]. It is now widely accepted that PD is an idiopathic, multifactorial disease, originating from the interaction between one or more susceptibility loci of the host and one or several environmental modifiers [5–8]. Since numerous PD-risk factors, including positive family history, toxicants exposure, and personal habits, have been identified [5, 6, 9], specific efforts should be made to further define the PD-risk status and, consequently, improve inclusion criteria for neuroprotective treatments. In this case-control study, we screened a large urban population from Italy to outline a population "at risk" of PD. Specifically, we examined the association between PD and risk factors, measured either as single items or in combination. In addition, in support to this PD-risk stratification, we measured serum levels of iron, copper, mercury, and manganese.

2. Methods

2.1. Study Population. We enrolled 300 consecutive PD patients afferent to *Centro di Riferimento Regionale per il Parkinson della Clinica Neurologica dell'Università "Tor Vergata,"* Rome, Italy, between 2012 and 2015. PD was diagnosed according to UK-PDSBB diagnostic criteria. Enrolled controls were age (±5 years) and sex matched non-blood relatives or friends of patients, not showing signs of parkinsonism or other extrapyramidal signs. Every participant came from the same geographical area (Rome or other cities of Lazio, Italy) and signed an informed consent. All subjects underwent a structured interview. Data collected regarded the following: (1) demographics (name, sex, birth, age at the interview, place of birth, and place of residence); (2) family history of PD (positive = at least one relative of first or second degree affected; negative); (3) occupational exposure (subjects declared the jobs they carried out, years of employment, and use or exposure to three types of toxicants: pesticides/herbicides, chemicals (cleaners, printing products, asbestos, paints, oils, glues, and others), and metals (lead, mercury, manganese, cadmium, chromium, nickel, iron, and copper); to facilitate the report of occupational exposure a list of jobs with the correlating risk of metals exposure has been provided (e.g., painter: lead, manganese, cadmium, etc.)); (4) Environmental exposure (subjects declared the distance between their living place and potential pesticides/herbicides or pollutants sources, toxicants use/exposure for leisure or hobbies; both occupational and environmental exposure were considered as categorical variables (exposed: ≥10 years of exposure); indeed, because of the nature of the data collection (self-reported, retrospective), it was not possible to quantify the exposure precisely [10]); (5) personal habits (subjects declared the smoking status (according the WHO definitions: never-smoker, former-smoker, and current-smoker [11]), the alcohol consumption (no consumption, up to 200 mL/day, and between 200 and 500 mL/day)).

Then, subjects were classified depending on single variables. (1) Family history of PD: it is positive or negative. (2) Toxicants exposure: it includes exposed or nonexposed (exposed = all subjects reporting at least 10-year history of exposure to pesticides/herbicides, chemicals, and metals). According to the cause of exposure, toxicants exposure has been classified into, occupational and environmental. We thus grouped (A) subjects with neither family history of PD or toxicants exposure; (B) subjects with only positive family history of PD; (C) subjects with only toxicants exposure; (D) subjects with "double hit" (positive family history + toxicants exposure). (3) Jobs have been organized into six main categories according to the work setting: agriculture, industry, construction, office, mechanical workers, and other. (4) Smoking status has been divided into current-smoker or non-current-smoker (never-smoker + former-smoker). (5) Alcohol consumption has been divided into nonconsumer and consumer. To avoid or limit any bias, the interviews were conducted by personnel unaware of case status, whereas data were analyzed blindly by distinct operators.

2.2. Biochemical Measurements. Compelling evidence demonstrated the role of iron, copper, manganese, and mercury in the pathogenesis of PD [12–17] and a number of studies showed abnormal metal serum levels in PD patients [18, 19]. Since both the environmental pollution and the eating habits may affect the metal concentrations [16, 20–23], such levels could be measured as an index of toxicants exposure. Here we explored serum levels of iron, copper, manganese, and mercury aimed at identifying further elements supporting the PD-risk stratification. We thus selected 65 PD patients and 65 controls, with similar gender and age distributions; normal weight; no history of blood, lung, liver, kidney, or bowel diseases; no previous/ongoing chemotherapy. From each subject we obtained a blood sample in standardized conditions (between 8 and 10 AM, after an overnight fast). Blood was collected in sodium-heparin tubes and centrifuged for 20 min at 2000 rpm at room temperature. After centrifugation, plasma samples were collected and stored at −80°C until analysis. Hemolyzed samples were excluded from the study. Metals serum levels were measured by Farmlab Srl (Guidonia Montecelio, Rome, Italy) through Inductively Coupled-Plasma-Mass-Spectrometry (ICP-MS) [24]. (The study was approved by the local Ethic Committee, number 98-09. All participants signed an informed consent.)

2.3. Statistical Analysis. Chi-square test was used to examine differences between groups in categorical variables. Binomial logistic regression was used to calculate the odds ratio (OR) and 95% confidence interval (CI) for the association between PD and each considered variable.

Regarding biochemical measurements, Shapiro-Wilk (W) test demonstrated that the distribution of metal serum levels could not be accurately modeled by normal distribution. Thus, the Mann-Whitney U test was used to examine the distribution of serum concentrations between the two groups. Sensitivity and specificity of each metal as biomarker of PD were determined by the receiver operating characteristic (ROC) curve analysis, calculating the area under the curve (AUC). Statistical significance was set at $p < 0.05$. Statistical analysis was performed by IBM SPSS Statistics 22.

3. Results

3.1. Demographics. PD patients and controls were similar on demographic characteristics, consistent with the matched study design (all the results are summarized in Table 1).

3.2. Risk Factors. PD patients showed significantly higher positive family history for PD and percentages of exposed subjects (details in Table 1). The distribution of A, B, C, and D categories (see Section 2) into the two groups was significantly different. Specifically PD patients have greater percentage of B, C, and D categories (PD: none = 45.67%, toxicant exposure 34.67%, positive family history 10.33%, and "double hit" 9.33%; controls: none = 64.3%, toxicant exposure 29.7%, positive family history 3%, and "double hit" 3%; $p < 0.00001$).

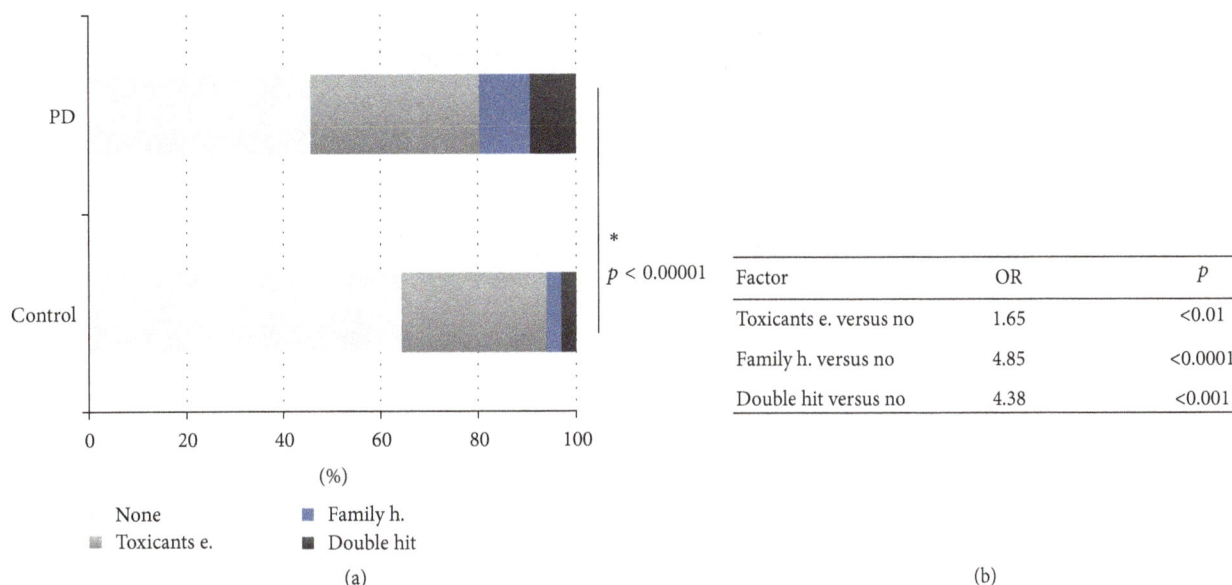

FIGURE 1: (a) Distribution of risk factors in the two groups (no factors, toxicants exposure, positive family history, "double hit," or positive family history + toxicants exposure). (b) OR of these risk factors. ∗ means statistical significance.

TABLE 1: Demographics and main risk factors in our study population.

Variable	Group			p
	Total $n = 600$	PD $n = 300$	Control $n = 300$	
Sex				ns
Male (%)	50.5	51	50	
Female (%)	49.5	49	50	
Age at interview				ns
Mean ± st. dev.	72.8±10.3	70.6±10.4	69.4±9.4	
40–70 y (%)	49.7	47	53	
71–100 y (%)	50.3	53	47	
Family history of PD				<0.000001
Negative (%)	87.2	80.3	94	
Positive (%)	12.8	19.7	6	
Toxicants exposure				<0.001
No (%)	62	56	67.3	
Yes (%)	38	44	32.7	
Smoking status				<0.00001
Never (%)	48.8	58.3	39.3	
Former (%)	15.7	8.7	22.7	
Current (%)	35.5	33	38	
Alcohol consumption				<0.05
No (%)	51.5	58.3	44.7	
<200 mL/day (%)	45.8	38.7	53.0	
200–500 mL/day (%)	2.7	3.0	2.3	

Among these conditions, positive family history and the "double hit" represent severe risk factors for PD (positive family history OR 4.852, 95% CI 2.238–10.519, and $p <$ 0.0001; "double hit" OR 4.383, 95% CI 2.005–9.583, and $p <$ 0.0001), whereas the only toxicants exposure is a milder risk factor (OR 1.646, 95% CI 1.151–2,354, and $p < 0.05$) (Figure 1).

3.3. External Risk Factors. We found, in both cases and controls, occupational exposure as main cause of toxicants exposure (PD: occupational = 77.3%, environmental = 22.7%; controls: occupational 81.6%; environmental = 18.4%; p = n.s.). Since the number of persons with occupational exposure was significantly higher in the PD group (PD = 34.3%; controls = 26.7%; $p < $ 0.05), this condition represents a PD-risk factor (OR 1.438, 95% CI 1.014–2.040; $p < 0.05$). Regarding toxicant substances, we observed a higher exposure to chemicals and, successively, to metals and herbicides/pesticides, although either PD patients or controls had a multiple exposure (PD: chemicals = 59.1%, metals = 44.7%, and herbicides/pesticides = 20.5%; controls: chemicals = 65.3%, metals = 16.3%, and herbicides/pesticides = 45.9%; p = n.s.) (Figure 2(a)). The distribution of job categories was roughly the same between the two groups (PD: agriculture = 4%, industry = 3.33%, construction = 8.67%, office = 24.33%, mechanical workers = 6.33%, and other = 53.33%; controls: agriculture = 2.33%, industry = 4.67%, construction: 7.33%, office = 33.33%, mechanical workers = 6%, and other = 46.33%; p = n.s.) (Figure 2(b)). None of these job categories was associated with an increased risk of PD; however some jobs had a higher risk of toxicants exposure (construction: OR 4.549, 95% CI 2.378–8.704, and $p <$ 0.0001; mechanical workers: OR 4.199, 95% CI 2.047–8.615, and $p <$ 0.0001; agriculture: OR 3.9, 95% CI 1.487–10.227, and $p <$ 0.05; industry: OR 3.791, 95% CI 1.6–8.981, and $p <$ 0.05).

3.4. Personal Habits. PD patients and controls showed different personal habits. The percentages of never-smokers,

(a)

(b)

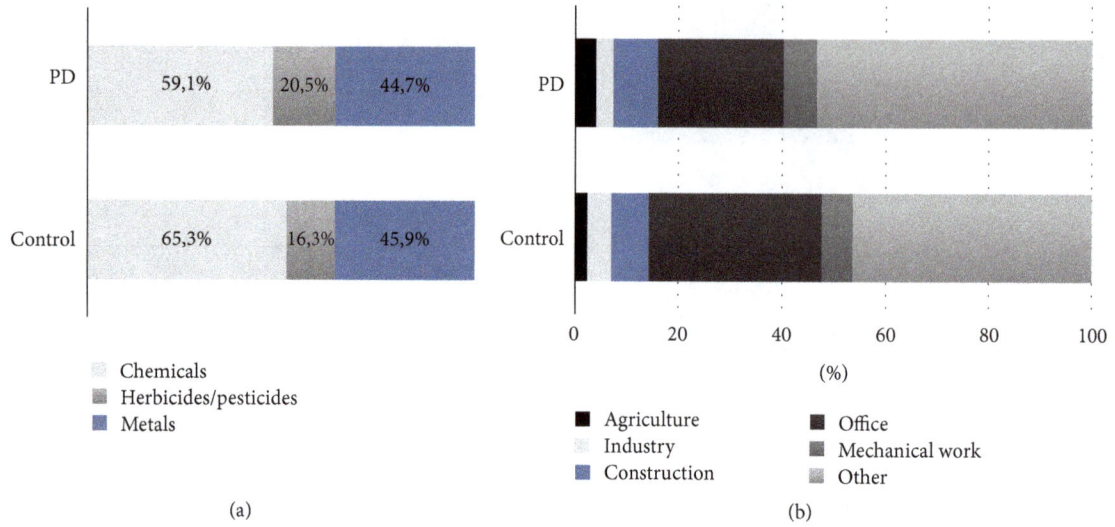

FIGURE 2: (a) Distribution of types of toxicants handled by the two groups. (b) Distribution of occupational categories in the two groups.

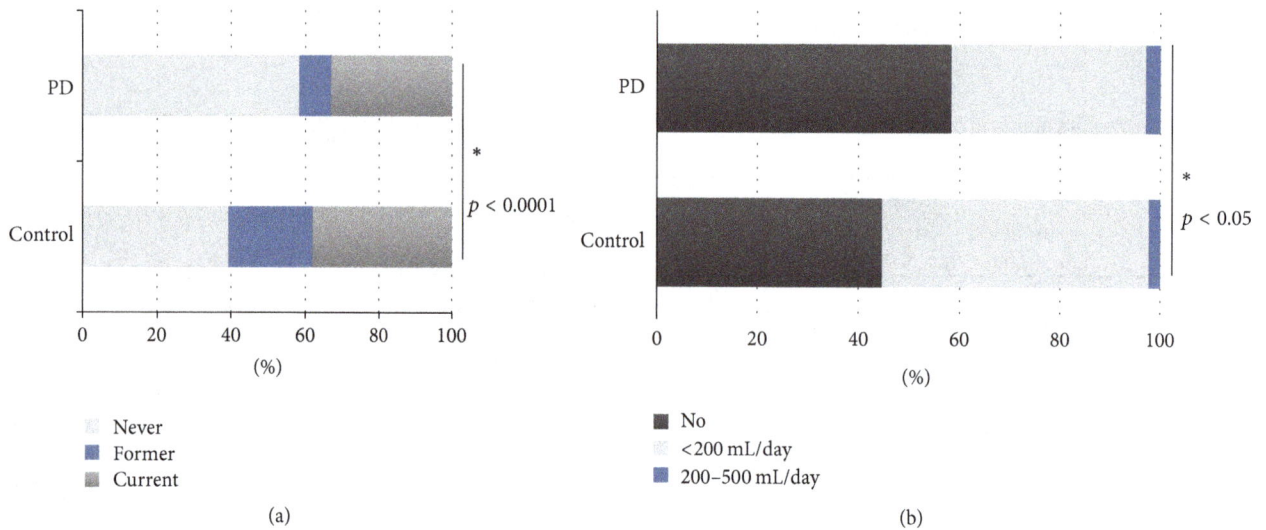

(a)

(b)

Factors	OR	p
Non-current-smoker	2.16	<0.0001
Alcohol nonconsumer	1.73	<0.001

(c)

FIGURE 3: (a) Smoking status in the two groups. (b) Alcohol consumption in the two groups. (c) OR of non-current-smokers and alcohol nonconsumer. ∗ means statistical significance.

former-smokers, and current-smokers were different between the groups ($p < 0.00001$) (data in Table 1, Figure 3(a)). Compared to current-smokers, never-smokers (OR 3.88, 95% CI 2.33–6.45, and $p < 0.0001$) and former-smokers (OR 2.27, 95% CI 1.34–3.84, and $p < 0.05$) resulted in having an increased risk of PD. Based on these data, the condition of non-current-smoker may, thus, represent a risk factor for PD (OR 2.16, 95% CI 1.56–2.99, and $p < 0.0001$) (Figure 3(c)). Also in alcohol consumption PD patients and controls behave differently ($p < 0.05$, data in Table 1,

Figure 3(b)). We calculated that consuming alcohol may have a protective effect on PD onset (OR 0.65, 95% CI 0.48–0.87, and $p < 0.05$). Therefore, the condition of nonconsumer could imply a risk for PD (OR 1.73, 95% CI 1.26–2.39, and $p < 0.001$) (Figure 3(c)).

3.5. Risk Combination. We identified four solid risk factors for PD (positive family history, toxicants exposure, non-current-smoker status, nonconsumer of alcohol) that can be variably expressed, singularly or in association, in each

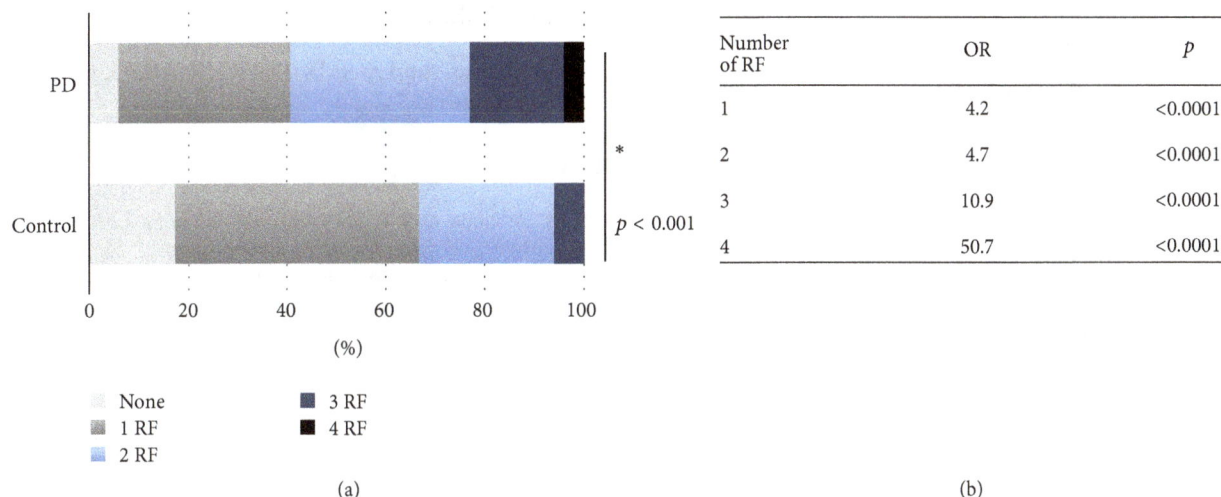

FIGURE 4: (a) Distribution of the number of concurrent risk factors (RF) in the two groups. (b) OR calculated for number of concurrent risk factors. * means statistical significance.

individual. Therefore, we calculated the number of risk factors present in each subject. In the PD group we observed 6% with no risk factors, 34.7% exhibiting one risk factor, 36.3% presenting two risk factors, 19% with three risk factors, and 4% with four risk factors. Conversely, in controls 17.3% had no risk factor, 49.3% had one risk factor, 27.3% had two risk factors, 6% had three risk factors, and none exhibited all four risk factors ($p < 0.001$) (Figure 4(a)). Binomial logistic regression demonstrated that the number of concurrent risk factors significantly predicts PD. Indeed, we measured that the presence of one factor has OR 4.22, 95% CI 2.36–7.55, and $p < 0.00001$; two factors OR 4.75, 95% CI 2.65–8.49, and $p < 0.00001$; three factors OR 10.94, 95% CI 5.37–22.28, and $p < 0.00001$; four factors OR 50.67, 95% CI 6.18–415.29, and $p < 0.00001$ (Figure 4(b)). These findings thus suggest that combination of three to four risk factors determines a statistically significant increase in the risk of developing PD.

3.6. Metal Serum Levels. By using the ICP-MS, we measured in the PD group a mean ± SD concentration of 926.04 ± 444.91 microg/L for iron, of 981.32 ± 273.56 microg/L for copper, of 28 ± 21 microg/L for mercury, and of 3.43 ± 1.77 microg/L for manganese. Instead, in the control group we detected a mean ± SD concentration of 965.39 ± 627.54 microg/L for iron, of 1061.11 ± 423.77 microg/L for copper, of 48 ± 33 microg/L for mercury, and of 1.78 ± 0.71 microg/L for manganese. Although the mean manganese concentration was higher in PD, the distribution of all the values was not normal. The Mann-Whitney U test excluded significant differences in the metals serum levels between the two groups and, accordingly, the ROC curve analysis failed to provide significant results. Therefore, in our population we did not observe relevant differences in the blood levels of iron, copper, mercury, and manganese excluding their function as toxicants exposure indexes or PD-risk factors. Indeed, it is likely that a remote exposure does not change the present

blood concentration of metals. However, it should be reminded that, because of either the biological variability of the elements or the variety of biochemical assays, the scientific literature did not yet provide univocal data on metals serum concentrations in PD [18].

4. Discussion

The results of this case-control study allow a clear and consistent PD-risk stratification based on pure anamnestic information obtained by counting the number of concurrent PD-risk factors.

As first step, we screened a large urban Italian population for few PD-risk factors. In agreement with previous reports, we confirmed the importance of a positive family history (OR 4.852) in the pathogenesis of PD [5, 6, 9]. Also the toxicants exposure (OR 1.646) has proven being PD-risk factor [9, 25], particularly when it occurs in subjects with a familiar predisposition (OR 4.383), supporting the well-established "double hit" pathogenic hypothesis [5, 26, 27]. In our population, the occupational exposure exceeds environmental exposure and represents a significant risk factor (OR 1.438). Although some professional categories have been historically considered at risk of PD (farmer, welder) [9, 25, 28], in our study we did not find a particularly dangerous occupation. However, we noticed that people working in constructions and mechanicals handle more frequently toxicants, which essentially consist in chemical products or metals. Regarding environmental exposure, in our geographical area the air pollution is a relevant matter [29] which acts as a source of multiple toxicants, including metals and chemicals, implicated in triggering the neurodegenerative diseases [30, 31]. Unfortunately, here we did not examine the eating habits and the taking of industrially derived foods, which may similarly contain traces of toxicants or abnormal concentrations of metals and minerals. However, since both the environmental pollution and nutrition can modify physiological body levels of metals [16, 20–23], we measured serum concentration of iron, copper, mercury, and manganese as indexes of environmental toxicants exposure, but we did not find significant differences between PD and controls.

The personal habits, such as smoking status and alcohol consumption, have been extensively studied in relation to the PD-risk. Specifically, regarding smoking, it has been demonstrated either that smokers have a lower prevalence of PD or that quitting smoking could represent a potential early nonmotor feature of PD [6, 9, 11, 32–34]. The evaluation of the smoking status in our population measured a consistent PD-risk for the non-current-smokers (OR 2.16). Instead, with regard to the alcohol consumption, several meta-analyses, despite many confounding factors, have reported an inverse correlation between alcohol intake and PD-risk [25, 35, 36]. Also in our case, we observed that PD patients are less prone to alcohol consumption, and coherently the nonconsumers have a significant PD-risk (OR 1.73).

Each of these four risk factors (positive family history, toxicants exposure, non-current-smoker, alcohol nonconsumer) has its own "risk power," the greatest belonging to the positive family history. However, many factors frequently overlap in the same person, increasing the PD-risk in direct proportion to their number. Precisely, we reported that in the presence of three or four of the mentioned risk factors, subjects are highly "at risk" of PD (resp., OR 10.94, OR 50.67). Our data thus suggest that it is possible to stratify the PD-risk by means of the recognition of the concurrent risk factors, allowing an early identification of populations "at risk" of PD. Currently, the adopted inclusion criteria for PD neuroprotective trials are idiopathic RBD (REM Behavior Disorder) and anosmia, which could both precede other neurodegenerative diseases and already underlie a neurodegeneration, inducing erroneous patients selection. [37–41]. Conversely, we profiled a simple PD-risk stratification, applicable to the general population, in order to select a group suitable for PD "primary prevention," as it has been commonly done with cardiovascular diseases. In fact, primary prevention in PD could be directed towards the external modifiable risk factors, as occupational toxicants exposure or environmental pollutants. Alternatively, other behaviors inversely associated with PD-risk and thus useful as primary preventive strategies are physical exercise [42], drinking green tea [43], and eating vitamins-rich aliment [16].

5. Conclusions

Simple and early stratification of PD-risk, helpful in identifying subjects suitable for neuroprotective strategies, can be achieved by counting the number of the main PD-risk factors (positive family history, toxicants exposure, non-current-smoker, and alcohol nonconsumer).

Acknowledgments

This work was supported by INAIL (INAIL G21-2/2009 to Antonio Pisani).

References

[1] D. Athauda and T. Foltynie, "The ongoing pursuit of neuroprotective therapies in Parkinson disease," *Nature Reviews Neurology*, vol. 11, no. 1, pp. 25–40, 2015.

[2] A. H. V. Schapira, C. W. Olanow, J. T. Greenamyre, and E. Bezard, "Slowing of neurodegeneration in Parkinson's disease and Huntington's disease: future therapeutic perspectives," *The Lancet*, vol. 384, no. 9942, pp. 545–555, 2014.

[3] F. Stocchi, "Therapy for Parkinson's disease: what is in the pipeline?" *Neurotherapeutics*, vol. 11, no. 1, pp. 24–33, 2014.

[4] J. Trinh and M. Farrer, "Advances in the genetics of Parkinson disease," *Nature Reviews Neurology*, vol. 9, no. 8, pp. 445–454, 2013.

[5] T. Kitada, J. J. Tomlinson, H. S. Ao, D. A. Grimes, and M. G. Schlossmacher, "Considerations regarding the etiology and future treatment of autosomal recessive versus idiopathic parkinson disease," *Current Treatment Options in Neurology*, vol. 14, no. 3, pp. 230–240, 2012.

[6] C. M. Tanner, "Advances in environmental epidemiology," *Movement Disorders*, vol. 25, supplement 1, pp. S58–S62, 2010.

[7] S. Petrucci, F. Consoli, and E. M. Valente, "Parkinson disease genetics: a 'continuum' from mendelian to multifactorial inheritance," *Current Molecular Medicine*, vol. 14, no. 8, pp. 1079–1088, 2014.

[8] P. De Rosa, E. S. Marini, V. Gelmetti, and E. M. Valente, "Candidate genes for Parkinson disease: lessons from pathogenesis," *Clinica Chimica Acta*, vol. 449, pp. 68–76, 2015.

[9] A. J. Noyce, A. J. Lees, and A. Schrag, "The prediagnostic phase of Parkinson's disease," *Journal of Neurology, Neurosurgery & Psychiatry*, vol. 87, no. 8, pp. 871–878, 2016.

[10] I. Litvan, P. S. J. Lees, C. R. Cunningham et al., "Environmental and occupational risk factors for progressive supranuclear palsy: Case-Control Study," *Movement Disorders*, vol. 31, no. 5, pp. 644–652, 2016.

[11] M. Moccia, R. Erro, M. Picillo et al., "Quitting smoking: an early non-motor feature of Parkinson's disease?" *Parkinsonism and Related Disorders*, vol. 21, no. 3, pp. 216–220, 2015.

[12] A. T. Jan, M. Azam, K. Siddiqui, A. Ali, I. Choi, and Q. M. R. Haq, "Heavy metals and human health: mechanistic insight into toxicity and counter defense system of antioxidants," *International Journal of Molecular Sciences*, vol. 16, no. 12, pp. 29592–29630, 2015.

[13] R. J. Ward, F. A. Zucca, J. H. Duyn, R. R. Crichton, and L. Zecca, "The role of iron in brain ageing and neurodegenerative disorders," *The Lancet Neurology*, vol. 13, no. 10, pp. 1045–1060, 2014.

[14] K. M. Davies, J. F. Mercer, N. Chen, and K. L. Double, "Copper dyshomoeostasis in Parkinson's disease: implications for pathogenesis and indications for novel therapeutics," *Clinical Science*, vol. 130, no. 8, pp. 565–574, 2016.

[15] S. Bouabid, A. Tinakoua, N. Lakhdar-Ghazal, and A. Benazzouz, "Manganese neurotoxicity: behavioral disorders associated with dysfunctions in the basal ganglia and neurochemical transmission," *Journal of Neurochemistry*, vol. 136, no. 4, pp. 677–691, 2016.

[16] Z. S. Agim and J. R. Cannon, "Dietary factors in the etiology of Parkinson's disease," *BioMed Research International*, vol. 2015, Article ID 672838, 16 pages, 2015.

[17] M. Chin-Chan, J. Navarro-Yepes, and B. Quintanilla-Vega, "Environmental pollutants as risk factors for neurodegenerative disorders: Alzheimer and Parkinson diseases," *Frontiers in Cellular Neuroscience*, vol. 9, article A124, 2015.

[18] H. W. Zhao, J. Lin, X. B. Wang et al., "Assessing plasma levels of selenium, copper, iron and zinc in patients of Parkinson's disease," *PLoS ONE*, vol. 8, no. 12, Article ID e83060, 2013.

[19] S. S. S. J. Ahmed and W. Santosh, "Metallomic profiling and linkage map analysis of early Parkinson's disease: a new insight to aluminum marker for the possible diagnosis," *PLoS ONE*, vol. 5, no. 6, Article ID e11252, 2010.

[20] S. Casjens, J. Henry, H.-P. Rihs et al., "Influence of welding fume on systemic iron status," *Annals of Occupational Hygiene*, vol. 58, no. 9, pp. 1143–1154, 2014.

[21] T. Fukushima, X. Tan, Y. Luo, and H. Kanda, "Relationship between blood levels of heavy metals and Parkinson's disease in China," *Neuroepidemiology*, vol. 34, no. 1, pp. 18–24, 2010.

[22] G. Logroscino, X. Gao, H. Chen, A. Wing, and A. Ascherio, "Dietary iron intake and risk of Parkinson's disease," *American Journal of Epidemiology*, vol. 168, no. 12, pp. 1381–1388, 2008.

[23] J. Hagemeier, O. Tong, M. G. Dwyer, F. Schweser, M. Ramanathan, and R. Zivadinov, "Effects of diet on brain iron levels among healthy individuals: an MRI pilot study," *Neurobiology of Aging*, vol. 36, no. 4, pp. 1678–1685, 2015.

[24] T. Konz, J. Alonso-García, M. Montes-Bayón, and A. Sanz-Medel, "Comparison of copper labeling followed by liquid chromatography-inductively coupled plasma mass spectrometry and immunochemical assays for serum hepcidin-25 determination," *Analytica Chimica Acta*, vol. 799, pp. 1–7, 2013.

[25] A. J. Noyce, J. P. Bestwick, L. Silveira-Moriyama et al., "Meta-analysis of early nonmotor features and risk factors for Parkinson disease," *Annals of Neurology*, vol. 72, no. 6, pp. 893–901, 2012.

[26] J. R. Cannon and J. T. Greenamyre, "Gene-environment interactions in Parkinson's disease: specific evidence in humans and mammalian models," *Neurobiology of Disease*, vol. 57, pp. 38–46, 2013.

[27] G. Martella, G. Madeo, M. Maltese et al., "Exposure to low-dose rotenone precipitates synaptic plasticity alterations in PINK1 heterozygous knockout mice," *Neurobiology of Disease*, vol. 91, pp. 21–36, 2016.

[28] M. van der Mark, R. Vermeulen, P. C. G. Nijssen et al., "Occupational exposure to solvents, metals and welding fumes and risk of Parkinson's disease," *Parkinsonism and Related Disorders*, vol. 21, no. 6, pp. 635–639, 2015.

[29] http://www.arpalazio.gov.it/.

[30] S. Levesque, M. J. Surace, J. McDonald, and M. L. Block, "Air pollution and the brain: subchronic diesel exhaust exposure causes neuroinflammation and elevates early markers of neurodegenerative disease," *Journal of Neuroinflammation*, vol. 8, article 105, 2011.

[31] C. L. Mumaw, S. Levesque, C. McGraw et al., "Microglial priming through the lung-brain axis: the role of air pollution-induced circulating factors," *The FASEB Journal*, vol. 30, no. 5, pp. 1880–1891, 2016.

[32] X. Li, W. Li, G. Liu, X. Shen, and Y. Tang, "Association between cigarette smoking and Parkinson's disease: a meta-analysis," *Archives of Gerontology and Geriatrics*, vol. 61, no. 3, pp. 510–516, 2015.

[33] F. Cicchetti, J. Drouin-Ouellet, and R. E. Gross, "Environmental toxins and Parkinson's disease: what have we learned from pesticide-induced animal models?" *Trends in Pharmacological Sciences*, vol. 30, no. 9, pp. 475–483, 2009.

[34] C. M. Tanner, S. M. Goldman, D. A. Aston et al., "Smoking and Parkinson's disease in twins," *Neurology*, vol. 58, no. 4, pp. 581–588, 2002.

[35] L. Ishihara and C. Brayne, "A systematic review of nutritional risk factors of Parkinson's disease," *Nutrition Research Reviews*, vol. 18, no. 2, pp. 259–282, 2005.

[36] S. S. Bettiol, T. C. Rose, C. J. Hughes, and L. A. Smith, "Alcohol consumption and Parkinson's disease risk: a review of recent findings," *Journal of Parkinson's Disease*, vol. 5, no. 3, pp. 425–442, 2015.

[37] A. Iranzo, J. L. Molinuevo, J. Santamaría et al., "Rapid-eye-movement sleep behaviour disorder as an early marker for a neurodegenerative disorder: a descriptive study," *Lancet Neurology*, vol. 5, no. 7, pp. 572–577, 2006.

[38] R. B. Postuma, A. Iranzo, B. Hogl et al., "Risk factors for neurodegeneration in idiopathic rapid eye movement sleep behavior disorder: a multicenter study," *Annals of Neurology*, vol. 77, no. 5, pp. 830–839, 2015.

[39] P. Mahlknecht, A. Iranzo, B. Högl et al., "Olfactory dysfunction predicts early transition to a Lewy body disease in idiopathic RBD," *Neurology*, vol. 84, no. 7, pp. 654–658, 2015.

[40] R. B. Postuma, J.-F. Gagnon, J.-A. Bertrand, D. Génier Marchand, and J. Y. Montplaisir, "Parkinson risk in idiopathic REM sleep behavior disorder: preparing for neuroprotective trials," *Neurology*, vol. 84, no. 11, pp. 1104–1113, 2015.

[41] Y. K. Kim, I.-Y. Yoon, J.-M. Kim et al., "The implication of nigrostriatal dopaminergic degeneration in the pathogenesis of REM sleep behavior disorder," *European Journal of Neurology*, vol. 17, no. 3, pp. 487–492, 2010.

[42] T. Paillard, Y. Rolland, and P. S. de Barreto, "Protective effects of physical exercise in Alzheimer's disease and Parkinson's disease: a narrative review," *Journal of Clinical Neurology*, vol. 11, no. 3, pp. 212–219, 2015.

[43] M. Caruana and N. Vassallo, "Tea polyphenols in Parkinson's disease," in *Natural Compounds as Therapeutic Agents for Amyloidogenic Diseases*, N. Vassallo, Ed., vol. 863 of *Advances in Experimental Medicine and Biology*, pp. 117–137, Springer, Berlin, Germany, 2015.

29

Phosphorylated α-Synuclein-Copper Complex Formation in the Pathogenesis of Parkinson's Disease

Juan Antonio Castillo-Gonzalez,[1] Maria De Jesus Loera-Arias,[1] Odila Saucedo-Cardenas,[1,2] Roberto Montes-de-Oca-Luna,[1] Aracely Garcia-Garcia,[1] and Humberto Rodriguez-Rocha[1]

[1]*Departamento de Histologia, Facultad de Medicina, Universidad Autonoma de Nuevo Leon, 64460 Monterrey, NL, Mexico*
[2]*Centro de Investigaciones Biomedicas del Noreste, Monterrey, NL, Mexico*

Correspondence should be addressed to Humberto Rodriguez-Rocha; humberto.rodriguezrc@uanl.edu.mx

Academic Editor: Jan Aasly

Parkinson's disease is the second most important neurodegenerative disorder worldwide. It is characterized by the presence of Lewy bodies, which are mainly composed of α-synuclein and ubiquitin-bound proteins. Both the ubiquitin proteasome system (UPS) and autophagy-lysosomal pathway (ALS) are altered in Parkinson's disease, leading to aggregation of proteins, particularly α-synuclein. Interestingly, it has been observed that copper promotes the protein aggregation process. Additionally, phosphorylation of α-synuclein along with copper also affects the protein aggregation process. The interrelation among α-synuclein phosphorylation and its capability to interact with copper, with the subsequent disruption of the protein degradation systems in the neurodegenerative process of Parkinson's disease, will be analyzed in detail in this review.

1. Introduction

Parkinson's disease (PD) is the second most frequent neurodegenerative disorder related to aging worldwide [1]. The clinical symptoms of this disease are resting tremor, rigidity, bradykinesia, akinesia, postural instability, difficulty in speech, and breathing problems [2]. Most PD cases appear to be sporadic, and only about 5–10% of the cases are due to genetic mutations [3]. Exposure to environmental pollutants such as herbicides (paraquat), pesticides (rotenone), and toxic substances during the manufacture of narcotic drugs ($MPTP^+$) and prolonged exposure to transition metals have been reported to be related to sporadic cases of PD [4–6]. PD is characterized by dopaminergic neuronal loss in the substantia nigra at the central nervous system (CNS), a significant reduction in dopamine levels, and the presence of Lewy bodies [7, 8]. Lewy bodies are composed of abnormal deposits of protein aggregates, particularly α-synuclein and ubiquitin-bound proteins [9]. Abnormal protein aggregation results from the UPS and ALS alteration, and the latter

includes disruption of lysosomal hydrolase trafficking [10–12]. Interestingly, some metal ions such as copper have shown to promote the protein aggregation process [13–15]. Additionally, phosphorylation of α-synuclein, along with copper, accelerates the protein aggregation process [16, 17].

Therefore, in order to have a better understanding of the mechanisms involved in the neurodegenerative process of PD, the interrelation among α-synuclein phosphorylation and its capability to interact with copper, as well as the consequent disruption of the protein degradation systems, will be analyzed in detail in this review.

2. α-Synuclein

The main histological hallmark of PD is the presence of eosinophilic cytoplasmic inclusions known as Lewy bodies, which are localized in the substantia nigra and are formed mostly by α-synuclein [18–20]. α-Synuclein is a thermostable, preserved, and unfolded cytosolic protein [21], belonging to a family of homologous proteins called synucleins, and

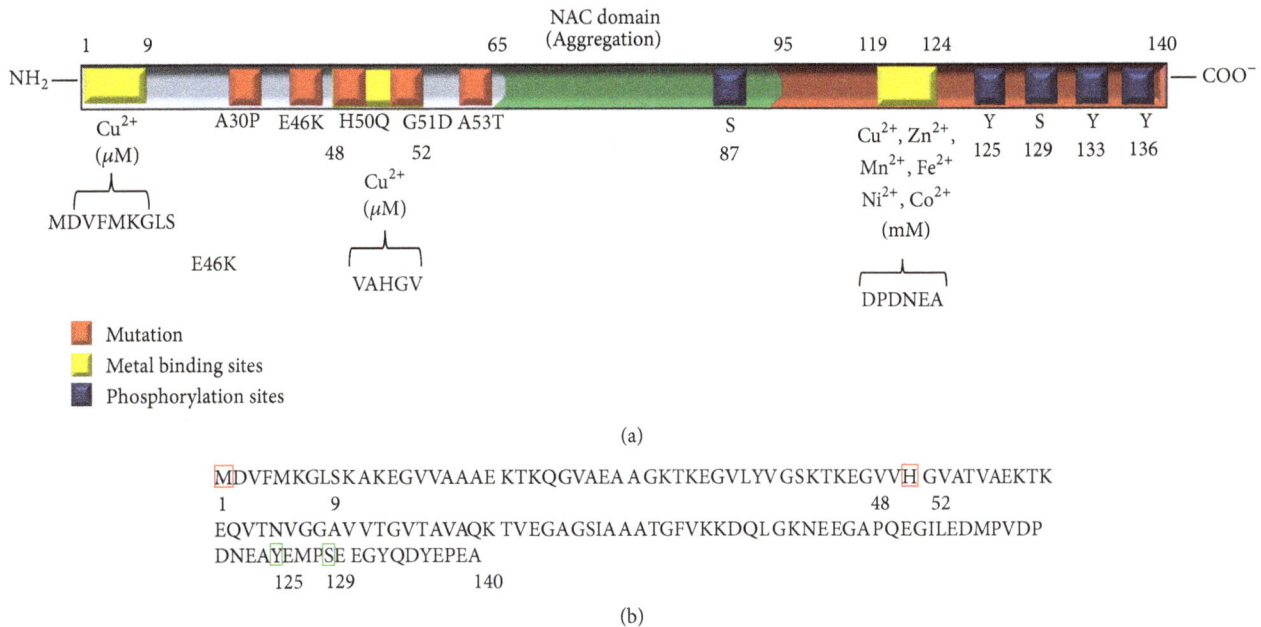

FIGURE 1: *Schematic structure of α-synuclein.* (a) α-Synuclein mutations related to familial PD are shown as red squares. Metal-binding sites are depicted as yellow squares. Seine (S) and threonine (Y) amino acid residues targeted by phosphorylation are indicated as blue squares. (b) Amino acid composition of α-synuclein. Residues in blue represent copper-binding sites. Red squares indicate methionine 1 and histidine 50, which are independent anchoring sites for copper binding. Green squares show phosphorylation sites (Y125 and S129) related to an increased copper-binding capability.

is expressed in approximately 80% of the total area of the human brain [22, 23]. α-Synuclein consists of 140 amino acid residues [24] organized in three structural regions: an amphipathic amino-terminal domain from 1 to 60 amino acid residues, responsible for the binding of α-synuclein to lipid vesicles [25, 26]; the NAC (non-amyloid-β component) region from 61 to 95 amino acid residues, also found in amyloid plaques of patients suffering from Alzheimer's disease [27] and responsible for α-synuclein aggregation and β sheets arrangement [28]; and the carboxy-terminal domain from 96 to 140 amino acid residues, which is the main target for the protein phosphorylation [29, 30] (Figure 1(a)). α-Synuclein is primarily expressed in neurons at cytosolic level and is abundant in presynaptic terminals [31]. However, it has also been linked to synaptic vesicles, plasma membrane lipid rafts and the nucleus [32]. Up to date, the main normal function of α-synuclein has not been well defined. α-Synuclein has been related to different functions, including inhibition of tyrosine hydroxylase [33], inhibition of dopamine release [34], dopamine uptake [35], neural plasticity, synaptic maturation and maintenance [36–38], and v-SNARE complex assembly [39, 40].

α-Synuclein has the capability to assemble into amyloid fibers, soluble oligomers, and/or aggregates. Once the accumulation of α-synuclein surpasses its degradation rate, it leads to the formation of Lewy bodies and the subsequent death of dopaminergic neurons in the substantia nigra [41]. It has been suggested that α-synuclein protofibrils are responsible for the neurotoxic effects induced by α-synuclein [42, 43]. Among the possible mechanisms involved in the neurotoxicity mediated by α-synuclein are the following:

mitochondrial dysfunction, oxidative stress [44], lysosomal leakage [45], cytoskeletal disruption [46], altered axonal transport, and subsequent synapses dysfunction, which are all related to neurodegeneration [47]. α-Synuclein is targeted for degradation by the UPS and the ALS including the chaperone-mediated autophagy (CMA) and macroautophagy (autophagy) [48–51]. Importantly, both degradation pathways are dysregulated or inhibited in PD [52].

The relationship between α-synuclein and PD was established with the identification of specific mutations in the SNCA gene encoding for α-synuclein, in families with PD. The specific mutations identified in α-synuclein were a substitution from alanine to threonine at amino acid residue 53 (A53T), a mutation of Greek origin [53]; a substitution from alanine to proline at amino acid residue 30 (A30P), a mutation of Germanic origin [54]; and a substitution from glutamic acid to lysine at amino acid residue 46 (E46K), a mutation of Spanish origin [55] (Figure 1(a)). Recently, two new mutations have been identified, a substitution from histidine to glutamine at amino acid residue 50 (H50Q) [56] and a substitution from glycine to aspartic acid at amino acid residue 51 (G51D), a mutation of French origin [57]. Additionally, SNCA gene duplication [58] and triplication also occur and are related to PD [59].

3. α-Synuclein Phosphorylation in Parkinson's Disease: Neuroprotective or Neurotoxic?

In the aggregation process of α-synuclein, its phosphorylation plays an important role [29, 60] by directing its localization and interaction [61] and by modifying its secondary

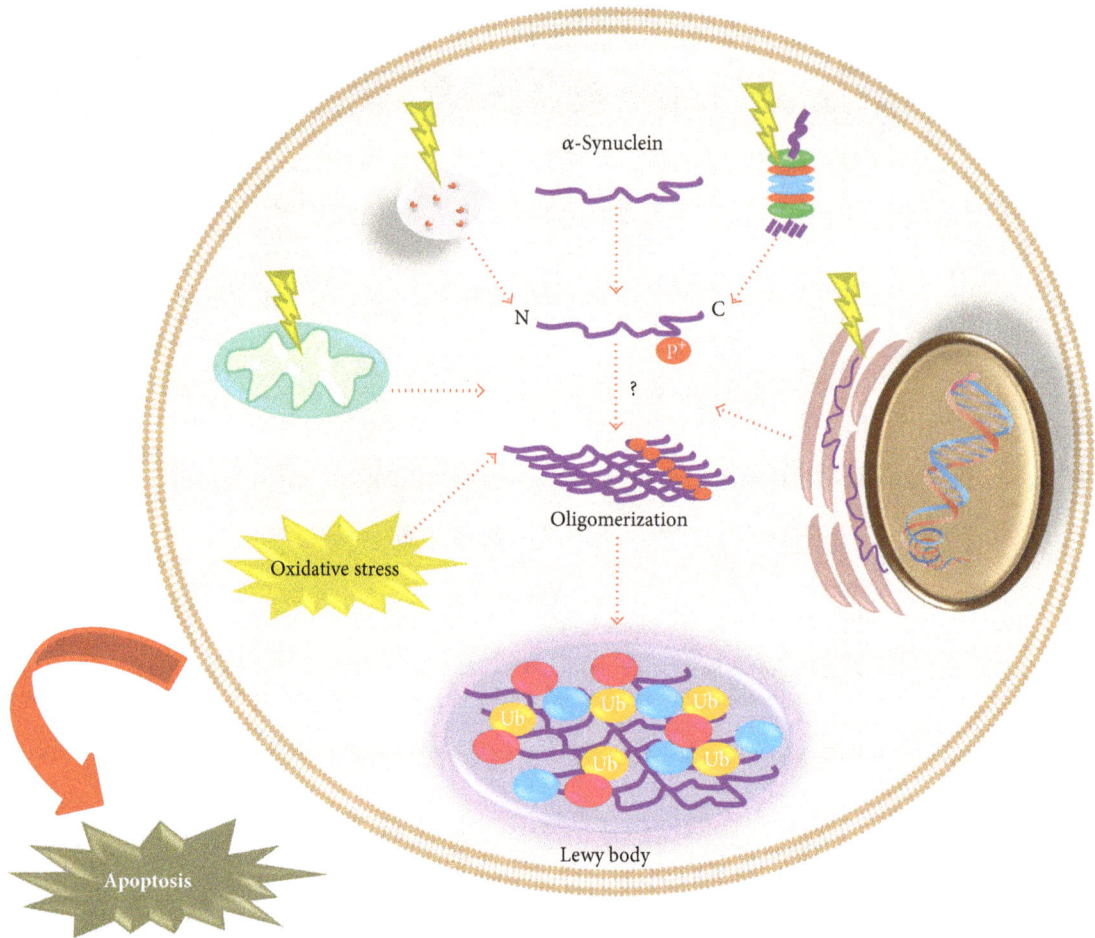

FIGURE 2: *Cell alterations involved in the aggregation process of α-synuclein*. Damaged or unrequired proteins are regulated by both the proteasomal and lysosomal degradation pathways. UPS disruption leads to activation of the ALS and vice versa, as a compensation mechanism. Both mechanisms are affected in PD, which results in protein accumulation including α-synuclein and ubiquitin-bound proteins. Accumulation of unfolded or misfolded proteins into the endoplasmic reticulum activates the unfolded protein response. Mitochondrial dysfunction and oxidative stress are also interrelated and linked to the pathogenesis of PD. All these alterations are associated with the phosphorylation process of α-synuclein and increase α-synuclein oligomerization, leading to Lewy body formation and subsequent apoptotic cell death.

and tertiary conformation [62–65]. α-Synuclein is targeted by phosphorylation on multiple sites located at its carboxy-terminal end (S87, S129, Y125, Y133, and Y136) [66–71] (Figure 1). Several kinases have been linked to α-synuclein phosphorylation, such as casein kinases 1 and 2 (CK1 and CK2), G protein-coupled receptor kinases 2 and 5 (GRK2 and GRK5), polo-like kinase 2 (PLK2) [29, 72, 73], Fyn [74], and more recently serine/threonine protein kinase (LK6) and MAP kinase-interacting kinase 2a (Mnk2a) [75].

Studies performed in cell cultures with neuronal phenotype have demonstrated that CK2-mediated α-synuclein phosphorylation, particularly at S129, increases the appearance of eosinophilic cytoplasmic inclusions resembling the Lewy bodies of PD [76]. A major component of these inclusions consists of C-terminally truncated α-synuclein, and lysosomal proteases, such as cathepsin D, may be involved in its production for α-synuclein oligomerization

[77]. Some mechanisms are triggered by the phosphorylation of α-synuclein, including the unfolded protein response (UPR) and disruption of lysosomal degradation pathways, which may lead to protein aggregation and subsequently to cell death (Figure 2) [78, 79]. Monomers and dimers of α-synuclein are degraded by ALS, specifically, CMA [79, 80]. In addition, it has been reported that a phosphorylated-like mutant version of α-synuclein (S129E), which mimics the biochemical and biophysical properties of α-syn phosphorylation observed in PD patients' brains [76] and remained "phosphorylated-like" after exposure to the lysosomal fraction, cannot translocate across the lysosomal membrane probably because of a conformational change induced by its phosphorylation, decreasing its interaction with the CMA receptor (LAMP-2A) at the lysosomal membrane [79, 80].

In addition, dysfunctional mitochondrial metabolism and increased ROS production are also related to the

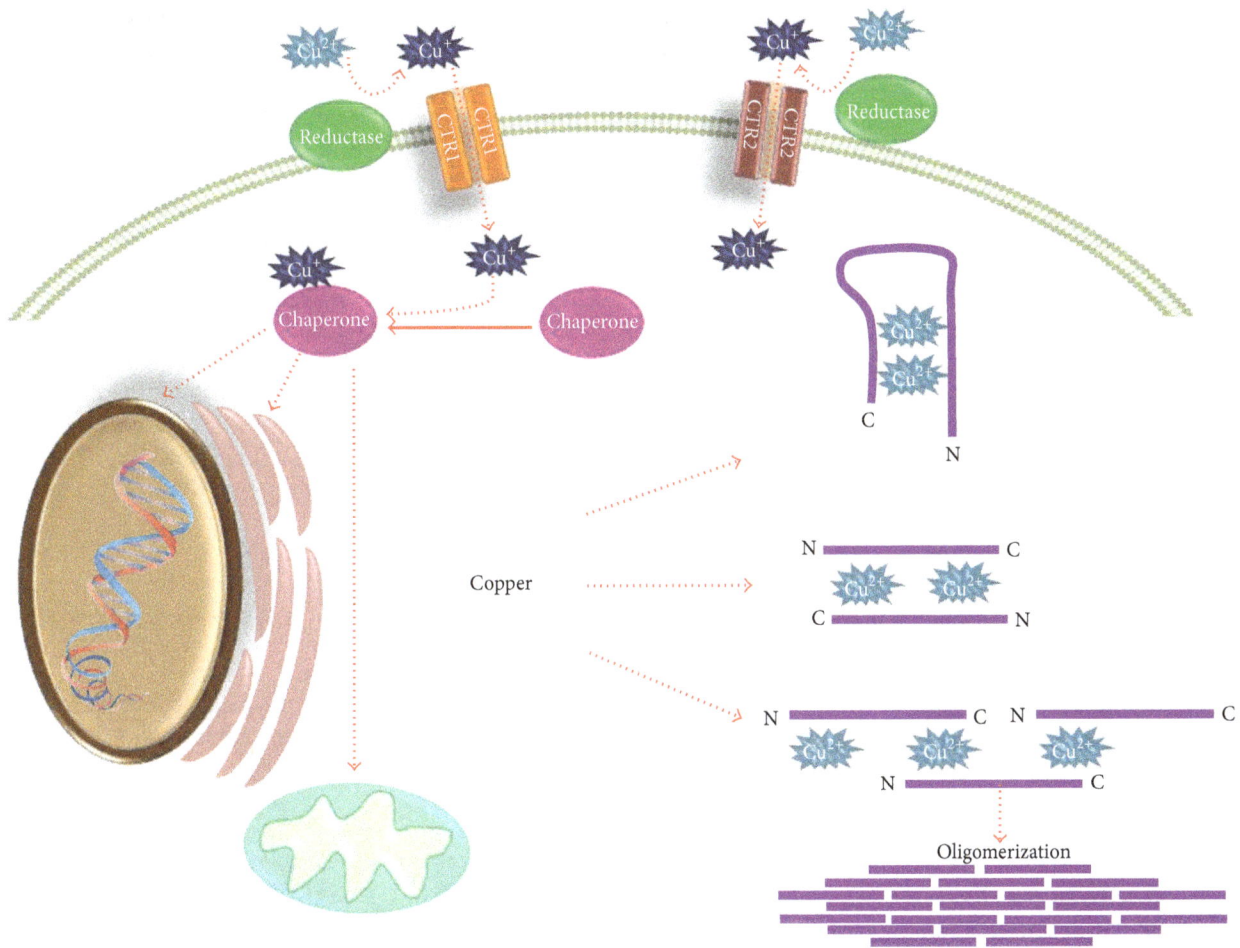

FIGURE 3: *α-Synuclein-copper complex formation process*. Copper can be found in living organisms in both forms, oxidized Cu^{2+} and reduced Cu^+, and enters into the cell as Cu^+ through CTR1 and CTR2. Afterwards, copper is transported to the nuclei, endoplasmic reticulum, and mitochondria via chaperone proteins. An overload of copper may lead to the α-synuclein-copper complex formation by three potential mechanisms. In the first one, a single α-synuclein molecule binds to Cu^{2+}, folding and bringing together the amino and carboxy-terminal ends. The second mechanism involves two molecules of α-synuclein with a head-to-tail arrangement, generating a copper-binding site at both ends. In the third mechanism, the carboxy-terminal region of one molecule of α-synuclein interacts with the amino-terminal region from another molecule of α-synuclein creating a Cu^{2+} binding site. Next, one of the two α-synucleins interacts with a third α-synuclein molecule, forming a second Cu^{2+} binding site. This process will eventually lead to α-synuclein oligomerization.

phosphorylation of α-synuclein (Figure 3) [81]. Hydrogen peroxide- (H_2O_2-) induced oxidative stress increases the phosphorylation of α-synuclein at S129 and the formation of cytoplasmic inclusions [76]. On the other hand, some neurotoxins and the UPS inhibition increase the activity of GRK5 and CK2, whose interaction with Ca^{2+}/calmodulin increases α-synuclein phosphorylation at S129 [82–84]. Rotenone, an inhibitor of mitochondrial complex I, along with iron, increases the levels of α-synuclein phosphorylation at S129, by inducing ROS production in dopaminergic cells [81].

So far, the role of α-synuclein phosphorylation is controversial. Some studies have shown a neuroprotective role of α-synuclein phosphorylation at S129 by preventing the binding of α-synuclein oligomers to membranes and, therefore, cellular disruption [85–88]. Additionally, phosphorylation at S129 blocked α-synuclein fibrillation *in vitro* [89]. Many studies had focused on the role of α-synuclein phosphorylation,

specifically at S129, and also at other residues such as S87. α-Synuclein mutant variants, capable of mimicking or inhibiting the phosphorylation process (S129D, S129E, and S129A), have contributed to the elucidation of its role [66, 70, 89–92]. Phosphomimic mutants S129D/E were not able to reproduce *in vitro* the structural and aggregation properties of α-synuclein. However, a nonphosphomimic mutant S129A showed a higher protein aggregation rate and neurotoxicity than the wild type form [70, 71, 89].

On the contrary, there is evidence showing that α-synuclein phosphorylation at S129 induces cytotoxicity [66, 77, 93, 94]. It has been demonstrated that α-synuclein phosphorylation at S129 mediated by CK2 is an important factor for its protein aggregation and toxicity, inducing UPR dysregulation, endoplasmic reticulum (ER) stress, and apoptosis [78]. Besides, phosphorylation at S129 is essential for interaction of α-synuclein with synphilin-1 and parkin, which form the ubiquitinated inclusions [76]. Recently, it has been reported that α-synuclein can also be phosphorylated by LK6 and Mnk2a, with subsequent dopaminergic neuronal death and formation of cytoplasmic inclusions, respectively [75]. Nonetheless, it has been suggested that malfunction of the UPS increases CK2 activity, resulting in hyperphosphorylation of the α-synuclein at S129 [95].

Approximately 90% of α-synuclein detected in Lewy bodies from postmortem PD samples is phosphorylated at S129. Conversely, only 4% of α-synuclein present in normal brains is phosphorylated [66, 70, 96, 97]. Importantly, a mass spectrometry study in human cerebrospinal fluid (CSF) of PD and other parkinsonian disorders determined a significantly higher concentration of phosphorylated α-synuclein at S129, as well as a significant increase in the ratio of phosphorylated α-synuclein at S129/total α-synuclein in PD compared to healthy controls [98]. More recently, a marked difference between PD patients and healthy controls was observed with a sensitive and specific Elisa test, by combining measurements of total, oligomeric, and phosphorylated (S129) α-synuclein in CSF [99].

4. Interaction of Phosphorylated α-Synuclein with Metal Ions

Proteins are the main biomolecules affected in most pathologies; posttranslational modifications of proteins suchlike oxidation, nitration, carbonylation, glutathionylation, and phosphorylation are related to protein inactivation. Phosphorylated proteins have a strong binding affinity to certain metals [16, 100, 101]. Multivalent metal ions, like manganese, cobalt, iron, and mainly aluminum and copper, increase α-synuclein fibril formation by inducing conformational changes [14, 102, 103]. α-Synuclein may interact with different metal ions at either its carboxy-terminal domain or its amino-terminal domain, depending on the metal ion concentration [13]. For instance, at low concentrations (40–100 μM) Cu^{2+} ion binds to the amino-terminal domain [13, 104], while at extremely high concentrations (0.5–5 mM), which are unlikely to occur in tissues, metal ions such as Fe^{2+}, Mn^{2+}, Ni^{2+}, Co^{2+}, and Cu^{2+} bind to the carboxy-terminal domain [105]. Cu^{2+} ion is a potent inducer and accelerator of α-synuclein aggregation, linked to the carboxy-terminal domain, which is required for its oligomerization [106]. Phosphorylation at both Y125 and S129 residues of α-synuclein, which are close to metal-binding sites, increments Cu^{2+}, Pb^{2+}, and Fe^{2+} binding capability to carboxy-terminal domain (Figure 1) [17, 105].

5. Copper Mediates α-Synuclein Aggregation

On the other hand, copper has the ability to inhibit the proteasomal chymotrypsin-like peptidase activity [107]. Copper enters into the cell through the copper transporters 1 and 2 (CTR1 and CTR2), which are located on the cell membrane (Figure 3) [108]. Two regions, [1]MDVFMKGLS[9] and [48]VVHGV[52] (Figure 1), with high-affinity binding sites for copper were identified at α-synuclein, and may be of

great biological importance in the pathogenesis of PD [104]. Within the α-synuclein sequence, methionine 1 and histidine 50 residues function as independent anchoring sites for copper binding (Figure 1) [104, 109, 110].

There are three models that have been suggested for copper binding to α-synuclein (Figure 3). In the first model, a single α-synuclein molecule binds to Cu^{2+}, folding and bringing together the amino and carboxy-terminal regions. The second model involves two molecules of α-synuclein with a head-to-tail arrangement, generating a copper-binding site at both ends. In the third model, α-synuclein oligomerization takes place by interaction of the carboxy-terminal region of one molecule of α-synuclein with the amino-terminal region from a second molecule of α-synuclein originating a Cu^{2+} binding site; then a second Cu^{2+} binding site is formed by interaction of one of the two α-synucleins with a third α-synuclein molecule [15].

Regarding the aggregation process of α-synuclein mediated by copper, two mechanisms have been proposed. In one of them, high levels of α-synuclein-copper complexes will cause instability of intramolecular interactions leading to self-assembling of α-synuclein into fibrillar complexes. In the second one, copper redox-mediated reactions induce oxidation of α-synuclein using electron donors (NADH, NADPH, glutathione, etc.), causing its oligomerization and precipitation [111–114].

Environmental exposure to metal ions (e.g., zinc and copper) induces α-synuclein aggregates and oxidative stress, which are also associated with dysregulation of the UPS in PD [82, 115, 116].

Copper plays a dual role in the neurotoxic effect of α-synuclein. Once intracellular copper concentration is raised, chaperone proteins (e.g., ATOX1, CCS, MT3, and COX17) are in charge to uptake this metal inside the cell, but an overload of copper might surpass the chaperone proteins available to regulate its levels. On the other hand, mutations affecting the ability of chaperones to bind copper might also increase its toxic effect [117]. Subsequently, free copper binds to the UPS to inhibit its activity; then α-synuclein is phosphorylated increasing its affinity to metals [71]. α-Synuclein-copper complex formation alters cell redox signaling, which results in ROS formation including H_2O_2. H_2O_2 oxidizes dopamine, which is toxic to dopaminergic neurons [118, 119].

6. Concluding Remarks

α-Synuclein is a highly relevant protein in PD etiopathology, and since the elucidation of α-synuclein-copper interactions, this transition metal was brought into the spotlight of neurodegeneration research. Although this complex formation is now subject of intense research, many open questions remain: How are levels of copper regulated by α-synuclein? Does copper influence α-synuclein phosphorylation and aggregation? How important is copper and α-synuclein interaction? Can we use phosphorylation of α-synuclein as a biomarker? Can we exploit the inhibition of phosphorylation of α-synuclein as a therapeutic approach? It is certain, that these therapies need to initiate promptly in order to address pathological changes in a less advanced stage. Regrettably, the diagnosis of PD nowadays is based on purely clinical signs, and these signs are manifested when more than half of dopaminergic neurons have died. Therefore, identification of early biomarkers such as α-synuclein phosphorylation may be a promising approach for diagnosis and subsequently for PD treatment and correlated with preclinical signs indicating incipient disease at a nonsymptomatic stage. Since α-synuclein and copper play such important roles in the aggregation process, a chelator administration is currently under investigation and may be a helpful approach against PD.

Acknowledgments

This work was supported by the National Council of Science and Technology (CONACYT) CB-2013-221615 (Aracely Garcia-Garcia) and Program for the Professional Development of the Professors (PRODEP) DSA/103.5/14/11175 (Humberto Rodriguez-Rocha). Juan Antonio Castillo-Gonzalez received a scholarship from CONACYT.

References

[1] K. Wirdefeldt, H. Adami, P. Cole, D. Trichopoulos, and J. Mandel, "Epidemiology and etiology of Parkinson's disease: a review of the evidence," *European Journal of Epidemiology*, vol. 26, supplement 1, pp. S1–S58, 2011.

[2] L. S. Forno, "Neuropathology of Parkinson's disease," *Journal of Neuropathology & Experimental Neurology*, vol. 55, no. 3, pp. 259–272, 1996.

[3] S. Lesage and A. Brice, "Parkinson's disease: from monogenic forms to genetic susceptibility factors," *Human Molecular Genetics*, vol. 18, no. R1, pp. R48–R59, 2009.

[4] B. C. L. Lai, S. A. Marion, K. Teschke, and J. K. C. Tsui, "Occupational and environmental risk factors for Parkinson's disease," *Parkinsonism & Related Disorders*, vol. 8, no. 5, pp. 297–309, 2002.

[5] J. Peng, L. Peng, F. F. Stevenson, S. R. Doctrow, and J. K. Andersen, "Iron and paraquat as synergistic environmental risk factors in sporadic Parkinson's disease accelerate age-related neurodegeneration," *The Journal of Neuroscience*, vol. 27, no. 26, pp. 6914–6922, 2007.

[6] K. Opeskin and R. M. Anderson, "Suspected MPTP-induced parkinsonism," *Journal of Clinical Neuroscience*, vol. 4, no. 3, pp. 366–370, 1997.

[7] C. W. Shults, "Lewy bodies," *Proceedings of the National Acadamy of Sciences of the United States of America*, vol. 103, no. 6, pp. 1661–1668, 2006.

[8] O. Hornykiewicz, "The discovery of dopamine deficiency in the parkinsonian brain," *Journal of Neural Transmission. Supplementa*, vol. 70, pp. 9–15, 2006.

[9] M. S. Pollanen, D. W. Dickson, and C. Bergeron, "Pathology and biology of the lewy body," *Journal of Neuropathology & Experimental Neurology*, vol. 52, no. 3, pp. 183–191, 1993.

[10] C. Cook, C. Stetler, and L. Petrucelli, "Disruption of protein quality control in Parkinson's disease," *Cold Spring Harbor Perspectives in Medicine*, vol. 2, no. 5, Article ID a009423, 2012.

[11] D. Ebrahimi-Fakhari, L. Wahlster, and P. J. McLean, "Protein degradation pathways in Parkinson's disease: curse or blessing," *Acta Neuropathologica*, vol. 124, no. 2, pp. 153–172, 2012.

[12] J. R. Mazzulli, F. Zunke, O. Isacson, L. Studer, and D. Krainc, "α-Synuclein-induced lysosomal dysfunction occurs through disruptions in protein trafficking in human midbrain synucleinopathy models," *Proceedings of the National Acadamy of Sciences of the United States of America*, vol. 113, no. 7, pp. 1931–1936, 2016.

[13] A. Binolfi, R. M. Rasia, C. W. Bertoncini et al., "Interaction of α-synuclein with divalent metal ions reveals key differences: a link between structure, binding specificity and fibrillation enhancement," *Journal of the American Chemical Society*, vol. 128, no. 30, pp. 9893–9901, 2006.

[14] L. Breydo and V. N. Uversky, "Role of metal ions in aggregation of intrinsically disordered proteins in neurodegenerative diseases," *Metallomics*, vol. 3, no. 11, pp. 1163–1180, 2011.

[15] D. R. Brown, "Metal binding to alpha-synuclein peptides and its contribution to toxicity," *Biochemical and Biophysical Research Communications*, vol. 380, no. 2, pp. 377–381, 2009.

[16] L. L. Liu and K. J. Franz, "Phosphorylation-dependent metal binding by α-synuclein peptide fragments," *Journal of Biological Inorganic Chemistry*, vol. 12, no. 2, pp. 234–247, 2007.

[17] Y. Lu, M. Prudent, B. Fauvet, H. A. Lashuel, and H. H. Girault, "Phosphorylation of α-synuclein at Y125 and S129 alters its metal binding properties: implications for understanding the role of α-synuclein in the pathogenesis of Parkinson's disease and related disorders," *ACS Chemical Neuroscience*, vol. 2, no. 11, pp. 667–675, 2011.

[18] A. J. Hughes, S. E. Daniel, Y. Ben-Shlomo, and A. J. Lees, "The accuracy of diagnosis of parkinsonian syndromes in a specialist movement disorder service," *Brain*, vol. 125, no. 4, pp. 861–870, 2002.

[19] P. T. Kotzbauer, J. Q. Trojanowski, and V. M.-Y. Lee, "Lewy body pathology in Alzheimer's disease," *Journal of Molecular Neuroscience*, vol. 17, no. 2, pp. 225–232, 2001.

[20] M. G. Spillantini, M. L. Schmidt, V. M. Lee, J. Q. Trojanowski, R. Jakes, and M. Goedert, "α-synuclein in Lewy bodies," *Nature*, vol. 388, no. 6645, pp. 839–840, 1997.

[21] M. Goedert, "Alpha-synuclein and neurodegenerative diseases," *Nature Reviews Neuroscience*, vol. 2, no. 7, pp. 492–501, 2001.

[22] E. Rockenstein, L. A. Hansen, M. Mallory, J. Q. Trojanowski, D. Galasko, and E. Masliah, "Altered expression of the synuclein family mRNA in Lewy body and Alzheimer's disease," *Brain Research*, vol. 914, no. 1-2, pp. 48–56, 2001.

[23] R. Jakes, M. G. Spillantini, and M. Goedert, "Identification of two distinct synucleins from human brain," *FEBS Letters*, vol. 345, no. 1, pp. 27–32, 1994.

[24] E. H. Norris, B. I. Giasson, and V. M.-Y. Lee, "α-Synuclein: Normal Function and Role in Neurodegenerative Diseases," *Current Topics in Developmental Biology*, vol. 60, pp. 17–54, 2004.

[25] J. P. Segrest, M. K. Jones, H. De Loof, C. G. Brouillette, Y. V. Venkatachalapathi, and G. M. Anantharamaiah, "The amphipathic helix in the exchangeable apolipoproteins: a review of secondary structure and function," *Journal of Lipid Research*, vol. 33, no. 2, pp. 141–166, 1992.

[26] W. S. Davidson, A. Jonas, D. F. Clayton, and J. M. George, "Stabilization of α-synuclein secondary structure upon binding to synthetic membranes," *The Journal of Biological Chemistry*, vol. 273, no. 16, pp. 9443–9449, 1998.

[27] K. Ueda, H. Fukushima, E. Masliah et al., "Molecular cloning of cDNA encoding an unrecognized component of amyloid in Alzheimer disease," *Proceedings of the National Acadamy of Sciences of the United States of America*, vol. 90, no. 23, pp. 11282–11286, 1993.

[28] A. M. Bodles, D. J. S. Guthrie, B. Greer, and G. Brent Irvine, "Identification of the region of non-Aβ component (NAC) of Alzheimer's disease amyloid responsible for its aggregation and toxicity," *Journal of Neurochemistry*, vol. 78, no. 2, pp. 384–395, 2001.

[29] M. Okochi, J. Walter, A. Koyama et al., "Constitutive phosphorylation of the Parkinson's disease associated α- synuclein," *The Journal of Biological Chemistry*, vol. 275, no. 1, pp. 390–397, 2000.

[30] M. P. Sang, Y. J. Han, T. D. Kim, H. P. Jeon, C.-H. Yang, and J. Kim, "Distinct roles of the N-terminal-binding domain and the C-terminal-solubilizing domain of α-synuclein, a molecular chaperone," *The Journal of Biological Chemistry*, vol. 277, no. 32, pp. 28512–28520, 2002.

[31] D. F. Clayton and J. M. George, "The synucleins: a family of proteins involved in synaptic function, plasticity, neurodegeneration and disease," *Trends in Neurosciences*, vol. 21, no. 6, pp. 249–254, 1998.

[32] M. C. Bennett, "The role of α-synuclein in neurodegenerative diseases," *Pharmacology & Therapeutics*, vol. 105, no. 3, pp. 311–331, 2005.

[33] R. G. Perez, J. C. Waymire, E. Lin, J. J. Liu, F. Guo, and M. J. Zigmond, "A role for alpha-synuclein in the regulation of dopamine biosynthesis," *The Journal of Neuroscience*, vol. 22, pp. 3090–3099, 2002.

[34] K. E. Larsen, Y. Schmitz, M. D. Troyer et al., "α-Synuclein overexpression in PC12 and chromaffin cells impairs catecholamine release by interfering with a late step in exocytosis," *The Journal of Neuroscience*, vol. 26, no. 46, pp. 11915–11922, 2006.

[35] C. Wersinger and A. Sidhu, "Disruption of the interaction of α-synuclein with microtubules enhances cell surface recruitment of the dopamine transporter," *Biochemistry*, vol. 44, no. 41, pp. 13612–13624, 2005.

[36] D. E. Cabin, K. Shimazu, D. Murphy et al., "Synaptic vesicle depletion correlates with attenuated synaptic responses to prolonged repetitive stimulation in mice lacking α-synuclein," *The Journal of Neuroscience*, vol. 22, no. 20, pp. 8797–8807, 2002.

[37] W. Dauer, N. Kholodilov, M. Vila et al., "Resistance of α-synuclein null mice to the parkinsonian neurotoxin MPTP," *Proceedings of the National Acadamy of Sciences of the United States of America*, vol. 99, no. 22, pp. 14524–14529, 2002.

[38] A. Abeliovich, Y. Schmitz, I. Fariñas et al., "Mice lacking α-synuclein display functional deficits in the nigrostriatal dopamine system," *Neuron*, vol. 25, no. 1, pp. 239–252, 2000.

[39] N. M. Bonini and B. I. Giasson, "Snaring the function of α-synuclein," *Cell*, vol. 123, no. 3, pp. 359–361, 2005.

[40] J. Burré, M. Sharma, T. Tsetsenis, V. Buchman, M. R. Etherton, and T. C. Südhof, "α-Synuclein promotes SNARE-complex assembly in vivo and in vitro," *Science*, vol. 329, no. 5999, pp. 1663–1667, 2010.

[41] J. E. Duda, V. M.-Y. Lee, and J. Q. Trojanowski, "Neuropathology of synuclein aggregates: New insights into mechanisms of neurodegenerative diseases," *Journal of Neuroscience Research*, vol. 61, no. 2, pp. 121–127, 2000.

[42] R. A. Fredenburg, C. Rospigliosi, R. K. Meray et al., "The impact of the E46K mutation on the properties of α-synuclein in its monomelic and oligomeric states," *Biochemistry*, vol. 46, no. 24, pp. 7107–7118, 2007.

[43] M. Periquet, T. Fulga, L. Myllykangas, M. G. Schlossmacher, and M. B. Feany, "Aggregated α-synuclein mediates dopaminergic neurotoxicity in vivo," *The Journal of Neuroscience*, vol. 27, no. 12, pp. 3338–3346, 2007.

[44] L. J. Hsu, Y. Sagara, A. Arroyo et al., "alpha-synuclein promotes mitochondrial deficit and oxidative stress," *The American Journal of Pathology*, vol. 157, no. 2, pp. 401–410, 2000.

[45] M. Hashimoto, K. Kawahara, P. Bar-On, E. Rockenstein, L. Crews, and E. Masliah, "The role of α-synuclein assembly and metabolism in the pathogenesis of Lewy body disease," *Journal of Molecular Neuroscience*, vol. 24, no. 3, pp. 343–352, 2004.

[46] M. A. Alim, Q.-L. Ma, K. Takeda et al., "Demonstration of a role for α-synuclein as a functional microtubule-associated protein," *Journal of Alzheimer's Disease*, vol. 6, no. 4, pp. 435–442, 2004.

[47] D. A. Scott, I. Tabarean, Y. Tang, A. Cartier, E. Masliah, and S. Roy, "A pathologic cascade leading to synaptic dysfunction in α-synuclein-induced neurodegeneration," *The Journal of Neuroscience*, vol. 30, no. 24, pp. 8083–8095, 2010.

[48] F. Yang, Y.-P. Yang, C.-J. Mao et al., "Crosstalk between the proteasome system and autophagy in the clearance of α-synuclein," *Acta Pharmacologica Sinica*, vol. 34, no. 5, pp. 674–680, 2013.

[49] Y. Machiya, S. Hara, S. Arawaka et al., "Phosphorylated α-Synuclein at Ser-129 is targeted to the proteasome pathway in a ubiquitin-independent manner," *The Journal of Biological Chemistry*, vol. 285, no. 52, pp. 40732–40744, 2010.

[50] T. Vogiatzi, M. Xilouri, K. Vekrellis, and L. Stefanis, "Wild type α-synuclein is degraded by chaperone-mediated autophagy and macroautophagy in neuronal cells," *The Journal of Biological Chemistry*, vol. 283, no. 35, pp. 23542–23556, 2008.

[51] A. M. Cuervo, L. Stafanis, R. Fredenburg, P. T. Lansbury, and D. Sulzer, "Impaired degradation of mutant α-synuclein by chaperone-mediated autophagy," *Science*, vol. 305, no. 5688, pp. 1292–1295, 2004.

[52] J. L. Webb, B. Ravikumar, J. Atkins, J. N. Skepper, and D. C. Rubinsztein, "α-Synuclein is degraded by both autophagy and the proteasome," *The Journal of Biological Chemistry*, vol. 278, no. 27, pp. 25009–25013, 2003.

[53] M. H. Polymeropoulos, C. Lavedan, E. Leroy et al., "Mutation in the α-synuclein gene identified in families with Parkinson's disease," *Science*, vol. 276, no. 5321, pp. 2045–2047, 1997.

[54] R. Krüger, W. Kuhn, T. Müller et al., "Ala30Pro mutation in the gene encoding α-synuclein in Parkinson's disease," *Nature Genetics*, vol. 18, no. 2, pp. 106–108, 1998.

[55] J. J. Zarranz, J. Alegre, J. C. Gómez-Esteban et al., "The new mutation, E46K, of α-synuclein causes Parkinson and Lewy body dementia," *Annals of Neurology*, vol. 55, no. 2, pp. 164–173, 2004.

[56] S. Appel-Cresswell, C. Vilarino-Guell, M. Encarnacion et al., "Alpha-synuclein p.H50Q, a novel pathogenic mutation for Parkinson's disease," *Movement Disorders*, vol. 28, no. 6, pp. 811–813, 2013.

[57] S. Lesage, M. Anheim, F. Letournel et al., "G51D α-synuclein mutation causes a novel Parkinsonian-pyramidal syndrome," *Annals of Neurology*, vol. 73, no. 4, pp. 459–471, 2013.

[58] M. Chartier-Harlin, J. Kachergus, C. Roumier et al., "α-synuclein locus duplication as a cause of familial Parkinson's disease," *The Lancet*, vol. 364, no. 9440, pp. 1167–1169, 2004.

[59] A. B. Singleton, M. Farrer, J. Johnson et al., "α-synuclein locus triplication causes Parkinson's disease," *Science*, vol. 302, no. 5646, article 841, 2003.

[60] J. P. Anderson, D. E. Walker, J. M. Goldstein et al., "Phosphorylation of Ser-129 is the dominant pathological modification of α-synuclein in familial and sporadic lewy body disease," *The Journal of Biological Chemistry*, vol. 281, no. 40, pp. 29739–29752, 2006.

[61] T. Hunter, "Signaling—2000 and beyond," *Cell*, vol. 100, no. 1, pp. 113–127, 2000.

[62] A. A. Bielska and N. J. Zondlo, "Hyperphosphorylation of tau induces local polyproline II helix," *Biochemistry*, vol. 45, no. 17, pp. 5527–5537, 2006.

[63] N. Errington and A. J. Doig, "A phosphoserine-lysine salt bridge within an α-helical peptide, the strongest α-helix side-chain interaction measured to date," *Biochemistry*, vol. 44, no. 20, pp. 7553–7558, 2005.

[64] R. S. Signarvic and W. F. DeGrado, "De novo design of a molecular switch: Phosphorylation-dependent association of designed peptides," *Journal of Molecular Biology*, vol. 334, no. 1, pp. 1–12, 2003.

[65] A. Tholey, A. Lindemann, V. Kinzel, and J. Reed, "Direct effects of phosphorylation on the preferred backbone conformation of peptides: A nuclear magnetic resonance study," *Biophysical Journal*, vol. 76, no. 1 I, pp. 76–87, 1999.

[66] L. Chen and M. B. Feany, "α-synuclein phosphorylation controls neurotoxicity and inclusion formation in a Drosophila model of Parkinson disease," *Nature Neuroscience*, vol. 8, no. 5, pp. 657–663, 2005.

[67] B.-H. Ahn, H. Rhim, Y.-M. S. Shi Yeon Kim et al., "α-synuclein interacts with phospholipase D isozymes and inhibits pervanadate-induced phospholipase d activation in human embryonic kidney-293 cells," *The Journal of Biological Chemistry*, vol. 277, no. 14, pp. 12334–12342, 2002.

[68] T. Nakamura, H. Yamashita, T. Takahashi, and S. Nakamura, "Activated Fyn phosphorylates α-synuclein at tyrosine residue 125," *Biochemical and Biophysical Research Communications*, vol. 280, no. 4, pp. 1085–1092, 2001.

[69] C. E. Ellis, P. L. Schwartzberg, T. L. Grider, D. W. Fink, and R. L. Nussbaum, "α-Synuclein Is Phosphorylated by Members of the Src Family of Protein-tyrosine Kinases," *The Journal of Biological Chemistry*, vol. 276, no. 6, pp. 3879–3884, 2001.

[70] H. Sato, S. Arawaka, S. Hara et al., "Authentically phosphorylated α-synuclein at Ser129 accelerates neurodegeneration in a rat model of familial Parkinson's disease," *The Journal of Neuroscience*, vol. 31, no. 46, pp. 16884–16894, 2011.

[71] H. Sato, T. Kato, and S. Arawaka, "The role of Ser129 phosphorylation of α-synuclein in neurodegeneration of Parkinson's disease: A review of in vivo models," *Reviews in the Neurosciences*, vol. 24, no. 2, pp. 115–123, 2013.

[72] K. J. Inglis, D. Chereau, E. F. Brigham et al., "Polo-like kinase 2 (PLK2) phosphorylates α-synuclein at serine 129 in central nervous system," *The Journal of Biological Chemistry*, vol. 284, no. 5, pp. 2598–2602, 2009.

[73] A. N. Pronin, A. J. Morris, A. Surguchov, and J. L. Benovic, "Synucleins are a novel class of substrates for G protein-coupled receptor kinases," *The Journal of Biological Chemistry*, vol. 275, no. 34, pp. 26515–26522, 2000.

[74] J. Kosten, A. Binolfi, M. Stuiver et al., "Efficient modification of alpha-synuclein serine 129 by protein kinase CK1 requires phosphorylation of tyrosine 125 as a priming event," *ACS Chemical Neuroscience*, vol. 5, no. 12, pp. 1203–1208, 2014.

[75] S. Zhang, J. Xie, Y. Xia et al., "LK6/Mnk2a is a new kinase of alpha synuclein phosphorylation mediating neurodegeneration," *Scientific Reports*, vol. 5, Article ID 12564, 2015.

[76] W. W. Smith, R. L. Margolis, X. Li et al., "α-synuclein phosphorylation enhances eosinophilic cytoplasmic inclusion formation in SH-SY5Y cells," *The Journal of Neuroscience*, vol. 25, no. 23, pp. 5544–5552, 2005.

[77] M. Takahashi, L.-W. Ko, J. Kulathingal, P. Jiang, D. Sevlever, and S.-H. C. Yen, "Oxidative stress-induced phosphorylation, degradation and aggregation of α-synuclein are linked to upregulated CK2 and cathepsin D," *European Journal of Neuroscience*, vol. 26, no. 4, pp. 863–874, 2007.

[78] N. Sugeno, A. Takeda, T. Hasegawa et al., "Serine 129 phosphorylation of α-synuclein induces unfolded protein response-mediated cell death," *The Journal of Biological Chemistry*, vol. 283, no. 34, pp. 23179–23188, 2008.

[79] M. Martinez-Vicente, Z. Talloczy, S. Kaushik et al., "Dopamine-modified α-synuclein blocks chaperone-mediated autophagy," *The Journal of Clinical Investigation*, vol. 118, no. 2, pp. 777-778, 2008.

[80] S. K. Mak, A. L. McCormack, A. B. Manning-Bog, A. M. Cuervo, and D. A. Di Monte, "Lysosomal degradation of α-synuclein in vivo," *The Journal of Biological Chemistry*, vol. 285, no. 18, pp. 13621–13629, 2010.

[81] R. Perfeito, D. F. Lázaro, T. F. Outeiro, and A. C. Rego, "Linking alpha-synuclein phosphorylation to reactive oxygen species formation and mitochondrial dysfunction in SH-SY5Y cells," *Molecular and Cellular Neuroscience*, vol. 62, pp. 51–59, 2014.

[82] K.-Y. Chau, H. L. Ching, A. H. V. Schapira, and J. M. Cooper, "Relationship between alpha synuclein phosphorylation, proteasomal inhibition and cell death: Relevance to Parkinson's disease pathogenesis," *Journal of Neurochemistry*, vol. 110, no. 3, pp. 1005–1013, 2009.

[83] A. N. Pronin, C. V. Carman, and J. L. Benovic, "Structure-function analysis of G protein-coupled receptor kinase-5: Role of the carboxyl terminus in kinase regulation," *The Journal of Biological Chemistry*, vol. 273, no. 47, pp. 31510–31518, 1998.

[84] T. T. Chuang, L. Paolucci, and A. De Blasi, "Inhibition of G protein-coupled receptor kinase subtypes by Ca2+/calmodulin," *The Journal of Biological Chemistry*, vol. 271, no. 45, pp. 28691–28696, 1996.

[85] G. S. Nübling, J. Levin, B. Bader et al., "Modelling Ser129 phosphorylation inhibits membrane binding of pore-forming alpha-synuclein oligomers," *PLoS ONE*, vol. 9, no. 6, Article ID e98906, 2014.

[86] T. Kuwahara, R. Tonegawa, G. Ito, S. Mitani, and T. Iwatsubo, "Phosphorylation of α-synuclein protein at ser-129 reduces neuronal dysfunction by lowering its membrane binding property in Caenorhabditis elegans," *The Journal of Biological Chemistry*, vol. 287, no. 10, pp. 7098–7109, 2012.

[87] V. Sancenon, S.-A. Lee, C. Patrick et al., "Suppression of α-synuclein toxicity and vesicle trafficking defects by phosphorylation at S129 in yeast depends on genetic context," *Human Molecular Genetics*, vol. 21, no. 11, Article ID dds058, pp. 2432–2449, 2012.

[88] B. Wu, Q. Liu, C. Duan et al., "Phosphorylation of α-synuclein upregulates tyrosine hydroxylase activity in MN9D cells," *Acta Histochemica*, vol. 113, no. 1, pp. 32–35, 2011.

[89] K. E. Paleologou, A. W. Schmid, C. C. Rospigliosi et al., "Phosphorylation at Ser-129 but not the phosphomimics S129E/D inhibits the fibrillation of α-synuclein," *The Journal of Biological Chemistry*, vol. 283, no. 24, pp. 16895–16905, 2008.

[90] N. R. McFarland, Z. Fan, K. Xu et al., "α-Synuclein S129 phosphorylation mutants do not alter nigrostriatal toxicity in a rat model of parkinson disease," *Journal of Neuropathology & Experimental Neurology*, vol. 68, no. 5, pp. 515–524, 2009.

[91] O. S. Gorbatyuk, S. Li, L. F. Sullivan et al., "The phosphorylation state of Ser-129 in human α-synuclein determines neurodegeneration in a rat model of Parkinson disease," *Proceedings of the National Acadamy of Sciences of the United States of America*, vol. 105, no. 2, pp. 763–768, 2008.

[92] K. E. Paleologou, A. Oueslati, G. Shakked et al., "Phosphorylation at S87 is enhanced in synucleinopathies, inhibits α-synuclein oligomerization, and influences synuclein-membrane interactions," *The Journal of Neuroscience*, vol. 30, no. 9, pp. 3184–3198, 2010.

[93] M. Yamada, T. Iwatsubo, Y. Mizuno, and H. Mochizuki, "Overexpression of α-synuclein in rat substantia nigra results in loss of dopaminergic neurons, phosphorylation of α-synuclein and activation of caspase-9: Resemblance to pathogenetic changes in Parkinson's disease," *Journal of Neurochemistry*, vol. 91, no. 2, pp. 451–461, 2004.

[94] A. L. McCormack, S. K. Mak, and D. A. Di Monte, "Increased a-synuclein phosphorylation and nitration in the aging primate substantia nigra," *Cell Death & Disease*, vol. 3, no. 5, article no. e315, 2012.

[95] E. A. Waxman and B. I. Giasson, "Specificity and regulation of casein kinase-mediated phosphorylation of α-synuclein," *Journal of Neuropathology & Experimental Neurology*, vol. 67, no. 5, pp. 402–416, 2008.

[96] H. Fujiwara, M. Hasegawa, N. Dohmae et al., "α-synuclein is phosphorylated in synucleinopathy lesions," *Nature Cell Biology*, vol. 4, no. 2, pp. 160–164, 2002.

[97] M. Hasegawa, H. Fujiwara, T. Nonaka et al., "Phosphorylated α-synuclein is ubiquitinated in α-synucleinopathy lesions," *The Journal of Biological Chemistry*, vol. 277, no. 50, pp. 49071–49076, 2002.

[98] Y. Wang, M. Shi, and K. A. Chung, "Phosphorylated α-synuclein in Parkinson's disease," *Science Translational Medicine*, vol. 4, no. 121, Article ID 121ra20, 2012.

[99] N. K. Majbour, N. N. Vaikath, K. D. Van Dijk et al., "Oligomeric and phosphorylated alpha-synuclein as potential CSF biomarkers for Parkinson's disease," *Molecular Neurodegeneration*, vol. 11, no. 1, article no. 7, 2016.

[100] L. L. Liu and K. J. Franz, "Phosphorylation of an α-synuclein peptide fragment enhances metal binding," *Journal of the American Chemical Society*, vol. 127, no. 27, pp. 9662-9663, 2005.

[101] A. Garcia-Garcia, H. Rodriguez-Rocha, N. Madayiputhiya, A. Pappa, M. I. Panayiotidis, and R. Franco, "Biomarkers of protein oxidation in human disease," *Current Molecular Medicine*, vol. 12, no. 6, pp. 681–697, 2012.

[102] A. Santner and V. N. Uversky, "Metalloproteomics and metal toxicology of α-synuclein," *Metallomics*, vol. 2, no. 6, pp. 378–392, 2010.

[103] V. N. Uversky, J. Li, and A. L. Fink, "Metal-triggered structural transformations, aggregation, and fibrillation of human α-synuclein: A possible molecular link between parkinson's disease and heavy metal exposure," *The Journal of Biological Chemistry*, vol. 276, no. 47, pp. 44284–44296, 2001.

[104] R. M. Rasia, C. W. Bertoncini, D. Marsh et al., "Structural characterization of copper(II) binding to α-synuclein: insights into the bioinorganic chemistry of Parkinson's disease," *Proceedings of the National Acadamy of Sciences of the United States of America*, vol. 102, no. 12, pp. 4294–4299, 2005.

[105] A. Binolfi, L. Quintanar, C. W. Bertoncini, C. Griesinger, and C. O. Fernández, "Bioinorganic chemistry of copper coordination to alpha-synuclein: Relevance to Parkinson's disease," *Coordination Chemistry Reviews*, vol. 256, no. 19-20, pp. 2188–2201, 2012.

[106] S. R. Paik, H.-J. Shin, J.-H. Lee, C.-S. Chang, and J. Kim, "Copper(II)-induced self-oligomerization of α-synuclein," *Biochemical Journal*, vol. 340, no. 3, pp. 821–828, 1999.

[107] Y. Xiao, D. Chen, X. Zhang et al., "Molecular study on copper-mediated tumor proteasome inhibition and cell death," *International Journal of Oncology*, vol. 37, pp. 81–87, 2010.

[108] N. K. Y. Wee, D. C. Weinstein, S. T. Fraser, and S. J. Assinder, "The mammalian copper transporters CTR1 and CTR2 and their roles in development and disease," *The International Journal of Biochemistry & Cell Biology*, vol. 45, no. 5, pp. 960–963, 2013.

[109] A. Binolfi, G. R. Lamberto, R. Duran et al., "Site-specific interactions of Cu(II) with α and β-synuclein: Bridging the molecular gap between metal binding and aggregation," *Journal of the American Chemical Society*, vol. 130, no. 35, pp. 11801–11812, 2008.

[110] A. Binolfi, E. E. Rodriguez, D. Valensin et al., "Bioinorganic chemistry of Parkinson's disease: Structural determinants for the copper-mediated amyloid formation of alpha-synuclein," *Inorganic Chemistry*, vol. 49, no. 22, pp. 10668–10679, 2010.

[111] H. R. Lucas and J. C. Lee, "Copper(ii) enhances membrane-bound α-synuclein helix formation," *Metallomics*, vol. 3, no. 3, pp. 280–283, 2011.

[112] T. Kowalik-Jankowska, A. Rajewska, E. Jankowska, and Z. Grzonka, "Products of Cu(II)-catalyzed oxidation of α-synuclein fragments containing M1-D2 and H50 residues in the presence of hydrogen peroxide," *Dalton Transactions*, no. 6, pp. 832–838, 2008.

[113] L. Guilloreau, S. Combalbert, M. Sournia-Saquet, H. Mazarguil, and P. Faller, "Redox chemistry of copper-amyloid-β: The generation of hydroxyl radical in the presence of ascorbate is linked to redox-potentials and aggregation state," *ChemBioChem*, vol. 8, no. 11, pp. 1317–1325, 2007.

[114] T. Kowalik-Jankowska, A. Rajewska, E. Jankowska, and Z. Grzonka, "Copper(II) binding by fragments of α-synuclein containing M 1-D2- and -H50-residues; a combined potentiometric and spectroscopic study," *Dalton Transactions*, no. 42, pp. 5068–5076, 2006.

[115] P. Jenner, "Oxidative stress in Parkinson's disease," *Annals of Neurology*, vol. 53, supplement 3, pp. S26–S38, 2003.

[116] H. Snyder, K. Mensah, C. Hsu et al., "β-Synuclein reduces proteasomal inhibition by α-synuclein but not γ-synuclein," *The Journal of Biological Chemistry*, vol. 280, no. 9, pp. 7562–7569, 2005.

[117] S. Montes, S. Rivera-Mancia, A. Diaz-Ruiz, L. Tristan-Lopez, and C. Rios, "Copper and copper proteins in Parkinson's disease," *Oxidative Medicine and Cellular Longevity*, vol. 2014, Article ID 147251, 2014.

[118] M. E. Rice and I. Russo-Menna, "Differential compartmentalization of brain ascorbate and glutathione between neurons and glia," *Neuroscience*, vol. 82, no. 4, pp. 1213–1223, 1997.

[119] J. Sian, D. T. Dexter, A. J. Lees et al., "Alterations in glutathione levels in Parkinson's disease and other neurodegenerative disorders affecting basal ganglia," *Annals of Neurology*, vol. 36, no. 3, pp. 348–355, 1994.

Permissions

All chapters in this book were first published in PD, by Hindawi Publishing Corporation; hereby published with permission under the Creative Commons Attribution License or equivalent. Every chapter published in this book has been scrutinized by our experts. Their significance has been extensively debated. The topics covered herein carry significant findings which will fuel the growth of the discipline. They may even be implemented as practical applications or may be referred to as a beginning point for another development.

The contributors of this book come from diverse backgrounds, making this book a truly international effort. This book will bring forth new frontiers with its revolutionizing research information and detailed analysis of the nascent developments around the world.

We would like to thank all the contributing authors for lending their expertise to make the book truly unique. They have played a crucial role in the development of this book. Without their invaluable contributions this book wouldn't have been possible. They have made vital efforts to compile up to date information on the varied aspects of this subject to make this book a valuable addition to the collection of many professionals and students.

This book was conceptualized with the vision of imparting up-to-date information and advanced data in this field. To ensure the same, a matchless editorial board was set up. Every individual on the board went through rigorous rounds of assessment to prove their worth. After which they invested a large part of their time researching and compiling the most relevant data for our readers.

The editorial board has been involved in producing this book since its inception. They have spent rigorous hours researching and exploring the diverse topics which have resulted in the successful publishing of this book. They have passed on their knowledge of decades through this book. To expedite this challenging task, the publisher supported the team at every step. A small team of assistant editors was also appointed to further simplify the editing procedure and attain best results for the readers.

Apart from the editorial board, the designing team has also invested a significant amount of their time in understanding the subject and creating the most relevant covers. They scrutinized every image to scout for the most suitable representation of the subject and create an appropriate cover for the book.

The publishing team has been an ardent support to the editorial, designing and production team. Their endless efforts to recruit the best for this project, has resulted in the accomplishment of this book. They are a veteran in the field of academics and their pool of knowledge is as vast as their experience in printing. Their expertise and guidance has proved useful at every step. Their uncompromising quality standards have made this book an exceptional effort. Their encouragement from time to time has been an inspiration for everyone.

The publisher and the editorial board hope that this book will prove to be a valuable piece of knowledge for researchers, students, practitioners and scholars across the globe.

List of Contributors

Rachael A. Lawson, Daniel Collerton, John-Paul Taylor and David J. Burn
Institute of Neuroscience, Newcastle University, Newcastle upon Tyne, UK

Katie R. Brittain
Department of Nursing, Midwifery and Health, Northumbria University, Newcastle upon Tyne, UK

Perla Massai, Francesca Colalelli, Marco Tofani and Michela Scuccimarri
Sapienza University of Rome, Rome, Italy

Julita Sansoni and Giovanni Galeoto
Department of Public Health and Infection Disease, Sapienza University of Rome, Rome, Italy

Donatella Valente and Andrea Fabbrini
Department Human Neurosciences, Sapienza University of Rome, Rome, Italy

Giovanni Fabbrini
Department Human Neurosciences, Sapienza University of Rome, Rome, Italy
IRCSS Neuromed Institute, Pozzilli, IS, Italy

Francescaelena De Rose, Paolo Solari, Simone Poddighe and Anna Liscia
Department of Biomedical Sciences, University of Cagliari, Cagliari, Italy

Valentina Corda
Department of Life and Environmental Sciences, University of Cagliari, Cagliari, Italy

Patrizia Sacchetti and Antonio Belcari
Department of Agricultural Biotechnology, Section of Plant Protection, University of Florence, Firenze, Italy

Sanjay Kasture
Pinnacle Biomedical Research Institute, Bhopal, India

Paolo Solla and Francesco Marrosu
Department of Public Health, Clinical and Molecular Medicine, University of Cagliari, Cagliari, Italy

Hector R. Martinez, Alexis Garcia-Sarreon, Carlos Camara-Lemarroy, Fortino Salazar and Marìa L. Guerrero-Gonzàlez
Tecnologico de Monterrey, Escuela de Medicina y Ciencias de la Salud, Ave. Morones Prieto 3000, 64710 Monterrey, NL, Mexico

Mirna Wetters Portuguez
Pontifical Catholic University of Rio Grande do Sul (PUCRS), Porto Alegre, RS, Brazil
Brain Institute of Rio Grande do Sul (InsCer), Porto Alegre, RS, Brazil

Valéria de Carvalho Fagundes
Pontifical Catholic University of Rio Grande do Sul (PUCRS), Porto Alegre, RS, Brazil
Brain Institute of Rio Grande do Sul (InsCer), Porto Alegre, RS, Brazil
Hospital de Clìnicas de Porto Alegre (HCPA), Porto Alegre, RS, Brazil

Bárbara Costa Beber
Hospital de Clìnicas de Porto Alegre (HCPA), Porto Alegre, RS, Brazil

Carlos R. M. Rieder
Hospital de Clìnicas de Porto Alegre (HCPA), Porto Alegre, RS, Brazil
Federal University of Health Sciences from Porto Alegre (UFCSPA), Porto Alegre, RS, Brazil

Aline Nunes da Cruz
Hospital de Clìnicas de Porto Alegre (HCPA), Porto Alegre, RS, Brazil
Federal University of Rio Grande do Sul (UFRGS), Porto Alegre, RS, Brazil

Lingjia Xu and Jiali Pu
Department of Neurology, 2nd Affiliated Hospital, School of Medicine, Zhejiang University, Hangzhou, Zhejiang 310009, China

Michele Fragola, Francesco Lena, Deborah Lanni, Marco Grano and Nicola Modugno
lstituto Neurologico Mediterraneo "Neuromed", Pozzilli, Italy

Giovanni Mirabella
lstituto Neurologico Mediterraneo "Neuromed", Pozzilli, Italy
Department of Anatomy, Histology, Forensic Medicine and Orthopedics, Sapienza University of Rome, Rome, Italy

Fulvia Dilettuso, Marta Iacopini, Raffaella d'Avella, Maria Concetta Borgese, Silvia Mazzotta, Sara Lubrani, Silvia Rampelli and Paolo De Vita
PARKIN-ZONE onlus, Roma, Italy

Wen Su, Shu-Hua Li, Ying Jin and Hai-Bo Chen
Department of Neurology, Beijing Hospital, National Center of Gerontology, No. 1 Dahua Road, Dong Dan, Beijing 100730, China

Kai Li
Department of Neurology, Beijing Hospital, National Center of Gerontology, No. 1 Dahua Road, Dong Dan, Beijing 100730, China
Department of Geriatric Medicine, Beijing Hospital, National Center of Gerontology, No. 1 Dahua Road, Dong Dan, Beijing 100730, China

Ndidi C. Ngwuluka, Yahya E. Choonara, Lisa C. du Toit, Pradeep Kumar and Viness Pillay
Wits Advanced Drug Delivery Platform Research Unit, Department of Pharmacy and Pharmacology, School ofTherapeutic Sciences, Faculty of Health Sciences, University of theWitwatersrand, Johannesburg, 7 York Road, Parktown 2193, South Africa

Girish Modi
Department of Neurology, Faculty of Health Sciences, University of theWitwatersrand, Johannesburg, 7 York Road, Parktown 2193, South Africa

Leith Meyer
Department of Paraclinical Sciences, Faculty of Veterinary Science, University of Pretoria, Pretoria, South Africa

Tracy Snyman
National Laboratory Services, Faculty of Health Sciences, University of theWitwatersrand, Johannesburg, 7 York Road, Parktown 2193, South Africa

D. McClurg, K. Walker, P. Aitchison, K. Jamieson and S. Hagen
Nursing, Midwifery, and Allied Health Professions, Research Unit, Glasgow Caledonian University, Glasgow G4 0BA, UK

L. Dickinson
Nursing, Midwifery and Allied Health Professions, Research Unit, Stirling University, Stirling, UK

L. Paul
School of Medicine, Dentistry and Nursing, Nursing and Health Care School, 59 Oakfield Avenue, Gilmorehill Campus, Glasgow University, Glasgow, UK

A.-L. Cunnington
Care of Elderly Department, Glasgow Royal Infirmary, 84 Castle Street, Glasgow G4 0SF, UK

Cheng Tan, Xiaoyang Liu and Jiajun Chen
Department of Neurology, China-Japan Union Hospital of Jilin University, Changchun, Jilin 130033, China

Jeremy Steinberger, Jeffrey Gilligan, Christopher A. Sarkiss and John M. Caridi
Department of Neurosurgery, Icahn School of Medicine at Mount Sinai, New York, NY, USA

Branko Skovrlj
Department of Neurosurgery, North Jersey Spine Group, Wayne, NJ, USA

Javier Z. Guzman and Samuel K. Cho
Department of Orthopaedics, Icahn School of Medicine at Mount Sinai, New York, NY, USA

Payam Saadat and Alijan Ahmadi Ahangar
Mobility Impairment Research Center, Health Research Institute, Babol University of Medical Sciences, Babol, Iran

Seyed Ehsan Samaei
Social Determinants of Health Research Center, Health Research Institute, Babol University of Medical Sciences, Babol, Iran

Alireza Firozjaie
Cellular and Molecular Biology Research Center, Health Research Institute, Babol University of Medical Sciences, Babol, Ira

Fatemeh Abbaspour and Azam Khoddami
Clinical Research Development Center, Ayatollah Rohani Hospital, Babol University of Medical Sciences, Babol, Iran

Sorrayya Khafri
Department of Statistic and Epidmiology, School of Medicine, Babol University of Medical Sciences, Babol, Iran Jinhua Zheng, Xinglong Yang, Quanzhen Zhao, Sijia Tian,

Hongyan Huang, Yalan Chen and Yanming Xu
Department of Neurology, West China Hospital, Sichuan University, 37 Guo Xue Xiang, Chengdu, Sichuan Province 610041, China

Sarah H. Millan, Mallory L. Hacker, Maxim Turchan, Anna L. Molinari, Amanda D. Currie and David Charles
Department of Neurology, Vanderbilt University Medical Center, 1611 21st Ave S., A-0118 Medical Center North, Nashville, TN 37223-2551, USA

Jie Fang, Xingkai An, Hongli Qu, Qing Lin and Min Bi
Department of Neurology, The First Affiliated Hospital of Xiamen University, Xiamen, China

Qilin Ma
Department of Neurology, The First Affiliated Hospital of Xiamen University, Xiamen, China
The First Clinical Medical College of Fujian Medical University, Fuzhou, China

Kehui Yi
The First Clinical Medical College of Fujian Medical University, Fuzhou, China

Mingwei Guo
Department of Neurology, The First Affiliated Hospital of Gannan Medical University, Ganzhou, China

Aparna Wagle Shukla and Pam Zeilman
Center for Movement Disorders and Neurorestoration, Department of Neurology, University of Florida, Gainesville, FL, USA

Hubert Fernandez
Center for Neurological Restoration, Cleveland Clinic, Cleveland, OH, USA

Jawad A. Bajwa
Parkinson's Disease, Movement Disorders and Neurorestoration Program, National Neuroscience Institute, King FahadMedical City, Riyadh, Saudi Arabia

Raja Mehanna
University of Texas Health Science Center, McGovern Medical School, Houston, TX, USA

Colleen D. Knoop
Ochsner Health System, Division of Movement Disorders, 1514 Jefferson Highway, New Orleans, LA 70121, USA

Robert Kadish and Kathrin LaFaver
Department of Neurology, University of Louisville, 220 Abraham FlexnerWay, Suite 606, Louisville, KY 40202, USA

Kathy Hager
BellarmineUniversity, 2001 Newburg Road, MilesHall 301, Louisville, KY 40205, USA

Michael C. Park
Department of Neurosurgery and Neurology, University of Minnesota, 420 Delaware Street SE, MMC 96, Minneapolis, MN 55455, USA

Paul D. Loprinzi
University of Mississippi, 229 Turner Center, Oxford, MS 38677, USA

Ota Gal, Martin Srp, Romana Konvalinkova, Martina Hoskovcova, Jan Roth and Evzen Ruzicka
Department of Neurology and Centre of Clinical Neuroscience, First Faculty of Medicine and General University Hospital, Charles University in Prague, Katerinska 30, 128 21 Prague, Czech Republic

Vaclav Capek
Applied Neurosciences and Brain Imaging, National Institute of Mental Health, Topolova 748, 250 67 Klecany, Czech Republic

Evelien Nackaerts and Alice Nieuwboer
Neuromotor Rehabilitation Research Group, Department of Rehabilitation Sciences, KU Leuven, Leuven, Belgium

Elisabetta Farella
E3DA Research Unit, ICT Center, Fondazione Bruno Kessler, Trento, Italy

Dongping Huang, Jinghui Wang, Jiabin Tong, Xiaochen Bai, Heng Li, Zishan Wang, Mei Yu and Fang Huang
The State Key Laboratory of Medical Neurobiology, The Institutes of Brain Science and the Collaborative Innovation Center for Brain Science, Shanghai Medical College, Fudan University, 138 Yixueyuan Road, Shanghai 200032, China

Jing Xu
School of Life Science and Technology, Tongji University, 1239 Siping Road, Shanghai 200092, China

Yulu Huang and Yufei Wu
School of Basic Medical Sciences, Fudan University, 138 Yixueyuan Road, Shanghai 200032, China

Kathrin Brockmann, Senait Ogbamicael, Ann-Kathrin Hauser, Claudia Schulte, Jasmin Fritzen and Thomas Gasser
Department of Neurodegeneration, Hertie Institute for Clinical Brain Research, University of Tübingen, Tübingen, Germany
German Research Center for Neurodegenerative Diseases (DZNE), University of Tübingen, Tübingen, Germany

Karin Srulijes
Department of Neurodegeneration, Hertie Institute for Clinical Brain Research, University of Tübingen, Tübingen, Germany
German Research Center for Neurodegenerative Diseases (DZNE), University of Tübingen, Tübingen, Germany

Department of Geriatrics and Clinic of Geriatric Rehabilitation, Robert-Bosch-Hospital, Stuttgart, Germany

Markus A. Hobert, Daniela Berg and Walter Maetzler
Department of Neurodegeneration, Hertie Institute for Clinical Brain Research, University of Tübingen, Tübingen, Germany
German Research Center for Neurodegenerative Diseases (DZNE), University of Tübingen, Tübingen, Germany
Department of Neurology, Kiel University, Kiel, Germany

Michael Schwenk
Department of Geriatrics and Clinic of Geriatric Rehabilitation, Robert-Bosch-Hospital, Stuttgart, Germany
Network Aging Research, Heidelberg University, Heidelberg, Germany

Michaela Karlstedt and Johan Lökk
Karolinska Institutet, Department of Neurobiology Care Sciences and Society, Division of Clinical Geriatrics, Floor 7 141 83 Huddinge, Stockholm, Sweden

Seyed-Mohammad Fereshtehnejad
Karolinska Institutet, Department of Neurobiology Care Sciences and Society, Division of Clinical Geriatrics, Floor 7 141 83 Huddinge, Stockholm, Sweden
Department of Neurology and Neurosurgery, McGill University, Montreal, QC, Canada

Dag Aarsland
Karolinska Institutet, Alzheimer Disease Research Center (KI-ADRC) Novum, Floor 5 SE-141 86, Stockholm, Sweden
Department Old Age Psychiatry, Kings College, London, UK

Marjolein A. E. van Stiphout
Foundation for Oral Health and Parkinson's Disease, 2340 BD Oegstgeest, Netherlands

Cees de Baat
Foundation for Oral Health and Parkinson's Disease, 1155, 2340 BD Oegstgeest, Netherlands
Department of Dentistry, Radboud university medical center, 6500 HB Nijmegen, Netherlands

Johan Marinus and Jacobus J. van Hilten
Department of Neurology, Leiden University Medical Center, Albinusdreef 2, 2333 ZA Leiden, Netherlands

Frank Lobbezoo
Department of Oral Kinesiology, Academic Centre for Dentistry Amsterdam (ACTA), University of Amsterdam and Vrije Universiteit Amsterdam, Gustav Mahlerlaan 3004, 1081 LA Amsterdam, Netherlands

A. M. Martínez-Martínez and C. A. Acevedo-Triana
Department of Psychology, Pontificia Universidad Javeriana, Bogotà, Colombia

O. M. Aguilar
Department of Brain Repair and Rehabilitation, University College London, London, UK

Jéssica Lopes Fontoura, Camila Baptista and Marcelo Machado Ferro
Department of Biology, Universidade Estadual de Ponta Grossa, Ponta Grossa, PR, Brazil

Flávia de Brito Pedroso, José Augusto Pochapski and Edmar Miyoshi
Department of Pharmaceutical Sciences, Universidade Estadual de Ponta Grossa, Ponta Grossa, PR, Brazil

Ji Young Yun
Department of Neurology, EwhaWomans University Mokdong Hospital, EwhaWomans University College of Medicine, Seoul, Republic of Korea

Young Eun Kim
Department of Neurology, Hallym University Sacred Heart Hospital, Hallym University College of Medicine, Anyang, Republic of Korea

Hui-Jun Yang
Department of Neurology, Ulsan University Hospital, Ulsan, Republic of Korea

Han-Joon Kim and Beomseok Jeon
Department of Neurology and Movement Disorder Center, Seoul National University Hospital, Seoul National University College of Medicine, Seoul, Republic of Korea

Tommaso Schirinzi, Alessio D'Elia, Giulia Di Lazzaro, Paola Imbriani, Graziella Madeo and Marta Maltese
Neurology, Department of Systems Medicine, University of Rome Tor Vergata, Via Montpellier 1, 00133 Rome, Italy

Giuseppina Martella and Antonio Pisani
Neurology, Department of Systems Medicine, University of Rome Tor Vergata, Via Montpellier 1, 00133 Rome, Italy
IRCCS Fondazione Santa Lucia, Via del Fosso di Fiorano, Rome, Italy

Leonardo Monaco
Psychiatry, Department of Systems Medicine, University of Rome Tor Vergata, Via Montpellier 1, 00133 Rome, Italy

Juan Antonio Castillo-Gonzalez, Maria De Jesus Loera-Arias, Roberto Montes-de-Oca-Luna, Aracely Garcia-Garcia and Humberto Rodriguez-Rocha
Departamento de Histologia, Facultad de Medicina, Universidad Autonoma de Nuevo Leon, 64460 Monterrey, NL, Mexico

Odila Saucedo-Cardenas
Departamento de Histologia, Facultad de Medicina, Universidad Autonoma de Nuevo Leon, 64460 Monterrey, NL, Mexico
Centro de Investigaciones Biomedicas del Noreste, Monterrey, NL, Mexico

Index

www.ingramcontent.com/pod-product-compliance
Lightning Source LLC
Chambersburg PA
CBHW080507200326
41458CB00012B/4121